TEXTBOOK OF OCCUPATIONAL MEDICINE PRACTICE

Fifth Edition

TEXTBOOK OF OCCUPATIONAL MEDICINE PRACTICE

Fifth Edition

Edited by

David Koh
Universiti Brunei Darussalam, Brunei Darussalam
National University of Singapore, Singapore

Wee Hoe Gan
Singapore General Hospital, Singapore
Changi General Hospital, Singapore

World Scientific

NEW JERSEY • LONDON • SINGAPORE • BEIJING • SHANGHAI • HONG KONG • TAIPEI • CHENNAI • TOKYO

Published by

World Scientific Publishing Co. Pte. Ltd.
5 Toh Tuck Link, Singapore 596224
USA office: 27 Warren Street, Suite 401-402, Hackensack, NJ 07601
UK office: 57 Shelton Street, Covent Garden, London WC2H 9HE

Library of Congress Cataloging-in-Publication Data
Names: Koh, David, 1956– editor. | Gan, Wee Hoe, editor.
Title: Textbook of occupational medicine practice / edited by David Koh, Wee Hoe Gan.
Description: Fifth edition. | Hackensack, NJ : World Scientific Publishing Co., [2022] |
Includes bibliographical references and index.
Identifiers: LCCN 2021043207 | ISBN 9789811245640 (hardcover) |
ISBN 9789811245657 (ebook) | ISBN 9789811245664 (ebook other)
Subjects: MESH: Occupational Diseases | Occupational Injuries |
Occupational Health | Occupational Medicine
Classification: LCC RC963 | NLM WA 400 | DDC 616.9/803--dc23
LC record available at https://lccn.loc.gov/2021043207

British Library Cataloguing-in-Publication Data
A catalogue record for this book is available from the British Library.

For any available supplementary material, please visit
https://www.worldscientific.com/worldscibooks/10.1142/12512#t=suppl

Typeset by Stallion Press
Email: enquiries@stallionpress.com

For Wan Tsyr, Nicola, Katherine, Elliot
and Drs Gregory and Mark

For our mentors and patients who taught us to be
doctors with compassion

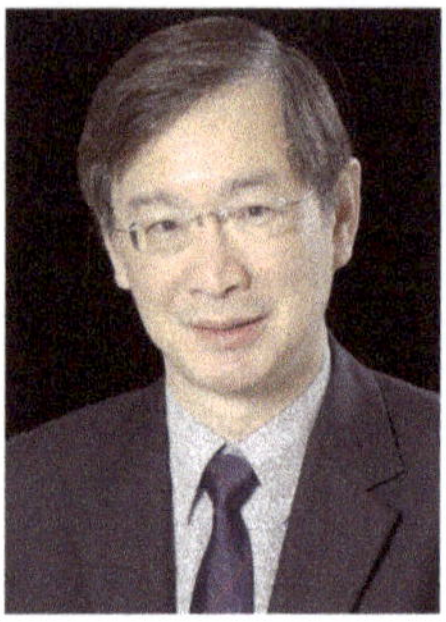

IN LOVING MEMORY OF PROFESSOR TAR CHING AW (1948–2017)

An Inspirational Teacher, Selfless Mentor and Great Advocate for the Discipline

Contents

Foreword

It gives me great pleasure to write the foreword to this fifth edition of the *Textbook of Occupational Medicine Practice*. Occupational Medicine Physicians work at the interface between work and health, and recent times have placed unprecedented demands on this medical specialty. Occupational medicine is crucial as it involves preventative programmes such as immunisations, health surveillance, rehabilitation of workers with an illness or disability, and advising organisations (governmental and business) on how to best optimise the health of their most important asset, their employees.

Work has an incredibly important impact on our health. We know that work in general has a positive effect in promoting overall health, with well proven mental, physical, social and economic benefits. However, adverse influences can also be seen; The International Labour Organization has estimated that over 2.3 million workers die from work-related causes annually. The majority (over 85%) succumb to cancer, as well as communicable, cardiovascular and respiratory diseases that are caused by work. The morbidity from occupational exposures is staggering, with over 300 million serious injuries annually. Worldwide, it is estimated that 37% of back pain, 16% of hearing loss, 13% of chronic obstructive pulmonary diseases, 11% of asthma, 10% of lung cancers and 2% of leukaemias are related to work. Much of these deaths, illnesses and injuries are preventable.

Given this background, it is unsurprising that occupational medicine has emerged as a specialty in its own right. The Royal College of Physicians of Ireland has been a global leader in the recognition and promotion of this important specialty. Its Faculty of Occupational Medicine, which was established in 1976, was one of the first faculties in the College, and the first such faculty in any Royal College of Physicians in the world. The Faculty has been an integral part of RCPI since its inception — as the national professional and training body for Occupational Medicine in Ireland, working to ensure the highest standards in health at work. Today, the College and Faculty continue to lead in advancing the science and practice of occupational medicine, and in promoting education, study and research in occupational medicine.

This textbook is a welcome addition to the educational resources available in the field of occupational medicine. Its focus on clinical aspects as well as integrative and multidisciplinary approaches required for the practice of occupational medicine is sensible and adds value to the competency training of occupational physicians and other occupational health practitioners. Previous editions have been very well-received internationally; Its most recent 4th edition was highly commended in the Primary Health Care category for the 2018 British Medical Association Medical Book Awards in 2018.

This book takes a particularly modern outlook; many workers are currently faced with new and deadly risks, which have to be managed appropriately. In tandem, the nature of work has changed in ways almost unimaginable from the past. This edition updates the practice of occupational medicine, which has been tremendously impacted by recent events such as the fourth industrial revolution, globalisation of work, the rise of workplace mental health issues and the COVID-19 pandemic. The disruptive effect of COVID-19 has brought into even greater focus the importance of work in the context of employee health and wellbeing, as well as the essential and central role of occupational medicine in supporting the health of employees. The book is a timely — and most welcome — addition as a medical resource of great range.

Professor David Koh and Dr Wee Hoe Gan are highly respected leaders and role models in occupational medicine on the world stage. They have both contributed heavily on research, teaching and policy making and greatly developed the discipline of occupational medicine wherever they have practised. They have a wealth of experience to share, and that experience is very evident in this, the 5th edition of their rightly celebrated *Textbook of Occupational Medicine Practice*. I think that the authors can be confident that their readers who will have gained a broader perspective on occupational medicine as a result of their efforts.

I congratulate the authors on the publication of this latest edition of the textbook, which I have no doubt will be as well received, and as indispensable, as its predecessor editions.

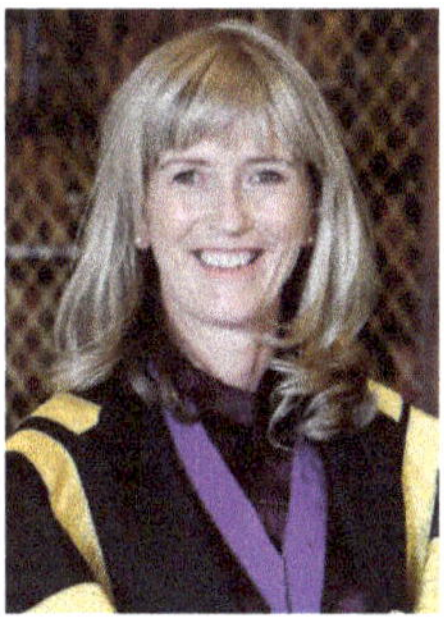

Professor Mary Horgan
President of the Royal College of Physicians of Ireland
and Consultant in Infectious Diseases at Cork University Hospital Ireland

Preface

Following the success of the fourth edition, which was highly commended in the primary health care category for the 2018 British Medical Association (BMA) Medical Book Awards, this fifth edition has been substantially revised and updated to reflect significant changes in health care practice and to incorporate the explosion of information since the advent of the fourth industrial revolution and the COVID-19 pandemic.

As before, the book covers target organ systems that can be affected by hazardous exposures in traditional industries and modern workplaces, both of which coexist in different parts of the world and present unique occupational health challenges for the medical practitioner. To this end, this reference textbook focuses on the clinical presentations, investigations and medical and work-centric management of affected individuals. We have retained consideration of some special issues relevant to occupational medicine practice in this new edition and included a new section relating to the multidisciplinary nature of occupational health practice.

The main emphasis continues to be prevention of disease and early detection of health effects caused by work exposures. This edition of the book has been updated to include new information and references. We have kept some of the previous case studies and illustrations, and introduced several new ones, some of which reflect the changes of practice due to the COVID-19 pandemic — for example, in risk communication, recognition and management of the risks of health care and frontline work.

We have again asked international experts in occupational medicine and cross disciplinary medical specialties to jointly author many of the chapters. Some of the authors are from Asia, and others from the United States, United Kingdom and Australia. All the authors have either clinical and/or academic experience in, or related to occupational medicine practice.

The book is targeted at all those who are interested in the interaction between work and health, and how occupational diseases and work-related disorders may present and be managed. It will be of interest to medical practitioners, especially those in primary care and doctors intending to pursue a career in occupational medicine. It would also be relevant for allied health and safety professionals wanting to know more about health effects resulting from occupational exposures. Other groups who may find this edition useful as a ready reference are medical students, occupational health nurses, or clinical specialists in diverse fields such as dermatology, respiratory medicine, infectious diseases or toxicology.

We wish to thank all our readers, especially those who have given valuable feedback on how we can improve this edition. In particular, thanks are also due to Ms Joy Quek from World Scientific for her encouragement and help in the production of this edition, and especially also to Dr Alvin Tan and Ms Akhwinder Kaur for their excellent editorial assistance and meticulous proofreading.

David Koh
Wee Hoe Gan
November 2021

About the Editors

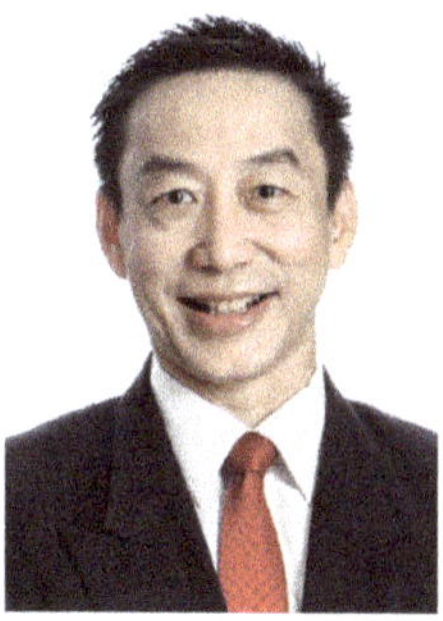

Professor David Koh qualified in medicine in Singapore and completed his postgraduate training in the United Kingdom. His main academic appointment is with the National University of Singapore (NUS), where he has served as Chair of the Department of Community, Occupational and Family Medicine and Director of the Centre for Environmental and Occupational Health Research. He joined the Universiti Brunei Darussalam (UBD) from 2012 to 2022, where he was Distinguished Professor of Occupational Health and Medicine, and Vice-President and Assistant Vice-Chancellor (2014–2018).

His research and teaching interests are in occupational and environmental health — with particular interests in salivary biomarkers, occupational dermatology, occupational infections and education and training in occupational health. He has authored several hundred peer-reviewed publications, edited several books and is listed among the top 2% of researchers in terms of research citation impact in the field of environmental and occupational health. Professor Koh serves on the advisory and editorial boards of major international occupational and environmental health journals, and has been a World Health Organization consultant in occupational health in several countries in the Asia-Pacific such as Vietnam, Myanmar, Indonesia, and the Solomon Islands.

In recognition of his international work in occupational and environmental health, he has been conferred the Smiley Medal from the Faculty of Occupational Medicine of the Royal College of Physicians Ireland, the Wilf Howe Memorial Prize from the Faculty of Occupational Medicine, Royal College of Physicians London, the Outstanding Volunteer Award from the Singapore International Foundation, and the Lifetime Achievement Award from the College of Public Health and Occupational Physicians, Academy of Medicine, Singapore.

ephkohd@nus.edu.sg
david.koh@u.nus.edu

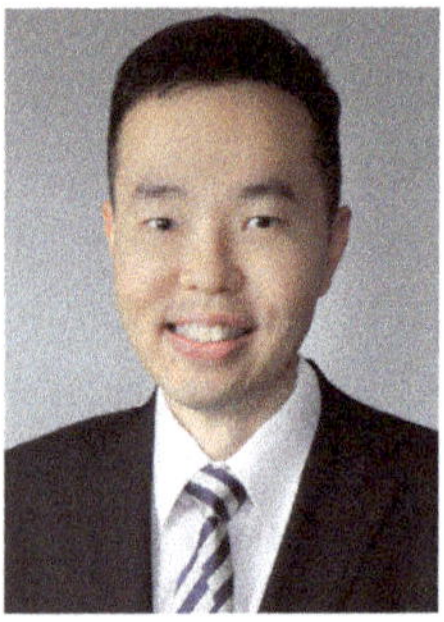

Dr Wee Hoe Gan is dually qualified and accredited in occupational medicine and aviation medicine. He completed his undergraduate medical training in Singapore, and postgraduate medical training in Singapore and the United Kingdom.

He started his career with the Singapore Armed Forces. In almost two decades of military service, his key appointments included Commander of the Military Medicine Institute, Chief Air Force Medical Officer and Assistant Chief of Medical Corps. For his distinguished service, he was awarded the Public Administration Medal (Silver) (Military) by the President of Singapore in 2014.

He is currently Head of the Department and Occupational and Environmental Medicine at the Singapore General Hospital, which is Singapore's largest hospital and listed by Newsweek as among the world's top ten best hospitals for three consecutive years (2019–2021). He also serves as Senior Consultant in Aviation Medicine at Singapore's Changi General Hospital. He is active in undergraduate and postgraduate medical education and training, and sits on the national specialist training committees in both occupational medicine and aviation medicine. He is appointed by the Ministry of Health and Ministry of Manpower as a member of Singapore's Workplace Safety and Health Council and Tripartite Oversight Committee for Workplace Safety and Health. He also leads specialist committees in formulating recommendations on national occupational health and safety policies and practices.

With a special interest in clinical informatics, he holds leadership roles as Deputy Group Chief Medical Informatics Officer (Acute Care) at Singapore's largest healthcare cluster, as well as at the Singapore General Hospital.

He is the current President-Elect of the College of Public Health and Occupational Physicians, Academy of Medicine, Singapore. He will assume the appointment of President of the College in mid-2022.

gan.wee.hoe@singhealth.com.sg

List of Contributors

Ken **Addley**
OBE, MB BCh, MD, FFOM, FFOM Hon (UK), FRCPI
Consultant Occupational Physician
Faculty of Occupational Medicine
Royal College of Physicians of Ireland
Dublin, Ireland
Visiting Professor
Department of Management, Leadership and Marketing
Ulster University Business School
Northern Ireland, United Kingdom

Adul **Bandhukul**
MD (Specialty Board Occupational Medicine, Thailand)
Director of Occupational Medicine
Institute of Nopparat, Rajathanee Hospital
Thailand

Chris **Barber**
BMBS, BMedSci, MD, FRCP, AFOM
Senior Medical Adviser
Centre for Workplace Health
Health and Safety Executive
Great Britain
Respiratory Consultant

Sheffield Teaching Hospitals
United Kingdom

Hathaichon **Boonhat**
MS
College of Public Health
China Medical University
Taichung, Taiwan

Ian **Brown**
OBE FRCP FFOM DDAM ERT
Consultant Physician in Occupational Health Medicine and Toxicology
Responsible Officer to NHS England and the General Medical Council
Member of the Oxford Epilepsy Research Group
Nuffield Department of Clinical Neurology
Oxford University and Oxford University Hospitals
United Kingdom

Doris T. **Chan**
MBBS, FRACP, PhD
Consultant Nephrologist
Department of Renal Medicine
Sir Charles Gairdner Hospital
Hospital Avenue
Nedlands, Western Australia, Australia

Gregory C.T. **Chan**
MBBS, MMed (Occup Med), Dip Geriatric Med, Dip FP Derm, PP
Medical Director
The Occupational and Diving Medicine Centre, Singapore
Visiting Consultant
Singapore General Hospital, Sengkang Health
Adjunct Assistant Professor
Saw Swee Hock School of Public Health
National University of Singapore, Singapore

Jeremiah **Chng**
MBBS, MPH (OM), FAMS
Head, Occupational Medicine
Woodlands Health Campus, Singapore
Adjunct Assistant Professor
Saw Swee Hock School of Public Health
National University of Singapore, Singapore

Paul **Cullinan**
MD, FRCP, FFOM
Professor of Occupational and Environmental Respiratory Disease
Department of Occupational and Environmental Medicine
Royal Brompton Hospital
London SW3 6LR, United Kingdom

Mikhail S. **Dzeshka**
PhD
Grodno State Medical University
Grodno, Belarus

David **Fishwick**
MBChB FRCP AFOM FFOM (Hon) MD
Chief Medical Adviser, Centre for Workplace Health
Health and Safety Executive
Great Britain
Respiratory Consultant
Sheffield Teaching Hospitals, United Kingdom
Honorary Professor of Occupational and Environmental Medicine
University of Sheffield
United Kingdom

Lin **Fritschi**
PhD, MBBS, FAFPHM
Professor of Epidemiology
School of Public Health
Curtin University
Western Australia, Australia

Wee Hoe **Gan**
MBBS, MPH, DAvMed (Lond), MRCP (UK), FRCP (Edin), FAMS
Head and Senior Consultant
Department of Occupational and Environmental Medicine, Singapore General Hospital, Singapore
Senior Consultant
Changi Aviation Medicine Centre, Changi General Hospital
Chief Medical Informatics Officer
Singapore General Hospital; Singapore
Deputy Group Chief Medical Informatics Officer (Acute Care)
Singapore Health Services

Chee Leok **Goh**
MBBS, MD, FRCP
Senior Consultant
National Skin Centre, Singapore
Clinical Professor
Yong Loo Lin School of Medicine
National University of Singapore, Singapore

Yue-Liang Leon **Guo**
MD, MPH, PhD
Professor and Clinical Staff
Environmental and Occupational Medicine
National Taiwan University College of Medicine and NTU Hospital
Adjunct Professor
Graduate Institute of Occupational Medicine and Industrial Hygiene
National Taiwan University College of Public Health
Taipei, Taiwan

Jayakumar **Gurusamy**
MBBS, MMed (OM), FFOMI, FRCPI, FAMM, FAOEMM
Dean
Professor of Community and Occupational Medicine
Faculty of Medicine
Manipal University College Malaysia

Li Yang **Hsu**
MBBS, MRCP (UK), DTMH, MPH (Harvard)
Vice Dean (Global Health), Programme Leader (Infectious Diseases) and Associate Professor
Saw Swee Hock School of Public Health
National University of Singapore, Singapore
Associate Professor
Yong Loo Lin School of Medicine
National University of Singapore, Singapore

Robert **Kerr**
DPhil BA (Hons), PG Dip FHEA Senior Lecturer
Department of Management, Leadership & Marketing
Ulster University Business School
Belfast, Northern Ireland
United Kingdom

David **Koh**
MBBS, MSc, PhD, FFOM, FFOMI, FRCPI, FFPH, FAOEMM, FAMS
Distinguished Professor of Occupational Health and Medicine
Universiti Brunei Darussalam
Professor
Saw Swee Hock School of Public Health and
Yong Loo Lin School of Medicine
National University of Singapore, Singapore

See Muah **Lee**
MBBS, MSc (Occup Med), FAMS (Occup Med), PG Dip Diab, LLB (Hons), LLM (Edin)
Adjunct Associate Professor
Saw Swee Hock School of Public Health
National University of Singapore, Singapore
Senior Consultant
Ng Teng Fong General Hospital
National University Health System, Singapore

Adjunct Associate Professor
Centre for Biomedical Ethics
National University of Singapore

Laurence Shen **Lim**
MBBS, FRCS (Ed)
Senior Consultant
Singapore National Eye Center and
Duke-NUS Graduate Medical School, Singapore

John Wah **Lim**
MB BCh (Hons) (UK), MPH (Occup Med), Dip Fam Med, FFOMI, FAMS (Occup Med)
Senior Consultant Occupational Physician
Singapore General Hospital, Singapore
Adjunct Assistant Professor
Saw Swee Hock School of Public Health
National University of Singapore, Singapore

Ro-Ting **Lin**
MSc, PhD
Associate Professor
Department of Occupational Safety and Health
College of Public Health
China Medical University
Taichung, Taiwan

Gregory Y.H. **Lip**
MD
Liverpool Centre for Cardiovascular Science
University of Liverpool and Liverpool Heart & Chest Hospital Liverpool, UK
Aalborg Thrombosis Research Unit
Department of Clinical Medicine, Faculty of Health
Aalborg University, Aalborg, Denmark

Max **Lum**
Ed.D MPA
Senior Advisor, e-Communication and Research Translation
Office of the Director
National Institute for Occupational Safety and Health
Center for Disease Control and Prevention
Washington, D.C., United States of America

Retneswari **Masilamani**
MBBS, MMed (OM), PhD, FFOMI, FRCPI, FAMM, FAOEMM, FPHMM
Professor of Community and Occupational Medicine
Faculty of Medicine and Health Sciences
Universiti Tunku Abdul Rahman
Selangor, Malaysia

Halim **Mohamed**
AM (Mal), MB ChB (UK), MMed (OM) (S'pore)
Health Manager
Karachaganak Petroleum Operating B.V.
Kazakhstan Branch, Aksai, Burlin Region
West Kazakhstan Oblast, Republic of Kazakhstan

Rosmawati **Mohamed**
MBBS, MRCP, MMed (Int Med), MD
Professor and Consultant Hepatologist
University of Malaya
Kuala Lumpur, Malaysia

Mark **Newson-Smith**
MB ChB, MMedSc, LLM, FFOM, FFOMI
Occupational Health Physician
Avon Partnership Occupational Health Services
Avon Partnership Occupational Health Services Centre
Bristol, United Kingdom

Wee Tong **Ng**
MB ChB (UK), MMed (OM) (S'pore), Dip Av Med (UK)
Dip Geriatric Med (S'pore)
Associate Professor
Saw Swee Hock School of Public Health
National University of Singapore, Singapore

John Nelson **Norman**
MD, DSc, PhD, FRCS (Glasg, Edin), CB, FRSB
Emeritus Professor of Environmental Medicine University of Aberdeen, United Kingdom
President, Institute of Remote Healthcare
United Kingdom

Krishna Gopal **Rampal**
MBBS, MPH, PhD, FFOMI, FFOM, FAOEMM, FAMM
Professor of Community and Occupational Medicine
Cyberjaya University College of Medical Sciences
Cyberjaya, Selangor DE, Malaysia

Ailin **Razali**
MBBS, MSc, PhD
Associate Professor
Department of ORL-HNS
International Islamic University Malaysia, Kuantan, Malaysia

Huw **Rees**
MB BCh, FFOM, MD, Registered Toxicologist
Course Director, MSc Occupational Health
College of Biomedical and Life Sciences
Cardiff University School of Medicine, United Kingdom
Principal Medical Adviser
South Wales Fire and Rescue Service, United Kingdom
Consultant Occupational Physician
Powys Teaching Health Board, United Kingdom

Alison **Reid**
BSc (Hons), MSc, PhD
Associate Professor of Epidemiology School of Public Health
Curtin University
Western Australia, Australia

Steve **Riley**
MD, FRCP, FAcadMed
Dean of Medical Education
Honorary Consultant Nephrologist
Director, Centre for Medical Education
Cardiff University School of Medicine
United Kingdom

Abu Hasan **Samad**
MD, FRCP (Glasg), MMed (OM) (S'pore), FAMM, FAOEMM
Occupational Health Physician
Twin Towers Medical Centre KLCC Sdn Bhd, Malaysia
President
Academy of Occupational and Environmental Medicine Malaysia
Malaysia

Brian **See**
MBBS (S'pore), MPH (Occup Environ Health), DAvMed (Lond), FAMS
Centre Head, Aeromedical Centre
Deputy Chief Air Force Medical Officer
Republic of Singapore Air Force
Director
Changi Aviation Medicine Centre, Changi Hospital, Singapore
Visiting Consultant
Changi General Hospital, Singapore
Adjunct Assistant Professor
Saw Swee Hock School of Public Health
National University of Singapore, Singapore

Arjune **Sen**
MA (Oxon), PhD, FRCP, FRSB
Consultant Neurologist and Associate Professor
Head, Oxford Epilepsy Research Group
Nuffield Department of Clinical Neurosciences
National Institute of Health Research Biomedical Research Centre
John Radcliffe Hospital
Oxford, United Kingdom

Alena **Shantsila**
PhD
Liverpool Centre for Cardiovascular Science
University of Liverpool, Liverpool, UK

Eduard **Shantsila**
PhD
Faculty of Health and Life Sciences and
Liverpool Centre for Cardiovascular Science
University of Liverpool, UK

Dominic **Tan**
MBBS (S'pore), MPH (Occup Environ Health), DAvMed (Lond)
Head
Certification and Standards Branch, Aeromedical Centre
Republic of Singapore Air Force

Livia **Teo**
MBBS, MMed (Ophth), FRCS (Ed), FAMS
Senior Consultant
General Cataract and Comprehensive Ophthalmology and
Oculoplastic Departments
Singapore National Eye Centre, Singapore and
Duke-NUS Graduate Medical School, Singapore

Eng Loon **Tng**
MBBS, MRCP (UK), MMed (S'pore), FAMS (Endocrinology), CFPS, DFD (CAW), SCE (Endocrinology and Diabetes), MSc (Endocrinology and Diabetes), Specialist Dip (Statistics and Data Mining)
Consultant
Department of Medicine, Division of Endocrinology
Ng Teng Fong General Hospital
National University Health Systems, Singapore

Jane Frølund **Thomsen**
MD, PhD
Consultant
Associate Professor
Department of Occupational and Environmental Medicine
Bispebjerg University Hospital
Copenhagen, Denmark

Karen **Walker-Bone**
BM, FRCP, PhD, Hon FFOM
Professor in Occupational Rheumatology and
Honorary Consultant in Rheumatology
Director
MRC Versus Arthritis Centre for
Musculoskeletal Health and Work
University of Southampton, United Kingdom

Nerys **Williams**
MSc, FRCP, FFOM, MRCGP(1988), DCH, DRCOG, DGM, DDAM, Adv Cert PR
Consultant Occupational Physician
Birmingham, England, United Kingdom

Tien Yin **Wong**
MBBS, MMed (Ophth), FRCSE, FRANZCO, MPH, PhD (Johns Hopkins)
Medical Director and Senior Consultant Ophthalmologist
Singapore National Eye Centre
Vice Dean, Office of Clinical Sciences and Head of AMRI
Duke-NUS Graduate Medical School, Singapore

Section 1 —

Clinical Occupational Medicine

Chapter 1

Work and Health

David Koh and Wee Hoe Gan†*

Occupational Health, Occupational and Environmental Medicine

The International Labour Office (ILO) and World Health Organization (WHO) define occupational health as 'the promotion and maintenance of the highest degree of physical, mental and social well-being of workers in all occupations' (Forsmann, 1983). Occupational health seeks to not only maintain and promote workers' health and working capacity, it also extends to the improvement of working environment and work to be conducive to safety and health (Coppee, 2011).

The global working age population comprised an estimated 5.7 billion people, of which 3.3 billion (57%) are employed (International Labour Office, 2020). Access to paid work is no guarantee of decent work, and hence protection of the worker against sickness, disease and injury arising out of his employment is one of the tasks assigned to

*PAPRSB Institute of Health Sciences, Universiti Brunei Darussalam, Brunei Darussalam *and* Saw Swee Hock School of Public Health and Yong Loo Lin School of Medicine, National University of Singapore, Singapore.
†Department of Occupational and Environmental Medicine, Singapore General Hospital; Changi Aviation Medicine Centre, Changi General Hospital and Duke-NUS Medical School, National University of Singapore, Singapore.
Corresponding author: David Koh (ephkohd@nus.edu.sg).

the International Labour Organization under its constitution (International Labour Organization, 1985). The provision of Occupational health services is a means to achieve this objective.

Occupational and environmental medicine, as defined by the American College of Occupational and Environmental Medicine, is 'the medical specialty devoted to the prevention and management of occupational and environmental injury, illness and disability, and promotion of health and productivity of workers, their families, and communities.

The role of the occupational and environmental physician has expanded to enhancing the productivity of the worker with absence management and increased emphasis on the overall health, wellness, and safety of the worker — not just at the work site but also at home and in the community (American College of Occupational and Environmental Medicine, 2011).

Relationship between Work and Health

A crucial concept in occupational health is the recognition of a two-way relationship between work and health.

WORK ⇔ HEALTH

Work may not only have an adverse impact on health, but it can also be beneficial to health and well-being. The health status of the worker will have an impact on work. The worker who is healthy is more likely to be productive than an unhealthy worker. Workers with impaired health are not only less productive but could also be a danger to themselves as well as other workers, the community and the environment. Hence the development of the "Total Worker Health" concept proposed by National Institute for Occupational Safety and Health (NIOSH, 2016).

Case Study 1: Accident While Drunk on Duty

An oil company has known for years that the captain of one of its oil tankers had a serious drinking problem, but nonetheless left him in command of oil tankers. On one of the tanker journeys, the captain was drunk on duty and left an inexperienced officer in charge of navigating the tanker through hazardous icy conditions. The tanker ran aground on a reef and spilled millions of litres of crude oil, which coated thousands of kilometres of coastline and killed thousands of birds and marine mammals.

History of Occupational Medicine

The discipline of occupational medicine is a relatively recent development in the history of modern medicine. In comparison to modern medicine which evolved from Hippocratic times over 2,500 years ago, occupational medicine only became a recognised discipline from the time of Ramazzini, in the 18th century (Franco and Franco, 2001). Certain historical features in the development of occupational medicine have had a major impact on health and work.

Firstly, its developmental direction was influenced by the fact that it was intimately linked to the legislative process, with legislation such as the Factories Act and Compensation Act in Great Britain, requiring greater consideration of measures to reduce injury and ill-health from workplace factors. Legislation remains an important component of occupational medicine practice today, and is a driver for change and implementation of preventive measures at workplaces.

During the Industrial Revolution from the mid-18th century, much attention was focused on workers in mines and factories, as these were situations where workers were at obvious health risk as a consequence of their work. This led to the discipline in the early days being known as Industrial Medicine or even Factory Medicine. With the recognition of other hazards in the workplace, however, the focus was enlarged to include all persons at work, and the term Occupational Medicine came into being.

The specialty has since evolved to be known as Occupational Health, for the reason that it is not only concerned with preventing disease but also promoting health among people who work. This also extended recognition to the contribution of non-medical professionals who made major contributions to health and safety in the workplace. The term occupational health recognises the multidisciplinary nature of the specialty, as well as covers the provision of health services for working populations.

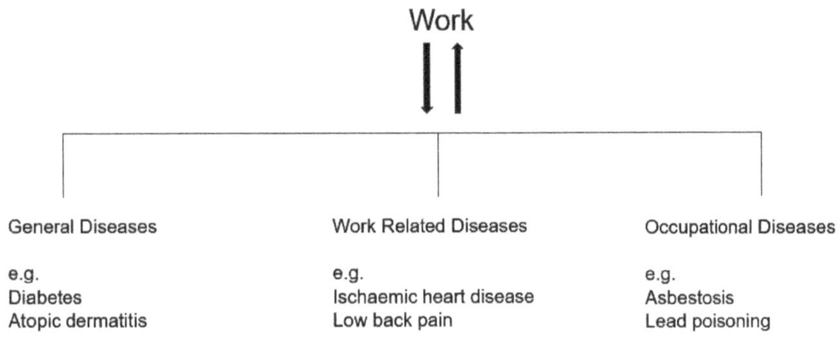

Fig. 1. Categories of disease at the workplace.

Work and Health

All workers may suffer from a spectrum of diseases, including: (i) diseases that affect the general population that are not caused by occupational factors, although prevalent in the community; (ii) work-related diseases; and (iii) occupational diseases (Fig. 1).

Any physician or clinician seeing an individual patient must recognise the possible relationship between work and disease. Non-occupational diseases may be worsened by work activities or workplace exposures; or diseases can occur mainly or solely because of workplace exposures. As an example of the former, many people who have diabetes mellitus may remain in the workforce. Their health condition could have an impact on work performance (as illustrated in Case Study 2) and equally, work may adversely affect the progression and/or prognosis of the diabetes.

Case Study 2: Diabetic Worker Requiring Shiftwork and Overseas Travel

Mr. B is a factory supervisor who has to be placed on shiftwork after the restructuring of his company's production and work processes. In addition, the recent acquisitions of new factories in overseas locations required him to travel abroad frequently.

Mr. B is an insulin-dependent diabetic and is concerned about his diabetic control in relation to the changes in the work situation.

He rightly expresses concern about the diabetic control with regard to travel through several time zones, access to medical care in the developing countries where the new factories are located, and vaccination requirements for the travel.

Disease Burden

Globally, 1.53 million deaths and 76.1 million disability adjusted life years (DALYs) were estimated to be attributable to the following occupational risk factors — carcinogens; asthmagens; particulate matter, gases and fumes (PMGF); secondhand smoke (SHS); noise; ergonomic risk factors for low back pain; and risk factors for injury. This accounted for 2.8% of deaths and 3.2% of DALYs from all causes in 2016.

Most deaths were attributable to PMGF, carcinogens (particularly asbestos), injury risk factors and SHS. Most DALYs were attributable to injury risk factors and ergonomic exposures. Men and persons 55 years or older were most affected. Population attributable fractions (PAFs) ranged from 26.8% for low back pain from ergonomic risk factors and 19.6% for hearing loss from noise to 3.4% for carcinogens (The Global Burden of Diseases 2016 Occupational Risk Factors Collaborators, 2020).

Occupational Diseases

The World Health Organization (2021) defines an "occupational disease" as any disease contracted primarily as a result of an exposure to risk factors arising from work activity.

Occupational diseases occur as a result of exposure to physical, chemical, biological or psychosocial factors in the workplace (Table 1).

These factors in the work environment are necessary in the causation of occupational diseases. For example, exposure to lead in the workplace is essential for lead poisoning, and exposure to silica is necessary for silicosis to occur. Other factors such as individual susceptibility may play a varying role in the development and progression of disease among exposed workers (i.e. workplace exposures are

Table 1. Occupational Health Hazards and Adverse Health Effects

Hazards	Adverse Health Effects
Physical Hazards	
Noise	Noise-induced hearing loss
Vibration	Vasospastic disease
Extreme of temperature	Heat stress
	Cold-induced disorders
Fire	Burns
Explosion	Injuries
Accidents	Injuries
Chemical Hazards	Poisoning
	Cancers
	Allergies
Biological Hazards	Infections
	Allergies
Ergonomic Hazards	
Repetitive movement	Repetitive strain injuries
Poor work organisation	Lowered productivity and work quality
Psychosocial Hazards	Stress
	Work dissatisfaction
	Conflicts
	Burnout
	Depression

necessary but not necessarily sufficient as the sole cause of an occupational disease).

Occupational diseases occur exclusively among workers exposed to specific hazards (Figs. 2 and 3) and are cause specific. However, in some situations these diseases may also occur among the general community as a consequence of contamination of the environment from the workplace, or from secondary exposure through contaminated

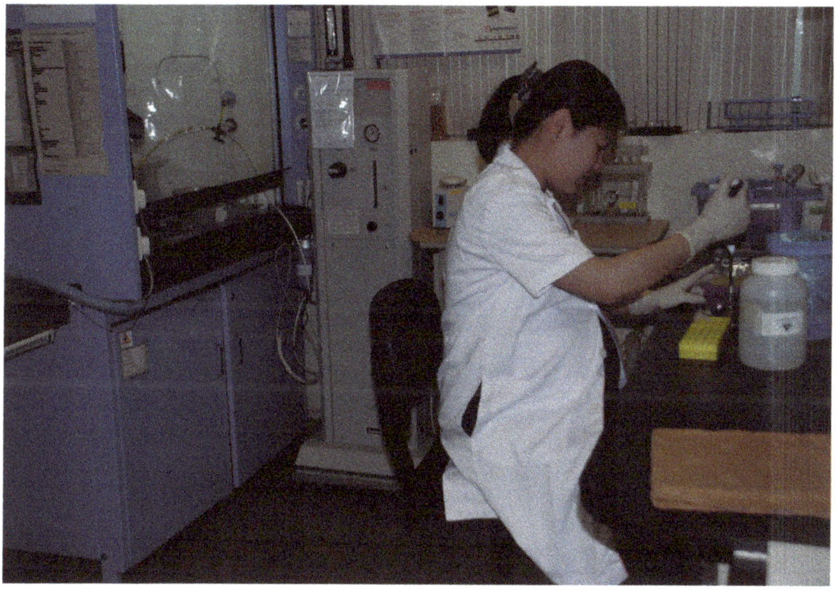

Fig. 2. A pregnant female laboratory technologist may be exposed to various chemicals (e.g. organic solvents) in her workplace.

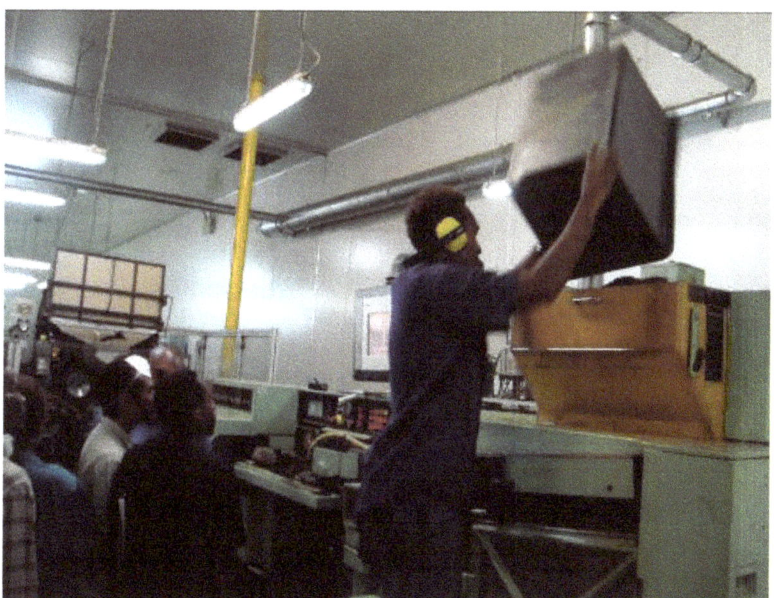

Fig. 3. This worker who has to repeatedly lift cartons above shoulder height may develop neck and shoulder complaints

work clothes brought home to cause exposure among family members, e.g. asbestos, lead, and pesticides.

Overt occupational diseases are often more commonly recognised in developing nations where the more hazardous occupations such as mining and traditional forms of agriculture are predominant, whereas work-related diseases generally become increasingly important as a country becomes more industrialised and phases out industries which are linked to an increased risk of the "traditional" occupational diseases. There is also a group of countries that underwent rapid economic growth in a short span of time, termed the Newly Industrialising Countries (NICs). Such countries face a unique blend of traditional occupational diseases, emerging occupational diseases as well as work-related diseases (Koh and Sng, 2009).

Work Related Diseases

The WHO categorises work-related diseases as "multifactorial" in origin, where factors in the work environment may play a role, together with other risk factors, in the development of such diseases. (WHO, 2021). These are diseases that are frequently seen in the general community. Such work-related diseases include (i) hypertension, (ii) ischemic heart disease, (iii) psychosomatic illness, (iv) musculoskeletal disorders, (v) chronic non-specific respiratory disease, and (vi) chronic bronchitis.

In these diseases, work may be associated in their causation or may aggravate a pre-existing condition. The main differences between occupational diseases and work-related diseases are shown in Table 2.

Table 2. Differences Between Occupational and Work-related Diseases

Work-related Diseases	Occupational Diseases
Occurs largely in the community	Occurs mainly among working population
"Multifactorial" in origin	Cause specific
Exposure at workplace may be a factor	Exposure at workplace is essential
Less likely to be notifiable and compensable	Likely to be notifiable and compensable

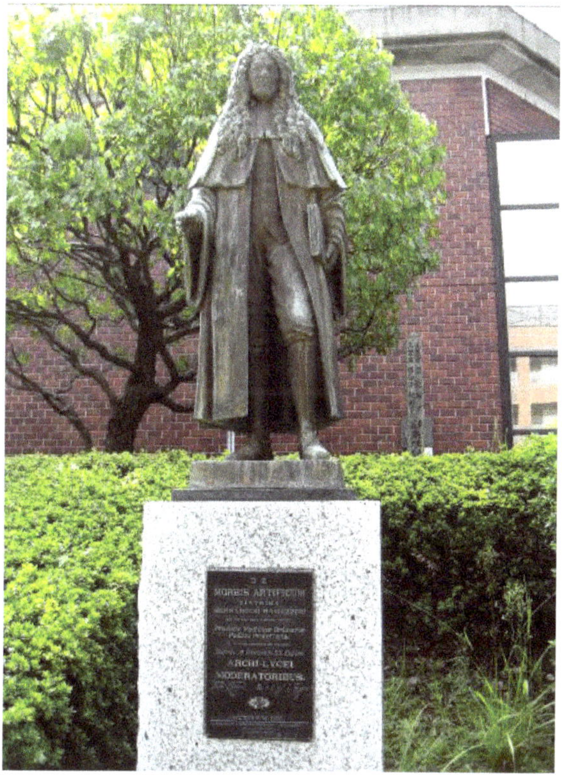

Fig. 4. Statue of Ramazzini at the University of Occupational and Environmental Health in Kitakyushu, Japan.

Clinical History Taking

It was only in 1700s that Bernadino Ramazzini (Fig. 4), physician and professor of medicine in Modena and Padua, Italy, recommended that physicians enquire about a patient's occupation. Previous to this, the standard three questions recommended by Hippocrates were to enquire of the patient's name, age and residence.

The routinely asked question "What is your job?" often provides inadequate information. It is important to obtain an adequate occupational history for the following reasons:

Firstly, to assess the extent to which the illness has been caused or is related to the patient's job. For example, the patient's anaemia may be consequent to exposure to lead; or the "malingering" patient may be in some way related to a highly stressful or hostile work environment.

Has Work Caused, or is it in Some Way Associated with the Disease?

Another reason for taking a good occupational history is to assess the patient's fitness to return to work. In this regard, the following four factors need to be considered:

1. What are the long-term effects of the disease?
2. What is the nature of the job the patient is returning to?
3. Is the return to work likely to cause a recurrence of disease or is it likely to aggravate the disease?
4. Is returning to work likely to cause damage or ill-health to other work colleagues or the general community?

For instance, if the patient was seen for a condition which was clearly the result of occupational exposure, e.g. occupational asthma; occupational dermatitis; musculoskeletal disorders due to poor ergonomic factors; then returning to the same work situation will only result in a recurrence of the condition. In this situation, corrective measures need to be taken at the workplace to prevent such recurrences.

There are other situations where return to some work may aggravate illness. For instance, a diabetic patient's regular meal times and medication may be adversely affected if he returns to shift work; particularly as a diurnal variation exists with medication and insulin. Similarly, a patient after suffering from a myocardial infarction may not be able to return to work requiring heavy physical exertion or returning to a high-stress environment.

Return to work may also have an impact on work colleagues or the general community. For example, a patient with chronic infectious disease returning to work, such as a healthcare worker with hepatitis B or HIV may pose a risk to colleagues and patients. Another example is where the worker's residual clinical condition may be a danger to himself and fellow workers; such as an epileptic (with poorly controlled seizures) working at a conveyor belt or at heights or alone at the worksite. Examples of ill-advised return to work affecting the public could be a worker with an infected wound on his finger returning to work as a food vendor, an airline pilot with psychological problems returning to fly, or the Case Study 3.

Case Study 3: Return to Work for a Taxi Driver after a Cerebrovascular Accident

Mr. C has just been discharged from the hospital after a cerebrovascular accident. He responded well to treatment and has only a mild residual left-sided paresis. He decides to return to work as a taxi driver after a further two weeks' rest. This is not in contravention of any law, as there are no legislative requirements for a return to work medical assessment, and no approved guidelines for medical assessments for fitness to work as a taxi driver in his country.

Finally, asking a patient his job may give an indication of the patient's educational and socio-economic status. This information is of value in providing holistic care as well as sensible practical advice to the patient for which compliance can be facilitated.

Occupational History

In summary, the components of an occupational history include:

- Job description/nature of job and work tasks
- Hours of work/shift work
- Types of hazards
- Past occupations
- Other concurrent jobs
- Domestic exposures
- Hobbies

In taking an occupational history, as much detail as possible must be obtained regarding the job. The detail required would depend on the circumstances. It is important to know the possible hazards the worker may be exposed to, the type of job, and the hours of work. Equally important would be to take a history of past occupations; as the present health problem may be the consequence of an earlier job, particularly if the disease has a long latent period between exposure and onset of disease, e.g. asbestosis, silicosis, toxic neuropathies, occupational cancers.

Additional information relevant to the occupational history should include:

- Smoking history/Alcohol intake/Drugs and medications
- Similar complaints among other workers
- Time relationship between work and symptoms
- Relationship of illness to periods away from work
- Extent of exposure to recognised hazards (i.e. intensity and duration of exposure)
- Use of protective devices
- Methods of materials handling.

These are additional items that may be useful in an occupational history. For instance, a history of smoking is of particular relevance. Workers who smoke are at higher risk of developing certain occupational diseases such as asbestosis and lead poisoning, as well as many cancers including of the lung and bladder. Similarly, alcohol consumption may increase the risk of hepatitis in a solvent-exposed worker.

It is important to note the temporal sequence of the onset of symptoms and exposure. This is of particular importance in occupational diseases of acute onset, such as pesticide poisonings, and occupational asthma. Occupational diseases also tend to improve when the patient is away from work, such as during long weekends, or on vacation.

Information on the use of protective devices such as masks or gloves is also useful. One issue to consider is that sometimes the workers may use such devices inappropriately or incorrectly, or that the devices are not well maintained. Thus, even if the worker reports that protective devices are used, it does not automatically exclude occupational disease.

Challenges

There are some common challenges to be aware of while obtaining an occupational history. Some of these issues include end occupations, uninformative job titles, multiple jobs and other concurrent environmental exposures, e.g. from hobbies.

End occupations

Most patients would give their current occupation when a healthcare worker asks about their job. However, the patient could have retired or changed job and his current health problems may be associated with a previous job. Therefore, it is important to ask a patient about their entire occupational history, as far as possible. In some situations, this may be tedious, but it is crucial so that proper diagnosis and management can be instituted, particularly if there is even the slightest likelihood of the illness being linked to an occupational exposure, as in the patient in Case Study 4.

Case Study 4: Chronic Respiratory Complaints in a Retiree

A 63-year-old retiree consults his general practitioner with chronic respiratory complaints which started 2 years ago, and had worsened since then. His case notes recorded that he had worked as a general worker for 20 years, before retiring 3 years ago. He is a non-smoker, and had no other past medical or surgical history of note. His previous consultations were infrequent and unremarkable.

At this consultation, further enquiry into his past occupations revealed that he had worked as a general worker in a shipyard, doing a variety of jobs. One of his main duties was sandblasting paint off the ships. The patient also recalled having to remove and replace the insulation on the ships' old boiler pipes several times a year in the course of his work.

Note: In this case an adequate occupational history points to a possibility of exposure to silica (from sandblasting) and asbestos (lagging in old boiler pipes) from his work. Either exposure may have caused his current respiratory symptoms.

Job titles

Patients may provide a job title that may not be of much value, unless the physician is familiar with the workplace and the potential hazards of the job. This is particularly so when a worker gives a job description as a factory worker. It is necessary to follow up with questions about the nature of the job hazards. Further, a job description that may appear free of exposure to workplace hazards may still have relevance to the causation of the illness.

For instance, a young lady was seen with a rash over the malar region of the face. She worked as a clerk. The rash had been persistent and was better during weekends and holidays, indicating a relationship to work. On detailed enquiry, it was revealed that her work desk was directly below the air-conditioner vent. Her rash was diagnosed as low humidity dermatitis — a condition that disappeared as soon as her desk position was changed.

Similarly, backache is a common problem. If an office worker or a nurse complains of it, the possibility of ergonomic factors contributing to the illness must be considered.

Multiple jobs

Another potential pitfall in taking an occupational history is that some patients may be holding more than one job. In such situations, patients may choose only to reveal what they consider to be their main occupation, and not inform the physician of other concurrent jobs. Thus, it is often appropriate to ask if an individual holds other jobs as well.

Walk Through Assessment of the Workplace

An occupational physician should be able to undertake, in a systematic way, a complete evaluation of a workplace for occupational hazards. In occupational health practice, such an evaluation may be needed because of concerns expressed by the workforce or management about possible health effects related to the work environment. Alternatively, it may arise in the course of a regular inspection to ensure compliance with health and safety legislation. It can also occur because of a request to audit a work area in order to identify potential problem areas, and to recommend appropriate preventive action to reduce occupational ill-health.

Most experienced occupational physicians have their own method for evaluating workplaces. This will have been developed over years of practical experience of visiting places of work. The methods include using a mental checklist, a written aide memoire, or a blank sheet of paper to record observations. In order to ensure that any evaluation is complete, some form of written checklist is needed. This allows for a reduced likelihood of error and/or omission. A standardised basic form can be used to record findings when evaluating workplaces for occupational hazards.

The form

The contents of the form are shown in Box 1. This requires the recording of identification data on the workplace visited. The analogy is to a hospital patient record where identification data is needed for future reference. Information about names and phone numbers of contacts is best recorded when they are provided. This avoids having to contact the workplace again to re-establish the identity of the key people met during the visit, but whose names and phone numbers have been forgotten or not written down by the end of the visit. If further contact with the factory is required, knowledge of the key names invokes a sense of concern and interest on the part of the caller.

Information on the history of the workplace — whether it has been recently built, if it is part of a larger conglomerate, what it does and how it has developed over time in relation to its activities and the surrounding community and environment, and its record on health and safety are useful as a background to understanding that particular workplace. The analogy in the clinical situation is a patient's social, family, personal and past history. The geographical location of the workplace can be made, for example, by obtaining a map that shows the way to the workplace. A site plan helps to ensure that any work area visited is put in the context of the rest of the worksite, and that all relevant areas are eventually visited and evaluated. Two other sections of importance are:

- Data on the workforce. The characteristics of the workforce (e.g. age, gender, ethnic group) give an indication of the population "exposed" to the work environment. This will also be of use if epidemiological investigations are contemplated.
- Services provided and available to the workforce. This enables an assessment of the health, safety and welfare provisions in relation to any workplace hazards that may be identified.

All the above information may be obtained before or during the visit to the workplace.

Box 1. Workplace Visit Checklist Contents (Aw *et al.*, 1990).

1. Identification Data
   - Name of workplace
   - Address and phone number
2. Contacts (Name and Telephone No.):
   - Personnel manager/managing director
   - Union representative
   - Doctor
   - Other, e.g. supervisor
3. Workplace
   - History
   - Geography and site plan
   - No. of workers (age, sex, race, shifts, turnover)
4. Services
   - Medical (staff, procedures)
   - Canteen/shower
   - Protective equipment
   - Hygiene and safety
5. Systematic Identification of Hazards and Assessment of Risks
   Raw materials → Finished product
   - Physical
   - Chemical
   - Biological
   - Mechanical/ergonomic
   - Psycho-social
   - Safety issues

Findings on whether an occupational hazard exists are recorded in the next section. This requires that the occupational physician using the format visits each section of the factory starting from raw materials to storage and distribution of the finished products.

Although it would be ideal to go systematically through the various stages of production, in practice because of the location of different parts of the processes, these may not necessarily be shown to the visiting physician in any systematic order. Hence the usefulness of a site plan to indicate what has been seen and what has not.

At each part of the process the occupational physician needs to determine and record the presence of any hazards according to whether these are physical, chemical, mechanical and ergonomic, biological or psychosocial. This is based on an aetiological classification of occupational hazards. The procedure allows a complete and thorough evaluation to be made; and it ensures that important hazards at each stage of the work activities are not missed out. The analogy to clinical medical practice is that in the examination of a patient, the doctor goes systematically through inspection, palpation, percussion, and auscultation.

Physical hazards would include exposure to extremes of temperature, poor lighting, noise, and pressure, vibration, electricity, and radiation.

Chemical hazards may be present in solid, liquid, semi-solid, or gaseous form. Identification of the presence of a chemical may require that the information on the label of the container or packaging be recorded, so that further checking on the chemical composition of a trade substance and its known health effects can be subsequently ascertained. Most of the necessary information about chemicals is available on Safety Data Sheets. If necessary, arrangements can then be made for industrial hygiene measurements to be taken to determine compliance with current airborne standards.

Mechanical hazards are often obvious to the trained safety professional, who will readily spot the unguarded sections of factory machinery. Ergonomic problems may be anticipated by observation of the way in which posture and repeated movements of limbs and joints occur in the course of work.

Biological hazards are relevant to workplaces such as laboratories and hospitals. These may be classified by aetiological agent into viruses, bacteria, fungi, and so on.

Psychosocial hazards in the workplace may be difficult to identify, and one approach is to gather information by talking to workers on the production line in the course of the factory visit, or to consider other indirect indicators such as labour turnover rate, industrial relations difficulties, poor quality control, or sickness absence.

An extended version of this form can be prepared to give further items to be recorded for an audit on occupational health services. The additional checklist is shown in Box 2.

Box 2. Additional Checklist for Occupational Health Services (Aw *et al.*, 1990).

1. Staff
   - Medical
   - Nursing
   - First aiders
   - Industrial hygiene staff
   - Safety officer/advisor
   - Welfare officer
2. Facilities
   - Rooms for OHS services
3. Equipment
   - Medical
   - Hygiene
   - Safety
4. OH records
   - (Computerised or files?)
5. Library or information source
6. Other amenities
   - Canteen
   - Showers/changing rooms
   - Laundry
7. Activities
   - Health examinations/assessments (periodic, special groups, statutory, non-statutory)

Box 2. (*Continued*)

- Immunisation
- Health education/counselling
- Treatment activities
- Rehabilitation
- Compensation
- Disaster planning
- Food hygiene
- Ergonomics
- Environmental health

8. Waste management
9. Waste disposal

The Future of Work

The nature of work is evolving in response to technological progress, globalisation, ageing populations and free movement of labour. New business models and relationships have also emerged, with an increasing trend for companies and independent workers to set short term and on-demand professional relationships which are flexible and skill based, the so-called "gig economy". Such changes can impact job quality positively and negatively. The diversity in employment contracts can provide flexibility for many firms and workers, but also result in challenges in ensuring the quality (including occupational health) of non-standard work. Occupational health practice will have to adapt and respond to these changes in work.

Advances in artificial intelligence, automation and robotics, and the shift in economies to adopt sustainable practices and clean technologies will create new jobs, but also render many other jobs obsolete. The OECD estimates that 14% of existing jobs could disappear as a result of automation in the next 15–20 years, and another 32% are likely to change radically as individual tasks are automated. (Organisation for Economic Co-operation and Development, 2019) Unfortunately, those who lose their jobs in this transition may be the least equipped to seize the new opportunities (International Labour Office, 2019).

The Coronavirus Disease 2019 (COVID-19) Pandemic

On 31 December 2019, the WHO China office was informed of cases of pneumonia of unknown aetiology detected in Wuhan city in Hubei Province, central China. By 9 January 2020, WHO released a statement on the cluster of cases, which stated that "Chinese authorities have made a preliminary determination of a novel (or new) coronavirus, identified in a hospitalised person with pneumonia in Wuhan. The virus was initially referred to as 2019-nCoV, but has since been re-named as SARS-CoV-2 by the WHO on 12 February 2020. The WHO declared this disease as a Public Health Emergency of International Concern (PHEIC) on 30 January 2020. By April 2021, there were over 130 million COVID-19 cases worldwide with over 3 million deaths.

Occupational Risks for COVID-19

Among the first 25 locally transmitted cases of COVID-19 reported in Singapore in early February 2020, 17 cases (68%) were highly likely to be related to occupational exposure. The cases included staff working in a retail store selling complementary health products primarily serving Chinese tourists, a jewellery store worker who attended to Chinese tourists, a tour guide who led tour group from China, casino and theme park workers and taxi and private hire car drivers. These workers were exposed to infected customers and clients (Koh, 2020a). Multinational company staff attending an international business meeting in Singapore were also infected from exposure to the virus at the meeting (Case Study 5). In the ensuing months, the vast majority of cases in Singapore were from migrant workers who lived together in close proximity in housing provided by their employers (Koh, 2020b).

Case Study 5: Occupationally Acquired COVID-19

An international business meeting for 109 staff was organised by a multinational company from 20–22 January 2020 in Singapore. At this event, healthy company workers interacted with other infected participants, which resulted in the transmission of the SARS-CoV2 to three employees based in Singapore. Besides those infected from Singapore, a company employee from Malaysia, two participants from South Korea and one staff member from the United Kingdom were also infected. They presented as COVID-19 patients after leaving Singapore.

Impact of COVID-19 on Work Practices

With movement restriction orders in place and lockdowns in most countries, working in split shifts and telecommuting became the norm. Workers in non-essential sectors were encouraged to stay away from work. In addition, there were unprecedented job losses because of the economic fallout. Important questions to address would include how, and at what speed, to manage a safe return to economic activity without a resurgence of new waves of infections. Most governments have provided support to businesses and workers, but these cannot continue indefinitely and have to be scaled down and adapted. Finally, provisions should also be made for the cohort of young people whose education and early work experience have been adversely impacted by the pandemic (Organisation for Economic Co-operation and Development, 2020). Even with effective vaccines and/or treatment available, it is likely that the work norms in the post COVID-19 era will feature aspects of telecommuting, working from home and social distancing.

From Occupational Health to Environmental Health

Previously, public interest in environmental health was not matched by a well-developed specialty in the health field which could respond to its needs and concerns. Occupational health practice today has gradually evolved to encompass environmental health issues. This is because of several reasons. Firstly, many sources of pollution originate from the workplace. Secondly, in many other instances, the distinction between the work environment and the home environment

Table 3. Comparison of Occupational Health and Environmental Health

Occupational Health	Environmental Health
Hazards in workplace environment	Hazards in community environment
Hazards largely in air	Hazards in air, soil, water and food
Hazards are physical, chemical, biological and psychosocial	Hazards are physical, chemical, biological and psychosocial
Route of exposure: inhalation and dermal	Route of exposure: ingestion, inhalation and dermal
Exposure period: 8 hrs/day for working life	Exposure period: lifelong
Exposed population: adults, usually healthy	Exposed population: children, adults, elderly, sick persons

may not be clearly defined. This is particularly seen in agriculture and small-scale industries, where some occupational activities may be done at home. There are several areas of common ground between occupational and environmental health. Table 3 compares factors in the work environment that influence the health of the working population (Occupational health) and that of the general environment affecting the health of the community (Environmental Health).

Occupational health practitioners and physicians have the necessary skills in clinical medicine, toxicology, hygiene, epidemiology and preventive health to position themselves for the management of environmental health concerns, as illustrated in Case Study 6.

Case Study 6: Skin Disorders Among Villagers Residing Near a Pulp and Paper Mill

Villagers living along a river began to complain of skin disorders a few months after a pulp mill was sited upstream from their villagers. The residents, who were mainly fishermen and farmers, bathed in the river and used river water for many of their domestic activities. They claimed that pollutants discharged from the pulp mill caused the skin disorders. An occupational health team was consulted to resolve the matter.

Workplace assessment revealed some occupational health and safety issues that needed to be addressed. The plant utilised modern "state of the art" technology, with a closed mill system. Monitoring of the effluent from the mill revealed that quality of the discharge was within internationally accepted limits.

Examination of a group of the most severely affected villagers revealed that the main skin disorders were fungal infections of the skin, endogenous eczema, and irritant contact dermatitis at specific sites (e.g. from application of topical medicaments, hand dermatitis from use of detergents).

A comparison of the existing health records of the village showed no increase in the proportion of cases of skin disorders before and after the pulp mill commenced operations. The main health problems were malaria and gastroenteritis.

The conclusion was that the villagers' health concerns (with regard to dermatological disorders) were unrelated to the pulp mill. The mill management however, provided supplementary community health care through its health care department, in conjunction with the local health authorities. This gesture was appreciated by the villagers.

Conclusion

This chapter introduces the concept of occupational health, emphasising that occupational health is concerned with the total health of all persons at work. The three categories of illnesses affecting the working population are: General diseases, Work-related diseases and Occupational diseases. General diseases and work-related diseases of working population are usually covered in the undergraduate and postgraduate training programmes of medical education.

In the practice of occupational health, prevention of work-related and occupational disease is a major objective. Primary prevention should be the main priority in occupational health practice. When this fails, secondary prevention activities are undertaken to contain damage.

However, health protection is not the only occupational health concern. Health promotion in the working population is another important activity. The workplace is an ideal setting for health promotion activities, and appropriate lifestyle interventions can prevent many of the common causes of morbidity in society.

As work practices evolve and new health challenges are faced, priorities in occupational health will change. However, as long as the majority of people continue to work, occupational health practice and quality care of workers will still be needed.

Finally, the practice of occupational health today has extended beyond the domain of the workplace, into the general environment. Hence the term occupational and environmental medicine might more accurately describe this important aspect of health care.

References

American College of Occupational and Environmental Medicine. (2011) Scope of occupational and environmental health programs and practice. [Online] Available from: https://acoem.org/acoem/media/News-Library/Scope-of-Occupational-and-Environmental-Health-Programs.pdf [Accessed on 17 Aug 2020].

Aw TC, Koh D, Harrington M.A. (1990) Format for systematic evaluation of the workplace. *J Occup Med* **2**(1): 40–43.

Coppee, G.H. (2011) Occupational health services and practice. In: Stellman, J.M. (ed.), *Encyclopedia of Occupational Health and Safety* (4th Ed), Geneva, Switzerland, International Labour Organization. Available from: https://www.iloencyclopaedia.org/ [Accessed 17 Aug 2020].

Forsmann, S. (1983) Occupational health. In: Parmeggiani, L (ed.), *Encyclopedia of Occupational Health and Safety* (3rd Ed), Geneva, Switzerland, International Labour Organization, pp. 1491–1492.

Franco G, Franco F. (2001) Bernardino Ramazzini: the father of occupational medicine. *Am J Public Health* **91**(9): 1382.

Koh D, Sng J. (2009) Occupational health and safety in newly industrializing countries. *Occup Health South Afr* **15**(Special ICOH issue): 12–16.

Koh D. (2020a) Occupational risks for COVID-19. *Occup Med* **70**(1): 3–5.

Koh D. (2020b) Migrant workers and COVID-19. *Occup Environ Med* **77**: 634–636.

Global Burden of Diseases 2016 Occupational Risk Factors Collaborators. (2020) Global and regional burden of disease and injury in 2016 arising from occupational exposures: a systematic analysis for the global burden of disease study 2016. *Occup Environ Med* 77: 133–141.

International Labour Organization. (1985) Occupational health services convention 1985. In: International Labour Organization. *The General Conference of the International Labour Organization, Issue 161, Geneva, Switzerland,* International Labour Organization. Available from: https://www.ilo.org/dyn/normlex/en/f?p=NORMLEXPUB:12100:0::NO::P12100_ILO_CODE:C161 [Accessed on 17 Aug 2020].

International Labour Office. (2019) *Work for a Brighter Future — Global Commission on the Future of Work.* ISBN 978-92-2-132795-0 (print) ISBN 978-92-2-132796-7(web pdf). Available from https://www.ilo.org/wcmsp5/groups/public/---dgreports/---dcomm/---publ/documents/publication/wcms_734455.pdf[Accessed on 17 Aug 2020].

International Labour Office. (2020) *World employment and social outlook trends 2020.* International Labour Office. ISBN 978-92-2-031408-1 (print) ISBN 978-92-2-031407-4 (web pdf). Available from https://www.ilo.org/wcmsp5/groups/public/---dgreports/---dcomm/---publ/documents/publication/wcms_734455.pdf [Accessed on 17 Aug 2020].

National Institute for Occupational Safety and Health. (2016) *NIOSH Total Worker Health® Program.* [Online] Available from: https://www.cdc.gov/niosh/twh/ [Accessed on 17 Aug 2020].

Organisation for Economic Co-operation and Development. (2019) *The Future of Work OECD Employment Outlook 2019.* [Online] Available from: https://www.oecd-ilibrary.org/employment/oecd-employment-outlook-2019_9ee00155-en [Accessed on 17 Aug 2020].

Organisation for Economic Co-operation and Development. (2020) *OECD Employment Outlook 2020 Worker Security and the COVID 19 Crisis.* [Online] Available from: https://www.oecd-ilibrary.org/docserver/1686c758-en.pdf?expires=1597636504&id=id&accname=guest&checksum=5B3C011BA4540BFDA1FC70A0242A5481 [Accessed on 17 Aug 2020].

World Health Organization. (2021) *Occupational and Work-related Diseases.* [Online] Available from: https://www.who.int/activities/occupational-and-work--related-diseases [Accessed on 17 Aug 2020].

Chapter 2

Diagnosis and Management of Occupational Diseases

Wee Hoe Gan and David Koh†*

Introduction

An occupational disease is a disorder primarily caused by an exposure to risk factors from work activity. Some authorities make a distinction between occupational diseases and work-related diseases, the latter of which have multi-factorial aetiologies not limited to work (World Health Organization (WHO), 2021). In a work-related disease, occupational hazards contribute to, but do not form the dominant factor in disease causation. The International Labour Organization (ILO) highlighted two main elements in the definition of an occupational disease, namely the causal relationship between exposure in a specific working environment or work activity and a specific disease, as well as the disease occurring among a group of exposed persons with a frequency above the average morbidity of the rest of the population

*Department of Occupational and Environmental Medicine, Singapore General Hospital; Changi Aviation Medicine Centre, Changi General Hospital and Duke-NUS Medical School, National University of Singapore, Singapore.
†PAPRSB Institute of Health Sciences, Universiti Brunei Darussalam, Brunei Darussalam *and* Saw Swee Hock School of Public Health and Yong Loo Lin School of Medicine, National University of Singapore, Singapore.
Corresponding author: Wee Hoe Gan (gan.wee.hoe@singhealth.com.sg).

(ILO, 2009). While such a distinction may have an impact on the extent of work injury compensation potentially claimable, it often does not affect the worker's clinical and occupational health management. They can both be considered part of a spectrum of clinical conditions where occupational factors are an important component.

Based on a systematic analysis of the Global Burden of Disease Study 2016, occupational risk factors accounted for 2.8% of global deaths and 3.2% of disability-adjusted life years (DALYs) from all causes (GBD, 2016; Occupational Risk Factors Collaborators, 2020). The top three contributors for global occupational-attributable deaths are particulate matter, gases and fumes (PMGF), carcinogens (mainly asbestos) and injury risk factors, whereas most DALYs were attributable to injury risk factors and ergonomic exposures. The significant burden of mortality and morbidity from occupational exposures compels occupational physicians and other health professionals to play key roles in the prevention, early detection and management of workers with occupational diseases.

Criteria for Diagnosis of Occupational Diseases

Clear criteria for diagnosing occupational diseases will facilitate consistency and fairness in terms of disease causation attribution and compensation. Key information needed for diagnosis are the symptoms and signs, any special diagnostic tests, and relevant exposures. However, the ability to definitively establish a work-related cause–effect relationship of a disease is not straightforward in all cases because other environmental, social and personal factors may confound the development and progression of a worker's medical condition. In the absence of clinical guidance and principles, the difficulty in making a causal link of a disease to work can lead to undesirable variations in practice and reporting.

A commonly used practical guidance to establish causality for occupational diseases is the set of principles presented by Sir Austin Bradford Hill, Professor Emeritus of Medical Statistics at the University of London, at the first meeting of the then-newly founded Section of Occupational Medicine under the Royal Society of Medicine, United Kingdom (UK) (Hill, 1965). This became known as the Bradford Hill's criteria (Box 1). To establish the causative link of diseases to work exposures, the first five criteria are generally considered the most important.

Box 1. Bradford Hill's Criteria (Adapted from International Labour Organization (2009))

1. **Temporality:** The occupational exposure of interest preceded the disease by a period of time consistent with any proposed biological mechanism.
2. **Biological plausibility:** From what is known of toxicology, chemistry, physical properties or other attributes of the occupational risk or hazard, a biologically plausible mechanism should be able to explain why the exposure leads to the disease.
3. **Consistency**: Different studies replicated in different populations and by different investigators have generally similar results and conclusions.
4. **Strength of association:** The greater the impact of an occupational exposure on the occurrence of development of a disease, the stronger the likelihood of a causal relationship. For example, the mortality from scrotal cancer is 200 times higher in chimney sweepers than in workers not exposed to tar.
5. **Biological gradient:** The greater the level and duration of occupational exposure, the greater the severity of diseases or their incidence. Such a dose–response relationship may not always be observed, such as for occupational diseases caused by allergens at work.
6. **Specificity:** Exposure to a specific occupational risk factor results in a clearly defined pattern of disease or diseases.
7. **Coherence:** A general synthesis of all the evidence (e.g. epidemiological studies, animal studies) should fit with the known facts of the natural history and biology of the disease to lead to the conclusion that there is a cause–effect relationship.
8. **Experiment (or interventional studies):** If a hazard control intervention has a beneficial effect, then removing the intervention will also negate the benefit of eliminating the development of a specific disease or reducing its incidence.

Another suggested algorithm for the diagnosis of an occupational disease is based on the following four essential criteria.

Relevant effect

The first criterion that should be met in diagnosing an occupational disease is the clinical presentation. The symptoms and signs of the case should be consistent with what is known about the disease. The health effects should fit what is described in the literature about the specific occupational illness. Vahabzadeh *et al.* (2016) reported a cluster of three professional gilders who developed neuro-psychiatric symptoms of anxiety, loss of memory and concentration, and sleep disturbances. All three workers were working on the same project to gild a shrine dome, which involved the mixing of liquid mercury with gold powder. The workers' clinical presentation is consistent with the manifestations of metallic mercury poisoning, and their work exposure points to an occupational causation of the disease.

Relevant exposure

A second essential criterion is confirmation of exposure. To diagnose an occupational disease requires that there should be sufficient exposure to a relevant agent at the workplace. For a chemically induced occupational illness, the exposure should be to an appropriate species of a chemical agent; in a suitable physical state (e.g. liquid, gas, or wax); and with sufficient intensity, frequency, and duration of exposure. Confirmation of exposure may be through ambient air monitoring and/or biological monitoring. For chronic exposures, a review of records from such monitoring, where available, may confirm a past history of workplace exposures that exceed occupational exposure standards. A single small excursion above an occupational exposure standard may in itself be insufficient to cause an occupational illness. If occupational exposures exceed the standards by a large margin on many occasions, this will indicate poor workplace control measures, and could constitute sufficient evidence regarding occupational causation. Where records of occupational hygiene assessments are not available, the diagnosis may have to depend on other evidence suggesting unacceptable exposure, such as acute incidents involving leak of chemicals, or where personal protective equipment is not available or not used when required.

Appropriate time sequence

The third essential criterion is that the exposure should precede the effect. The time interval between initial exposure and the development of disease should also be consistent with what is known about the latent period for the disease. For example, most occupational cancers usually appear after a long latent period which may be decades. Conversely, the concept of minimum induction period describes the shortest period from the start of exposure to the disease onset, below which the exposure would have been unlikely to have caused the disease (Directorate-General for Employment, Social Affairs and Inclusion (European Commission), 2009). Hence, lung cancer developing within a year after the first exposure to asbestos is unlikely to be attributed to that exposure. Other factors such as intensity of exposure, age, health status and genetic susceptibility may also be relevant.

For some acute occupational poisonings, the longer the interval between exposure and development of signs and symptoms, the less likely is the link between exposure and effect. The concept of the maximum latent period is used to refer to the length of time from cessation of exposure beyond which it is unlikely that any resulting disease can be attributed to that exposure (Directorate-General for Employment, Social Affairs and Inclusion (European Commission), 2009). An example is that of delayed pulmonary oedema due to exposure to phosgene, an industrial chemical used in the manufacturing of plastics and pesticides. There is usually a delay of 24 to 48 hours after exposure to phosgene gas before respiratory effects occur. However, if pulmonary oedema appears more than a month after exposure to phosgene, it will be difficult to conclude that phosgene was responsible for the respiratory effects.

Differential diagnosis

A fourth criterion is to consider the differential diagnosis. Whether or not there is occupational exposure to a suspected causative agent, it is possible that some other non-occupational factor is responsible for the symptoms and signs. For example, a worker in a pharmaceutical plant presenting with peripheral neuropathy may be a result of exposure to n-hexane (a solvent and a recognised neuropathic agent with commercial applications such as the manufacture of pharmaceuticals) at work. It may also be due to diabetes mellitus. Hence, focussing on possible diabetes without asking about occupational exposure to n-hexane or other neuropathic agents would be inappropriate. And so would focusing on possible occupational aetiology without remembering that diabetes is common in the general population and can be managed and controlled if diagnosed early. Hence, both occupational and non-occupational factors should be considered in the differential diagnosis, and the conclusion would depend on the balance of probability. Is the patient's illness more likely to be due to a non-occupational condition, or is it a result of occupational exposure, or both? If both factors exist, then managing one without considering the other may well result in continuation of the patient's illness despite clinical and/or occupational health intervention.

Additional considerations

The aforementioned criteria are by no means exhaustive. There are other factors that have been suggested to help in diagnosing occupational diseases. These additional considerations include whether there are special clinical or histological features that are unique to occupationally caused diseases, and whether there is the occurrence of clusters of cases in a particular workplace. However, these characteristics do not always exist.

For example, the cell type of respiratory or skin cancers due to occupational exposures may be more common with certain exposures, but are not unique to specific exposures. Squamous cell carcinomas, small cell carcinomas, and adenocarcinomas occur in both occupational and non-occupational lung cancers. Even for mesotheliomas, it is difficult to conclude that asbestos is the only cause of this malignancy. The detection of ferruginous bodies in sputum or in post-mortem lung tissue only confirms asbestos exposure, but does not necessarily prove conclusively a cause and effect link. Asbestos may presently be the primary known cause, but there are some cases where it is difficult to establish definite exposure to asbestos. Environmental exposure to erionite, a naturally occurring mineral fibre belonging to the zeolite family, has also been attributed as a cause malignant mesothelioma (Metintas *et al.*, 2019).

In general, the clustering of cases of a particular disease at a workplace should trigger a clinical suspicion of work-related causation. The rarer the cases, the more likely it is that some common aetiological factor exists. However, a cluster is not necessary to diagnose an occupational disease. The special circumstances of exposure relevant to one individual may cause an occupational disease in a single worker without producing a cluster.

ILO's Criteria and Classification of Occupational Diseases

ILO (2009) adopts a similar set of principles taking into consideration the following general criteria for the identification of occupational diseases:

1. There is a causal relationship with a specific agent, exposure or work process.
2. The disease occurs in connection with the work environment and/or in specific occupations.
3. The disease occurs among the groups of persons concerned with a frequency which exceeds the average incidence within the rest of the population.
4. There is scientific evidence of a clearly defined pattern of disease following exposure and plausibility of cause.

At the time of writing, ILO's list of occupational diseases was last updated in 2010 (ILO, 2010). This reference is often used by national labour authorities and other legislative bodies to derive country-specific categorisation of occupational diseases for the purposes of occupational disease surveillance, reporting and compensation.

Classification is by occupational diseases that are:

1. Caused by exposure to agents arising from work activities (chemical, physical, biological and infectious agents).
2. By target organ systems (respiratory diseases, skin diseases, musculoskeletal disorders, mental and behavioural disorders).

3. Occupational cancers.
4. Other diseases.

While a specified number of occupational conditions are covered in the ILO list, there is a "catch-all" category referring to "other specific diseases caused by occupations or processes not mentioned in this list where a direct link is established scientifically, or determined by methods appropriate to national conditions and practice, between the exposure arising from work activities and the disease(s) contracted by the worker". This therefore covers entities that have been inadvertently left out, and newer conditions that are identified, such as the health effects of engineered nanomaterials on the pulmonary and cardiovascular systems (Schulte *et al.*, 2019).

Challenges in Diagnosing Occupational Diseases

Unlike work-related traumatic injuries which are usually well-defined by an antecedent event, establishing the diagnosis of occupational diseases may not be straightforward in all cases because of the less clear cause–effect relationship between occupational exposure and disease.

Multifactorial causation, where occupational exposure can either be a dominant (occupational disease) or contributing (work-related disease) component, is commonly encountered in clinical practice. Symptoms may be compounded or blunted by factors such as personal health, age-related symptoms or non-occupational exposures. Hearing loss, for instance, may be contributed by both ageing and occupational noise exposure. Pregnancy and repetitive strain at work are independently associated with a higher risk of the development of carpal tunnel syndrome. Occupational sitting (i.e. sedentary behaviour) has been associated been various health risks, including cardiovascular diseases and diabetes mellitus (van Uffelen *et al.*, 2010; Koh, 2018).

However, logical reasoning will bring us to the conclusion that avocational factors also have a part to play, and it will be difficult for these chronic diseases to be primarily attributed to work. In almost every circumstance when managing a disorder in a worker, physicians will have to carefully evaluate and make a determination whether the work factor is a dominant one in disease causation.

Occupational diseases may also have clinical manifestations very similar or undifferentiable from the condition arising from non-occupational cause. For example, without a careful occupational history of work exposure to wood dust, the woodworker may simply be managed as any other patients with adult-onset asthma where interventions to eliminate wood dust exposure would not be thought of and implemented. Inhalation of beryllium, an important material used in industries ranging from electronics, telecommunications to aerospace, can cause granulomatous lung disease mimicking sarcoidosis.

It has also been suggested that the relationship between occurrence of symptoms and time at work or away from work may help differentiate occupational from non-occupational disorders. The premise is that work-related conditions tend to occur at work, and improve at weekends, on holidays, or other times away from the workplace. However, there are limitations to having this as an essential criterion. Many non-occupational disorders improve on weekends or on holidays. Most people generally feel better when they go away on holidays. Also, some occupational disorders can manifest when the affected individuals are away from work. An occupational cancer may be detected long after the person has retired and left the industry where exposure to the carcinogen occurred. Occupational asthma may present as delayed, dual, or episodic respiratory effects, such that some instances of airway obstruction could occur away from work, during weekends, or even during holidays.

Additionally, clinical manifestations of the same occupational disease may present differently in, for example, tropical countries compared to temperate countries (Bandhukul, 2018). One example is hand-arm vibration syndrome (HAVS) from the use of vibrating hand tools. Workers with HAVS in both tropical and temperate environments have a similar degree of peripheral neuropathy symptoms such as numbness, tingling and loss of dexterity. However, unlike the latter group, those working in the tropics generally do not experience any marked vascular manifestation of secondary Raynaud's phenomenon of the hands (Su *et al.*, 2013).

Given the centrality of the need to establish the role that work plays in disease causation, an occupational health consultation cannot be limited to the confines of the clinic. More information on the work environment, processes and exposures from the employer, co-workers and/or the company's safety officer are often required to supplement the patient's account. Where available, exposure records, environmental and biological surveillance reports, as well as a survey of epidemiological studies, other published literature and the workplace will facilitate the comprehensive evaluation of the work-relatedness by the attending physician (Greaves *et al.*, 2018).

Underreporting and Underrecognition of Occupational Diseases

Despite the availability of guidance on diagnosis, and reference lists of occupational diseases by ILO and national legislations, it is generally accepted that occupational diseases are underreported in many countries. ILO (2013) describes this phenomenon as a "hidden epidemic". The underlying causes are often multifactorial.

An obstacle is the perceived or real fear by workers of job loss and reprisal by employers (Fagan and Hodgson, 2017). Authorities are often unable to follow up and interview workers because they may no longer be under employment, having quit or being terminated by their employers. Even for occupational diseases which are reported, there is common underreporting of severity indicators such as the period of medical absenteeism and the omission of reporting such occurrences in itinerant workers (Wuellner and Phipps, 2018; Alaguney *et al.*, 2020).

Other oft-cited reasons for underreporting are the result of the lack of training or appreciation of the importance of recognising and notifying occupational diseases. Clinicians are well placed to have a high index of suspicion as to the possibility of an occupational disease, and to report the cases when they occur. However, this avenue is not used often. The number of hours dedicated to teaching occupational medicine to medical undergraduates is very limited (Eu *et al.*, 2020), hence doctors in practice may not fully appreciate the relevance of the subject nor the importance of recognising an occupational disease.

When clinically reviewing patients, the lack of or a suboptimal occupational history by doctors and other healthcare professionals impedes the establishment of an important occupational link to disease causation or aggravation (Alex *et al.*, 2013). Less than half of family physicians surveyed routinely obtained an occupational history from their patients. Those who did were more likely to discuss their patients' clinical management with an occupational physician (Yildiz *et al.*, 2019). This affects the consequent holistic management of the patient in terms of medical treatment, the preventive control or elimination of the hazards at the workplace, and the patient's work disposition.

Interesting underreporting trends can also be gleaned over time and across different occupational sectors. While studies found more than half of all occupational injuries and illnesses were routinely underreported at the turn of the century (Rosenman *et al.*, 2006; Samant *et al.*, 2012), there has been improvement in the reporting compliance over the last decade or so. A Swedish study by Orellana *et al.* (2021) showed that approximately one in four occupational injuries were not reported. Stricter legislations, facilitation of notification through electronic reporting platforms, and a greater awareness on the link between reporting and the eligibility for work injury compensation are all contributory factors in improving the compliance of occupational disease notification. Underreporting tends to be more prevalent in smaller work establishments (Wuellner *et al.*, 2016), where occupational health and safety regulations may not be as well enforced. Workplaces and employers may also deem unnecessary to report injuries and illnesses of lesser severity.

Underreporting of occupational diseases and injuries is a major obstacle that will otherwise enable a greater emphasis on occupational health and safety on the political agenda, especially in developing countries. The lack of accurate data misrepresents the extent and burden of work-related disorders, resulting in lesser resources being allocated to preventive programmes and measures. To address this, certain principles must first be acknowledged and agreed upon by the tripartite of government, employer and worker bodies.

1. Occupational diseases are preventable. Reduction or removal of the causative factor/s will benefit the affected individual. Appropriate treatment can also be provided to the affected individual if the correct diagnosis is reached.

2. Recognition of a case of occupational disease can indicate poor workplace conditions that may affect other workers with similar work tasks and therefore similar exposure to workplace hazards (a "sentinel event").
3. Adequate data on the extent of occupational disease can facilitate the tracking of trends of disease, and provides an indication of the success of control measures. It can also help when trying to make a case for resources to support occupational health initiatives.
4. A diagnosis of occupational disease will enable suitable advice to be provided to the affected worker with regard to issues such as period of sickness absence, prognosis, return to work, change of job, compensation and benefit entitlements, and other queries that the individual and/or the employer could raise.

Accurate reporting is also instrumental in the early identification of previously uncharacterised or emerging occupational diseases. These can arise as a result of the transformation of work, the increasing use of novel and synthetic materials, the changing context and circumstances of occupational exposures, and even the effects of climate change on worker health and safety. Trends of emerging and re-emerging occupational diseases reflect the wider shifts in the employment landscape and changes in work hazard exposure.

For example, in the United States (US), the growth of the healthcare and service sectors has given rise to cleaning products as an important cause of occupational lung diseases. Cleaning disinfectants containing alcohol, bleach, hydrogen peroxide, glutaraldehye and quarternary ammonium compounds, well known to be linked to occupational asthma, has recently been shown to be associated with an increased risk of chronic obstructive lung disease. Women who cleaned at home and professionally were found to have an accelerated decline in both forced expiratory volume in one second (FEV_1) and forced vital capacity (FVC), correlated with the frequency of cleaning and independent of other respiratory diseases such as asthma (Svanes *et al.*, 2018). Another noteworthy trend is silica-related lung diseases (Case Study 1).

Case Study 1: Silicosis from Exposure to Artificial Stone Dust

Inhalation of respirable crystalline silica dust in industries such as masonry, stonework and the coal mining sector expose workers to an increased risk of silicosis, lung cancer and tuberculosis. For decades, the progressive offshoring of such hazardous industries in many developed countries has resulted in a decline in the incidence of silica-related lung diseases. However, in recent years, there have been reports of the re-emergence of more advanced silicosis cases in these countries. The trend is epidemiologically investigated and linked to the manufacture of artificial stone countertops, which have substantially higher silica content than natural stone such as granite (Fazen et al., 2020). A national audit in Australia identified silicosis in more than 12% of artificial stone workers (Kirby, 2019).

Beyond underreporting, there are still diseases linked to work hazard exposures, especially novel agents, that are under-recognised and which we do not yet know at this point in time. In striving to achieve the vision of total workplace safety and health, our ultimate goal is to pre-empt hazards and prevent disease. A key strategy is to form a network of partners which will allow reported data to be pooled and shared for the investigation of trends in work-related ill health, and the identification of new or emerging health risks from work. One such network is Monitoring trends in Occupational Diseases and tracing new and Emerging Risks in a NETwork (MODERNET). Founded in 2008, this is a collaboration among academic centres in European Union countries to investigate occupational disease trends, validate new occupational health risks through analysing workers' and physicians' reporting with novel statistical techniques, and share the information timely through multiple media platforms (MODERNET, 2021). Another strategy is to build the capacity to predict new hazards through techniques such as quantitative structure–activity relationships (QSAR). QSAR is a computational modelling approach to study the relationships between chemical structures and their biological activities. This method is useful especially for the predictive analyses of novel work materials, where there may be relatively scarce information on their medium- to long-term occupational health effects. QSARs have been developed to forecast the biological effects of nanoparticles, as well as lesser known chemicals as potential asthmagens (Agius *et al.*, 2015).

Notification of Occupational Diseases

Who to Report to?

In many countries, different governmental agencies have the responsibility for receiving notifications about occurrence of disease. In England, notification of infectious diseases is to a responsible officer at a local council or local health protection team (responsibility of Public Health England), whereas notification of occupational diseases and injury is to the Health and Safety Executive (part of the Department for Work and Pensions). In other countries the responsible agency is often the Ministry of Health and/or the Ministry of Labour or equivalent. Even if the correct department is identified, finding the correct section responsible may not always be an easy task.

How to Notify?

The mechanism for notification might not be widely known or understood by key stakeholders in some cases. Can one notify by phone, or e-mail? Is there an official form to be used? If a form exists, should it be completed and posted, or completed on-line, or completed, scanned, and e-mailed? Is there a deadline for notification? These are some questions that may cross the mind of someone intending to notify a case of occupational disease.

What Cases Should Be Notified?

Statutory provisions usually require notification of a limited list of occupational disorders. This does not mean that only conditions that are listed are recognised as being occupational in origin. It only indicates that the responsible agencies have a particular interest in data on the specified conditions. Agencies could otherwise be inundated with notifications if, for example, all cases of low back pain with a possible occupational factor have to be notified. This is because low back pain is a common entity, with a reported real-world prevalence of up to 20% among adults of working age (Fatoye *et al.*, 2019). There can also be a difference between a notifiable disease and a compensable disease. The former deals with provision of information, usually with a view to prevention, and the latter addresses possible entitlement to special benefits as a means of redress for loss of earnings, pain and suffering, discomfort and inconvenience.

Who Has the Responsibility for Notifying?

It would seem that the obvious person to be given the responsibility to notify should be the physician making the diagnosis. For a period of time, this was the system in the UK but it did not work even when some financial incentive was provided for notifying. Part of the reason for poor notification rates was insufficient availability of doctors with some level of training in occupational medicine, and the absence of agreed diagnostic criteria for specific occupational diseases. The onus for notification was then transferred to the "employer", and this remains the legal requirement under the Reporting of Injuries, Diseases, and Dangerous Occurrences Regulations 2013 in the UK (Health and Safety Executive, 2021a). However, this does not necessarily improve the notification rates.

What Happens if One Notifies?

A major concern is the consequence of notification. Employers may worry that notification would lead to the visit of an inspector followed by prohibition of work processes, or an improvement notice, or a prosecution. In countries where occupational physicians are contracted by companies to provide a clinical service and occupational health advice, the concern may be about possible non-renewal of the contract if notification leads to inconvenience or costs to the company. Individual workers may request that notification of their occupational illness should not proceed, for fear of losing their jobs or being transferred to a lower-paying job.

Managing Occupational Diseases

Following the diagnosis of a case of occupational disease, action is required on at least two fronts. There should be immediate measures to treat the individual and alleviate his/her symptoms, with advice to prevent recurrence. Concurrently, there should be interventions at the workplace to eliminate or reduce exposures to the hazard(s) responsible for the disease.

Management at the Workplace

Prevention of recurrence of illness in the affected individual, or of disease occurring in other workers working in the same environment, requires the strict control of risks. The hierarchy of controls (Fig. 1) is a widely adopted framework to help industries and work places develop and implement feasible and effective control solutions (National Institute for Occupational Safety and Health, 2021).

Where total hazard elimination is not feasible, the ALARP (As Low As Reasonably Practicable) and the ALARA (As Low As Reasonably Achievable) principles advocate control to levels that are either practicable or possible, the difference being a matter of degree.

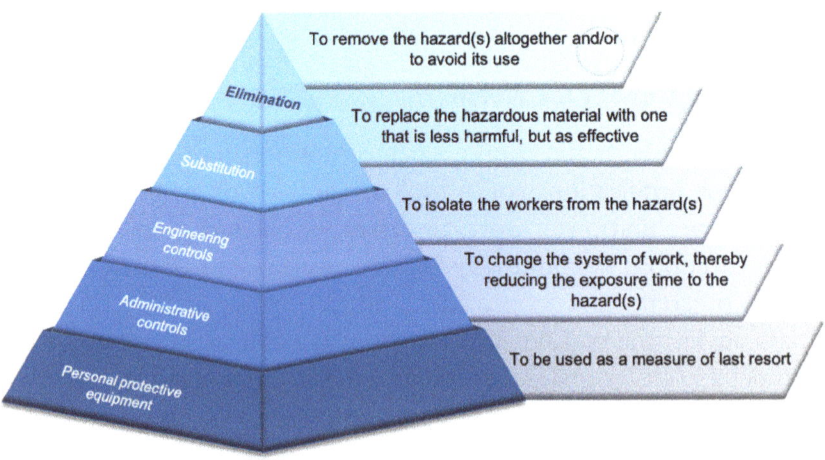

Fig. 1. Hierarchy of controls.

Occupational exposure to cosmic radiation in flight crew is often used to illustrate the ALARA principle (Case Study 2).

Case Study 2: Control of Cosmic Radiation Exposure Among Flight Crew

Given that exposure to cosmic radiation is inevitable and cannot be eliminated in the aviation industry, the International Commission on Radiological Protection (International Commission on Radiological Protection, 2016) recommends that occupational exposure to ionising radiation, including in flight crew, not exceed an effective dose of 20 mSv per year (averaged over 5 years), with a maximum exposure dose of 50 mSv in any given year.

As low as reasonably achievable (ALARA) levels of exposure is attained through regulating the amount of flight time annually allowable for a flight crew, taking into consideration factors such as flight duration and flight sector. Flight crew operating long haul flights spend more time at cruising altitudes compared to those on short hops with multiple take-offs and landings. There is also a greater exposure to cosmic radiation for flights over the polar routes.

With such administrative control measures, there is no conclusive evidence of an increased risk of melanoma, thyroid and gynaecological cancers in flight crew (Pinkerton et al., 2018). One study observed an increase in breast cancer incidence in flight attendants, but this could be explained by the lower parity and older age at first birth of the cohort compared to the general population (Schubauer-Berigan et al., 2015).

After introducing control measures, there should be a process of regular monitoring to ensure that these measures continue to be effective. In addition, health surveillance can also complement these measures as a method of ensuring that no further ill-health occurs. Ensuring compliance with current occupational exposure standards, e.g. the US Threshold Limit Values and Biological Exposure Indices (American Conference of Governmental Industrial Hygienists, 2021) or UK Workplace Exposure Limits (Health and Safety Executive, 2021b), would provide some reassurance of limiting exposure to workplace hazards. Assessment of ambient exposure to chemicals and analysis of blood and/or urine samples for substances and their metabolites are ways of determining exposure.

Measurement of exposure to some hazards can pose a challenge in linking the levels measured to the cause of the disease. This is particularly true for agents that are carcinogenic or allergenic, where the necessary dose required to produce an effect is uncertain. Genotoxic carcinogens may act at very small levels of exposure. Respiratory sensitisers may require a large dose to cause sensitisation, but may only need a small re-exposure to elicit a reaction.

Genotoxicity may arise from occupational exposure to high levels of particulate matter and volatile organic compounds emitted by photocopiers, and to carbon black, iron, silicon, magnetite and other elements in photocopier toners. Studies comparing photocopier operators and maintenance personnel with controls showed increased DNA damage in the former group (Kasi *et al.*, 2018). However, the correlation between occupational exposure limits and the extent of genetic damage, or the type of mutation that can result in disease, remains unclear.

Targeted Treatment of Occupational Diseases

Other than provision of supportive measures or medications to relieve symptoms, there is only a limited number of effective specific antidotes that can be used for occupational diseases. These are mainly restricted to acute occupational poisonings. Three case studies are covered below (Case Studies 3–5).

Case Study 3: Organophosphate Poisoning

A 20-year-old male presented to a rural hospital's urgent care clinic with chest heaviness, muscle weakness, fatigue and nausea for two weeks. He also complained of intermittent abdominal cramps with loose stools, but was otherwise clinically stable. A careful history-taking revealed that he had just been employed as a farm hand in a crop farm for about a month. Prior to this, he took on odd jobs as a general worker, mainly helping to load and unload goods. At the farm, one of his tasks was to mix organophosphorus pesticide granules with water in a container with a hose apparatus, and spray the crops with this device. He uses a cloth wrapping to cover his nose and mouth when spraying the pesticide but not during the preparation process. He was not provided with any gloves, respirator or other personal protective equipment by his supervisor.

Organophosphorous (OP) compounds are most commonly encountered as pesticides or ectoparasiticides (e.g. sheep dip). Commercial pesticide formulations may also contain surfactants and organic solvents which contribute to their toxicity. The inactivation of the acetylcholinesterase enzyme occurs by the formation of a stable OP–cholinesterase compound. This may slowly regenerate, but may also subsequently become re-inhibited by the ongoing exposure of the worker to the OP compound.

Inhibition of acetylcholinesterase results in a build-up of acetylcholine at synapses within the autonomic and central nervous systems, and at neuromuscular junctions. This results in overstimulation of both nicotinic and muscarinic receptors. While the farm hand worker in the case study presented with symptoms suggestive of subacute OP poisoning, acute toxicity can result in more florid dermatological (e.g. burning sensation, excessive sweating), neurological (e.g. headache, mood disturbances), neuromuscular (e.g. muscle twitching, seizures), ocular (e.g. excessive tearing), respiratory (e.g. cough, pulmonary oedema, respiratory failure), cardiovascular (e.g. arrhythmias) and gastrointestinal (e.g. vomiting, diarrhoea) manifestations.

The mainstay of medical therapy in OP poisoning involves the use of atropine, oximes (e.g. pralidoxime) and benzodiazepines (e.g. diazepam). Atropine (an anti-muscarinic agent) decreases the excess secretions from glands, reducing salivation and lacrimation and reverses bradycardia. Oximes act primarily by reactivating the acetylcholinesterase–OP complex, regenerating active cholinesterase and thereby decreasing acetylcholine. Some OP–cholinesterase complexes undergo a process called 'ageing' during which an alkyl group is removed from the phosphate. Once ageing has occurred, oximes are much less effective in reactivating the enzyme. The rate of ageing varies hugely between oximes. Acetylcholinesterase effectors and even atropine have been demonstrated to retard ageing in OP poisoning.

Re-alkylation of aged acetylcholinesterase by alkylators such as sulphonates has been proposed for post-ageing treatment, but this strategy is not widely used clinically (Zhuang *et al.*, 2016). Benzodiazepines such as diazepam are effective as an anticonvulsant. It is helpful in treating OP-induced seizures and pronounced muscle fasciculations. In animal studies, the combination of atropine and diazepam significantly reduced mortality compared to atropine alone (Marrs, 2003). In severe acute OP poisoning, the administration of benzodiazepine can be considered even before the onset of complications such as convulsions.

Case Study 4: Lead Poisoning

A 45-year-old migrant worker developed symptoms of colic, constipation, malaise, and lethargy six months after beginning work replacing lead linings from an old church. His work required him to burn away some lead strips from the church roof, almost on a daily basis. No respiratory protective equipment was used in the process. He had done similar restorative and demolition work on old buildings in his previous jobs. Significant physical examination findings included conjunctival pallor and mild peripheral motor weakness of upper limbs without sensory loss. Haematological investigation showed anaemia and a raised blood lead level, confirming the diagnosis of inorganic lead poisoning.

Workers can be exposed to inorganic lead compounds in a variety of industries, such as in the manufacture of lead-acid storage batteries and lead-based paints, and when burning, welding and cutting of lead-coated structures, as in this case study. Lead poisoning can produce a variety of features depending upon the severity of the exposure. Apart from anaemia and paresis, often of the extensors of the hands and feet without sensory loss, acute lead poisoning can also affect the gastrointestinal (e.g. Burton's line, abdominal colic), renal (e.g. chronic interstitial nephritis) and central nervous (e.g. behavioural changes, encephalopathy) systems. Lead can also cross the placental barrier and result in neurological damage to the foetus.

The initial requirement in treatment is to establish the diagnosis and determine the severity of the exposure. Removal from further exposure to lead is a priority. Patients with high concentrations of lead with accompanying severe symptoms should be considered for chelation therapy.

A chelating agent binds to lead, creating a compound that can be excreted in the bile and urine. Both parenteral (Ethylenediaminetetraacetate, or EDTA; and edetate calcium disodium, or CaNa2EDTA) and oral (dimercaptosuccinic acid, or DMSA) chelating agents are available. However, chelation therapy is not without risks. Potential adverse effects associated with CaNa2EDTA chelation therapy are renal failure, hypocalcaemia and arrhythmia (Flora and Pachauri, 2010). Therefore, chelation is best undertaken in units familiar with its use and with the facilities for monitoring therapy. It is not recommended in asymptomatic individuals with slight raised blood lead levels (Kosnett *et al.*, 2006).

Case Study 5: Carbon Monoxide Poisoning

A worker in a coffee processing plant was brought to the Emergency Department with loss of consciousness. He was found by another co-worker unresponsive in a coffee storage tank within the plant. He was last seen by his co-workers about an hour ago towards the end of the lunch break. Carboxyhaemoglobin level was found to be 38%. He was hypotensive, had clinical and radiological signs of bilateral pulmonary oedema, and raised B-type natriuretic peptide suggestive of severe myocardial dysfunction. He was resuscitated and arrangement made to undergo hyperbaric oxygen therapy (Hawley et al., 2017).

Carbon monoxide (CO) is generally encountered as a product of combustion. Workers working in boiler rooms, petrochemical refineries, steel production and other jobs that require working around combustion sources are at risk. CO acts as a poison by several different mechanisms. It binds to haemoglobin with a high affinity to produce carboxyhaemoglobin, which decreases the ability of the blood to transport oxygen to the tissues. In addition, CO produces a conformational change in the remaining haemoglobin which results in more avid binding of oxygen with a left-shift in the oxygen dissociation curve and decreased delivery of oxygen to the tissues from the remaining haemoglobin. It is also thought to inhibit mitochondrial cytochrome oxidase impairing aerobic metabolism, and bind to other intracellular targets to produce cellular damage and inflammation by the formation of free radicals.

Carboxyhaemoglobin levels greater than 5% in non-smokers and 10% in smokers are abnormal and should lead the physician to suspect CO poisoning in the presence of symptoms and the relevant occupational or environmental exposure. Carboxyhaemoglobin levels of 20% may result in nausea, headache or dizziness; 30% in impaired vision and judgement; 40% in confusion and syncope; and 50% in seizure and coma. Levels higher than 60% may be lethal.

The first-line for acute carbon monoxide poisoning is to provide high-flow oxygen via a rebreather mask or endotracheal tube. Oxygen works by competing with CO for binding to red blood cells, thereby alleviating tissue hypoxia. Where hyperbaric oxygen treatment facility is available, it should be considered in cases of severe CO poisoning. Studies have shown that hyperbaric oxygen therapy could improve the clinical outcome and reduce long-term cognitive impairment in those whose carboxyhaemoglobin level is at least 25%, of age 36 years and older, and present with loss of consciousness (Hampson *et al.*, 2012).

Conclusion

The accurate and timely diagnosis of occupational diseases is one of the most important first steps in occupational medicine practice. The ability to recognise that a disease condition is attributed to hazards at work is not straightforward in all cases. It requires a level of training in occupational medicine that should be incorporated as part of the standard curricula for medical students. In addition, the ability of the physician to interpret environmental surveillance data and biological monitoring data is advantageous as they are instructive for diagnosis and management. Taken together, the complement of clinical and occupational inputs facilitates the assessment, treatment and prevention of occupational diseases in the context of work and the work ecosystem.

References

American Conference of Governmental Industrial Hygienists. (2021) *TLV/BEI guidelines.* [Online] Available from: https://www.acgih.org/science/tlv-bei-guidelines/. [Accessed on 20 May 2021].

Agius R, Lenderink A, Colosio C. (2015) Finding 'new' occupational diseases and trends in 'old' ones. *Occup Med (Lond)* **65**(8): 607–609.

Alaguney ME, Yildiz AN, Demir AU, Ergor OA. (2020) Physicians' opinions about the causes of underreporting of occupational diseases. *Arch Environ Occup Health* **75**(3): 165–176.

Alex R, Francis M, Prashanth HR, Kundavaram A. (2013) Occupational history: A neglected component of history taking. *Indian J Occup Environ Med* **17**(1): 29–30.

Bandhukul A. (2018) Mini symposium for ASEAN diagnostic criteria or occupational diseases. *Occup Environ Med* **75**(Suppl 2): A1–A650.

Directorate-General for Employment, Social Affairs and Inclusion (European Commission). (2009) *Information Notices on Occupational Diseases: A Guide to Diagnosis.* [Online] Luxembourg, Office for Official Publications of the European Communities.

Eu E, Soo M, Gan WH. (2020) A short review of undergraduate occupational medicine training. *Occup Med (Oxford, England)* **70**(7): 485–489.

Fagan KM, Hodgson MJ. (2017) Under-recording of work-related injuries and illnesses: An OSHA priority. *J Safety Res* **60**: 79–83.

Fatoye F, Gebrye T, Odeyemi I. (2019) Real-world incidence and prevalence of low back pain using routinely collected data. *Rheumatol Int* **39**(4): 619–626.

Fazen LE, Linde B, Redlich CA. (2020) Occupational lung diseases in the 21st century: The changing landscape and future challenges. *Curr Opin Pulm Med* **26**(2): 142–148.

Flora SJS, Pachauri V. (2010) Chelation in metal intoxication. *Int J Environ Res Public Health* 7(7): 2745–2788.

GBD 2016 Occupational Risk Factors Collaborators. (2020) Global and regional burden of disease and injury in 2016 arising from occupational exposures: A systematic analysis for the Global Burden of Disease Study 2016. *Occup Environ Med* 77(3): 133–141.

Greaves WW, Das R, McKenzie JG, Sinclair DC, 2nd. Hegmann KT. (2018) Work-relatedness. *J Occup Environ Med* **60**(12): e640–e646.

Hampson NB, Piantadosi CA, Thom SR, Weaver LK. (2012) Practice recommendations in the diagnosis, management, and prevention of carbon monoxide poisoning. *Am J Resp Crit Care Med* **186**(11): 1095–1101.

Hawley B, Cox-Ganser JM, Cummings KJ. (2017) Carbon monoxide exposure in workplaces, including coffee processing facilities. *Am J Respir Crit Care Med* **196**(8): 1080–1081.

Health and Safety Executive. (2021a) *Reporting Accidents and Incidents at Work.* [Online] Available from: https://www.hse.gov.uk/pubns/indg453.htm. [Accessed on 17 May 2021].

Health and Safety Executive. (2021b) *Work Exposure Limits.* [Online] Available from: https://www.hse.gov.uk/pubns/books/eh40.htm. [Accessed on 20 May 2021].

Hill AB. (1965) The environment and disease: Association or causation? *Proc R Soc Med* **58**(5): 295–300.

International Commission on Radiological Protection. (2016) *ICRP Publication 132: Radiological Protection from Cosmic Radiation in Aviation.* Ottawa, ILO.

ILO. (2009) *Identification and recognition of occupational diseases: Criteria for incorporating diseases in the ILO list of occupational diseases.* [Online] Geneva, ILO.

ILO. (2010) *ILO List of Occupational Diseases (revised 2010).* [Online] Available from: https://www.ilo.org/safework/info/publications/WCMS_125137. [Accessed on 24 June 2021].

ILO (International Labour Organization). (2013) *The Prevention of Occupational Diseases.* [Online] Available from: https://www.ilo.org/safework/info/WCMS_208226. [Accessed on 24 June 2021].

Kasi V, Elango N, Ananth S, Vembhu B, Poornima JG. (2018) Occupational exposure to photocopiers and their toners cause genotoxicity. *Hum Exp Toxicol* **37**(2): 205–217.

Kirby T. (2019) Australia reports on audit of silicosis for stonecutters. *Lancet* **393**(10174): 861.

Koh D. (2018) Sedentary behaviour at work – An underappreciated occupational hazard? *Occup Med (Lond)* **68**: 350–351.

Kosnett MJ, Wedeen RP, Rothenberg SJ, Hipkins KL, Materna BL, Schwartz BS, Hu H Woolf A. (2006) Recommendations for medical management of adult lead exposure. *Environ Health Perspect* **115**(3): 463–471.

Marrs TC. (2003) Diazepam in the treatment of organophosphorus ester pesticide poisoning. *Toxicol Rev* **22**(2): 75–81.

Metintas S, Ak G, Metintas M. (2019) A review of the cohorts with environmental and occupational mineral fiber exposure. *Arch Environ Occup Health* **74**(1–2): 76–84.

MODERNET. (2021) *Monitoring Occupational Diseases and Tracing New and Emerging Risks in a Network.* [Online] Available from: https://www.modernet.info/about-us/. [Accessed on 16 May 2021].

National Institute for Occupational Safety and Health. (2021) *Hierarchy of controls.* [Online] Available from: https://www.cdc.gov/niosh/topics/hierarchy/default.html. [Accessed on 17 May 2021].

Orellana C, Kreshpaj B, Burstrom B, Davis L, Frumento P, Hemmingsson T, Johansson G, Kjellberg K, Wegman DH, Bodin T. (2021) Organisational factors and under-reporting of occupational injuries in Sweden: A population-based study using capture-recapture methodology. *Occup Environ Med* oemed-2020-107257.

Pinkerton LE, Hein MJ, Anderson JL, Christianson A, Little MP, Sigurdson AJ, Schubauer-Berigan MK. (2018) Melanoma, thyroid cancer, and gynecologic cancers in a cohort of female flight attendants. *Am J Ind Med* **61**(7): 572–581.

Rosenman KD, Kalush A, Reilly MJ, Gardiner JC, Reeves M, Luo Z. (2006) How much work-related injury and illness is missed by the current national surveillance system? *J Occup Environ Med* **48**(4): 357–365.

Samant Y, Parker D, Wergeland E, Lund J, Westin S. (2012) Estimating work-related amputations in the Norwegian manufacturing section: A 10-year retrospective study based on two-source capture-recapture method. *Int J Occup Environ Health* **18**(4): 292–298.

Schubauer-Berigan MK, Anderson JL, Hein MJ, Little MP, Sigurdson AJ, Pinkerton LE. (2015) Breast cancer incidence in a cohort of U.S. flight attendants. *Am J Ind Med* **58**(3): 252–266.

Schulte PA, Leso V, Niang M, Lavicoli I. (2019) Current state of knowledge on the health effects of engineered nanomaterials in workers: A systematic review of human studies and epidemiological investigations. *Scand J Work Environ Health* **45**(3): 217–238.

Su TA, Fukumoto J, Darus A, Hoe CWV, Miyai N, Isahak M, Takemura S, Bulgiba A, Yoshimasu K, Maeda S, Miyashita K. (2013) A comparison of hand-arm vibration syndrome between Malaysian and Japanese workers. *J Occup Health* **55**(6): 468–478.

Svanes Ø, Bertelsen RJ, Lygre SHL, Carsin AE, Anto JM, Forsberg B, Garcia-Garcia JM, Gullon JA, Heinrich J, Holm M, Kogevinas M, Urrutia I, Leynaert B, Moratalla JM, Moual NL, Lytras T, Norback D, Nowak D, Olivieri M, Pin I, Probst-Hensch N, Schlunssen V, Sigsgaard T, Skorge TD, Villani S, Jarvis D, Zock JP, Svanes C. (2018) Cleaning at home and at work in relation to lung function decline and airway obstruction. *Am J Respir Crit Care Med* **197**(9): 1157–1163.

Vahabzadeh M, Balali-Mood M. (2016) Occupational metallic mercury poisoning in gilders. *Int J Occup Environ Med* 7(2): 116–122.

van Uffelen JGZ, Wong J, Chau JY, van der Ploeg HP, Riphagen I, Gilson ND, Burton NW, Healy GN, Thorp AA, Clark BK, Gardiner PA, Dunstan DW, Bauman A, Owen N, Brown WJ. (2010) Occupational sitting and health risks: A systematic review. *Am J Prev Med* **39**(4): 379–388.

WHO. (2021) *Occupational and Work-related Diseases.* [Online] Available from: https://www.who.int/occupational_health/activities/occupational_work_diseases/en/. [Accessed on 9 May 2021].

Wuellner S, Phipps P. (2018) Employer knowledge of federal requirements for recording work-related injuries and illnesses: Implications for occupational injury surveillance data. *Am J Ind Med* **61**(5): 422–435.

Wuellner SE, Adams DA, Bonauto DK. (2016) Unreported workers' compensation claims to the BLS survey of occupational injuries and illness: Establishment factors. *Am J Ind Med* **59**(4): 274–289.

Yildiz AN, Piskin TM, Alaguney ME, Kurt OK, Ozlu A, Basarali MK. (2019) Attitudes and behaviours of family physicians regarding occupational diseases. *Arch Environ Occup Health* **74**(1–2): 85–92.

Zhuang Q, Young A, Callam CS, McElroy CA, Ekizi OD, Yoder RJ, Hadad CM. (2016) Efforts towards treatments against aging of organophosphorus-inhibited acetylcholinesterase. (2017) *Ann N Y Acad Sci* **1374**(1): 94–104.

Chapter 3

Respiratory Disorders

David Fishwick[*,†] *and Chris Barber*[*]

Introduction

Inhaled occupational exposures remain an important global cause of lung disease. In certain circumstances, occupational exposures may be the sole cause of a respiratory problem, for example, when respirable crystalline silica exposure over several years causes silicosis. In other circumstances, occupational exposures may be considered as contributing to the development of a respiratory problem, along with contributions from one or more other risk factors. An example of the latter is the development of chronic obstructive pulmonary disease (COPD), where inhaled workplace agents may contribute, along with tobacco smoking and other factors, to its development.

Much more is now known about the causation of both common and rare occupational lung disorders; and the understanding of occupational attribution of causation continues to improve. These issues will be dealt with later in this chapter.

---

*Centre for Workplace Health, Health and Safety Executive and Respiratory Consultant, Sheffield Teaching Hospitals, Great Britain.
†Occupational and Environmental Medicine, University of Sheffield, Sheffield, England, United Kingdom.
Corresponding author: David Fishwick (d.fishwick@sheffield.ac.uk).

Regardless of the nature of the lung disease in question, it is important for the practicing clinician to be suspicious of an occupational cause for almost all respiratory diseases. This awareness will lead on to taking an appropriate clinical and occupational history from the patient, in order to confirm or exclude occupation as a cause, or partial cause, of their particular condition. A confirmed diagnosis of an occupational respiratory disease not only allows proactive management of the case itself, but also potentially can influence the reduction of harmful exposures at the worksite that may be posing risks to others. Excluding a diagnosis in an exposed worker may be equally important, preventing unnecessary changes in the workplace that may be associated with loss of income or employment.

This chapter summarises the main occupational diseases of the airway and interstitium using case studies, appropriate investigation, results and radiology where indicated, and more typical descriptive text.

Respiratory Problems — Making the Link to Work

Making the link back to the workplace, when assessing a case of potential occupational lung disease, may be relatively straightforward, or relatively difficult to verify. In diseases with longer latency such as COPD and lung cancer, distant exposures may be very difficult to quantify and link to current health outcomes. In practice, each case differs in its presentation to clinicians, and in terms of the amount of workplace information that is available. For example, some workers will be able to give a good account of the nature and duration of inhaled exposures, whereas others may not have any such information available. Clearly the latent period of the disease has a big impact on this, as historic exposures may be less accurately recalled than recent ones.

Even within an exposure type, the links to disease may require differing considerations. For example, benign pleural disease may be relatively easily linked to a historic exposure to asbestos, and most would not doubt a link between mesothelioma and such exposure, but a patient presenting 30 years after such exposure may not recall this in the context of a diagnosis, for example, of pulmonary fibrosis, that might otherwise be labelled as a case of idiopathic pulmonary fibrosis (IPF). There is some evidence to suggest that job title itself, and not recalled exposures, may be a better marker of previous occupational hazard and risk. Similarly, a worker who develops acute irritant induced asthma (AIIA) following an inhalational accident may be able to recall accurate details of exposure to high levels of ozone, but a worker in a complex printing process may not even be aware that they are potentially exposed to reactive dyes that can cause asthma.

Thus the extent to which clinicians make this link will be a function of the nature of the information supplied by the worker during the consultation, the worker's and clinician's knowledge about associated hazards and risks during these work processes. Importantly, retaining a heightened awareness that occupational exposures contribute significantly to many common respiratory diseases is important; particularly when workers themselves may not have made this link.

A series of cases follow linked to various types of occupational lung diseases. They are a mix of real cases and cases constructed in order to emphasise certain learning points.

Obstructive Lung Disease

The airway, as opposed to the lung tissue or parenchyma, appears vulnerable to the effects of many inhaled occupational agents. Although the links are now well understood between various historic inhaled exposures and diseases, such as flour dust and asthma, cadmium and emphysema, workers continue to present to clinicians with a wide range of classical and novel occupational airway problems. This section deals with some of the common occupational airway conditions, focusing on the management of specific cases.

Case Study 1: Acute Irritant Induced Asthma

A 28-year-old man has been diagnosed with adult-onset asthma that is difficult to control despite standard asthma therapy. His persistent symptoms of uncontrollable coughing were interfering with his ability to do his job, and he has needed time off work. His attacks of coughing were precipitated by exercise, strong smells, cold air, and car exhaust fumes.

He is finding it difficult to accept his condition, as he was previously a very fit and well marathon runner. He has never smoked, has no pets and no history of childhood illness.

He worked for a chemical company maintaining and repairing ventilation equipment. Six-months ago, he was admitted with an acute asthma attack from a workplace following an accidental exposure to chlorine gas that leaked from a damaged pipe. He had noticed an unusual smell when he entered the workplace, and within fifteen minutes started to feel unwell. He left the work area as he developed a burning sensation in his eyes, a tight feeling in his chest and couldn't stop coughing. He was seen by the occupational health nurse who called an ambulance. He was admitted to hospital for 48 hours and treated with nebulised bronchodilators, oxygen, and oral steroids. A chest x-ray was normal. He was discharged on inhaled bronchodilators and corticosteroids, but there has been very little if any improvement in his condition despite stepwise increases in asthma medication.

His spirometry and gas transfer were at the lower end of the normal predicted range. Serial peak flow testing confirmed a high level of diurnal variation (>20% variation). A mannitol challenge four months after the accident confirmed severe non-specific airway responsiveness (Fig. 1).

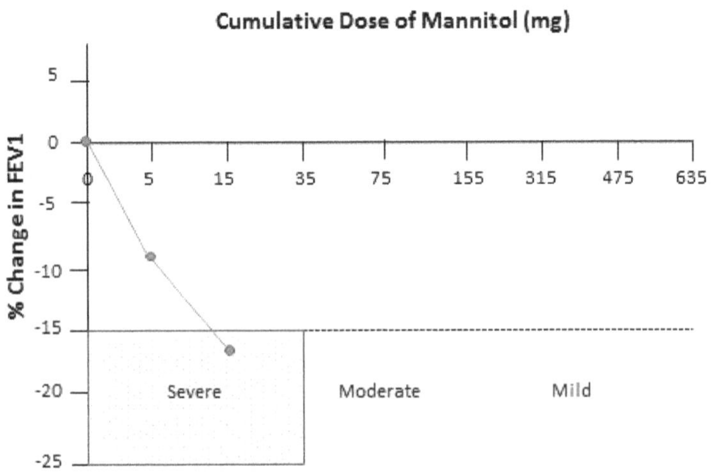

Fig. 1. Dry powder mannitol challenge test.

Case commentary

The occupational history is classical for a diagnosis of acute irritant induced asthma (AIIA), formerly known as reactive airway dysfunction syndrome (RADS). In this case an individual without any history of chest problems was admitted with an asthma attack following an accidental workplace exposure to an irritant gas. Symptoms persisted for many months, due to increased levels of airway hyper-responsiveness. In this case, it was not possible for the patient to continue in his work, as he continued to have very disabling bouts of coughing despite high dose asthma treatment. Losing his job and the impact of his illness on his family life had an additional affect in terms of prolonged depression.

Case summary

Around 10% of occupational asthma is caused by an acute high-dose inhalation injury in the workplace, with no latency (or time lag between first exposure and first attributable symptom). The history is usually very clear, as the majority of affected individuals are admitted to hospital or seek an emergency primary care consultation soon after the exposure. A wide range of exposures have been reported to cause AIIA, most commonly irritant gases, isocyanates, cleaning agents and concentrated acids.

Individual patients with AIIA should be treated with standard asthma medication, and there is some evidence that inhaled corticosteroids improve outcomes. Clinical improvements may be seen up to 2–3 years following the inhalation accident, but in general the condition has a poor prognosis, with many individuals requiring long-term asthma medication for persistent symptoms of airway hyper-responsiveness. Patients with AIIA commonly also report high levels of anxiety and depression many years after the acute event, and have associated psychosocial and financial problems.

Case Study 2: Allergic Occupational Asthma

A 57-year-old man was referred to a hospital clinic following a visit to his GP. He had recently had a lower respiratory tract infection, and had discussed with his doctor a two year history of wheeze and intermittent chest tightness. He was a woodworker and had changed jobs about 4 years ago. His current work was to make furniture from medium density fibreboard (MDF), a mix of soft and hard woods bound with a urea formaldehyde resin. His wheeze was described as worse at work, particularly when sawing through MDF, and improving on his days away from work. He borrowed his sister's salbutamol inhaler and felt better after taking this. He had never smoked, had no nasal symptoms, no family history, and no previous medical history and was not taking any regular medication.

His baseline lung function was normal, with a forced expiratory volume in one second (FEV$_1$) of 99% predicted, and an forced vital capacity (FVC) of 98% predicted. His FEV$_1$/FVC ratio was 0.83, excluding airways obstruction. His workplace had also measured his FEV$_1$ before and after the working shift; there was no significant fall over the shift. His serial peak flow readings (sPEF) were taken for five weeks (Fig. 2) and showed a clear work effect; that is, the pattern of peak flow readings confirmed their general improvement away from work, and worsening at work. The OASYS 2 software used to analyse these peak flow readings identified a significant work effect score; associated with high sensitivity and specificity for a diagnosis of occupational asthma (OASYS, 2021).

Immunological investigations were unhelpful in this case; serum IgE to both soft and hard work mixes were negative. He was subsequently challenged to wood dust as part of a Specific Inhalation Challenge (SIC), as MDF was not a well characterised cause of occupational asthma. This showed no response to control exposures of pine dust, but a typical early and late asthmatic response was seen following MDF dust inhalation. A diagnosis of occupational asthma to MDF was made and he was advised to discuss this with his employer. This conversation resulted in successful relocation away from MDF exposure and he continues to work productively whilst enrolled into a health surveillance programme. The latter monitors his symptoms and lung function each year.

Case commentary

The diagnosis in this case of allergic occupational asthma was based on a combination of medical history, knowledge of exposures likely to cause asthma, sPEF measures demonstrating better asthma control

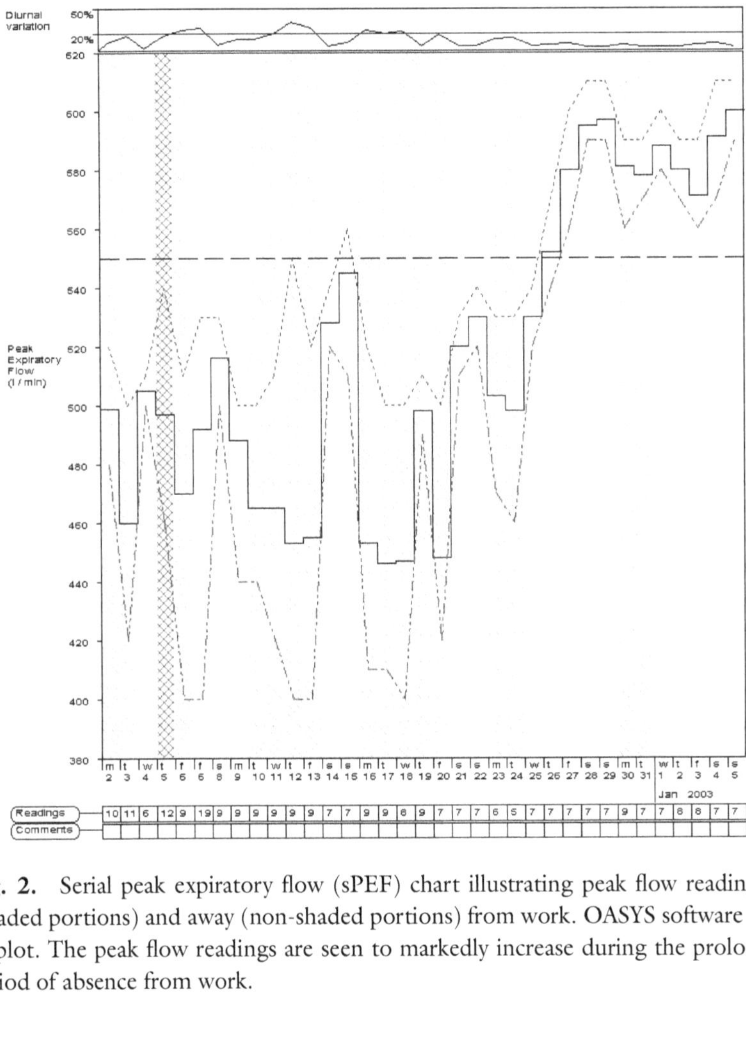

Fig. 2. Serial peak expiratory flow (sPEF) chart illustrating peak flow readings at (shaded portions) and away (non-shaded portions) from work. OASYS software used to plot. The peak flow readings are seen to markedly increase during the prolonged period of absence from work.

away from work and finally a positive SIC. Such serial measures are generally regarded as the best initial validation of a possible work effect on asthma control. They require worker training from a skilled operator, and should be carried out for at least 3 weeks, with a minimum of four readings per day. Various software packages are available to assist with their analysis, and sPEF are preferred to cross shift changes in FEV_1 because (as in this case) they lack sensitivity to identify occupational asthma (Fishwick *et al.*, 2012).

This patient remained well, under surveillance at work and under medical follow up in the outpatient clinic. Removal from the offending allergen, in this case MDF, has led to a rapid and sustained improvement in his asthma symptoms and overall control.

Case summary

Occupational causes of asthma remain common. Recent estimates suggest that 15% of the burden of adult asthma is attributable to occupational exposures. Consequently, the clinician requires vigilance to this possibility when assessing patients of working age with asthma. Wood dust exposure is one of the most commonly reported causes of occupational asthma in the United Kingdom (UK) (Centre for Occupational and Environmental Health, 2021).

The diagnosis of occupational asthma relies on piecing together clinical information, and this process will differ between individual workers. Wherever possible, a suggestive history of occupational asthma must be confirmed by objective tests, as making a diagnosis based on clinical history alone can be misleading (Nicholson *et al.*, 2005).

Objective tests aim to confirm changes in physiology between periods of work and rest (for example sPEF, bronchial reactivity measures) or confirmation of a response to a specific inhalation challenge. The latter can be helpful when making a diagnosis, although are not required in many cases and may have a significant false negative outcome rate. The European Respiratory Society recently reviewed their utility for making a diagnosis of occupational asthma (Vandenplas *et al.*, 2014), and concluded that the sensitivity and specificity of SICs were high, but not easily quantified, as this method is usually used as the reference standard for diagnosing the condition.

Whilst in this case immunological investigations were negative, these may also assist in the diagnosis of occupational asthma, particularly if the causative agent is a high molecular weight allergen (for example, laboratory animal protein, flour, bakery enzymes). It must also be borne in mind that IgE testing to occupational allergens are neither totally sensitive nor specific, and false negative and false positive tests do occur. Their interpretation must be placed in the context of the entire case, and also in knowledge of the atopic status of the worker.

Case Study 3: Work Aggravated Asthma

A 47-year-old woman with long-standing asthma was seen in primary care. She had just returned from a 2-week holiday during which she reported feeling 'fantastic' and 'hardly need to use my salbutamol inhaler.' Overall, however, her asthma has been more difficult to control recently with frequent episodes of wheeze during the working day. She also reported that her symptoms were better on days off work. She had noticed this ever since she had moved to her current job two years ago.

She worked day shifts as a warehouse worker for a large food company. This involved moving in and out of a cold storage facility, a large 'walk-in room' that is used as a chiller for keeping foodstuffs cool prior to their dispatch. She estimated that the temperature was kept at a constant 4°C and that the room adjoined to this was kept at a standard 19°C. All foodstuffs were fully packaged before they arrived at the department. She said that she had been a little worried about discussing these symptoms at work because the company was looking to reduce staff numbers. No definite allergen exposure could be identified from her history.

Her sPEF values were recorded plotted using the OASYS software (Fig. 3). These readings are just variable enough to support a diagnosis of asthma, but the work effect index of 2.5 (a value automatically calculated by the software that allows interpretation of the results, and >2.51 deemed a positive value) was equivocal.

Case commentary

The occupational history suggests that the most likely exposure at work relates to changes in workplace temperature, and that this may well be responsible for the increased asthma symptoms. The occupational history does not suggest that it is likely that she is exposed to an asthmagen capable of causing her asthma. The likely diagnosis

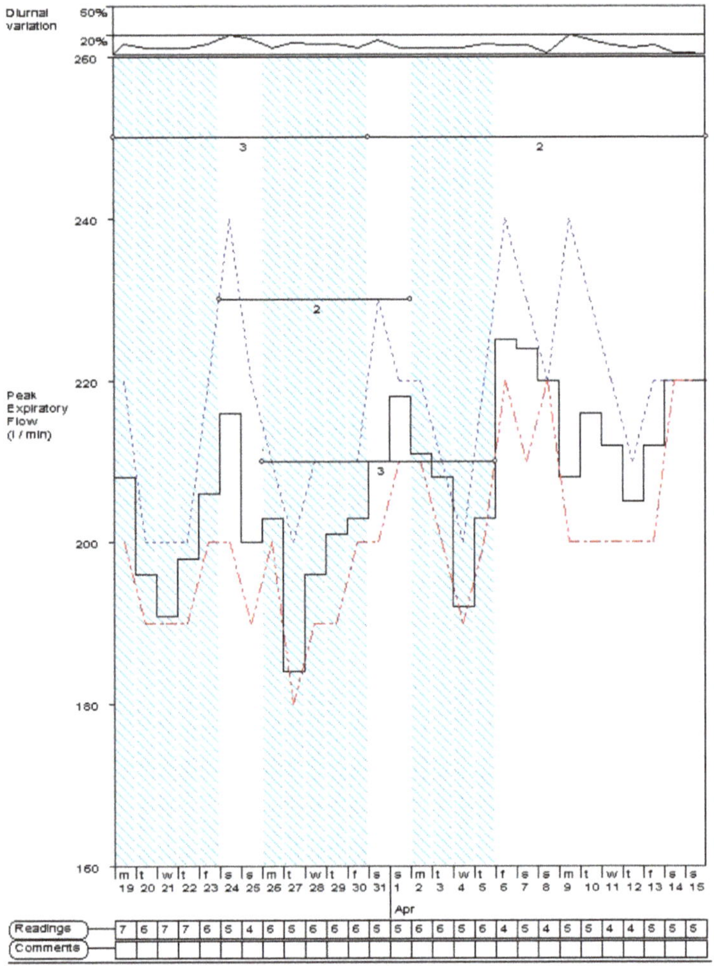

Fig. 3. sPEF chart illustrating peak flow readings at (shaded portions) and away (non-shaded portions) from work. OASYS software used to plot. The peak flow readings are seen to vary between periods of work and rest.

is therefore work-aggravated asthma. This information is key to the future management of this patient.

In this case the employer moved her to a standard temperature environment warehouse, which resulted in improved asthma control and reduced symptoms.

Case summary

Worsening of asthma symptoms at work, or work-aggravated asthma (WAA), is often reported, and must be distinguished from occupational asthma where possible. There are a large variety of inhaled and other aggravants that need consideration. Often the workplace can adjust the environment to reduce the risk of aggravating asthma. The interested reader can find more information in recent comprehensive reviews of this subject (Fishwick, 2014; Henneberger *et al.*, 2011).

Case Study 4: Lobar Pneumonia in a Welder

A 33-year-old man presented to the accident and emergency department with cough and fever. He had been unwell for 3 days and had also developed muscle aches. His weight was normal and stable, and he had no significant previous medical or surgical history. He lived with his wife and young daughter and was a lifelong never smoker.

He worked as a welder for a local fabrication firm. His regular work tasks included both MIG and MMA welding on to a mild steel base. His workplace was not a modern site, and he described dirty, dusty and noisy conditions. He was provided with a UV welders mask, but no respiratory protection. After long days welding, he described his facial skin and overalls were very stained from the welding fume.

He was unwell and dehydrated on admission. Physical examination noted a reduced percussion note at the left lung base and bronchial breathing. His temperature was measured at 38.2 degrees Celsius.

His chest radiograph noted evidence of a left lower lobe pneumonia, with no clear evidence of a pleural effusion or other abnormality. There were no features to suggest an underlying malignancy. He was negative for a full viral screen; including influenza and SARS-CoV-2. His sputum and blood cultures grew a fully sensitive Streptococcus pneumoniae. He had already been commenced on oral amoxicillin and intravenous fluids and made a full clinical recovery over a few days. A follow up chest radiograph at 6 weeks was normal.

Case commentary

His presentation and subsequent progress are entirely consistent with a lobar pneumonia caused by streptococcus. He improved rapidly on the appropriate treatment, fluids added as he was clinically and biochemically dehydrated on admission. His radiology normalised after an appropriate period of time.

His occupation was not considered relevant by the admitting team and no further consideration was given to this; was this correct?

His general practitioner saw him with the result of his 6-week radiograph and raised the issue of his work. She was familiar with the link between welding and the development of pneumonia. What had prompted her attention was a recent article in the peer reviewed press, that had identified a link between welding and invasive pneumococcal disease (Torén *et al.*, 2020).

Case summary

The link between welding and the development of pneumococcal pneumonia and invasive disease is now well established (Coggon and Palmer, 2016). The paper identified by the GP was a summary of data from a Swedish Registry of invasive infections. Torén *et al.* (2020) studied 4,438 cases of invasive pneumococcal infection, and non-cases were identified from the same population using a population registry. Welders had an increased risk of this infection; an OR of 2.99, with a 95% CI of between 2.09 and 4.30. The authors concluded that welders, and "potentially others with relevant exposures" should be offered pneumococcal vaccination. The recent American Thoracic Society (ATS)/*European Respiratory Journal* (*ERJ*) official statement on the occupational attribution of common respiratory problems (Blanc *et al.*, 2019) also stressed this link. The statement team reviewed 15 relevant publications, including 6 population based and nine cohort studies. Depending on the study type, PAF values between 10% and 52.5% were identified for welding. Various authorities suggest the vaccination of welders against pneumococcal infection.

Case Study 5: Chronic Obstructive Pulmonary Disease

A 62-year-old man presented to his GP with a long history of mild shortness of breath on exercise. He also developed chest tightness and wheezed occasionally, but the latter two symptoms were not precipitated by any single exposure. His weight was stable, and he could walk 100 meters on the flat slowly before needing to stop.

He lived with his wife and disabled son, for whom he cared. He had no relevant hobbies and received as required salbutamol that did not appear to help his shortness of breath but did help relieve his wheeze. He was a smoker and had a previous medical history of argyria. His father had emphysema.

He worked as a wire extruder for 5 years before retiring. His occupational history prior to this was as a metal smelter in a variety of workplaces over 25 years, exposed regularly to cadmium and silver fumes.

Physical examination noted a reduced body mass index, skin pigmentation associated with argyria, and occasional expiratory wheezes.

His chest radiograph noted evidence of hyper-expansion, and his high resolution Computed Tomography (HRCT) scan, showed features of emphysema (Fig. 4). His lung function identified his FEV$_1$ to be 35%

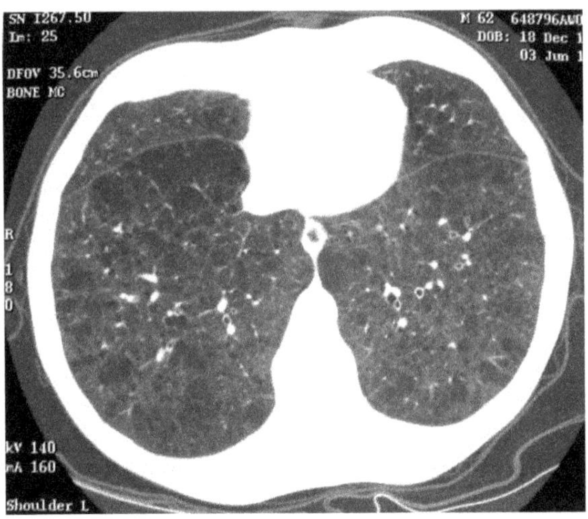

Fig. 4. Showing predominant emphysema on this HRCT of the patient.

of the predicted value, with a corresponding value of 85% predicted for his FVC. His ratio between the FEV_1 and FVC was 0.45, confirming the presence of airways obstruction. His carbon monoxide transfer factor was 34% of predicted.

Case commentary

His medical history, physiology and imaging are consistent with a diagnosis of COPD. He had smoked 10 pack years in total. Whilst this could have been responsible for the total clinical picture, the relatively low tobacco consumption suggests that other risk factors for COPD should be considered. In addition to the family history of emphysema, he has worked in environments exposed to fumes, dusts and gases. Cadmium in particular has been associated with the development of emphysema which would alert the clinician to a possible occupational contribution to his COPD.

Sadly, this man was admitted to hospital a year later with an exacerbation of his COPD associated with respiratory failure. He died during this admission, and a postmortem revealed congested lungs (483 g and 512 g in weight, right and left respectively), and histological evidence of bronchopneumonia with moderate emphysema. Tissue cadmium analysis was performed because of his occupational history and noted the following; Liver Cadmium; 27 mg/kg (measured by ICPMS) (for guidance a typical non-exposed value of 1.3 mg/kg would be seen, not normally >4 mg/kg) and Renal Cadmium 59 mg/kg (non-exposed 18–24 mg/kg). It was concluded that his cadmium exposure contributed to the overall severity of his COPD.

Case summary

The link between COPD and inhaled workplace exposures is now increasingly understood (Omland *et al.*, 2014). The previous American Thoracic Society Statements in 2005 (ATS, 2005) identified that on average occupational exposures account for 10–15% of the total burden of COPD. Whilst multiple risk factors may be present in each case of COPD, and including the predominance of tobacco smoking, various inhaled workplace exposures have more evidence to support a link to the development of COPD in workers. These include agricultural dusts (from poultry, animal and arable farming products and practices), asbestos, cadmium, carbon black, (refractory) ceramic fibres, coal mine dust, other dusts (from rubber, cotton, wood, iron/steel and smelting), endotoxin, flour, isocyanates and other chemicals, silica and welding fumes (Fishwick *et al.*, 2015). More recent work from the Biobank data in the UK has also used a lifetime job history approach in order to identify at risk occupations (De Matteis, 2019).

Attribution of the individual effects of multiple cause of COPD in the patient is often difficult, but clinicians should ideally be vigilant not only to previous exposures that may have contributed to the development of existing COPD, but current exposures in workers with COPD (or at risk of COPD) that may have the potential to cause this disease. The latter scenarios may be identified by accelerated annual decline in FEV_1 in individual workers, leading on to interventions in the workplace to reduce the risk to other workers.

Case Study 6: Obliterative Bronchiolitis in a Coffee Bean Worker

A 46-year-old non-smoking male worked in a local coffee flavouring facility close to his home. It was a small company that was carrying out several coffee bean related tasks; including coffee roasting and flavouring. He worked on the shop floor, and no respiratory protection was supplied or used. The working conditions were described as poor. He was responsible for adding liquid flavourings into a barrel that was then rotated in order to flavour coffee beans. He had noted a dry cough and shortness of breath on exertion, gradually worsening over the last 6 months.

He was concerned about the rapidity of these symptoms, and although he was a current smoker of 20 cigarettes per day, he felt these symptoms could not be caused by his smoking alone. He saw his GP and was immediately referred to a respiratory specialist.

His lung function showed a reduced FEV1 (55% of predicted) and FVC (75% of predicted), with a reduced transfer factor. An HRCT showed changes consistent with an obliterative bronchiolitis. An open lung biopsy was carried out given the uncertain nature of his condition, and its possible occupational cause. This revealed chronic and subacute small airways injury morphologically consistent with a bronchiolitis.

Given his work, and the potential relationship between coffee bean work and the development of bronchiolitis, he was advised not to be exposed in that work environment and ceased that work. At follow up one year later, he remained unchanged. His cough and shortness of breath on exertion were both similar in severity.

Case commentary

His medical history, physiology, imaging and biopsy are consistent with a diagnosis of obliterative bronchiolitis. Occupational associations and causes are described, and predominantly attributed to diacetyl exposure in the initial outbreaks in the US. In fact, flavourings in general are increasingly implicated.

For example, Bailey *et al.* (2015) published a summary paper describing their experiences relating to coffee processors given their concerns about potential exposures both to diacetyl and the related flavouring 2,3-pentanedione. They assessed 75 workers with lung function, and also devised exposure groups based on work history. They identified an excess of respiratory symptoms and reduction in lung function associated with flavouring exposures. In addition, however, they identified problems in non flavouring areas also. The authors suggested that 2,3-pentanedione may well also be responsible for bronchiolitis given its structural similarities to diacetyl (2,3 butanedione). In addition, animal studies have shown that 2,3-pentanedione also is toxic to the respiratory epithelium (Hubbs *et al.*, 2012; Morgan *et al.*, 2012).

Case summary

This case describes the presentation and brief history of obliterative bronchiolitis relating to a coffee bean worker. The presentation was typical for such a diagnosis, and the occupational exposure must be regarded as potentially relevant, given that other causes of obliterative bronchiolitis were not easily identifiable. Keeping these types of exposure at the front of your mind when dealing with this diagnosis, and unexplained airways obstruction, would be a sensible approach. This case of course has similarities to other flavouring related cases that have been described, for example, in microwave popcorn manufacture (Kanwal *et al.*, 2006) and cookie dough workers (Cavalcanti *et al.*, 2012).

Restrictive Lung Disorders

Case Study 7: Hypersensitivity Pneumonitis Due to Metalworking Fluids

A 56-year-old man reported work-related cough and mild exertional breathlessness during routine health surveillance. He was normally fit and well, had never smoked, and has no pets. His symptoms had worsened slowly over the previous two-years. Six months ago, his GP had prescribed a salbutamol inhaler for possible asthma. He had no other medication. He reported that his symptoms did not vary much at work, but did feel progressively more tired through the working week. He had not lost weight. His wife recently noticed he coughed less, and was able to walk further than normal, at the end of a two-week walking holiday. His cough returned within two days of returning to work. He noted that several other workers also had a cough.

He worked as a machine setter and operator operating four Computer Numeric Control (CNC) cutting and grinding machines. He had been at this company for five years, making a range of steel components for the automobile industry. The machines used a water-soluble coolant that was recirculated via a large shared sump, shared by 18 other machines. The coolant is regularly dip-slide tested, and he reported that there had been a problem with high levels of microbial contamination on one of his machines. Each machine has a timed lock and most had local exhaust ventilation. He has noticed some chest tightness when using compressed air, to clean the coolant from metal components. Workers were not required to wear respiratory protective equipment.

On examination he appeared well but had fine end inspiratory crackles at his lung bases on chest auscultation. His spirometry taken at health surveillance was within the normal range, with an FEV1 of 86% predicted and FVC 84% predicted. No previous results were available for comparison. Full lung function testing however showed his transfer factor to be reduced at 65% predicted. An HRCT was reported as showing widespread ground glass change with sparing of secondary pulmonary lobules, gas trapping and early sub pleural fibrosis compatible with hypersensitivity pneumonitis (Figs. 5 and 6).

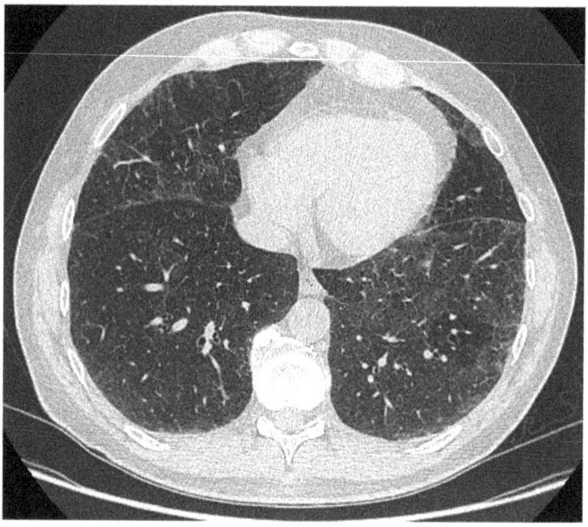

Fig. 5. Inspiratory HRCT view showing ground glass change with sparing of the secondary pulmonary lobules and early subpleural fibrosis.

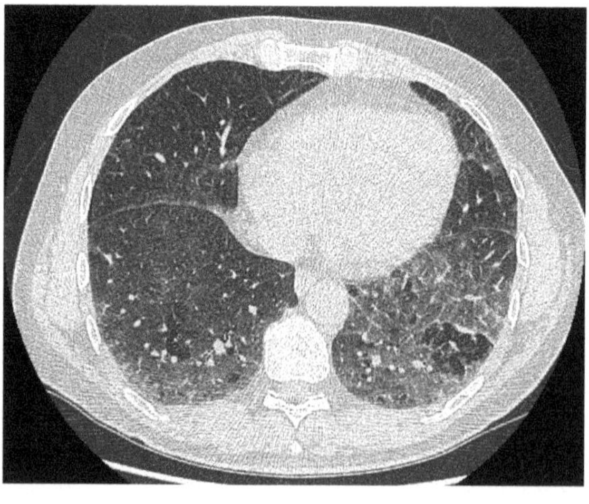

Fig. 6. Expiratory HRCT view confirms widespread air trapping due to bronchiolitis.

A bronchoscopy with broncho alveolar lavage found no evidence of infection, but a marked lymphocytosis on differential cell count. Routine blood tests were normal apart from a mildly raised C-reactive protein. Specific immunoglobulin G tests were negative to avian proteins, Aspergillus fumigatus, Micropolysporium faenii and Thermoactinomycetes vulgaris.

Case commentary

This case is fairly typical of hypersensitivity pneumonitis (HP) due to metalworking fluid (MWF) exposure. His symptoms were non-specific but included work-related respiratory and constitutional symptoms. He was a non-smoker and had been earlier misdiagnosed with asthma. In this case the radiological features were typical, and the diagnosis was confirmed by the bronchoalveolar lavage (BAL) lymphocytosis. No other potential causative exposures (e.g. domestic bird exposures or household damp) were identified in this case. Following the diagnosis, this patient was relocated to a non-exposed inspection role in a different building at the same workplace. Over the next twelve months he was carefully monitored, with some improvement in his symptoms. In addition, his physiology improved; his FVC rising to 96% of the predicted value, and gas transfer to 82% of predicted. In this case the HRCT findings had confirmed a mixed picture of reversible ground glass inflammation, and permanent fibrotic scarring.

A detailed health survey of the other workers at this workplace with the potential for MWF exposure revealed two other case of HP, and one case of occupational asthma. Although no specific single microbiological cause could be identified in this workplace, a range of workplace improvements resulted in no further cases. These improvements included extensive cleaning of the machines and central sump, replacement of the MWF, improved exhaust ventilation, reduced use of compressed air, and use of appropriate respiratory protective equipment (RPE) for high risk work processes.

Case summary

Over the last decade, exposure to water-soluble MWFs has become the leading cause of occupational HP in the UK. Disease occurs as single cases, but "outbreaks" have also been reported in the United States and Europe, with several individuals affected in the same workplace. As with other causes of HP, the majority of exposed workers are not affected, suggesting an underlying genetic predisposition. Despite extensive investigations the exact cause of the outbreaks remains elusive. Although a wide range of bacterial, fungal and environmental mycobacterial contaminants have been reported, immunological tests have not yet been able to reliably confirm causation.

Symptoms of MWF HP are often non-specific and commonly misdiagnosed in primary care as asthma or viral infections. In some situations, the predominant symptoms may be constitutional with unexplained weight loss. No single diagnostic test is available, and a diagnosis is usually reached based on a combination of clinical features, physiology, and radiology. Spirometry typically shows a restrictive pattern, but may also show airflow obstruction or remain within the normal range. Serial measures of spirometry may be more useful in highlighting excessive annual decline, and gas transfer estimates are more sensitive tests in confirming impaired gas exchange.

The most useful diagnostic test is an HRCT, with inspiratory and expiratory views, taken whilst the patient is symptomatic. Radiological features may be typical, but HP may also "mimic" a wide range of other types of interstitial disease including idiopathic NSIP and IPF. Many centers also utilise BAL to confirm the diagnosis. Unlike other common causes of occupational HP, particularly farming and bird-breeding, no established IgG panel of allergens is routinely available.

Prognosis in HP is improved where a cause can be identified, and further exposure can be prevented. Recent work (Barber *et al.*, 2019) however notes that it is not possible to identify a cause in the majority of cases. In general, the degree of established fibrosis at the time of diagnosis is the other main prognostic factor. Treatment with oral prednisolone is indicated for severe hypoxic acute cases and chronic progressive disease. The latter are also commonly treated with a range of other immunosuppressants, although evidence is lacking in this area. Selected patients may also be suitable for lung transplantation.

Case Study 8: Complicated Silicosis in a Stonemason

A 46-year-old man presented to his general practitioner with mild shortness of breath. His previous medical history was unremarkable, and he had never smoked. There was no significant family history and he was not taking any regular medication. He had no relevant hobby exposure to fumes, dusts or gases. He had noticed mild, but progressive, shortness of breath on exercise over the previous 18 months. There were no other symptoms, and he denied previous ocular problems and rashes.

He worked as a stonemason and had done this job since the age of 18 years. He reported very poor workplace conditions from the age of 18 years to 40 years, with some reported reduction in dust exposure in the last 6 years. He had never really consistent been supplied with, or worn, RPE. There was no periodic health surveillance, using lung function and chest radiography, offered at work.

Physical examination was unremarkable, noting a man with a normal body mass index who was mildly short of breath on minimal exercise. There was no lymphadenopathy, and no evidence of skin rashes. There were very minor but persistent crackles on auscultation of the chest.

Lung function testing revealed an FEV_1 and FVC respectively of 78% and 83% of the predicted values, and his carbon monoxide transfer factor was 65% of the predicted value. His plain chest radiograph was consistent with the findings of the HRCT (Fig. 7).

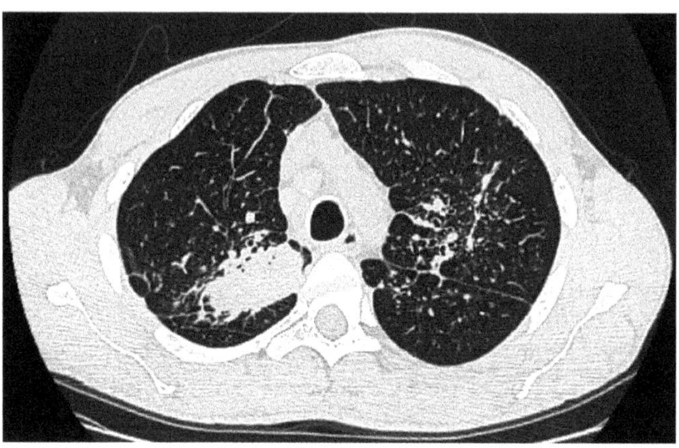

Fig. 7. HRCT showing both small nodules and a conglomerate mass consistent with complicated silicosis.

Case commentary

A diagnosis of complicated silicosis was made, based on a supportive medical and occupational history with no extra-thoracic features to suggest sarcoidosis. He is now under regular review, and was advised to cease silica exposure at work. He has managed to achieve a job task change within the same employment, now in a role where there is no significant silica exposure.

His FEV_1 has remained relatively stable over the 2-year period of follow up, and he has not developed any new clinical features to suggest an alternate diagnosis.

Case summary

The risk of silicosis is finite when working for a lifetime at the current, for example, GB and US, workplace exposure limits. Dose-response in silica exposed workers is a complicated area, but in general terms previous estimates have suggested a lifetime risk of developing silicosis to be in the order of 2.5–10% if working at a level of 0.1 mg/m^3 (Finkelstein, 2000). Although not relevant (yet) in this case, additional previous work has estimated that silica exposure not sufficient to cause silicosis may be associated with an increased risk of developing COPD (Hnizdo and Vallyathan, 2003). This worker decided to stay at work, in a much lesser exposed job.

There is little evidence concerning outcomes in silicosis in relation to continued, or reduced exposure once a diagnosis has been made although a pragmatic approach to reduce exposures once a diagnosis is made appears sensible and precautionary. There is however general agreement that health surveillance programmes with periodic lung function and chest radiograph assessment are required to identify early workers who are developing silicosis or airways obstruction. The details of each programmes will differ according to risk assessments at work, and local requirements.

Both Health and Safety Executive (HSE), UK and National Institute for Occupational Safety and Health (NIOSH) have web-based resources that the reader may find useful (HSE, 2021; NIOSH, 2020).

Case Study 9: Asbestosis

A 66-year-old man consulted primary care with progressive exertional breathlessness. He had been a lifelong smoker with a 40 pack-year history, but had stopped 2 years earlier. He started to notice problems with his breathing 4–5 years ago, but thought it was a combination of smoking and his increasing age. Despite stopping smoking, his breathing had deteriorated, and he reported breathlessness walking uphill, upstairs, and carrying his work tools. Apart from taking bendrofluamethazide for hypertension, he was taking no regular medication, and was normally fit and well. He has no symptoms of arthritis or connective tissue disease, had no pets, and no relevant family history. A chest x-ray was reported as showing pleural plaques, and bi-basal interstitial change.

He had worked since leaving school as an electrician, and for the last 20 years was self-employed working on domestic properties. Prior to this, he worked for several different companies providing electrical services to industry. For approximately 12 years (late 1960s to early 1980s) he had worked in a number of power stations, steel works and rolling mills. This work involved direct contact with asbestos containing materials whilst installing electrical cables. Regular additional exposure occurred working alongside laggers who were applying insulation to pipework. Their work involved emptying bags of asbestos powder into large open containers and mixing it with water by stirring it with a stick. Insulation was then hand applied to the pipework. This process generated a lot of dust, and waste insulation was swept up at the end of the shift. No RPE was provided.

On examination he appeared well. He did not have finger clubbing but had marked bi-basal fine end inspiratory crackles at his lung bases on chest auscultation. His spirometry was restrictive, with an FEV_1 *of 75% predicted and FVC of 78% predicted. His gas transfer was more severely reduced at 58% predicted. A HRCT (Fig. 8) confirmed upper zone pleural plaques and bi-basal pulmonary fibrosis with a pattern in keeping with usual interstitial pneumonitis (UIP).*

Case commentary

This patient has developed slowly progressive interstitial lung disease, with classical clinical and physiological findings. The HRCT has

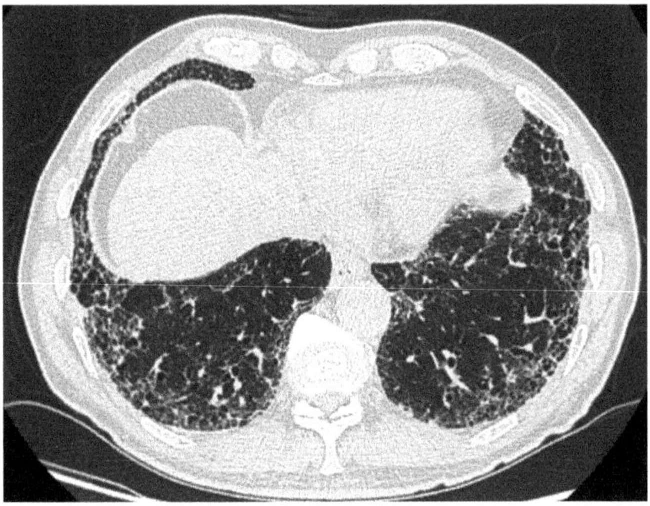

Fig. 8. HRCT image of asbestosis showing sub pleural bi-basal honeycombing typical of UIP pattern disease.

shown a UIP pattern of disease that may be seen in IPF, connective tissue diseases, chronic HP, and asbestosis. In this case, the occupational history and presence of calcified pleural plaques confirmed previous exposure to asbestos. This exposure occurred regularly over a prolonged period, up to around 30 years prior to the onset of breathlessness.

These findings are typical of asbestosis, a long latency disease. Treatment is supportive, with benefits and compensation advice provided. This patient had already quit smoking, which is important due to the at least additive risk of future lung cancer.

Case summary

Asbestosis is a form of pneumoconiosis that occurs due to the inhalation and retention of significant numbers of asbestos fibres within the lung. Asbestos fibres reaching the alveolus are difficult for the body to clear as the fibres are longer than the macrophage attempting to engulf it. The resultant release of cytokines attracts other immune cells, and results in chronic inflammation. Over many years, this process results in permanent scarring of the lung due to fibrosis. It is a disease that generally only occurs with higher lifetime doses of exposure, most commonly at least 5–10 years of regular exposure. Very high historical exposures, for only a few months, have also previously resulted in disease.

This condition can be very difficult to differentiate from IPF, as both may have a typical UIP-pattern on HRCT. The presence of pleural plaques confirms exposure, but not the duration or lifetime dose inhaled. An absence of pleural plaques makes asbestosis less likely, but does not exclude the disease. Diagnostic guidelines vary internationally in terms of the lifetime dose required for diagnosis, and how frequently invasive tests such as BAL or biopsy are performed. In the UK, the majority of patients are diagnosed based on radiological findings, and a compatible history of exposure with a suitable latent period. Obtaining a reliable estimate of exposure is commonly difficult however, as it relies on patient recall of events several decades in the past. In other cases, individuals were significantly exposed to asbestos without their knowledge, either through handling materials they didn't know contained asbestos, or being exposed indirectly by others working around them.

Management of asbestosis is currently supportive, as there is no proven therapy, and no published trials of anti-fibrotic drugs. If asbestosis is diagnosed whilst an individual has the potential to be exposed, measures to avoid further exposure should be taken where possible. Smoking cessation is of particular importance in individuals with asbestosis due to the increased risk of lung cancer.

The long latency seen in asbestosis means that the number of deaths due to the condition in developed countries has continued to rise in recent years despite the introduction of asbestos bans. As asbestos continues to be produced and utilised in developing countries, the global burden from asbestosis and asbestos-related malignancy remains high.

Case Study 10: Artificial Stone Silicosis

A 43-year-old man was admitted to hospital with acutely increasing shortness of breath associated with a productive cough, producing green sputum. He had also noted that for the last 6 months that he had been gradually developing shortness of breath on exercise, although this was mild, and he had ignored these symptoms.

He denied other breathing problems more generally. He was a never smoker, and had no relevant hobby, pet or environmental exposures. He had no significant previous medical history. In particular, he had no previous diagnosed respiratory history, no ocular, joint or skin complaints. He was not taking any longer-term medication.

On examination he was tachypnoeic, tachycardic and febrile. He had a chest x ray that confirmed a likely right lower lobe pneumonia, but also raised the possibility of a significant nodular lung disease. His sputum grew H Influenzae, and he was treated with an appropriate antibiotic and improved. During early convalescence from this illness, he had a HRCT scan to assess the nodular lung disease.

By way of occupational background, he reported that he worked as a kitchen fitter and had done this work for the last 7 years. Before this, he worked for a local council as a labourer but had developed some expertise using a variety of power tools and handheld grinders. He had never worked as a stone mason. He described his kitchen fitting work as often dusty and dirty, and the provision of respiratory protective equipment was rather intermittent. Even when it was provided, it was generally of the simple surgical face mask type that did not require a fit testing.

His HRCT scan and chest radiograph are shown in Figs. 9 and 10. This shows typical features of silicosis with prominent nodules, some of which are coalescent and forming larger masses.

Case commentary

Kitchen fitters and artificial stone workers are at an increased risk of developing silicosis as a consequence of exposure to high levels of respirable crystalline silica. Initial case reports of silicosis in artificial stone workers were described in Israel. 25 cases were described in association with work with artificial stone. There were a range of exposure histories, but most workers were dry cutting the product whilst fitting countertops into domestic kitchens (Kramer *et al.*, 2012).

Artificial stone is a relatively new product, which is increasingly popular in the marketplace. It consists of a mix of finely crushed stone and a polymeric resin. Its silica content may be as high as 90%; clearly

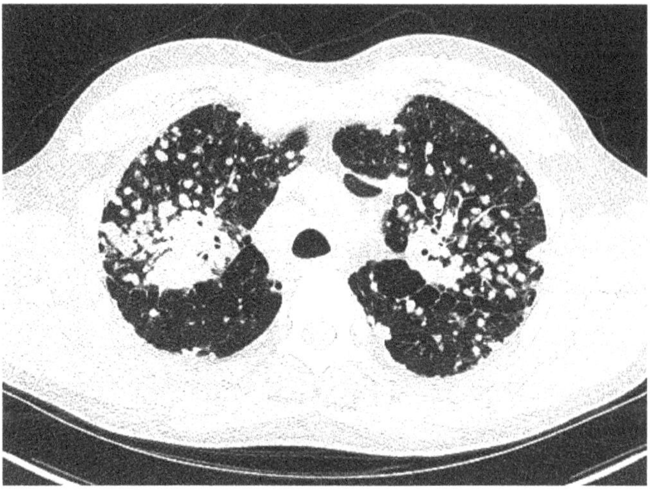

Fig. 9. HRCT of this case.

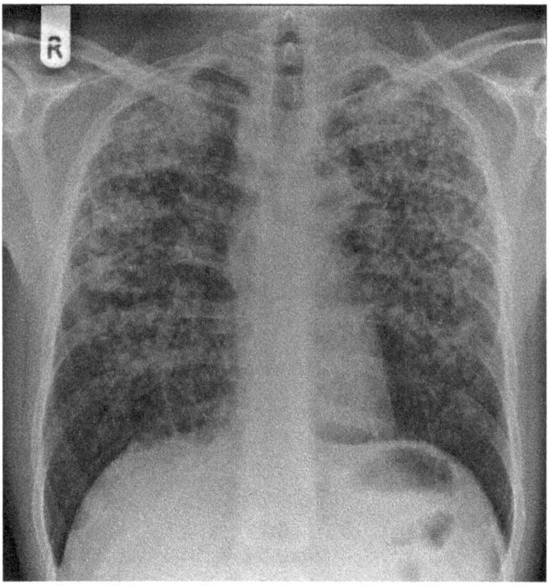

Fig. 10. Chest X-ray of this case.

exceeding the majority of natural stone RCS content. Some exposure information does exist about this type of exposure in real life workplaces. Rosengarten (Rosengarten *et al.*, 2017) cites data from the Israel Ministry of Labor suggesting that dry cutting of the artificial stone could generate RCS levels of 1 mg/m^3; a value that is 10-fold excess above the legal limit for exposure in Israel at that time (and also, for example, 10 times the current UK workplace exposure limit). It may well be that these workers are developing silicosis purely because of such high RCS exposures; although work continues to identify if there are other characteristics of the exposure that enhance its ability to cause this disease.

It is interesting that many countries have now identified cases of artificial stone silicosis including Australia (Hoy *et al.*, 2018) but some have not. For example, the UK has yet to identify such a case (Barber *et al.*, 2018).

Case summary

This gentleman developed accelerated silicosis as a direct result of high RCS exposure to work whilst working with artificial stone as a kitchen fitter. The international literature contains now many such cases. Vigilance is required when assessing the risks posed by not only new exposures, but also typical and well characterised exposures such as RCS that appear in different materials and workplaces.

Less Common Conditions

Rarer Pneumoconioses

Whilst silica, coal and asbestos exposures are probably responsible for the majority of global pneumoconioses seen today, other less common but nevertheless notable causes of pneumoconiosis include iron (siderosis), tin (stannosis) and barium (baritosis). These are dealt with briefly here.

Siderosis; caused by iron fume exposure, siderosis is typically associated with widespread soft pulmonary nodules and a general lack of physiological impairment. Its presence may not be associated with any respiratory symptoms, and it may only come to light following a routine chest radiograph. In general terms, it is regarded as a non-fibrogenic pneumoconiosis, and does not normally progress to cause symptoms or physiological impairment.

Stannosis; caused by tin exposure, stannosis is again typically associated with marked radiological small nodules. As tin has a high atomic number, these nodules appear rather striking on a plain chest radiograph. In a similar fashion to siderosis, tin associated stannosis does not generally cause symptoms or impairment of physiology.

Baritosis; caused by barium exposure, the situation is similar to that caused by tin. Again, as a reflection of its high atomic number, marked radiological abnormalities are often seen in the absence of significant symptoms or physiological impairment. The regression of these appearances has been described following cessation of exposure to dusts containing barium.

Epidemiology of Occupational Lung Diseases

According to the 2005 study of global burden of occupational diseases, the annual number of deaths for occupational lung diseases is estimated at 318,000 for COPD, 38,000 for asthma, 30,000 for pneumoconiosis, 102,000 for lung cancer and 43,000 for malignant mesothelioma. The corresponding DALY (or "disability adjusted life years," a weighted estimate of the number of years lived with disability for which weight refers to the severity of the disability) is 3.73 million for COPD, 1.62 million for asthma, 1.29 million for pneumoconioses, 0.97 million for lung cancer and 0.56 million for malignant mesothelioma (Driscoll *et al.*, 2005a; Driscoll *et al.*, 2005b). More recently, attempts have been made to map the burden of asbestos disease in individual countries, based on past per capita asbestos usage and suitable latency (Lin *et al.*, 2007).

2013 data of all cases of COPD and asthma globally show little change, although no data are supplied on the occupational cases within each category in the most recent data (Global Burden of Disease Study, 2013).

The ATS and ERS have recently repeated (Blanc *et al.*, 2019) the assessment of occupational attribution for non-malignant lung diseases and also expanded the remit of the original 2003 document (Balmes *et al.*, 2003). This official statement summarises pertinent literature where an occupational cause has been sought or estimates how much of the total burden of a particular lung disease can be attributed to occupational. Its remit included asthma Incidence, COPD and Chronic Bronchitis, IPF, pulmonary alveolar proteinosis, HP, sarcoidosis and other granulomatous lung diseases, tuberculosis and community acquired pneumonia.

Occupational asthma is regarded as the most common occupational lung disease in industrialised countries, and the second most common occupational lung disease reported after pneumoconioses in developing countries (Schuitemaker *et al.*, 2007). One such example was given in Case Study 2. There is increasing clinical and research recognition that a substantial proportion of adult onset asthma is attributable to occupational exposures. The population attributable fraction (PAF) is calculated in order to identify the proportion of the total burden of a particular condition that would be prevented if the occupational exposure was removed. A review of papers published during 1999–2007 reported the PAF to be 16.3% (Toren and Blanc, 2009). Earlier estimates had suggested that a PAF of 9% to 15% for asthma in industrialised countries (Mapp *et al.*, 2005) and 29% for men and 17% for women in Finland (Karjalainen *et al.*, 2001). The ATS/ERS official statement also concluded similarly. Based on just the longitudinal studies assessing asthma incidence, given the high number of cross-sectional studies now in this area, a PAF of 16% (95% CI 10–22) was calculated for asthma. In other words, 16% of incident asthma could be prevented in the future if all contributing and relevant exposures ceased today.

A similar view is now being adopted for COPD, although contribution of occupational factors is often more difficult to differentiate from the effects of tobacco smoking. This was illustrated in Case Study 5. Other than smoking, occupational exposures have been listed among the important risk factors for COPD together with indoor (e.g. smoke from biomass fuel) and outdoor air pollution and infections (Mannino and Buist, 2007; Salvi and Barnes, 2009). More recent data from GB identify occupations associated with COPD from a very large population database (De Matteis *et al.*, 2016). The body of evidence continues to grow here, and many authorities regard this as a strong indicator that these relationships are now more than associations but represent causation.

Data in the most recent European Lung White Book confirm these assertions and also concluded that "systematic under-reporting and difficulties in attributing causation both contribute to under-appreciation of the burden of occupational respiratory diseases" (*European Lung White Book*, 2012)

The ATS/ERS official statement findings concord with these figures. The pooled PAF for the occupational contribution to the burden of COPD, adjusted for smoking, was 14% (95% CI, 10–18%). This figure increased to 31% in never smokers. Figures were similar for chronic bronchitis; 13% (95% CI, 6–21%). Taken as read, these suggest that a substantial proportion of these conditions are contributed to by the harmful effects of occupational exposures. This clearly supports the development of interventions in workplaces to reduce these.

The ATS/ERS official statement, in brief, also identified significant PAF values for workplace contribution to other respiratory diseases that may be seen relatively commonly in clinical practice. Outcomes were identified as follows; IPF (for vapours, gases, dust and fumes exposure (VGDF); a PAF of 26%, 95% CI 10–41%), HP (weighted meta-proportion 19%, 95% CI 12–28%), sarcoidosis (weighted meta-proportion of 30%, 95% CI 17–45%) and tuberculosis (the median health care worker associated burden of TB was 1.0%, range, 0.8–9%). Community acquired pneumonia attribution was discussed in Case Study 4.

PAF values have been derived for other, for example, malignant, respiratory conditions with causative links to the workplace. For example, the link between carcinogen exposure at work and the development of lung cancer has been assessed. Based on 31 epidemiologic studies which evaluated occupational exposures to suspected or known lung carcinogens among men, and controlled for smoking, PAF values ranged between 0% and 40%. The wide range in time and place was primarily thought to be due to the variable prevalence of hazardous industries in each of the individual studies (De Matteis *et al.*, 2008). For example, it can be expected that countries and regions which record high level of asbestos use will eventually shoulder a proportionate burden of asbestos-related diseases. Such relationships have been demonstrated as plausible correlations using national level data, accounting for latency time. This supports the need to eliminate asbestos use as a national policy (Lin *et al.*, 2007). Indeed, World Health Organization (WHO) recognises that asbestos is one of the most important occupational carcinogens causing about half of the deaths from occupational cancer.

Clinical History in the Investigation of Respiratory Disorders

A complete history should include a careful review of respiratory symptoms, the smoking history, history of atopy and allergies including family history, occupational and environmental exposures and exposures related to hobbies. Review of symptoms should include questions on cough, sputum production, shortness of breath, chest tightness, wheezing and chest pain. Other related symptoms such as rhinitis, eye irritation, rashes, fever, weight loss and muscular pains may also be relevant.

For reported symptoms, details of their onset, duration, severity, aggravating or relieving factors and time relationship to work or any particular exposures or activities should be sought. For occupational asthma, it is particularly useful to ask how symptoms vary between works and rest without asking direct leading questions. Certain workers may not describe improvement on rest days but will nominate that symptoms are worse at work. Similarly, certain patients with asthma may use more medication during periods of work in comparison to when they are not at work. All these patterns should alert the clinicians to a possible diagnosis of an occupational lung disorder.

Furthermore, some workers may even be able to identify the particular substance or activity which provokes their asthmatic symptoms (for example, high levels of flour dust, or a particular type of wood dust exposure). Safety Data Sheets, or international equivalents, are useful to obtain for exposures that are known about, as these may offer clues in relation to the nature of exposures. For chronic diseases such as silicosis and asbestosis, it is important to document a detailed and accurate occupational history starting from their very first job. Both the intensity and duration of exposure should be documented as far as possible. It is also useful to ask whether other workers have been similarly affected with an occupational respiratory disease.

Use of personal protective equipment (and specifically RPE) is important to document as this practice may reduce exposures.

Physical Examination

General and respiratory examinations are carried out in normal clinical practice and may assist by identifying general (shortness of breath, cyanosis, finger clubbing) and specific (crackles, wheeze) features consistent with respiratory disease and more particularly airways obstruction or interstitial lung disease. In general, examination findings need to be put into the context of the entire clinical picture, and not interpreted in isolation.

It is unusual to identify features on examination that may suggest specific occupational respiratory disease, but an example relatively commonly seen is coal pigmentation in the skin of miners presenting with either coal worker's pneumoconiosis or coal dust related COPD.

Imaging

Chest Radiograph

The chest radiograph has been for many decades the basic investigation for detection and characterisation of occupational lung disease. Its role is primarily in the screening for, and diagnosis of, interstitial and pleural occupational respiratory diseases. Its role in the assessment of airways diseases, and in particular asthma and COPD, is best left to the judgement of the clinician, although is of course a very useful investigation for workers with unexplained respiratory symptoms such as increasing shortness of breath and or cough.

Its advantages include its relatively portable nature, as chest radiographs can be performed at the workplace itself, and additionally the relatively low dose of ionising radiation used to capture a good quality digital image. A full sized postero-anterior (PA) chest radiograph is particularly useful in the diagnosis of early asbestosis or silicosis. Comparison with the standard films for pneumoconiosis (for example, the International Labour Organization (ILO) Classification of Radiographs of Pneumoconiosis) is very helpful when looking for evidence of nodular or linear profusions suggesting silicosis or asbestosis. An excellent resource concerning ILO is available on the NIOSH website, and the ILO classification system has been extensively validated by comparison with duration and intensity of dust exposure, and outcome.

Additionally, the chest radiograph can give certain detail of the lung hilae and the pleura. Examples include hilar lymph node calcifications (i.e. "egg-shell calcifications") seen in some cases of silicosis and various pleuro-pulmonary changes such as pleural plaques, thickening, calcification or fluid seen in asbestos exposed workers. Pleural effusions generally require further active investigation in this context. Whilst benign asbestos effusions are a possible outcome, it is clearly advisable to exclude malignancy such as mesothelioma as a cause. Further characterisation of all these changes is best carried out by computed tomography (CT) scanning.

Other useful radiological features can be seen on the chest radiograph, including features of complicated pneumoconiosis (confluent areas of fibrosis and mass like structures), features that might suggest active or previous tuberculosis, and even pneumothorax. Equally, absence of changes consistent with a pneumonitis, or indeed pulmonary edema, may also assist with a definitive diagnosis in the acute setting.

Both individual, and serial chest radiographs may be indicated for the assessment of established or possible occupational respiratory diseases. Workers exposed to respirable crystalline silica may require surveillance over a number of years with serial chest radiographs in order to identify early ILO grades of silicosis.

Despite their central role, however, the sensitivity and specificity of chest radiograph for the diagnosis of occupational respiratory diseases are generally considered to be relatively low (Akira, 2008) in comparison to other more modern imaging modalities. In reality, most abnormalities identified on a chest radiograph that may relate to occupational exposures are normally better defined using CT.

CT Scanning

Modern CT scanning produces very detailed images that may offer very significant additional diagnostic information over a plain chest radiograph. Depending on the settings used, they can accurately define the pleural, parenchyma, bones and mediastinal structures.

It is now widely recognised that CT is more sensitive than a chest radiograph in certain occupational contexts. For example, when considering the detection of pleuro-parenchymal abnormalities in pneumoconiosis, CT is able to demonstrate plaques along the mediastinum, paravertebral areas, and diaphragm which are difficult to assess by conventional techniques. Indeed, chest radiograph has a generally low sensitivity (in one study 8.3–40.3%; depending on the detection criteria and population) for pleural plaque detection, and particularly so for non-calcified pleural plaques.

CT has a central role in diagnosis and staging of pleural and lung malignancy associated with occupational exposures. Figure 11 shows a

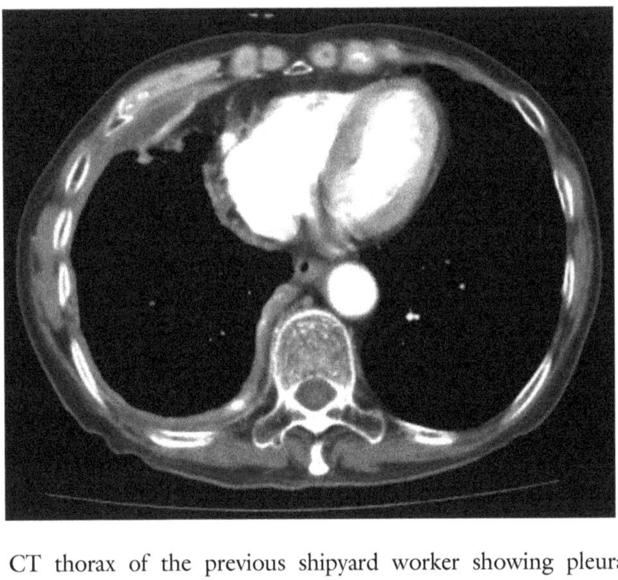

Fig. 11. CT thorax of the previous shipyard worker showing pleural thickening encasing the lung, with mediastinal pleural thickening, within the smaller right hemi thorax, associated with pleural calcification (arrows). Video-assisted thoracoscopic biopsy of the pleura confirmed the diagnosis of a sarcomatoid (desmoplastic) mesothelioma.

CT scan of a worker with a sarcomatoid (desmoplastic) mesothelioma. Features that have previously been shown to be more associated with malignant as opposed to benign disease included; (i) circumferential pleural thickening, (ii) nodular pleural thickening, (iii) parietal pleural thickening greater than 1 cm, and (iv) mediastinal pleural involvement (Leung's Criteria).

HRCT is also a more sensitive diagnostic tool to demonstrate parenchymal abnormalities. Work in silica exposed populations has identified its superiority to a chest radiograph for identifying small opacities associated with early silicosis, although as yet there is no agreed ILO system for grading CT abnormalities against an agreed standard set of films.

For example, Sun *et al.* (2008) identified that HRCT was more sensitive than a standard chest radiograph when detecting small opacities in the mid zones of the lung, but not in the lower zones. HRCT, as anticipated, also identified detail of other abnormalities including bullae, emphysema, pleural, mediastinal and hilar changes. Similar work in asbestos exposed workers supports its sensitivity in identifying earlier changes of pneumoconiosis. This is an interesting area of development, and clinicians are increasingly required to interpret more early and subtle findings from ever increasingly sensitive imaging. A recent excellent review summarises the utility of CT scanning in these areas (Weissman, 2015).

Similarly, HRCT is increasingly used to assist differentiating types of interstitial lung disease where historically lung biopsy would have been undertaken. An example is the distinction between HP and IPF.

The application of CT to screening for early changes consistent with occupational pneumoconioses, or indeed lung cancer, is as yet an area of uncertainty. McCunney concluded that it is unclear whether Low Dose CT reduces mortality from lung cancer in view of the absence of randomised, controlled studies needed to address biases commonly encountered in observational and population based studies (McCunney, 2006).

The American Thoracic Society has subsequently released clinical guidelines (Jaklitsch *et al.*, 2012) relating to lung cancer screening. These guidelines suggested that a proactive approach to screening should be adopted in individuals over 55 years old and more than a 30 pack year history of smoking. Subsequently, the ATS have issues guidance on how best to implement these guidelines into clinical practice (Wiener *et al.*, 2015).

Magnetic Resonance Imaging

Magnetic resonance imaging (MRI) has a very limited role in diagnosing or staging occupational respiratory disease, with one main exception. It is used to assist with the diagnosis and staging of malignant mesothelioma, as this modality is superior to CT in identifying local invasion by mesothelioma into the diaphragm, endothoracic fascia, and mediastinum or chest wall, in selected patients who have potentially resectable mesothelioma (Nickell *et al.*, 2014). Additionally, T2-weighted MRI may discriminate between pleural plaques and malignant mesothelioma.

One relatively small study (Tsim *et al.*, 2020) compared CT and MRI in the assessment of malignant mesothelioma and identified that different mesothelioma tumour volumes were identified with each technique, but that tumour volumes identified with MRI were larger than with CT, and also independently associated with survival. It was also noted that MRI tumour volume assessment was quicker and more reproducible than for CT.

Positron Emission Tomography

Positron emission tomography (PET) imaging with flurorodeoxyglucose may be useful in distinguishing benign from malignant asbestos-related pleural disease, although this may be positive in folded lung. PET in conjunction with CT scanning has improved the diagnosis and staging of pleural mesothelioma (Fig. 12). Specifically, PET/CT can accurately demonstrate intrathoracic and extra thoracic lymphadenopathy and metastatic disease.

PET is increasingly used to define the nature of the solitary pulmonary nodule, which may be used to investigate nodules incidentally identified in workers that are being investigated for potential

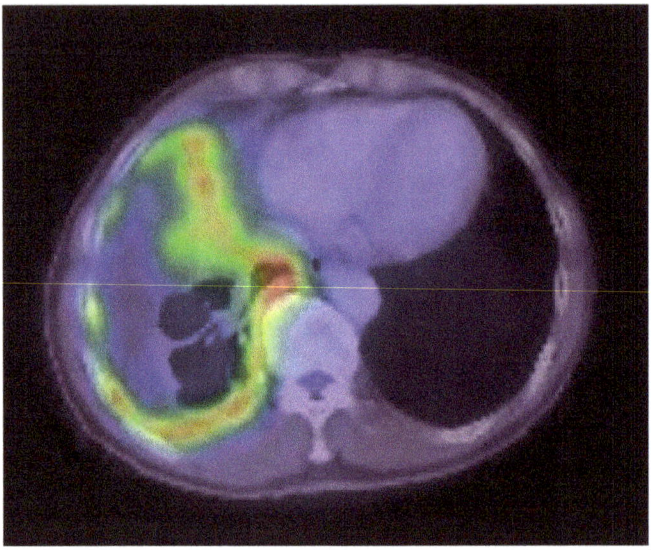

Fig. 12. F-18 fluorodeoxyglucose PET imaging with contrast enhanced CT showing fluorodeoxyglucose-avid enhancing nodular thickening of the right pleura with pleural effusion. Pleural biopsy confirmed the diagnosis of sarcomatoid mesothelioma.

occupational respiratory diseases. Individual case reports of occupational lung diseases have also incorporated PET images as a marker of metabolic activity of tissue (Barnes *et al.*, 2019).

Pulmonary Function Tests

Basic Lung Function Testing

Lung function tests are used commonly in the assessment of workers with possible occupational respiratory disease. They are also useful to give the clinician a guide about levels of impairment and respiratory disability. The lung function tests results should not, of course, be used solely to define disability, as the latter will also be a function of levels of reported symptoms and the reported impact these symptoms have on a worker's ability to carry out tasks.

Spirometry is probably the most common physiology test carried out either in the workplace, or in workers attending a laboratory when being assessed for a possible occupational respiratory disease. The FEV_1 is an excellent marker of lung health when compared to the predicted value for each worker. The latter is calculated using predicted equations, and is predominantly influenced by gender, height and age. Various sets of equations exist, and modern spirometers normally integrate these into the operating software. If the population under study has an ethnic mix, it will be necessary to consider how predicted values may vary between ethnic groups.

The FVC is also recorded using the same forced expiration. The technology is developing in this area, with devices that now measure flow using rotating systems or ultrasound probes.

While predicted normal values have been established for various populations, such values may need to be re-established from time to time. With improvements in the socio-economic and developmental status, succeeding generations would be expected to have higher normal values for FEV_1 and FVC. Where baseline or serial measurements are available for the individual, comparison with previous results is also informative. Based on the American Thoracic Society (ATS) and European Respiratory Society (ERS) task force 2005 recommendations (Pellegrino *et al.*, 2005) on the interpretation of lung function tests, for each lung function index, values below the 5th percentile of the frequency distribution of values measured in the reference population are considered to be below the expected "normal range" (i.e. below the lower limit of the reference range). The practice of using 80% predicted as a fixed value for the lower limit of normal may lead to important errors when interpreting lung function in adults. There are relatively newly generated prediction equations that are being increasingly used and permit a comprehensive consideration of differences between ethnic groups (Quanjer *et al.*, 2012). These prediction equations are for parameters in patients between 3 and 95 years old and include lower limit of normal values. The latter are increasingly used over a fixed percentage predicted cut off to define likely abnormality.

In order to be able to rely on the results of this test, it is essential to develop a protocol or operating procedure that allows technicians or operators to achieve the best results either in the clinic or in the workplace. This is an extensive and complicated area, made accessible by excellent summary positions such as that written by the American College of Occupational and Environmental Medicine (Townsend, 2011) and also that by Redlich *et al.* (2014). The latter stresses the importance of a set of approaches to ensure that any measures taken in the workplace are of the highest quality. These approaches are essential to consider in workplaces, if lung function measures are to be recorded accurately. This is because errors of measurement may cause significant untended consequences for workers and their occupational health care professionals. In broad terms, these important considerations include equipment maintenance and where appropriate calibration, testing techniques and also technician training and feedback.

In terms of the tests themselves, in brief, at least three technically acceptable forced expiratory maneuvers (or "blows") must be recorded from each individual, after starting from total lung capacity. The highest two FEV_1 values, and the highest two FVC values must be within 150 mL of each other (or within 100 mL if the absolute FEV_1 value is less than a liter). Once these have been recorded reproducibly, each is compared to the predicted value for that individual.

Change in lung function over time; is also an important occupational consideration as accelerated, or faster than expected, decline in lung function over time may well be an indicator of an occupational lung disease (such as asthma, COPD or silicosis). Whilst beyond the remit of this brief article, various ways of assessing decline in comparison to expected levels are discussed in Redlich *et al.* (2014), and include (i) a 15% decline from baseline FEV_1 (plus expected age-related loss), (ii) use of limits of longitudinal decline and (iii) linear regression analyses. The freely available SPIROLA software is useful here (NIOSH, 2014), to permit the entry and plotting of spirometry values over time; and their subsequent interpretation. If workers are undergoing repeated lung function measures over time, it is essential that these are interpreted not just for normality each time the test is performed, but how the values are changing over time.

Airways obstruction; the FEV_1/FVC ratio is used to diagnose airways obstruction. In certain conditions where airways obstruction is more common, for example, COPD and asthma, the FEV_1 may be affected (reduced) more than the FVC, and consequently the ratio of FEV_1/FVC, which is normally more than 70%, is reduced. In practice, both a fixed value of less than 0.7, or using the lower limit of normal for each individual (based on the 5th percentile), are used to define this. Both these methods are commonly used. Airways obstruction may be relatively fixed, or irreversible, often seen in emphysema, or may be reversible as seen in certain workers with asthma. Bronchodilator testing with inhaled β_2 agonists is used to identify whether airways obstruction is partly or fully reversible, although this is not generally carried out in the workplace. The technical details are beyond the scope of this text, although results should be interpreted with caution, as absence of reversibility does not exclude asthma as a cause.

Pulmonary restriction; diseases which cause inflammation and thickening of the interstitial tissue (for example, the alveolar walls) such as seen in pulmonary fibrosis associated with asbestos exposure (asbestosis) generally cause reduction in lung volume and reduction in carbon monoxide gas transfer as they progress. The reduction in total lung capacity (or in practice most commonly measured is a reduction in the FVC) is used to define airways restriction, although many definitions are used. Additionally, the FEV_1/FVC ratio is often greater than normal (>90%) because FVC is reduced to a greater degree than FEV_1.

Airways obstruction and restriction can co-exist in the same patient. For example, a worker with chronic HP related to metal working fluid exposure may have evidence of both airways obstruction (with a reduced FEV_1/FVC ratio due to small airway involvement) and also a reduced FVC (due to the pulmonary fibrosis component of this illness seen in the chronic phase).

More Complex Testing

In certain circumstances, more extended physiology testing may be needed. For example, a carbon monoxide transfer estimate may be useful when dealing with conditions that may have altered the normal capillary alveolar interface. Examples include emphysema and interstitial lung diseases.

Challenge Testing

Non-specific bronchial provocation is often carried to assess workers with possible asthma and specifically occupational asthma. Availability and experience will largely dictate the inhaled agent used, although these include methacholine, histamine and, increasingly, mannitol. The results are not directly comparable, although all measure non-specific bronchial hyperactivity. This is often quantified, if present, as concentration (PC_{20}) or dose (PD_{20}) of an agent that causes a 20% fall in the pre-test FEV_1, although the mannitol endpoint is often taken as a 15% fall in FEV_1.

These tests are not without their risks, although generally considered safe in experienced hands. Because of this, the test is generally only done in those with a normal or near normal baseline FEV_1.

In the appropriate clinical setting, a positive test is strongly suggestive of asthma, although this test can be negative in asthma and occupational asthma. A negative histamine or methacholine test result does not exclude sensitiser-induced occupational asthma if performed when the patient is off work and free of symptoms. As has been shown in studies of diisocyanate asthma, both methacholine reactivity and symptoms can resolve in workers who have been away from active work exposure for just a brief period. It may be necessary to re-expose workers to the causative agent at work before asthma and methacholine reactivity return. A negative histamine or methacholine test result has a good negative predictive value, i.e. a negative test excludes active asthma in an actively exposed worker. Results must therefore be considered in light of the clinical context of a case, and they should not be sole relied upon to make or exclude a particular diagnosis.

Serial changes in non-specific bronchial hyper reactivity following removal of exposure may be used to support the diagnosis of sensitiser-induced occupational asthma. Certain, although not all, guidelines for the diagnosis of sensitiser-induced occupational asthma have recommended a methacholine or histamine challenge be performed toward the end of a working week. It is then suggested that this is repeated at the end of a period (usually 10 to 14 days) away from the exposure. Worsening of the PC_{20} at work, versus off work, beyond the normal variability of the test (defined as threefold or greater change in PC_{20}) would provide additional evidence to support the diagnosis of sensitiser-induced asthma (Tarlo *et al.*, 2008).

Specific inhalation challenge (SIC)

SIC normally involves exposing workers who are suspected of sensitiser-induced occupational asthma to suspected agents in a safe and controlled manner. It is also used in other less common scenarios such as investigation of response to agents suspected of causing HP. SIC is intended to demonstrate a direct relationship between exposure to a suspected agent and an asthmatic response. SIC is considered to be a "reference standard" and is performed in only a few centers with specialised facilities and expertise. SIC may also be useful in confirming new workplace agents as a cause of sensitiser-induced asthma, and may confirm the diagnosis of sensitiser-induced occupational asthma when other testing has been non-conclusive, may make the diagnosis more quickly, or may identify the specific agent if the worker is exposed to more than one occupational asthma-causative agent.

The ERS has recently produced a consensus statement relating to SICs. They conclude that such testing "should only be carried out in hospitals where physicians and healthcare professionals have appropriate expertise. Tests should always include a control challenge, a gradual increase of exposure to the suspected agent, and close monitoring of the patient during the challenge and for at least 6 h afterwards. In expert centers, excessive reactions provoked by SIC are rare."

The consensus also makes the point that the sensitivity and specificity of SIC are high, but not easily quantified, as the method is usually used as the reference standard for the diagnosis of occupational asthma.

Workplace challenges

Workplace challenges are an alternative to SIC, and useful particularly when it is difficult to re- create workplace conditions in a laboratory setting, and/or the job task involves multiple exposures. It may be possible in these contexts to learn more about the physiological and symptom response to these exposures by carrying out a workplace challenge. These can either be supervised by a technician, or indeed carried out by the worker themselves.

It is ordinary to collect serial measures of FEV_1 (or PEF) during days with and without exposure, and to compare the response between periods of exposure and no exposure.

Newer Tests of Lung Function and Response to Inhaled Agents

The use of exhaled nitric oxide is described in both research and clinical studies of workers with possible occupational lung disorders, as a marker of eosinophilic airways inflammation. Additionally, sputum eosinophil levels are used by certain centers to quantify patients. Changes in both these parameters are also used to assess the workplace or SIC response to inhaled agents suspected of causing asthma. Sputum eosinophilia is of course particularly important in the diagnosis of eosinophilic bronchitis. Still in its experimental phase, various researchers are beginning to develop the evidence relating to the examination of exhaled breath condensate, and how the findings may assist in the diagnosis of occupational respiratory diseases.

Specific Testing Circumstances

Cross shift lung function changes; A pre- and post-work shift FEV_1 and FVC can be measured in the same individual to study any cross-shift changes resulting from occupational exposures, e.g. byssinosis and occupational asthma. However, it may not be sensitive enough to detect those cases where the reaction is delayed beyond the normal shift. Serial PEF measurements done during periods at work and away from work have been found useful in the investigation of occupational asthma.

sPEF Monitoring; this is now an established tool in the investigation of possible occupational asthma. Patients should be given instruction on the proper use of a portable PEF meter, and asked to record their PEF every two to three hours during the waking hours for at least three weeks. Each time a recording is taken, the best of three readings is taken as the value to record. The period of recording should include periods at work and away from work.

The results can be graphed and assessed. In particular, it is important to look for evidence of PEF improvement during the period the patient is away from work, and deterioration during the period at work. Deterioration is shown by the falling mean and the widening diurnal variation, as demonstrated in the serial PEF recording of Case Study 2, Fig. 2.

Serial PEF recordings also allow the diurnal variation to be calculated; a diurnal variation of 20% or more is supportive evidence of asthma. Diurnal variation can be calculated as the difference between the maximum and minimum PEF expressed as a percentage of the maximum for each day, although the mean or predicted values can also be used as the denominator.

As in Case Study 2, a software such as OASYS can be used to assist interpretation of sPEF, as this will also calculate the degree to which workplace exposure influence the PEF values (the so-called "work effect"). More information for the interested reader is found on the dedicated software website (OASYS, 2016).

In essence, a minimum of four PEF readings taken each day, for at least three week, on both work and rest days is required. These data are inputted into the software which then produces a high-quality graphic of the changes in PEF between periods of work and rest, and also produces a discriminant analysis of the recordings. A work effect score (amongst other metrics including an ABC score) is calculated, which assists the clinician to make, or exclude, a diagnosis of asthma and also occupational asthma. As with all tests used to assist making a diagnosis of occupational asthma, the findings must be interpreted in the overall context of the case; as no single test in isolation is diagnostic for this condition.

Lung function changes over time

As a guiding principle, more accurate spirometry assessment (that is minimising errors when measuring in an individual worker) will allow earlier detection of significant declines, in comparison to lung function programmes at work that are measuring lung function less accurately. Similarly, the longer the follow up period, the more certain a clinician can be that a given lung function decline is accelerated.

Conclusion

This chapter has discussed the major airway, parenchymal and pleural occupational respiratory disorders. Their natures are broad, and these can result from exposure to a diverse set of inhaled agents. Developing a high level of suspicion that your patient may have an occupational respiratory disease is key to identifying occupational links where they exist. Failure to consider this link during history taking may lead to missing the diagnosis of a potentially preventable condition that will have adverse consequences not only for the individual worker but also for other workers similarly exposed.

References

American Thoracic Society. (2005) *COPD*. [Online] Available from: https://www.thoracic.org/statements/copd.php. [Accessed on 30 May 2021].

Akira M. (2008). Imaging of occupational and environmental lung disease. *Clin Chest Med* **29**: 117–131.

Bailey RL, Cox-Ganser JM, Duling MG, LeBouf RF, Martin SB, Jr, Bledsoe TA, Green BJ, Kreiss K. (2015) Respiratory morbidity in a coffee processing workplace with sentinel obliterative bronchiolitis cases. *Am J Indust Med* **58**(12): 1235–1245.

Balmes J, Becklake M, Blanc P, Henneberger P, Kreiss K, Mapp C, Milton D, Schwartz D, Toren K, Viegi G, Environmental and Occupational Health Assembly, American Thoracic Society. (2003) American Thoracic Society Statement: Occupational contribution to the burden of airway disease. *Am J Respir Crit Care Med* **167**(5): 787–797.

Barber CM, Burge PS, Feary JR, Parfrey H, Renzoni EA, Spencer LG, Walters GI, Wiggans RE, GB HP Survey Participants. (2019) Identifying causation in hypersensitivity pneumonitis: A British perspective. *BMJ Open Respir Res* 6(1): e000469.

Barber CM, Fishwick D, Seed MJ, Carder M, van Tongeren M. (2018) Artificial stone-associated silicosis in the UK. *Occup Environ Med* **75**(7): 541.

Barnes H, Goh N, Leong T, Hoy R. (2019) Silica-associated lung disease: An old-world exposure in modern industries. *Respirology (Carlton, Vic.)* **12**(24): 1165–1175.

Blanc PD, Annesi-Maesano I, Balmes JR, Cummings KJ., Fishwick D, Miedinger D, Murgia N, Naidoo RN, Reynolds CJ, Sigsgaard T, Torén K, Vinnikov D, Redlich CA. (2019) The occupational burden of nonmalignant respiratory diseases. An Official American Thoracic Society and European Respiratory Society Statement. *Am J Respir Crit Care Med* **199**(11): 1312–1334.

Cavalcanti Z, Albuquerque Filho AP, Pereira CA, Coletta EN. (2012) Bronchiolitis associated with exposure to artificial butter flavoring in workers at a cookie factory in Brazil. *Jornal brasileiro de pneumologia: Publicacao oficial da Sociedade Brasileira de Pneumologia e Tisilogia* **38**(3): 395–399.

Centre for Occupational and Environmental Health. (2021) *Surveillance of Work-related and Occupational Respiratory Disease (SWORD)*. [Online] Available from: https://sites.manchester.ac.uk/thor/reports-and-publications/ [Accessed on 30 May 2021].

Coggon D, Palmer KT. (2016) Are welders more at risk of respiratory infections? *Thorax* **71**(7): 581–582.

De Matteis S, Consonni D, Bertazzi PA. (2008) Exposure to occupational carcinogens and lung cancer risk. Evolution of epidemiological estimates of attributable fraction. *Acta Biomed* **79**(1): 34.

De Matteis S, Jarvis D, Hutchings S, Darnton A, Fishwick D, Sadhra S, Rushton L, Cullinan P. (2016) Occupations associated with COPD risk in the large population-based UK Biobank cohort study. *Occup Environ Med* **73**(6): 378–384.

De Matteis S, Jarvis D, Darnton A, Hutchings S, Sadhra S, Fishwick D, Rushton L, Cullinan P. (2019) The occupations at increased risk of COPD: Analysis of lifetime job-histories in the population-based UK Biobank Cohort. *Eur Respir J* **54**(1): 1900186.

Driscoll T, Nelson DI, Steenland K, Leigh J, Concha-Barrientos M, Fingerhut M, Prüss-Ustün A. (2005a) The global burden of non-malignant respiratory disease due to occupational airborne exposures. *Am J Ind Med* **48**(6): 432–445.

Driscoll T, Nelson DI, Steenland K, Leigh J, Concha-Barrientos M, Fingerhut M, Prüss-Ustün A. (2005b) The global burden of disease due to occupational carcinogens. *Am J Ind Med* **48**(6): 419–431.

European Lung White Book. (2012) *Occupational Lung Diseases.* [Online] Available from: http://www.erswhitebook.org/chapters/occupational-lung-diseases/. [Accessed on 30 May 2021].

Finkelstein MM. (2000) Silica, silicosis, and lung cancer: A risk assessment. *Am J Ind Med* **38**(1): 8–18.

Fishwick D, Barber CM, Bradshaw LM, Ayres JG, Barraclough R, Burge S, Corne JM, Cullinan P, Frank TL, Hendrick D, Hoyle J, Curran AD, Niven R, Pickering T, Reid P, Robertson A, Stenton C, Warburton CJ, Nicholson PJ. (2012) Standards of care for occupational asthma: An update. *Thorax* **67**(3): 278–280.

Fishwick D. (2014) Work aggravated asthma; a review of the recent evidence. *Br Med Bull* **110**(1): 77–88.

Fishwick D, Sen D, Barber C, Bradshaw L, Robinson E, Sumner J, COPD Standard Collaboration Group. (2015) Occupational chronic obstructive pulmonary disease: A standard of care. *Occup Med (Oxford, England)* **65**(4): 270–282.

Global Burden of Disease Study. (2013) Global, regional, and national age–sex specific all-cause and cause-specific mortality for 240 causes of death, 1990–2013: A systematic analysis for the Global Burden of Disease Study 2013. *Lancet* **385**: 117–171.

Henneberger PK, Redlich CA, Callahan DB, Harber P, Lemière C, Martin J, Tarlo SM, Vandenplas O, Torén K, ATS Ad Hoc Committee on Work-Exacerbated Asthma. (2011) An official american thoracic society statement: work-exacerbated asthma. *Am J Respir Crit Care Med* **184**(3): 368–378.

Hnizdo E, Vallyathan V. (2003) Chronic obstructive pulmonary disease due to occupational exposure to silica dust: A review of epidemiological and pathological evidence. *Occup Environ Med* **60**(4): 237–243.

HSE. (2021) *Silicosis.* [Online] Available from: http://www.hse.gov.uk/lung-disease/silicosis.htm. [Accessed on 30 May 2021].

Hoy RF, Baird T, Hammerschlag G, Hart D, Johnson AR, King P, Putt M, Yates DH. (2018) Artificial stone-associated silicosis: A rapidly emerging occupational lung disease. *Occup Environ Med* **75**(1): 3–5.

Hubbs AF, Cumpston AM, Goldsmith WT, Battelli LA, Kashon ML, Jackson MC, Frazer DG, Fedan JS, Goravanahally MP, Castranova V, Kreiss K, Willard PA, Friend S, Schwegler-Berry D, Fluharty KL, Sriram K. (2012) Respiratory and olfactory cytotoxicity of inhaled 2,3-pentanedione in Sprague-Dawley rats. *Am J Pathol* **181**(3): 829–844.

Jaklitsch MT, Jacobson FL, Austin JH, Field JK, Jett JR, Keshavjee S, MacMahon H, Mulshine JL, Munden RF, Salgia R, Strauss GM, Swanson SJ, Travis WD, Sugarbaker DJ. (2012) The American Association for Thoracic Surgery guidelines for lung cancer screening using low-dose computed tomography scans for lung cancer survivors and other high-risk groups. *J Thorac Cardiovasc Surg* **144**(1): 33–38.

Kanwal R, Kullman G, Piacitelli C, Boylstein R, Sahakian N, Martin S, Fedan K, Kreiss K. (2006) Evaluation of flavorings-related lung disease risk at six microwave popcorn plants. *J Occup Environ Med* **48**(2): 149–157.

Karjalainen A, Kurppa K, Martikainen R, Klaukka T, Karjalainen J. (2001) Work is related to a substantial portion of adult-onset asthma incidence in the Finnish population. *Am J Respir Crit Care Med* **164**(4): 565–568.

Kramer MR, Blanc PD, Fireman E, Amital A, Guber A, Rhahman NA, Shitrit D. (2012) Artificial stone silicosis [corrected]: Disease resurgence among artificial stone workers. *Chest* **142**(2): 419–424.

Lin RT, Takahashi K, Karjalainen A, Hoshuyama T, Wilson D, Kameda T, Chan CC, Wen CP, Furuya S, Higashi T, Chien LC, Ohtaki M. (2007) Ecological association between asbestos-related diseases and historical asbestos consumption: An international analysis. *Lancet (Lond)* **369**(9564): 844–849.

Mannino DM, Buist AS. (2007) Global burden of COPD: Risk factors, prevalence, and future trends. *Lancet* **370**: 765–773.

Mapp CE, Boschetto P, Maestrelli P, Fabbri LM. (2005) Occupational asthma. *Am J Respir Crit Care Med* **172**: 280–305.

McCunney RJ. (2006) Should we screen for occupational lung cancer with low-dose computed tomography? *J Occupa Environ Med* **48**(12): 1328–1333.

Morgan DL, Jokinen MP, Johnson CL, Price HC, Gwinn WM, Bousquet RW, Flake GP. (2016) Chemical reactivity and respiratory toxicity of the α-diketone flavoring agents: 2,3-butanedione, 2,3-pentanedione, and 2,3-hexanedione. *Toxicol Pathol* **44**(5): 763–783.

Nickell LT, Jr, Lichtenberger JP, 3rd, Khorashadi L, Abbott GF, Carter BW. (2014) Multimodality imaging for characterization, classification, and staging of malignant pleural mesothelioma. *Radiographics* **34**(6): 1692–1706.

Nicholson PJ, Cullinan P, Taylor AJ, Burge PS, Boyle C. (2005) Evidence based guidelines for the prevention, identification, and management of occupational asthma. *Occup Environ Med* **62**(5): 290–299.

NIOSH. (2020) *Silica, Crystalline.* [Online] Available from: http://www.cdc.gov/niosh/topics/silica/. [Accessed on 30 May 2021].

NIOSH. (2014) Spirometry Longitudinal Data Analysis (SPIROLA) Software. [Online] Available from: http://www.cdc.gov/niosh/topics/spirometry/spirola-software.html. [Accessed on 30 May 2021].

OASYS. (2016) *Oasys and Occupational Asthma.* [Online] Available from: http://www.occupationalasthma.com/oasys.aspx. [Accessed on 30 May 2021].

Omland Ø, Würtz ET, Aasen TB, Blanc P, Brisman JB, Miller MR, Pedersen OF, Schlünssen V, Sigsgaard T, Ulrik CS, Viskum S. (2014) Occupational chronic obstructive pulmonary disease: A systematic literature review. *Scand J Work Environ Health* **40**(1): 19–35.

Pellegrino R, Viegi G, Brusasco V, Crapo RO, Burgos F, Casaburi R, Coates A, van der Grinten CP, Gustafsson P, Hankinson J, Jensen R, Johnson DC, MacIntyre N, McKay R, Miller MR, Navajas D, Pedersen OF, Wanger J. (2005) Interpretative strategies for lung function tests. *Eur Respir J* **26**(5): 948–968.

Quanjer PH, Stanojevic S, Cole TJ, Baur X, Hall GL, Culver B.H, Enright PL, Hankinson JL, Ip MS, Zheng J, Stocks J, ERS Global Lung Function Initiative. (2012) Multi-ethnic reference values for spirometry for the 3-95-yr age range: The global lung function 2012 equations. *Eur Respir J* **40**(6): 1324–1343.

Redlich CA, Tarlo SM, Hankinson JL, Townsend MC, Eschenbacher WL, Von Essen SG, Sigsgaard T, Weissman DN, American Thoracic Society Committee on Spirometry in the Occupational Setting. (2014) Official American Thoracic Society technical standards: Spirometry in the occupational setting. *Am J Respir Crit Care Med* **189**(8): 983–993.

Rosengarten D, Fox BD, Fireman E, Blanc PD, Rusanov V, Fruchter O, Raviv Y, Shtraichman O, Saute M, Kramer MR. (2017) Survival following lung transplantation for artificial stone silicosis relative to idiopathic pulmonary fibrosis. *Am J Ind Med* **60**(3): 248–254.

Salvi SS, Barnes PJ. (2009) Chronic obstructive pulmonary disease in non-smokers. *Lancet* **374**: 733–743.

Schuitemaker A, van Berckel BN, Kropholler MA, Veltman DJ, Scheltens P, Jonker C, Lammertsma AA, Boellaard R. (2007) SPM analysis of parametric (R)-[11C]PK11195 binding images: Plasma input versus reference tissue parametric methods. *NeuroImage* **35**(4): 1473–1479.

Sun J, Weng D, Jin C, Yan B, Xu G, Jin B, Xia S, Chen J. (2008) The value of high resolution computed tomography in the diagnostics of small opacities and complications of silicosis in mine machinery manufacturing workers, compared to radiography. *J Occup Health* **50**(5): 400–405.

Tarlo SM, Balmes J, Balkissoon R, Beach J, Beckett W, Bernstein D, Blanc PD, Brooks SM, Cowl CT, Daroowalla F, Harber P, Lemiere C, Liss GM, Pacheco KA, Redlich CA, Rowe B, Heitzer J. (2008) Diagnosis and management of work-related asthma: American College Of Chest Physicians Consensus Statement. *Chest* **134**(3 Suppl): 1S–41S.

Toren K, Blanc PD. (2009) Asthma caused by occupational exposures is common. *BMC Pulm Med* **9**: 7.

Torén K, Blanc PD, Naidoo RN, Murgia N, Qvarfordt I, Aspevall O, Dahlman-Hoglund A, Schioler L. (2020) Occupational exposure to dust and to fumes, work as a welder and invasive pneumococcal disease risk. *Occup Environ Med* 77(2): 57–63.

Townsend MC. (2011) Occupational and Environmental Lung Disorders Committee. Spirometry in the occupational health setting — 2011 update. *J Occup Environ Med* **53**: 569–584.

Tsim S, Cowell GW, Kidd A, Woodward R, Alexander L, Kelly C, Foster JE, Blyth KG. (2020) A comparison between MRI and CT in the assessment of primary tumour volume in mesothelioma. *Lung Cancer (Amsterdam, Netherlands)* **150**: 12–20.

Vandenplas O, Suojalehto H, Aasen TB, Baur X, Burge PS, de Blay F, Fishwick D, Hoyle J, Maestrelli P, Muñoz X, Moscato G, Sastre J, Sigsgaard T, Suuronen K, Walusiak-Skorupa J, Cullinan P, ERS Task Force on Specific Inhalation Challenges with Occupational Agents. (2014) Specific inhalation challenge in the diagnosis of occupational asthma: Consensus statement. *Eur Respir J* **43**(6): 1573–1587.

Weissman DN. (2015) Role of chest computed tomography in prevention of occupational respiratory disease: Review of recent literature. *Semin Respir Crit Care Med* **36**(3): 433–448.

Wiener RS, Gould MK, Arenberg D. A, Au DH, Fennig K, Lamb CR, Mazzone PJ, Midthun DE, Napoli M, Ost DE, Powell CA, Rivera MP, Slatore CG, Tanner NT, Vachani A, Wisnivesky JP, Yoon SH, ATS/ACCP Committee on Low-Dose CT Lung Cancer Screening in Clinical Practice. (2015) An official American Thoracic Society/American College of Chest Physicians policy statement: Implementation of low-dose computed tomography lung cancer screening programs in clinical practice. *Am J Respir Crit Care Med* **192**(7): 881–891.

Chapter 4

Skin Disorders

David Koh and Chee Leok Goh†*

Introduction

Occupational skin diseases (OSDs) are defined as any pathological condition of the skin for which job exposure can be shown to be a major direct or contributory factor. Although such disorders are rarely life threatening, they can cause much morbidity and suffering to the workers. OSD are a significant cause of decreased productivity and sickness absence in industry.

Skin Structure and Function

The skin is the largest organ in the body, constituting about 10% of the normal body weight. It comprises the epidermis, dermis, and a subcutaneous fat layer (Fig. 1). The outermost layer consists of a keratin layer and the stratum corneum which forms the skin barrier. The rest of the epidermis consists of layers of keratinocytes, scattered

* PAPRSB Institute of Health Sciences, Universiti Brunei Darussalam, Brunei Darussalam *and* Saw Swee Hock School of Public Health and Yong Loo Lin School of Medicine, National University of Singapore, Singapore.
† National Skin Centre, Singapore *and* Yong Loo Lin School of Medicine, National University of Singapore, Singapore.
Corresponding author: Goh Chee Leok (clgoh@nsc.com.sg).

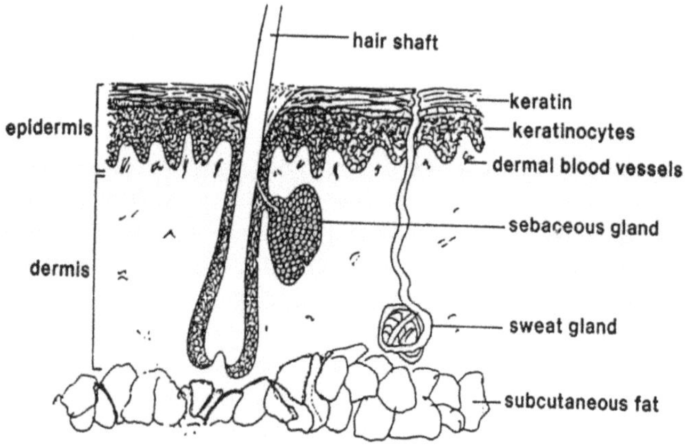

Fig. 1. Structure of the skin (Goh, 1990).

melanocytes along the basal layer and other cells, including immunocompetent cells such as the Langerhans cells. The dermis contains connective tissue consisting of collagen and elastic bundles. It contains blood vessels and lymphatics in which immunocompetent cells such as macrophages, mast cells and lymphocytes are transported to the dermis. Cutaneous appendages such as hair follicles, sebaceous glands, eccrine and apocrine sweat glands, hair, and erector pilorum muscle are found in the dermis. Nerves and tactile neuronal structures carry pain and tactile sensation from the skin to the central nervous system. Such tactile sensations serve as an important warning for skin injury and damage. Beneath the dermis is a layer of subcutaneous fat, which acts as a cushion between the epidermis/dermis and the internal body structures. Any layer and structure of the skin can be damaged and become diseased from environmental insults. Examples include contact dermatitis, skin cancers and skin infections.

The skin forms an important protective layer for the internal melieu of the body. Its high tensile strength and resilience provides defence against physical injury, especially shearing stress. The keratin layer and stratum corneum acts as a barrier against irritants and sensitisers, systemic poisons, and micro-organisms. The melanocytes secrete melanin which help to protect the skin against the damaging effects of ultraviolet light. The skin is also a responsible for thermoregulation of the body through sweating. Other functions of the skin include Vitamin D synthesis and immunoregulation. The keratinocytes possess a multitude of receptors, and secrete regulatory cytokines to modulate immune reactions. Environmental factors can cause immediate or delayed derangement of functions of these activities. Mutations of cellular tissue are also responsible for the manifestation of skin disorders.

Skin Barrier Functions

Skin barrier integrity plays an important role in contact dermatitis. As the body's skin surfaces are exposed to the environment, the skin's tough mechanical barrier serves as a first line of defence, sequestering the internal milieu from the harsh external environment. Keratinocytes are immunologically active cells. Traumatic barrier disruption alone, in the absence of signals from immune cells, stimulates both keratinocyte proliferation and cytokine production, which begin the process of wound repair and initiate skin inflammation.

The stratum corneum is a thin sheet of fully differentiated, enucleated corneocytes embedded in a lipid-rich matrix of sphingosine and ceramide. The stratum corneum has been referred to as the bricks of the barrier and the lipid matrix as the mortar. Any derangement in the brick or mortar due to genetic or environmental factors may initiate the process of skin inflammation (Fig. 2).

Workers with a background of atopic dermatitis (AD) are predisposed to injury by contact irritants. Atopic food handlers with repeated exposure to mild irritants, e.g. acetic acid had barrier disruption and significant trans-epidermal water loss (TEWL) increase; while no significant differences were found after the same exposure in healthy controls. Repeated exposure to sodium lauryl sulfate (SLS) and the irritant in tandem enhanced the reactions and resulted in a significantly higher increase in TEWL in the AD group compared to the control group. Cumulative irritant exposure reduced the natural moisturising factor (NMF) levels in both groups (Angelova-Fischer *et al.*, 2015).

The skin of AD patients is relatively deficient in ceramide and has a defective skin barrier. This lack of hydrophobic 'mortar' is associated

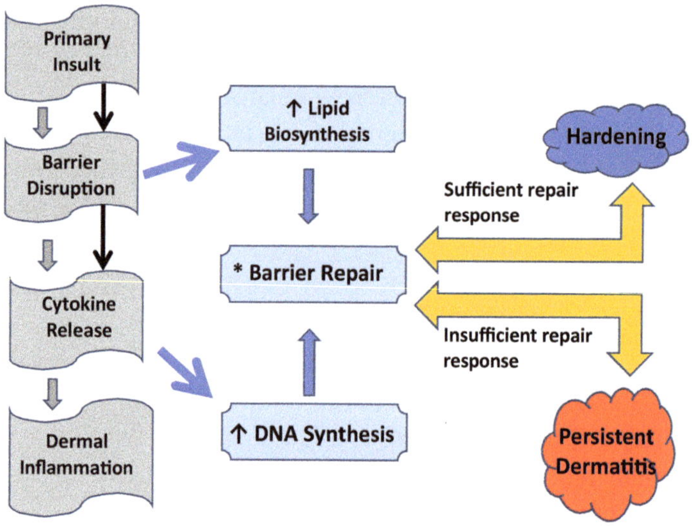

Fig. 2. Skin responses to irritation.

with increased TEWL which leads to xerosis and increased susceptibility to contact irritants penetration. Patients with AD have barrier function impairment even on non-eczematous looking skin. This defect is associated with enhanced aeroallergen sensitisation. Improving barrier function (e.g. by application of skin moisturisers such as ceramide-containing creams) can help to restore barrier function and prevent contact dermatitis. The understanding of these molecular derangements in the stratum corneum has important implications in the prevention and management of patients with contact dermatitis.

Many genes encode for protein products integral to the proper assembly of the layers of the skin. Identification of these genes helps determine risk factors for contact dermatitis. PPARα agonist has been reported to improve barrier function of filaggrin deficient skin models. This underlines the potential of PPAR agonists for the treatment of filaggrin-associated skin diseases (Wallmeyer *et al.*, 2015).

Atopics may also be particularly susceptible to sensory irritation induced by airborne chemicals compared to healthy individuals (van Kampen *et al.*, 2020).

Epidemiology of Occupational Skin Diseases

The reported incidence of OSD varies in different countries depending on their health care systems, legislation and reporting requirements. An estimate of the incidence in Europe is 0.7–1.5 cases per 1,000 per year, with higher rates in specific high risk occupational groups (Diepgen, 2003). The United Kingdom (UK) has The Health and Occupation Reporting (THOR) network, a voluntary surveillance scheme. The average annual incidence rates of work-related skin disease reported from 2002 to 2005 were different for dermatologists and occupational physicians (Turner *et al.*, 2007). For dermatologists, the incidence rate was 91.3 [95% confidence interval (CI) 81.8–101.1] per million, while among occupational physicians, the incidence rate was 316.6 (95% CI 251.8–381.3) per million. Most reports were of contact dermatitis.

In comparison, a voluntary surveillance scheme of OSD in the Netherlands, started in 2001 showed a decline in the number of notifications from 2001 to 2005. The highest number of notifications, recorded in the first year of the scheme, was probably due to reporting of a mixture of incident and prevalent cases. In the following years, the annual number of notifications declined. Hairdressers, nurses, metalworkers, mechanics and cleaners were the most commonly affected professions with wet work and irritants the most frequently reported causative agents. Most patients with occupational contact dermatitis were not absent from work (Pal *et al.*, 2009).

A more recent report from the Finnish Register of Occupational disease studying the risk occupations to contact dermatitis showed that the largest number of OSD cases included farmers, hairdressers, nurses, cooks, cleaners and machinists (Aalto-Korte *et al.*, 2020a). Epoxy compounds and acrylates were common causes of ACD (Aalto-Korte *et al.*, 2020b).

A report from Finland showed contact urticaria (CU) constituted 11% of all OSD studied between 2005 and 2016. Occupations with the highest incidence included bakers, chefs and cooks, farmers, veterinarians, gardeners and hairdressers. The most common causative agents were cow dander, flour and grain followed by rubber latex. (Pesonen *et al.*, 2020).

Under-reporting, under-recognition and misclassification of cases obscure the true magnitude of the problem. The true incidence has been estimated to be as much as 10–50 times higher than the reported figures. The reasons for the under-reported incidence include employees' fear of loss of job and limitation of future job prospects; and employer concerns over involvement in potential legal disputes and reimbursement. Other reasons include limited disability caused by the skin condition, which allows affected persons to continue working; and the multifactorial causes of OSD, which may complicate diagnosis.

It was estimated that 20–25% of all reported OSD resulted in time lost from work, averaging 10–12 lost work days per episode. A US report in 2004 on the Burden of Skin Disease Study indicated an economic impact of US$37 billion for 21 skin diseases (including costs of physician visits, hospitalisations, missed work, and medications). The estimate burden from contact dermatitis alone was 72.29 million episodes involving 9.2 million visits to clinics and 1.6 million visits to emergency rooms, costing about US$1.9 billion.

The impact of occupational skin disorders on Quality of Life has been studied increasingly (Rabin and Fraidlin, 2007; Nienhaus *et al.*, 2008; Lan *et al.*, 2008; Matterne *et al.*, 2009). In a study of over a thousand nurses in a university hospital, 22% of respondents reported occurrence of hand eczema. Occurrence of hand eczema was significantly associated with nursing for >10 years (27% prevalence) and working in a special care unit (29% prevalence). Hand eczema was associated with suboptimal life quality. Among such persons, pruritus or burning sensations were associated with a lower quality of life (Lan *et al.*, 2008).

Another major area of ignorance is that of risk factors for OSD. Although it is known that the work environment plays a major role in the development of OSD, genetic and other indirect factors (such as skin hygiene, age and work experience of workers and presence of coexisting skin disease) may also contribute to OSD development.

Some genes may be associated with an increased risk for OSD. In a study of 153 workers exposed to cement, sensitivity to chromate was significantly associated with TNF alpha promoter-308 heterozygous

(GA) as compared with GG genotype (OR 3.9, 95% CI 1.1–13.2) or GST-T1 null genotype (OR 5.5, 95% CI 1.4–36.2) (Wang *et al.*, 2007). In a case-control study, subjects who were intermediate or slow acetylators of NAT2 had a 2.01 fold (95% CI = 1.14–3.54) higher risk for hypersensitivity dermatitis induced by trichloroethylene (TCE) exposure compared to fast acetylators. When non-fast NAT2 phenotype (interme diate and slow acetylators) and a slow NAT1 phenotype were combined, the risk for the disease was significantly increased (OR = 2.71, 95% CI 1.29–5.70) to a level higher than that for NAT2 non-fast acetylators phenotype alone (Dai *et al.*, 2009).

Types of Occupational Skin Diseases

Occupational contact dermatitis is the most frequent OSD. It comprises irritant contact dermatitis (ICD), allergic contact dermatitis (ACD), CU and protein contact dermatitis. Contact dermatitis accounts for over 90% of all OSD cases seen at the secondary and tertiary levels of care. Other conditions such as CU, disorders of pigmentation, skin cancers and infections are much less commonly encountered.

In the USA, 310 workers' compensation independent medical examinations were evaluated for suspected work-related contact dermatitis. Hand dermatitis was the most common presentation (47.7%). Prevalent occupations included health care workers (16.5%), custodial staff (13.2%), and machinists (11.6%). ACD (47.5%) was more common than ICD (38.9%) among those diagnosed as having OSD. The highest-frequency work-related allergens were thiuram mix (23.9%), carba mix (22.7%), potassium dichromate (10.2%), and epoxy resin (10.2%). The authors reported that blue collar work and wet work were risk factors for the development of ACD and ICD (Coman *et al.*, 2015).

In Australia, a retrospective review of 2,894 patients seen at the Occupational Dermatology Clinic in Melbourne between 1993 and 2010, showed that 75% were diagnosed with OSD. The most common diagnosis in those with OSD was ICD (44%), followed by ACD (33%) and endogenous eczema (11%). Women were significantly more likely to have soaps and detergents ($P < 0.001$) and water/wet work ($P<0.001$) as causes of their ICD than men. Men were significantly more likely to have oils and coolants ($P<0.001$) and solvent exposures ($P<0.001$) as causes of their ICD. Occupational groups with the highest incidence of OSD were the hair and beauty professions (70 per 100,000), followed by machine and plant operators (38 per 100,000) and health-care workers (21 per 100,000) (Cahill *et al.*, 2015). A study on health care workers in Australia between 1993 and 2014 showed 81% were diagnosed to have OSD. ICD (79%) was the most common diagnosis followed by ACD (49%). Common allergens included natural rubber latex (13%) and rubber additives, preservatives. Common irritants included water/wet work and hand cleansers (Higgins *et al.*, 2016).

In Finland, 42% of 5,265 OSD between 2005 to 2016 had ICD, 35% ACD and 11% had CU. The incidence of OSD in the total labour force was 18.8 cases/100,000 person years. Resins and plastic related chemicals were the top allergens (Aalto-Korte *et al.*, 2020b).

In Singapore, ICD is the most common OSD seen among patients at its tertiary dermatological facility. This is followed by ACD. Table 1 shows irritants and allergens causing contact dermatitis among patients seen at the National Skin Centre in Singapore from 1984 to 2004. A recent report in 2020 from Singapore showed that ICD accounted for 55% of 264 patients with OSD vs. 43% with ACD and CU accounting for 1.5% with proportions of ICD and ACD almost identical what was previously seen (Kho *et al.*, 2020). The incidence of OSD has declined from 262.5 cases/year (1984–1985) to 26.4 cases per year (2009–2018), possibly due to the numerous preventive measures introduced over the years.

Dermatitis

Dermatitis is an inflammation of the skin with characteristic morphology but varied causes. Dermatitis is characterised by redness, swelling, small fluid filled blisters, and oozing in the acute state, and by scaly lichenified, thickened, fissuring with pigmentary changes in the chronic stage.

Table 1. Irritants and Allergens Causing Contact Dermatitis Among Patients Seen at the National Skin Centre, Singapore

Year	2009–2018	2003/2004	1989–1998	1984/1985
Irritants				
No. of cases	*N* = 146	*N* = 78	*N* = 591	*N* = 310
Wet work/detergents	58 (40%)	25 (32%)	133 (23%)	37 (12%)
Oil/grease	23 (16%)	22 (28%)	74 (13%)	27 (13%)
Solvents	14 (10%)	14 (18%)	133 (23%)	53 (17%)
Cement	5 (3%)	11 (14%)	NA	NA
Coolants/soluble oil	12 (8%)	7 (9%)	68 (12%)	62 (20%)
Food	NA	4 (5%)	NA	NA
Resins	NA	3 (4%)	NA	NA
Allergens				
No. of cases	*N* = 114	*N* = 47	*N* = 347	*N* = 215
Chromate	39 (34%)	28 (60%)	132 (38%)	106 (49%)
Rubber Chemicals	14 (12%)	7 (15%)	65 (19%)	35 (16%)
Cobalt	NA	6 (13%)	41 (12%)	28 (13%)
Resins	23 (20%)	6 (13%)	44 (13%)	13 (6%)
Nickel	8 (7%)	3 (6%)	46 (13%)	27 (13%)
Colophony	8 (7%)	2 (4%)	11 (3%)	3 (1%)
Food	5 (4%)	2 (4%)	33 (10%)	5 (2%)

Endogenous dermatitis such as atopic, seborrhoeic, varicose and discoid dermatitis, are genetically inherent skin disorders. They are not caused by environmental agents, although environmental factors can aggravate or precipitate flare ups among those with underlying endogenous dermatitis.

Contact dermatitis (Fig. 3) is skin inflammation caused by direct skin contact with an environmental contactant. Contact dermatitis can occur among persons without, or with pre-existing skin disorders, e.g. underlying endogenous eczema. Hence it is important to identify the various causative factors when managing patients with occupational contact dermatitis.

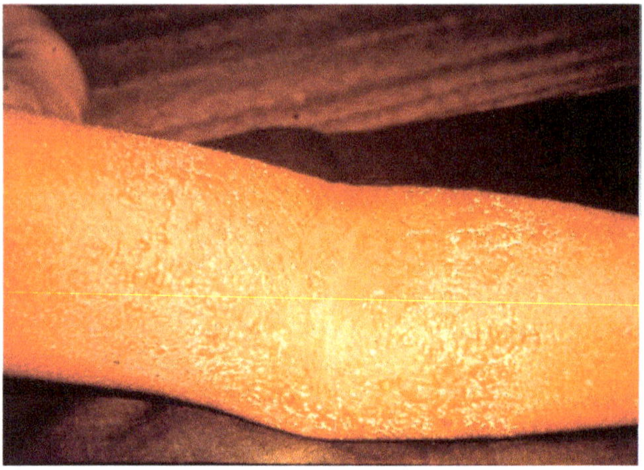

Fig. 3. Subacute contact dermatitis.

Contact dermatitis caused by airborne particles, also known as airborne contact dermatitis, usually presents with more intense dermatitis on exposed parts as compared to covered parts of body. Photosensitive chemicals may manifest as exposed part dermatitis. Some contact allergens may sometimes cause non-eczematous skin lesions such as erythema multiforme like eruptions.

Irritant contact dermatitis

Irritants are substances which directly damage the skin and can lead to skin inflammation termed ICD. Interaction between an irritant and the skin depends on several factors. These include the properties and nature of the irritant, specific individual factors, and environment-related variables.

The pathological mechanisms in skin irritation involve skin barrier disruption, induction of a cytokine cascade and involvement of the oxidative stress network. This results in a subclinical, then visible inflammatory reaction. There are several non-invasive parameters for the evaluation of skin irritation and irritant potential of compounds and their specific formulations. Among these are epidermal barrier function (e.g. TEWL measurement), skin hydration (e.g. corneometer measurement), surface pH, lipid composition, skin colour and skin blood flow (Fluhr *et al.*, 2008).

ICD is more common than ACD and can present as acute, chronic and cumulative irritant dermatitis, delayed acute irritant dermatitis, irritant reaction, pustular irritant dermatitis, suberythematous irritation, sensory irritation, friction dermatitis and airborne dermatitis. Hand dermatitis is the most frequent manifestation of occupational ICD (Chew and Maibach, 2003; Quah *et al.*, 2012).

In some instances, ICD resolves despite continued exposure. This process is known as "hardening," and this mechanism allows such patients to continue working. Those unable to develop hardening may progress to a chronic ICD (Watkins and Maibach, 2009).

Acute irritant dermatitis

Strong irritants, for example, concentrated acids, alkalis or solvents cause an acute ICD following a single exposure or repeated exposures. The skin barrier and underlying cellular structures are damaged directly by the caustic irritant. The cause of acute ICD is often obvious.

Strong irritants cause ICD in almost all individuals. In contrast, weak irritants such as water and mild detergents tend to cause ICD in susceptible individuals (e.g. individuals with history of AD or endogenous hand eczema) often only after repeated skin contact. In a study from Singapore 35% of patients with OSD had atopy whereas the prevalence in the general population is about 13%. In Australia 45% of those with OSD were considered atopic.

In the workplace, acute ICD often occurs from accidents or as a result of workers' poor work habits, or from careless handling of caustic irritants. It can also result from a failure to recognise the hazards of corrosive work materials. Acute irritant dermatitis can very often be prevented and affected workers need not require a job change. Health education is very important as a preventive measure. Where practicable, the use of impervious gloves, aprons and boots during work can prevent acute ICD.

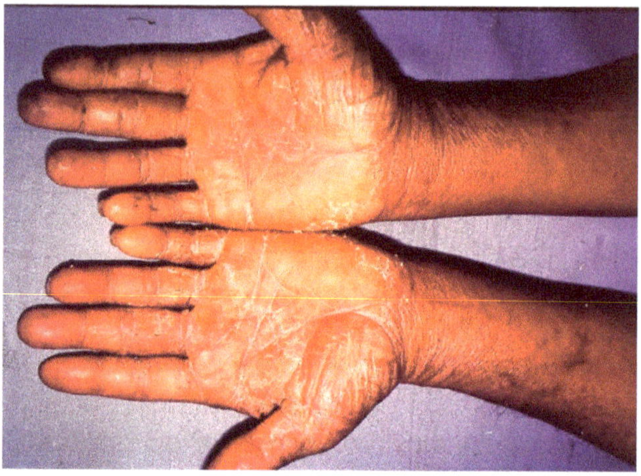

Fig. 4. Cumulative insult dermatitis.

Cumulative insult irritant contact dermatitis

This type of ICD is caused by repeated skin contact with weak irritants. Weak irritants cause ICD in susceptible individuals only. The duration from first exposure to the irritant and the appearance of dermatitis varies from weeks to years, depending on the nature of the irritant, frequency of contact, and host susceptibility. The clinical presentation is usually a chronic dermatitis (Fig. 4).

Cumulative insult dermatitis is exemplified by the chronic hand dermatitis caused by water and detergents among dishwashers and housewives, and by cutting fluid dermatitis among metalworkers. Solvents such as thinners and kerosene, when used inappropriately as skin cleansers, often cause cumulative insult dermatitis. Repetitive exposure to hand hygiene products and procedures is a significant factor in the development of occupational irritant hand dermatitis in healthcare workers.

Case Study 1: Irritant Contact Dermatitis

Five out of 15 newly employed persons in metalworking factory complained of itchy rashes over the hands and forearms within two months of starting work. All five workers had a history of atopy, and examination of the skin showed that the five had a contact dermatitis of the dorsum of the hands and distal half of the forearms. Patch testing of the workers with the standard series of allergens and the metalworking fluid battery was negative. The provisional diagnosis was an ICD to metalworking fluid, and symptomatic treatment was initiated.

A workplace inspection showed that the hands and forearms of the workers were heavily contaminated with the machine cutting oils in the course of their work. The use of gloves was not feasible because of the risk of accidental entrapment by the moving parts of the machine and injury.

The workers were shown how to improve their work habits and how to minimise contact with the cutting oils by their supervisors. Advice was also given to improve personal hygiene, to avoid other irritants in domestic and other non-work situations, and to use after work emollient cream. The condition of four of the workers improved, and they could continue with their work. The fifth worker, who had hand eczema previously, continued to have problems and left the job.

Allergic contact dermatitis (ACD)

ACD is an immunologic inflammatory reaction of the skin due to contact with an allergen. In contrast to ICD, the inflammatory reaction is mediated through an immunological process. An individual does not develop any reaction to the allergen during initial exposure to the allergen. Often repeat contacts are necessary before an individual becomes sensitised to an allergen. The expression "I have been in contact with the substance for many months and never had any rash with it previously and therefore the substance cannot be the cause of my rash" is a misconception.

Different substances have different sensitising potential. Individual susceptibility to sensitisation by an allergen also varies. Once an individual becomes sensitised to an allergen, further contact with the allergen will trigger a type IV hypersensitivity reaction, during which mediators are released from immunocompetent cells, leading to the manifestation of dermatitis. The dermatitis usually appears 36–48 hours after contact with the allergen. The dermatitis may be acute, subacute or chronic depending on the sensitivity of the worker.

Allergy to a substance is usually specific (although there may be cross reactivity), and once developed, is usually life-long.

Every year, new chemicals with sensitising potential are introduced into industry. Between 2008 and 2015, 172 such compounds were reported in the Contact Dermatitis and Dermatitis Journal; 119 of which induced ACD. About one third of the new allergens were ingredients of cosmetics, followed by drugs causing occupational ACD (18%), chemicals in rubber, plastics, and paints (9%), drugs causing a drug eruption (9%), as well as chemicals used in laboratories inducing occupational ACD (8%). It is important that physicians keep themselves updated on new allergens so that their patients can be patch tested to them where indicated (De Groot, 2015).

As an example, there was an outbreak of occupational and non-occupational of contact allergy to isothiazolinone, a preservative found in cosmetics and industrial products in Europe and around the world, despite initial legislative control in Europe when it was first introduced. Reported allergic contact reactions are primarily eczematous, most commonly in women from use of cosmetics and toiletries, e.g. wet wipes. Occupational exposure occurred during workplace use of healthcare hygiene (e.g. handrubs) and beauty products (used by hairdressers, beauticians) and water-based paints and other aqueous solutions such as cutting fluids. Legislation to improve labelling of industrial materials and reducing its concentration and use has helped to reduce the incidence of ACD.

Case Study 2: Allergic Contact Dermatitis

About 5% of female electronics workers involved in microcomputer assembly work complained of rashes of their wrists. The workers were required to wear an anti-static 'earthing' wrist strap while at work (Fig. 5).

All the affected workers gave a history of allergy to costume jewellery, and had dermatitis of varying severity at the site of contact with the wrist strap. The metal stud of the wrist strap was examined, and a dimethylglyoxime test demonstrated the presence of nickel. The provisional diagnosis was that of ACD to nickel. The problem was resolved by changing the wrist strap to another type that did not contain nickel.

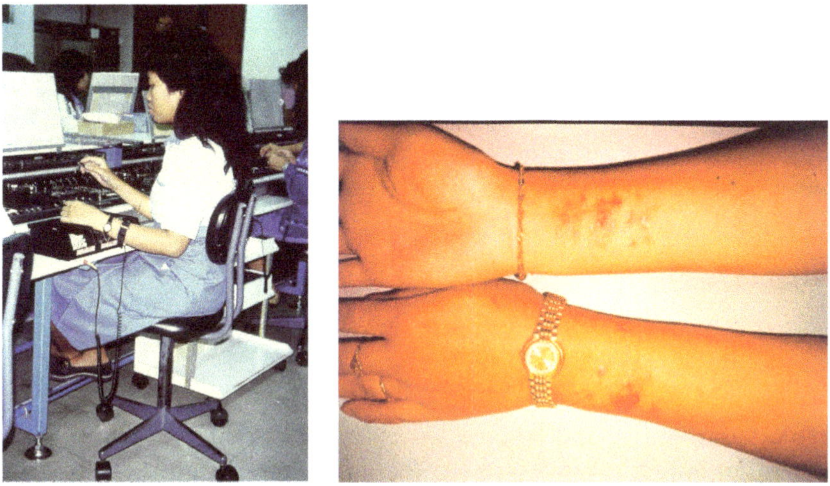

Fig. 5. Worker in an electronics company wearing an "earthing" wrist strap and ACD due to nickel in wrist strap.

Unlike a worker with ICD, a worker who develops ACD to a work substance may require a job change. Hence, it is important to differentiate ICD from ACD. Once an allergen has been identified as the cause of occupational dermatitis, it is necessary to inform the worker of the sources of the allergen and advise the patient to avoid contact with these substances permanently. One should also be aware that "automated processes" require maintenance. Workers performing maintenance of such processes are exposed to chemicals used in the automated machines and may also develop contact allergy to the chemicals.

Patch testing

Patch testing (Fig. 6) is the definitive test for ACD, which allows identification of the allergen responsible for the ACD. The patch test procedure consists of applying a set of suspected allergens under occlusion on the skin of the upper back for 48 hours simulating a miniature ACD. The reaction to the test allergens is scored after the allergens are removed at 48 hours. A second scoring is made at 96 hours. Patch testing results must be read by an experienced dermatologist to

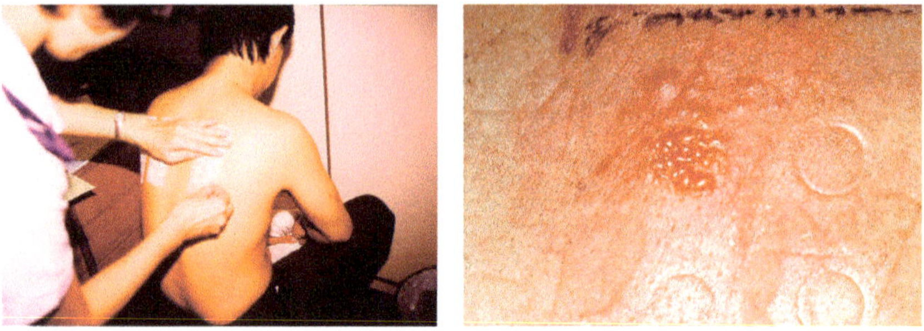

Fig. 6. Patch test being conducted and positive patch test result.

avoid false positive and false negative tests. For example, a false positive reaction may result if an irritant concentration of the test allergen is applied on the skin under occlusion and a false negative patch test recording may result if the concentration of the test allergen is too low to provoke a positive reaction. Patch testing should be carried out in a standardised procedure with appropriate patch test chambers and proper patch test allergen in the correct concentration. Interpretation of the patch test result is based generally on the International Contact Dermatitis Research Group recommended guidelines. The relevance of a positive patch test should be considered after reading the patch test reaction.

Other Types of Environmentally Induced Skin Disorders

Phototoxic and Photoallergic Contact Dermatitis

A phototoxic substance is a substance which becomes toxic when exposed to light and causes a sunburn-like-skin inflammation. Phototoxic substances absorb ultraviolet light, and the absorbed energy produces molecular changes that cause skin inflammation. It is not an immunologically mediated reaction. Examples of phototoxic substances include medicaments (e.g. phenothiazines, and tetracyclines), industrial chemicals (e.g. tars) and plant resins. The reaction is dose related. Phototoxic substances tend to cause reactions in almost all individuals.

Photoallergic contact dermatitis, like ACD, is mediated through an immunological mechanism. The allergen becomes activated only in the presence of ultraviolet light. There is individual susceptibility to photoallergy. Examples of photoallergens include medicaments, fragrances, sunscreens and antiseptics. Photoallergic contact dermatitis can be confirmed by a photopatch test.

Phototoxic and photoallergic contact dermatitis have a characteristic clinical presentation where only the sun exposed parts of the body such as the face, back of neck, the V of the anterior neck/chest and lateral forearms and dorsum of the hands are affected. The shaded areas including the area under the chin, eyelids, back of the ear and covered parts of the body are not affected.

Contact Urticaria

CU is an immediate wheal and flare reaction of the skin caused by contact with an urticant. Unlike contact dermatitis, which tends to develop several days after skin contact, CU develops very soon after skin contact with the urticant. The clinical presentation is usually immediate urticarial eruption (within 30 minutes of contact) manifesting as pruritic, raised skin wheals. It has been reported in 11% of OSD in Finland.

Another form of CU is protein contact dermatitis (PCD), which presents as chronic hand eczema. The characteristic of PCD is chronic eczematous dermatitis, possibly exacerbated by work with immediate erythema and pruritis upon exposure to the causative agent. PCD can be caused by contact with certain plants, latex, hydrolysed proteins or animal proteins (Barbaud *et al.*, 2015). Prick tests with the suspected protein-containing material are essential, as patch tests have negative results. A history of atopy is present in 56–68% of the patients. Food handlers are an occupational group at risk.

CU is not uncommon. Occupational contact urticaria (OCU) is an OSD that can cause serious health consequences and disability at work. In a report of 251 cases of OCU from France between 2001 and 2010, half were due to natural rubber latex, in particular in the health and social work activity sector (HSW). The number of these cases declined significantly over the study period (19% per year), and particularly after 2006. The other causes of OCU did not decrease. There was a significant decline in OCU due to natural rubber latex, particularly in HSW, after powdered latex gloves were banned from French hospitals (Bensefa-Colas *et al.*, 2015).

CU may be immunologically mediated (type I hypersensitivity reaction, usually IgE mediated) or non-immunologically mediated. Non-immunologically mediated CU is often due to a localised release of histamines and cytokines by mast cells following a local stimulus. The latter reaction is usually localised and not life-threatening, unlike immunologically mediated CU which can be generalised and life-threatening. Hence, there is a need to differentiate immunologically mediated from non-immunologically mediated CU. Immunologically-mediated CU can be confirmed by a skin prick test (Fig. 7) or by the detection of circulating antibodies.

The diagnosis of CU should include a relevant and physical examination combined with a relevant specific skin tests, and specific IgE determinations (e.g. the radioallergosorbent test (RAST) where available. Occasionally a provocation test may be carried out under medical supervision. A recent update of the various diagnostic test for IgE mediated

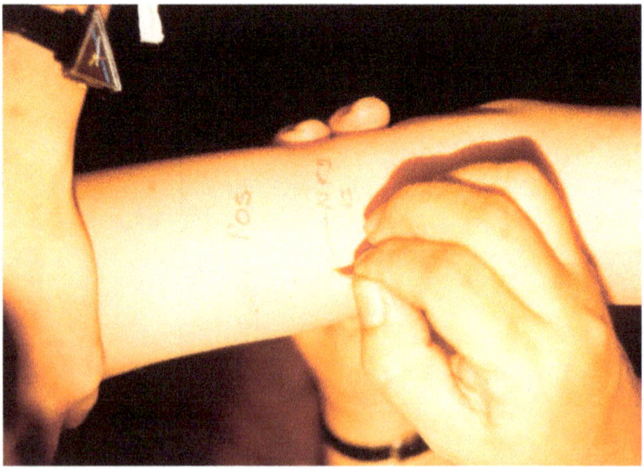

Fig. 7. Skin prick testing.

allergy provides useful guidelines on the selection of the appropriate tests (Ansotequi *et al.*, 2020).

Causes of CU include foodstuff (e.g. meats, eggs, seafood, vegetables), animal dander and secretions (e.g. from caterpillars and other arthropods), plants and spices (e.g. seaweed, thyme and cayenne pepper), fragrances and flavourings such as Balsam of Peru and cinnamon oil, several types of medicaments (e.g. some antibiotics), metals (e.g. cobalt), some preservatives (e.g. formaldehyde and benzoic acids), and rubber latex (e.g. gloves).

In Finland, of 2,759 workers with allergic contact reactions, 29.5% were due to CU (Kanerva *et al.*, 1996). It was much more common in women (70%) than in men (30%). The most common causes were cow dander (44.4%), natural rubber latex (23.7%), flour/grains (11.3%) and proteinaceous foodstuff. The occupations with the highest numbers of occupational CU were farmers, domestic animal attendants, bakers, nurses, chefs and dental assistants.

Contact urticaria to natural rubber latex proteins

Hand eczema and atopy are the main risk factors for NRL allergy. Therefore, skin prick testing (SPT) with NRL allergen is recommended in all suspected to have CU to NRL. Prohevein (20 kD) and hevein (4.7 kD) have been verified to be the major NRL allergens in sensitised persons. Patients allergic to NRL may be crossed sensitised to birch, alder, hazel and oak pollens, hazel nut, almond, apple, pear, peach, kiwi fruit, plum, potato, tomato, paprika, carrot, celery, parsnip and several spices.

In the health care environment, NRL proteins are probably the most important agents which cause CU. A study of rubber gloves used in among health care workers (HCWs) indicated that NRL proteins which can cause CU are higher in powdered (as compared to non-powdered) gloves, and in non-sterile examination gloves (as compared to sterile surgical gloves) (Koh *et al.*, 2005). As frequent glove users, healthcare workers are more likely to experience glove-related hand urticaria (Hawkey and Ghaffar, 2016).

The prevalence of NRL sensitisation among HCWs ranges from 3% to 17% (Ahmed *et al.*, 2004, Tang *et al.*, 2005). Among sensitised persons, contact with NRL can cause itch, eczematous hand rash, urticaria, rhinitis, asthma, or even anaphylaxis. There may be concurrent food allergy to bananas, avocados and kiwi fruit. Skin prick testing (SPT), using a commercial extract of NRL, can be performed to confirm the diagnosis. Blood tests can also be done for latex specific IgE antibody detection.

There is a need to increase the awareness of this condition among HCWs. Management of this condition includes health education and screening of workers with suspicious symptoms. Sensitised persons should be provided with latex free alternatives at work, such as vinyl gloves. Measures should also be taken to minimise other sources of latex exposure. The prevalence of CU to NRL has declined over the years due to better education and preventive measures introduced.

Whilst CU to latex is commonly suspected when immediate and local urticarial reactions develop, it is also important to consider other forms of glove-related hand urticaria. Rubber gloves have been reported to cause irritant contact reactions manifesting as symptomatic dermographism. This is thought to be caused by a combination of shearing forces associated with recurrent application and removal of gloves, as well as physical pressure exerted by the glove itself.

Case Study 3: Contact Urticaria

A restaurant chef complained of itch and rash over the fingers and hands whenever he prepared raw seafood. He noticed that the symptoms started within 15 minutes of handling the materials. On examination, there was a mild dermatitis of the hands. Patch testing with the standard series of allergens, the rubber gloves he used, and the food handlers series did not produce any positive reactions. Prick testing was performed, using the materials that he believed were responsible for the symptoms. A strong wheal and flare reaction was noted for squid and shellfish. The diagnosis was contact urticaria. The chef was advised to avoid handling these contact urticants as far as possible, and to use gloves while at work. This resulted in a reduction of his skin symptoms.

OSD due to Personal Protective Equipment for Infection Control

The use of PPE (which includes a mask, cap, goggles, face shield, gloves, gown and boots) and enhancement of hand hygiene practice have become a norm for many workers during the coronavirus disease 2019 (COVID-19) pandemic. Adverse reactions from prolonged PPE can and do occur. Such reactions to PPE should be identified early, treated immediately and preventive measures introduced, or it may affect PPE use compliance, staff morale and staff productivity. It may impair staff quality of life and expose at risk workers to microbial infections.

Adverse Skin Reactions from Masks and Goggles

Prolonged use of tightly fitting masks and goggles may result in facial bruising and abrasions (Dugdale and Walensky 2020). During the 2003 SARS outbreak in Singapore, 35.5% of staff using N95 masks regularly for an average duration of eight hours/day (mean period: 8.4 months) reported adverse skin reactions, including acne (59.6%), facial itch (51.4%) and rashes (35.8%) (Foo *et al.*, 2006). In comparison, 97% of frontline HCWs in China reported PPE-related skin reactions during the COVID-19 pandemic. Those who wore medical devices (N95 mask and goggles) longer than six hours had higher risk of skin damage than those who did for a shorter duration. Wearing a face shield for a longer duration (>6 hours) was not a significant risk factor in causing forehead skin damage (Lan *et al.*, 2020, Lin *et al.*, 2020).

Cutaneous adverse reactions to masks include the following:

- **Acne:** Existing acne and new acne lesions may appear due to pilosebaceous ductal occlusion from repetitive occlusions and friction.
- **Skin indentations and Pressure injuries (PIs):** Tight mask and goggles exert constant pressure to the same sites continually causing indentations and erythema which may progress to blisters, erosions and ulcers. The nasal bridge and cheeks are common sites of pressure.

Prevention include measures to relieve pressure by minimising the duration of pressure. HCWs should take frequent breaks of about 10–15 minutes during work and liberal use of moisturiser when off duty may help to restore and maintain skin barrier integrity.

- **Contact and Delayed Pressure Urticaria:** This may occur in tight fitting masks and goggle especially in those with dermographism. They can be treated or prevented with oral non-sedative antihistamines.
- **Cheilitis:** This is attributed to frequent licking of lips due to dehydration and limited fluid intake. Regular application of vaseline lip balm and regular hydration is recommended.
- **Other skin reactions:** ACD due to PPE components including rubber chemicals (elastic bands) and metals (metal clips and wires) and textile resins, dyes or chemicals have been reported. Patch tests may be needed to confirm the diagnosis and appropriate treatments instituted.

Skin Reactions Related to Hand Hygiene and Gloves

Hand hygiene is advocated in the prevention of infection transmission. Overzealous hand-hygiene without regular hand protection and skin barrier repair often results in contact dermatitis. During hand washing, the skin is exposed to friction, rubbing, water, surfactants and defatting chemicals which damage the skin barrier. Atopics are more susceptible to such irritant processes. 84.6% of HCWs reported the hands as the most common site affected in terms of PPE-related dermatoses. The majority washed their hands more than 10 times/day, but only 22.1% applied emollients after washing (Lin *et al.*, 2020).

Alcohol-based hand rubs (ABHRs) (>60% ethanol or 70% isopropanol) are recommended over soap and water unless there is visible soilage. ABHRs have been shown to inactivate the virus, are more convenient and improves compliance to hand hygiene amongst HCWs (Kratzel *et al.*, 2020). They are reported to cause less skin damage than hand washing (Traore *et al.*, 2007) Hand hygiene practices must be complemented with regular use of moisturisers to repair, restore and maintain skin barrier functions. However, the possibility of ACD from ingredients of skin moisturisers should be recognised. Common allergens include tocopherol, fragrance, preservatives, propylene glycol, benzoates and cetyl stearyl alcohol.

Glove-related skin reactions

ICD is the most common skin reaction to gloves amongst HCWs. Prolonged occlusion and hyperhydration may lead to skin maceration damaging the skin barrier. ACD to rubber chemicals and CU to natural rubber latex when they appear should be confirmed with the patch tests and skin prick test/RAST test respectively, treated and the allergens avoided permanently. Contact allergy to rubber additives in medical gloves is the most common cause of occupational allergic hand dermatitis in HCWs. Free formaldehyde and formaldehyde textile resins in disposable gowns and masks may cause ACD.

Other Types of Occupational Skin Diseases

Other environmental agents, including physical agents (e.g. ionising radiation, mechanical factors, ultraviolet light, heat, and cold) can damage the skin. Some chemicals are absorbed percutaneously and can cause systemic toxicity (e.g. dioxins causing chloracne). Oils and greases can cause oil acne. Phenolic compounds such as para-tertiary butyl-phenol formaldehyde resins may cause skin depigmentation.

Table 2 summarises the causes of non-eczematous presentations of OSD. Non-eczematous presentations of OSD are uncommon, accounting for <10% of all OSD.

Other examples include grain mite infestation (Fig. 8), leukoderma from exposure to chemicals (Fig. 9), and skin ulceration from metals such as chrome (Fig. 10).

Table 2. Examples of Non-Eczematous Occupational Skin Diseases

Category	Examples
Non-eczematous occupational skin diseases caused by physical agents	
Mechanical injury	Frictional callosity, abrasions/ lacerations
Localised vibration	Raynaud's phenomenon
Temperature	Miliaria from heat, frostbite from cold
Ultraviolet light	Photodermatitis, actinic damage
Ionising radiation	Radiation burns, skin cancers
Skin infections and infestations	
Viral	Herpetic Whitlow
Bacterial	Pyoderma, pitted keratolysis
Fungal	Superficial and deep mycoses
Parasitic	Larva migrans, mite infestations
Other skin disorders	
Acne and folliculitis	Caused by oil and grease, aggravated by heat
Skin ulceration	Caused by chromic and other acids
Hyperpigmentation	Post-inflammatory, such as those caused by tar and pitch
Hypopigmentation	Caused by phenolic compounds
Lichen planus like eruptions	Caused by paraphenylenediamine dyes
Scleroderma	Caused by exposure to silica or vinyl chloride monomer
Acquired porphyria cutanea tarda	Caused by hexachlorobenzene
Skin cancers	Caused by UV radiation, polycyclic aromatic hydrocarbons, arsenic

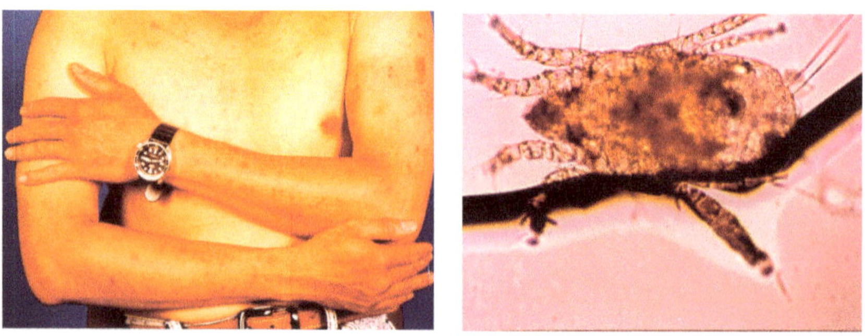

Fig. 8. Grain mite infestation in a chef. The mite was identified as *Pyemotes ventricosus*.

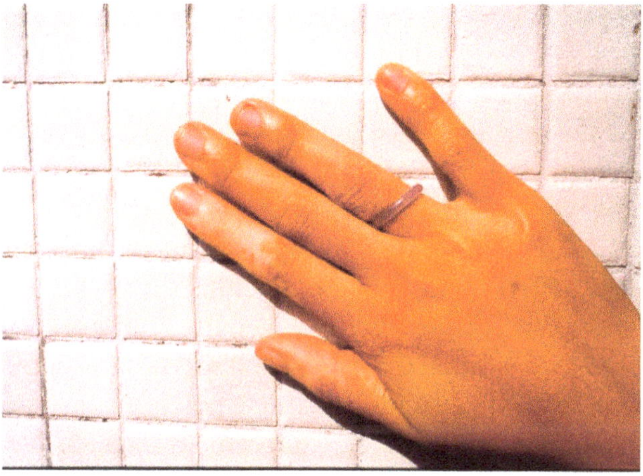

Fig. 9. Leukoderma in an electronics worker. The worker previously used a rubber finger cot (which contained an antioxidant) that caused the leukoderma.

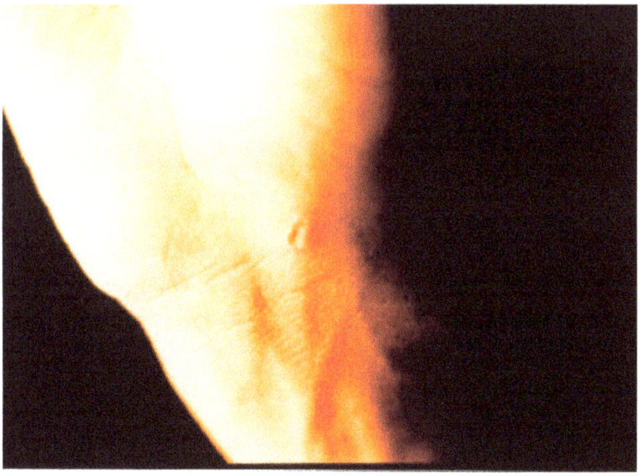

Fig. 10. Chrome ulcer at the base of the thenar eminence in an electroplater.

Skin Cancers

Skin cancers from environmental carcinogens (such as ultraviolet light, polycyclic aromatic hydrocarbons, and arsenic) are often induced after many years following exposure. They are uncommon in developed countries at present.

Outdoor work is a well-recognised risk factor for skin cancer especially in fair skinned individuals. In a study of data from a population based cancer registry in Bavaria, outdoor workers were found to have a higher risk for basal cell carcinoma (BCC) males [(RR, 2.9; 95% CI, 2.2–3.9) and females (RR, 2.7; 95% CI, 1.8–4.1)] as well as squamous cell carcinoma (SCC) [males (RR, 2.5; 95% CI, 1.4–4.7) and females (RR, 3.6; 95% CI, 1.6–8.1)] but not for cutaneous malignant melanoma (CMM). (Radespiel-Tröger *et al.*, 2009).

In some countries such as in Singapore, statutory regulations require designated workplace doctors to undertake medical examinations of the skin to screen for skin cancers in workers exposed to skin carcinogens such as arsenic, tar, pitch, bitumen and creosote.

Industries and Occupations at Risk

Workers in some occupations are at higher risk of developing OSD than others. Table 3 lists some industries with risks of OSD and some of the commonly encountered occupational irritants and allergens.

Table 3. Common Irritants and Allergens in Selected Industries

Category	Examples
Agriculture and horticulture	
Allergens	Plants, gloves (rubber, chromates), animal feeds (antibiotics, preservative, vegetables), antibiotics, pesticides, disinfectants, wood and its preservatives
Irritants	Animal feeds, fertilisers, solvents, plants, oils, disinfectants, pesticides
Chemical and pharmaceutical Industries	
Allergens	All chemicals and medicaments, gloves and masks (rubber chemicals)
Irritants	Chemicals, acids, alkalis, solvents, water, detergents, surfactants
Construction and building	
Allergens	Cement (chromates, cobalt), rubber gloves/boots, leather gloves/boots chromates, para-tertiary-butylphenol-formaldehyde (PTBPF) resins, epoxy resins, woods, paints
Irritants	Cement (alkalis), wood dust, wood preservatives, fibreglass, solvents, oils, pitch, tar, paints

Table 3. (*Continued*)

Category	Examples
Electronics and electrical industries	
Allergens	Resins (e.g. epoxy, acrylates, isocyanates, formaldehyde resins), soldering fluxes (amines and colophony), metals (nickel, chromates, and cobalt), gloves/cots
Irritants	Solvents, soldering fluxes, acids, alkalis, resins, fibreglass, metallic salts
Electroplating	
Allergens	Metals and their salts, gloves, boots, aprons
Irritants	Acids and alkalis (metal cleaners, pickling and plating solutions), chromic acid fumes, cleansers
Metal and engineering industries	
Allergens	Cutting fluids (metals, biocides, antioxidants, fragrances, resins), barrier creams, gloves
Irritants	Cutting fluids, solvents, abrasives, metal slivers, grease, oils, hand cleansers
Food and catering	
Allergens	Foods (vegetables, seafood, salad dressings, meat, fruits, flavouring agents), gloves, antioxidants, preservatives, utensils (nickel)
Irritants	Vegetables and fruit juices (enzymes, acids, alkalis), water and detergents, polishing agents
Hairdressing	
Allergens	Nickel, formaldehyde, hair dyes, fragrances and preservatives, gloves
Irritants	Shampoos, permanent wave solutions, water
Healthcare	
Allergens	Gloves, medicaments, antiseptics, disinfectants, metals, formaldehyde, preservatives, resins
Irritants	Water, soaps, detergents, solvents, resins, disinfectants, antiseptics, medicaments
Transport and shipbuilding	
Allergens	Cutting fluids and oils, gloves/boots, welding fumes, resins, metals, barrier creams, woods
Irritants	Cutting fluids, oils, grease, solvents, resins, metals, hand cleansers, fibreglass
Woodworking and furniture making	
Allergens	Woods, plants, gloves, resins, formaldehyde, wood preservatives, turpentine
Irritants	Wood dust, resins, soaps and detergents solvents, oils, turpentine, lacquer, polishes

Management of Occupational Skin Diseases

Diagnosis

The diagnosis of an OSD requires not only a good knowledge of dermatology, but also a working knowledge of the patient's work process, materials, practice and habits. The clinical appearance of an OSD (for example, dermatitis, acne, skin cancer) is exactly the same as a non-occupational related skin disorder. The danger of overlooking an OSD is that the patient's skin problem will likely recur when he returns to work. The failure to identify and avoid the causative agent of OSD at a workplace may also result in failure to recognise similar skin problems in other workers.

It is essential that an occupational history be obtained during any dermatological consultation. OSD should always be suspected when a worker presents with hand dermatitis and dermatitis on other exposed parts, as this is the most common presentation of an OSD. It is often necessary to enquire about the worker's job tasks, and details of the patient's work exposure and contact with various work chemicals should be elicited. A simple way to go about doing this is to ask the worker to describe his daily work activities. Important elements to look out for in the occupational history and during clinical examination are listed in Box 1.

Occupational factors in relation to the skin disorder

The history of the skin disorder, for example, duration of the rash, primary location, secondary spread (if any), should be correlated with the occupational history, for example, the duration of employment. The relationship of the appearance of the skin disorders to any recent change of work duties, new processes or materials, or even to different batches of raw materials, may give a clue to the occupational aetiology of the skin disorder. Off days, weekends or vacations are usually associated with an improvement of an OSD. A past history of the occurrence of similar skin disorders in other workers in the workplace may be another valuable piece of information which points to an occupational origin of the skin disorder.

Box 1. Checklist of Considerations During History Taking and Clinical Examination

Occupational History

- Place of Employment, Job Title
- Typical workday activities, Materials handling techniques
- Protective clothing and equipment, Hygiene facilities and practice

Occupational Factors in Relation to the Skin Disorder

- New job, materials, processes
- Health and safety information on materials handled
- Whether other workers affected, Improvement on weekends or holidays
- Sick leave taken for skin disorder
- Past occupational history
- Past history of occupational skin disease
- Concurrent occupation(s)

Other General History

- Atopic background (personal and familial)
- Skin allergies, other skin disorders
- Treatment for skin disorder
- Domestic exposure, Hobbies

Clinical Examination

- Is it dermatitis? Is it contact (exogenous) dermatitis?
- If it is contact dermatitis, is it irritant or allergic?
- Are additional factors involved (e.g. sunlight)?
- Is it a non-dermatitic occupational skin disease?

Are there any predisposing and aggravating factors for the OSD and are these preventable?

Personal occupational factors

Incorrect material handling techniques may cause OSD. The worker should be asked about the way he handles work materials. Protective devices are often worn by workers. The type of protective equipment, the material it is made of, how it is used and maintained (to determine if this is improperly done) should be recorded. The availability of cleansing facilities, the types of skin cleansers used and the cleansing habits of the worker should be enquired. Good personal hygiene reduces the risk of OSD. However, extremely effective cleansers (e.g. strong solvents) are often skin irritants.

A personal history of similar skin problems should be obtained. A worker may have experienced a similar skin disorder in his previous employment. Exposure to the same work chemical or process in his present job may then cause a recurrence of the OSD. The time off or sick leave taken by the patient for the skin disorder should also be recorded. Sick leave from OSD may be compensable. Seek the opinion of the worker regarding his skin problem. The worker can often help ascertain the cause of his skin disease.

Other aspects of history taking

A history of treatment received (medicaments can cause or aggravate a skin disorder), skin allergies (the patient may be exposed to the same allergen previously), a personal or family history of atopy (atopics are more susceptible to contact dermatitis), and a history of other skin disorders or other general illnesses should be recorded.

Other occupational or environmental exposures

The cause of a skin disorder may not be apparent from the worker's work environment. It may be due to chemicals handled during a secondary or part-time job elsewhere. This information may be more difficult to obtain, especially if the patient is apprehensive that his main employer may disapprove of his other job. Skin disorders may also result from hobbies (e.g. from contact with solvents, resins and other materials used in Do-It-Yourself kits) or from domestic exposure (e.g. copious amounts of water/detergents during housework) and cosmetics.

Case Study 4: "Hidden" Allergen Detected by Patch Testing

A 45 year old female developed finger dermatitis. She does most of her domestic chores herself including cooking, washing and cleaning up her place. She seldom wears gloves at work. She also does part-work as a nail manicurist at a beauty parlour 4 times a week. She was diagnosed to have ICD from wet work and frequent contact detergents. She was treated with topical steroids but her dermatitis did not improve despite avoiding wet work and wearing gloves. A patch test done showed that she was allergic to several acrylates. These acrylates were present in the nail resin that she comes into contact with as a manicurist. The hidden allergen would not have been detected if a patch test was not done to the substances that she handled in the part-time work.

The previous occupations of the worker should be obtained. Sensitisation from exposure to chemicals in the previous job may have occurred. A record of past occupations may also be important for OSD with long latent periods between work exposure to the chemicals and manifestation of disease, for example, skin cancers and ultraviolet light exposure.

Difficulties in obtaining occupational history

Often, difficulties are encountered during occupational history taking. The physician needs to understand various work processes. Workers performing similar work tasks in the same type of industry may work under different work conditions. A technical dictionary or reference book, such as the ILO Encyclopaedia of Occupational Health and Safety may provide useful information about work processes. Alternatively, the help of an experienced occupational health colleague may be sought. The physician needs to have a knowledge of the common industries and their work processes in the country, and a knowledge of the common causes of OSD in the various industries (see Table 3).

Occasionally, further information on the nature of the chemicals which are handled by the worker may be required. The usual way of obtaining such information is to ask the worker for the Safety Data Sheets (SDS) which may be available for the work chemical which is used. The SDS provides information on the nature of the substance and its possible health effects. Chemical safety and health databases (available either at a Poisons Centre, Occupational Health Centre or on the Internet) are other sources of information.

Where indicated, samples of the work materials handled by the worker should be obtained for patch testing or for chemical analysis.

This may be necessary for the detection of impurities which may not be specified in the information sheet, or detection of decomposition products. The physician may need to arrange for a workplace visit to better assess the worker's work conditions, to screen other workers for similar OSD or to learn more about the work process.

Clinical Examination

A well taken clinical and occupational history will often allow the physician to determine if the worker's skin disorder is work related. Clinical examination, patch tests and laboratory tests will help the physician to confirm the diagnosis and ascertain the cause of the skin disorder. The physician should always look for non-occupational skin disorders which may be present in a background of OSD e.g. AD or psoriasis.

Case Study 5: Scabies Infestation

An outbreak of skin rashes occurred in a woodworking factory. Thirteen workers in two adjacent sections had the rashes, and the workers believed that their skin disorder was due to wood dust and poor working conditions of the factory, such as poor ventilation and heat. The workers were concerned about the rashes because some of their family members were also affected. A workplace investigation showed that the work environment was generally satisfactory. Examination of the affected workers showed papular rashes and excoriation marks with typical skin burrows at the finger webs and flexor surfaces of the wrists. The diagnosis was skin infestation by Sarcoptes scabiei. The problem was resolved when the workers and their families were treated for scabies.

During examination of a patient presenting with a possible work-related skin disorder, the following questions can help the physician in the management of the case.

Is the skin disorder a dermatitis?

Most OSD present as eczematous eruptions secondary to a contact dermatitis. An ability to recognise the features of dermatitis is important as well as an ability to differentiate skin diseases with similar manifestation, e.g. psoriasis and drug eruptions.

Is the dermatitis a contact dermatitis?

Occupational contact dermatitis refers to dermatitis arising from contact with a work chemical. It should be distinguished from non-occupational contact dermatitis which are contact dermatitis arising from contact with non-occupational substances such as cosmetics, costume jewellery, or medicaments. Contact dermatitis should also be distinguished from endogenous dermatitis (for example, atopic, seborrhoeic, discoid or hand and feet dermatitis), which is genetic in origin. It should be noted that workers with endogenous dermatitis are more susceptible to develop ICD. It is not uncommon for contact dermatitis to coexist with endogenous dermatitis.

Is the contact dermatitis irritant or allergic in nature?

ICD results from direct skin injury from an irritant for example, solvents or detergents. ACD is an immunological skin reaction and tends to be more severe. Unlike an irritant, an allergen tends to trigger a dermatitis readily, even if the allergen is present in minute quantity and in low concentration.

Over three-quarters of occupational contact dermatitis cases are of ICD. The remainder are ACD or concomitant ICD and ACD. Sometimes more than one irritant or allergen may be the cause of the contact dermatitis. It is important to differentiate irritant from ACD, as the type of dermatitis affects rehabilitation and future job placements. While patch testing is the definitive test for ACD, there is no specific skin test to confirm ICD. The diagnosis of ICD is often based on clinical history, examination and after exclusion of ACD (by patch testing). In general, all workers with contact dermatitis should be patch tested.

Are there aggravating factors (e.g. sunlight)?

If a photoallergic contact dermatitis is suspected, a photopatch test may be indicated. One should also look for evidence of endogenous dermatitis.

Case Study 6: Chronic Actinic Dermatitis

An electrician presented with hand dermatitis, forearms dermatitis and facial dermatitis (Fig. 11). He noticed that his dermatitis was aggravated by sun exposure and while doing work outdoors. He wears rubber gloves at work.

Patch test showed that he was allergic to thiuram mix (present in his rubber gloves). His hand dermatitis improved after he switched to leather gloves but the dermatitis on his forearms and his face did not improve. A photopatch test was negative and phototest showed that he was sensitive to UV light.

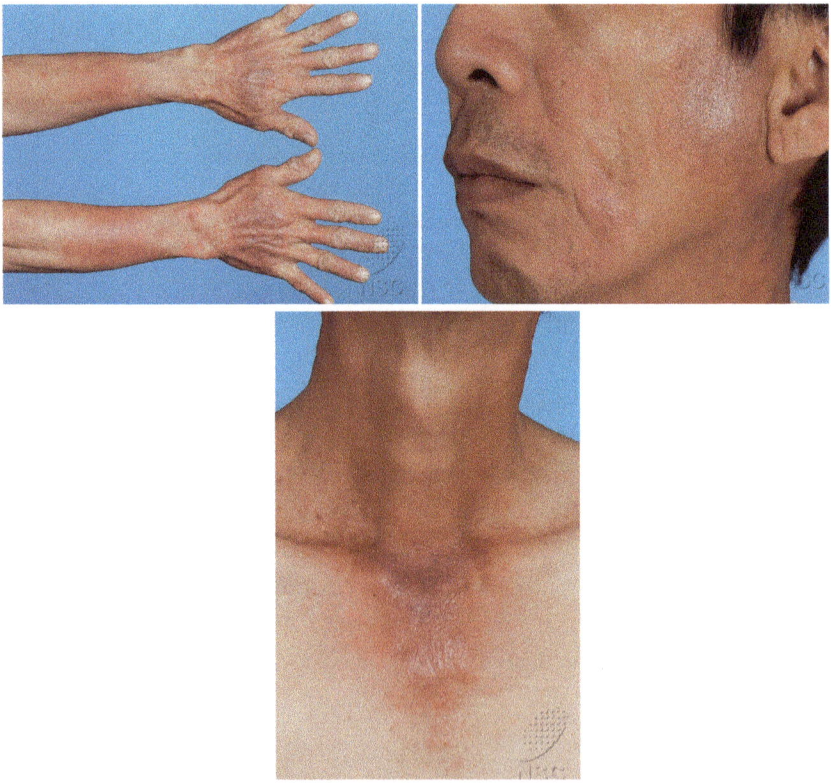

Fig. 11. An outdoor worker with chronic actinic dermatitis.

The patient had chronic actinic dermatitis. UV light exposure during his outdoor work was the cause of his persistent exposed parts dermatitis. Sun avoidance and changing to indoor work can help control his dermatitis.

Is there a Non-Eczematous Occupational Skin Disease?

About 5–10% of OSD present as non-eczematous skin lesions. These include physical or mechanical injuries (e.g. heat, friction) and infections (see Table 2). When such disorders are suspected relevant tests including skin scrapings for microscopy, prick tests, skin biopsy and serology may be necessary.

Are there any predisposing factors for the OSD? Are these preventable?

Several factors are known to predispose an individual to develop OSD. Individuals with constitutional predisposition, e.g. atopics are generally more susceptible to irritants. Damaged skin, such as lacerated or abraded skin may predispose to contact dermatitis. Workers who are ignorant of work hazards, and who do not observe good work habits and hygiene, are at higher risk of OSD.

Environmental conditions may also contribute to the development of OSD. For example, a poorly ventilated and hot workplace induces workers to perspire excessively and aggravate heat induced skin disorders and intertrigo. Sweat may also act as a solvent to enhance skin penetration of contact irritants and allergens.

Management of Occupational Skin Diseases

The management of OSD depends on its morphological presentation and cause. An accurate diagnosis is essential. The causative agent must be identified. A detailed history, thorough physical examination, and where indicated, relevant investigations including patch tests and laboratory tests together with a workplace visit, will often enable the physician to arrive at a correct diagnosis.

Specific Treatment

The worker should avoid contact with the causative agent immediately, especially if the dermatitis is severe. A temporary job change may be necessary. Severely affected workers should be given medical leave or hospitalised. Workers with mild dermatosis should be encouraged to resume work with proper protective garments and advised to observe good work habits.

Dermatitis is treated according to its severity. Acute dermatitis should be treated with wet compresses of normal saline or potassium permanganate (1:10,000) lotions until the dermatitis dries up. Chronic dermatitis should be treated with topical steroid creams or ointments of mild to moderate potency (e.g. hydrocortisone, betamethasone valerate, fluocinolone acetonide). Potent steroids such as clobetasol dipropionate should be avoided or used for short periods only because of their potential side effects. It is advisable to avoid combination steroid/antibiotic/antifungal preparations as they may pose problems of sensitisation. Contact allergy to neomycin and quinolines found in such preparations is not uncommon. Oral antibiotics should be administered where secondary bacterial infection is suspected. Oral antihistamines should be given to relieve pruritus.

Other OSD are treated according to diagnosis; for example, cutaneous larva migrans with cryotherapy and/or oral antihelminthics, and chromomycosis with oral antifungal agents.

Causes of chronicity of occupational skin diseases

Occasionally, the patient with an OSD may not respond to treatment. Chronicity of an OSD can be due to one or more of the following:

- Continuing exposure to the offending agent.
- Severe long standing dermatitis which generally takes longer to recover because the barrier functions of the skin are severely impaired.
- Complications of treatment, such as superimposed contact allergy to medicaments.

- Untreated complications, for example, secondary bacterial infection.
- Underlying endogenous factors, e.g. AD.
- Medico-legal problems. In some settings, a worker may malinger or even cause self-inflicted injury in attempts to seek compensation.

These conditions have to be considered and managed accordingly in a patient with chronic OSD.

Rehabilitation

The primary consideration of rehabilitation in OSD is to get the worker back to work as soon as possible, and at the same time prevent a relapse. The worker should be taken off work during the acute stage of the disease, but the physician should not encourage a long absence from work.

Permanent job change should be avoided wherever possible. A job change will require the worker to retrain for another job which may be expensive for both the employee and the employer. It will also mean social adjustment for the worker and adaptation to a new working condition, colleagues and workplace, and possibly even a salary reduction. The physician should therefore consider the worker's age, skills, capability, intellect and available preventive measures before recommending a job change. Job change is usually indicated only for workers with ACD and rarely for those with ICD. This is because in ACD, relapses tend to be more severe with each subsequent episode and even brief exposures to the allergen will trigger a reaction. A job change may not be necessary if substitution of the allergen is possible, or contact with the allergen can be totally avoided by changing work procedures.

Another important factor to consider before recommending a job change is whether a personal history of atopy is present. Job counselling is important for these workers, and they should be encouraged to perform jobs which do not involve exposure to wet conditions.

Prognosis of occupational contact dermatitis

Prognosis of occupational contact dermatitis refers to the course of dermatitis over a period of time with and without medical intervention. Understanding the prognosis of occupational contact dermatitis is important because it enables physicians to:

- Predict the course of the dermatitis in patients;
- Implement risk management for patients exposed to contact irritants and allergens;
- Plan preventive measures against contact and occupational dermatitis;

It also helps the relevant authorities to prioritise implementation of preventive measures. The long term outcome of occupational contact dermatitis has important medico-legal implications. It helps to determine the quantum of compensation for patients with such skin disorders.

The physician must also distinguish between medical and social prognosis in workers with OSD. Many workers with OSD are able to continue work despite their dermatosis. Indeed, many may prefer to remain in their current job despite their skin disorder, in order to avoid a salary reduction or a change to a less interesting or challenging job. Some who continue to be exposed to the work irritants or allergens may develop tolerance and hardening.

Complete clearance of occupational contact dermatitis has been reported to range from 8% to 77% over follow-up periods ranging from one year to more than 10 years. Studies done between 1961 and 1989 indicated that total clearance of occupational contact dermatitis occurred in only 8% to 33% of patients. In a study of 555 patients who completed a follow-up questionnaire 2–3 years after initial consultation, 26% of women had complete healing, 22% had continual problems, and 52% had recurrence. Among the men, 31% had complete healing, 29% had continual problems, and 40% had recurrence (Fregert, 1975). The prognosis was the same for those who changed their work or stopped working compared to those who continued their eczema-inducing work.

Of 230 patients with OSD surveyed by a telephone interview at least two years after diagnosis, 78% of the workers were working. However, 57% of those working had changed jobs, 67% because of their skin problem. Workers who changed their job tended to have better outcome than those who did not (Holness and Nethercott, 1995). Wall and Gebauer (1991) reported that 61% of patients with occupational contact dermatitis lost time from work. 6% of these patients were off work for more than one year. The economic cost can thus be considerable.

In another study of prognosis, a change in work and the presence of easily avoidable work-related allergens were associated with a good prognosis (Mälkönen *et al.*, 2009). Six months after diagnosis, the skin disease had healed in 27% of patients. The OSD had cleared in 17% in those with no changes at work, compared to 34% among those who had changed their job/occupation. The best clearing had occurred in patients with CU (35%), while the healing of allergic (27%) and irritant (23%) contact dermatitis was marginally lower.

As for long term prognosis, a 12-year Swedish follow-up study (from 1987 to 1999) of 2,897 patients with OSD showed that 70% had persistence of skin symptoms (Meding *et al.*, 2005). Skin atopy was the strongest factor for poor prognosis, followed by contact allergy and female gender. Most of the patients (82%) changed their work situation, and 44% changed their jobs. While the majority (62%) experienced no change in income, and 6% had better income, 32% had a reduced income. In the group with reduced income, 45% of persons had a reduction in income of greater than a quarter. The prognosis of hand eczema was poor, as in 60% of patients the eczema became chronic.

Prevention

All OSD are theoretically preventable. Standard principles of prevention include substitution or removal of the offending agent, isolation of the worker and enclosure of the work process. A well ventilated workplace is desirable when volatile solvents and irritant dusts and fibres are used in the work process.

Reports have indicated that good preventive measures and health education of workers and employers are able to reduce the incidence of OSD. It is cost effective and helps improve the quality of life of workers (Andrees *et al.*, 2020, Reich *et al.*, 2020).

Pre-employment medical examinations and advice to workers and employers on job suitability (e.g. advising atopics to avoid wet work) and regular health education and training of workers (for hazard awareness, proper handling techniques, and to stress the importance of good personal hygiene) play important roles in prevention.

The availability of conveniently sited washing and drying facilities at the workplace will encourage workers to utilise these facilities during breaks and after work. Proper skin cleansers should be provided, while abrasive detergents and solvents should be removed. The choice of cleanser will depend on the nature of the chemicals handled. A mild soap is usually adequate for office work. Non-aqueous cleansers may be needed to remove grease and oils. Unfortunately, strong cleansers tend to be corrosive and are more likely to cause ICD.

The habit of using organic solvents and abrasive detergents as skin cleansers must be discouraged. The most more sensible preventive approach is to avoid skin contamination during work. It may be better to have slightly dirtied hands than to suffer from chronic dermatitis from vigorous cleansing. Disposable towels should be provided for drying. Emollients or moisturising creams applied after work may help to restore the barrier function of the skin.

Barrier Creams

The efficacy of barrier creams against occupational dermatitis is questionable. Most studies have found them to provide limited protection. Workers using barrier creams may have a false sense of security. However, the use of barrier creams has the advantage of increasing the worker's awareness for cleaning their skin during breaks and after work. It also facilitates skin cleansing.

Gloves

Personal protective equipment (e.g. gloves, sleeves, aprons and boots), if properly maintained and correctly used can be a very effective means to prevent OSD. One limitation of using gloves is the risk of accidents. The correct type of gloves should be used. The choice of the type of gloves is based on the type of chemical handled and the type of work process. They should cover the distal third of the forearm to be effective. Where dripping of liquid towards the elbow is inevitable, elbow length gloves should be used. Alternatively, the dripping may be prevented by lowering the workbench or elevating the work platform.

Impervious gloves are occlusive, and may cause skin maceration. Gloves with a cotton lining may act as a wick and absorb sweat, enhancing a high humidity microclimate adjacent to the skin. Workers should remember to remove gloves periodically and to change them when they become moist or when the inner lining is contaminated. Workers should be provided with several pairs of gloves to change.

Workers can occasionally become sensitised to rubber chemicals in rubber gloves, or chromates and resins in leather gloves. ACD to gloves and boots is characteristic and should not be overlooked. The use of clean work clothes is also advisable. Skin contact with clothing contaminated by irritants or allergens may cause dermatitis.

Surveillance

The company safety officers, nurses and physician should maintain a vigilant surveillance on the occupational health of their workers so that prompt investigation and management of any outbreaks of OSD can be undertaken.

Legislation

Different countries have different medico-legal legislation regulating OSD. This may include regulatory laws on environmental standards for cutaneous hazards, the provision of skin hygiene and washing facilities at workplace, notification of OSD, statutory medical examinations, and workmen's compensation. Occupational health physicians and nurses, safety officers, general practitioners and anyone responsible for the health care of workers should be familiar with the occupational laws and regulations in their countries.

Case Study 7: Prevention of Chromate Dermatitis From Cement

Chromate allergy from cement still remains a predominant OSD in developing countries but is less encountered in European Union (EU) countries. In the EU legislative measures that reduced the hexavalent chromate contents in cement have been enacted. In January 2005, following EU legislation (EU Directive 2003/53/EC), the use or supply of cement containing >2 ppm of chromate was prohibited in the UK. There was a significant decline in the incidence of both ACD attributed to chromate (incidence rate ratio 0.48, 95% CI 0.36 to 0.64) between the time period preceding the EU legislation (2002–2004) and the post-legislation period (2005–2009). The majority of the decline in incidence occurred during 2005 (Stocks et al., 2012).

Percutaneous Absorption of Toxins

In addition to being a direct target organ for environmental chemicals, the skin is an important portal of entry for some environmental toxins into the body. The amount and rate of percutaneous absorption of substances in contact with the skin depends on several factors. Different body sites have different skin permeability to chemicals. There is also individual variation. Permeability also depends on the state of the skin barrier. Absorption is enhanced through damaged skin or when substances under placed under occlusion. Another factor which affects skin absorption rate is the physical and chemical nature of the substance, for example, whether it is lipid or non-lipid soluble.

Skin notation in environmental standards

The "skin notation" is sometimes encountered in environmental standards for toxic agents. This notation serves to highlight the skin as an important portal of entry for the toxin. For example, in the American Conference of Governmental Industrial Hygienists (ACGIH) guidelines for threshold limit values (TLVs), this notation is described to "refer to the potential contribution to the overall exposure by the cutaneous route including mucous membranes and eye — either by airborne, or more particularly, direct contact with the substance" (ACGIH, 2020). There is a need to have appropriate measures to prevent cutaneous absorption of substances having a "skin notation." Thus, for chemicals having a skin notation (e.g. solvents and pesticides), respiratory protection alone may be inadequate, even for exposure levels within the prescribed TLVs.

The skin notation of a chemical only refers to its potential for percutaneous absorption being an important portal of entry into the systemic circulation, and not to the capacity of the substance to cause skin irritation or sensitisation in workers.

Conclusion

The skin is an organ which is commonly affected by work-related disorders. As such, a good working knowledge of the epidemiology, aetiology, diagnosis, management, and rehabilitation of OSD is required for the practising occupational health professional. OSD are preventable. The principles of prevention, which is a major part of the ethos of occupational health practice, should be applied to safeguard the skin of the worker wherever possible.

References

Aalto-Korte K, Koskela K, Pesonen M. (2020) 12-year data on skin diseases in the Finnish Register of Occupational Diseases II: Risk occupations with special reference to allergic contact dermatitis. *Contact Derm* **82**(6): 343–349.

Aalto-Korte K, Koskela K, Pesonen M. (2020) 12-year data on dermatologic cases in the Finnish Register of Occupational Diseases I: Distribution of different diagnoses and main causes of allergic contact dermatitis. *Contact Derm* **82**(6): 337–342.

ACGIH. (2020). *Threshold Limit Values for Chemical Substances and Physical Agents and Biological Exposure Indices.* ACGIH, Cincinnati.

Ahmed SM, Aw TC, Adisesh A. (2004) Toxicological and immunological aspects of occupational latex allergy. *Toxicol Rev* **23**(2): 123–134.

Andrees V, John SM, Nienhaus A, Skudlik C, Brans R, Augustin M, Krensel M, ROQ-Study Group. (2020) Economic evaluation of a tertiary prevention program for occupational skin diseases in Germany. *Contact Derm* **82**(6): 361–369.

Angelova-Fischer I, Hoek AK, Dapic I, Jakasa I, Kezic S, Fischer TW, Zillikens D. (2015) Barrier function and natural moisturizing factor levels after cumulative exposure to a fruit-derived organic acid and a detergent: Different outcomes in atopic and healthy skin and relevance for occupational contact dermatitis in the food industry. *Contact Derm* **73**(6): 358–363.

Ansotegui IJ, Melioli G, Canonica GW, Caraballo L, Villa E, Ebisawa M, Passalacqua G, Savi E, Ebo D, Gómez RM, Luengo Sánchez O, Oppenheimer JJ, Jensen-Jarolim E, Fischer DA, Haahtela T, Antila M, Bousquet JJ, Cardona V, Chiang WC, Demoly PM, Zuberbier T. (2020) IgE allergy diagnostics and other relevant tests in allergy, a World Allergy Organization position paper. *World Allergy Organ J* **13**(2): 100080.

Barbaud A, Poreaux C, Penven E, Waton J. (2015) Occupational protein contact dermatitis. *Eur J Dermatol* **25**(6): 527–534.

Bensefa-Colas L, Telle-Lamberton M, Faye S, Bourrain JL, Crépy MN, Lasfargues G, Choudat D, RNV3P members, Momas I. (2015) Occupational contact urticaria: Lessons from the French National Network for Occupational Disease Vigilance and Prevention (RNV3P). *Br J Dermatol* **173**(6): 1453–1461.

Cahill JL, Williams JD, Matheson MC, Palmer AM, Burgess JA, Dharmage SC, Nixon RL. (2016) Occupational skin disease in Victoria, Australia. *Aust J Dermatol* **57**(2): 108–114.

Chew AL, Maibach HI. (2003) Occupational issues of irritant contact dermatitis. *Int Arch Occup Environ Health* **76**(5): 339–346.

Coman G, Zinsmeister C, Norris P. (2015) Occupational contact dermatitis: Workers' compensation patch test results of Portland, Oregon, 2005–2014. *Dermatitis* **26**(6): 276–283.

Dai Y, Leng S, Li L, Niu Y, Huang H, Liu Q, Duan H, Cheng J, Liu Q, Zheng Y. (2009) Effects of genetic polymorphisms of N-Acetyltransferase on trichloroethylene-induced hypersensitivity dermatitis among exposed workers. *Ind Health* **47**(5): 479–486.

De Groot AC. (2015) New contact allergens: 2008 to 2015. *Dermatitis* **26**(5):199–215.

Diepgen TL. (2003) Occupational skin-disease data in Europe. *Int Arch Occup Environ Health* **76**(5): 331–338.

Dugdale CM, Walensky RP. (2020) Filtration efficiency, effectiveness, and availability of N95 face masks for COVID-19 prevention. *JAMA Intern Med* **180**(12): 1612–1613.

Fluhr JW, Darlenski R, Angelova-Fischer I, Tsankov N, Basketter D. (2008) Skin irritation and sensitization: Mechanisms and new approaches for risk assessment. 1. Skin irritation. *Skin Pharmacol Physiol* **21**(3): 124–135.

Foo CC, Goon AT, Leow YH, Goh CL. (2006) Adverse skin reactions to personal protective equipment against severe acute respiratory syndrome — a descriptive study in Singapore. *Contact Derm* **55**(5): 291–294.

Fregert S. (1975) Occupational dermatitis in a 10-year material. *Contact Derm* **1**: 96–107.

Goh CL. (1990) *Occupational Skin Diseases.* Singapore, PG Publishing.

Hawkey S, Abdul Ghaffar S. (2016) Glove-related hand urticaria: An increasing occupational problem among healthcare workers. *Br J Dermatol* **174**(5): 1137–1140.

Higgins CL, Palmer AM, Cahill JL, Nixon RL. (2016) Occupational skin disease among Australian healthcare workers: A retrospective analysis from an occupational dermatology clinic, 1993–2014. *Contact Derm* **75**(4): 213–222.

Holness DL, Nethercott JR. (1995) Work outcome in workers with occupational skin disease. *Am J Ind Med* **27**: 807–815.

Kanerva L, Toikkanen J, Jolanki R, Estlander T. (1996) Statistical data on occupational contact urticaria. *Contact Derm* **35**(4): 229–233.

Kho F, Leow YH, Goon A, Teo S, Cheng S. (2020) Ten-year trends in occupational skin diseases in Singapore, 2009 to 2018: Experience of a tertiary referral center. *Contact Derm* **83**(6): 531–533.

Koh D, Ng V, Leow YH, Goh CL. (2005). A study of natural rubber latex allergens in gloves used by healthcare workers in Singapore. *Br J Dermatol* **153**(5): 954–959.

Kratzel A, Todt D, V'kovski P, Steiner S, Gultom M, Thao T, Ebert N, Holwerda M, Steinmann J, Niemeyer D, Dijkman R, Kampf G, Drosten C, Steinmann E, Thiel V, Pfaender S. (2020) Inactivation of severe acute respiratory syndrome coronavirus 2 by WHO-recommended hand rub formulations and alcohols. *Emerg Infect Dis* **26**(7): 1592–1595.

Lan CC, Feng WW, Lu YW, Wu CS, Hung ST, Hsu HY, Yu HS, Ko YC, Lee CH, Yang YH, Chen GS. (2008) Hand eczema among University

Hospital nursing staff: Identification of high-risk sector and impact on quality of life. *Contact Derm* **59**(5): 301–306.

Lan J, Song Z, Miao X, Li H, Li Y, Dong L, Yang J, An X, Zhang Y, Yang L, Zhou N, Yang L, Li J, Cao J, Wang J, Tao J. (2020) Skin damage among health care workers managing coronavirus disease-2019. *J Am Acad Dermatol* **82**(5): 1215–1216.

Lin P, Zhu S, Huang Y, Li L, Tao J, Lei T, Song J, Liu D, Chen L, Shi Y, Jiang S, Liu Q, Xie J, Chen H, Duan Y, Xia Y, Zhou Y, Mei Y, Zhou X, Wu J, Li H. (2020) Adverse skin reactions among healthcare workers during the coronavirus disease 2019 outbreak: A survey in Wuhan and its surrounding regions. *Br J Dermatol* **183**(1): 190–192.

Mälkönen T, Jolanki R, Alanko K, Luukkonen R, Aalto-Korte K, Lauerma A, Susitaival P. (2009) A 6-month follow-up study of 1048 patients diagnosed with an occupational skin disease. *Contact Derm* **61**(5): 261–268.

Matterne U, Apfelbacher CJ, Soder S, Diepgen TL, Weisshaar E. (2009) Health-related quality of life in health care workers with work-related skin diseases. *Contact Derm* **61**(3): 145–151.

Meding B, Lantto R, Lindahl G, Wrangsjö K, Bengtsson B. (2005) Occupational skin disease in Sweden — a 12-year follow-up. *Contact Derm* **53**(6): 308–313.

Nienhaus A, Kromark K, Raulf-Heimsoth M, van Kampen V, Merget R. (2008) Outcome of occupational latex allergy--work ability and quality of life. *PloS one* **3**(10): e3459.

Pal TM, de Wilde NS, van Beurden MM, Coenraads PJ, Bruynzeel DP. (2009) Notification of occupational skin diseases by dermatologists in The Netherlands. *Occup Med (Lond)* **59**(1): 38–43.

Pesonen M, Koskela K, Aalto-Korte K. (2020) Contact urticaria and protein contact dermatitis in the Finnish register of occupational diseases in a period of 12 years. *Contact Derm* **83**(1): 1–7.

Quah C, Koh D, How CH, Quah J. (2012) Approach to hand dermatitis in primary care. *Singapore Med J* **53**(11): 701–705.

Rabin B, Fraidlin N. (2007) Patients with occupational contact dermatitis in Israel: Quality of life and social implications. *Soc Work Health Care* **45**(2): 97–111.

Radespiel-Tröger M, Meyer M, Pfahlberg A, Lausen B, Uter W, Gefeller O. (2009) Outdoor work and skin cancer incidence: A registry-based study in Bavaria. *Int Arch Occup Environ Health* **82**(3): 357–363.

Reich A, Wilke A, Gediga G, Baurecht H, Rodríguez E, Jakasa I, Geier J, Mempel M, Buhl T, Weidinger S, Kezic S, John SM, Schön MP,

Brans R. (2020) Health education decreases incidence of hand eczema in metal work apprentices: Results of a controlled intervention study. *Contact Derm* **82**(6): 350–360.

Stocks SJ, McNamee R, Turner S, Carder M, Agius RM. (2012) Has European Union legislation to reduce exposure to chromate in cement been effective in reducing the incidence of allergic contact dermatitis attributed to chromate in the UK?. *Occup Environ Med* **69**(2): 150–152.

Tang MB, Leow YH, Ng V, Koh D, Go CL. (2005) Latex sensitisation in healthcare workers in Singapore. *Ann Acad Med Singap* **34**(5): 376–382.

Traore O, Hugonnet S, Lübbe J, Griffiths W, Pittet D. (2007) Liquid versus gel handrub formulation: A prospective intervention study. *Crit Care (Lond)* **11**(3): R52.

Turner S, Carder M, van Tongeren M, McNamee R, Lines S, Hussey L, Bolton A, Beck MH, Wilkinson M, Agius R. (2007) The incidence of occupational skin disease as reported to The Health and Occupation Reporting (THOR) network between 2002 and 2005. *The Br J Dermatol* **157**(4): 713–722.

van Kampen V, Hoffmeyer F, Monsé C, Raulf M, Brüning T, Bünger J, Sucker K. (2020) Discrimination between atopic, allergic, and asthmatic volunteers for human exposure studies on sensory irritaion. *Adv Exp Med Biol* **1279**: 27–35.

Wall LM, Gebauer KA. (1991) A follow up study of occupational skin disease in Western Australia. *Contact Derm* **24**: 241–243.

Wallmeyer L, Lehnen D, Eger N, Sochorová M, Opálka L, Kováčik A, Vávrová K, Hedtrich S. (2015) Stimulation of PPARα normalizes the skin lipid ratio and improves the skin barrier of normal and filaggrin deficient reconstructed skin. *J Dermatol Sci* **80**(2): 102–110.

Wang BJ, Shiao JS, Chen CJ, Lee YC, Guo YL. (2007) Tumour necrotizing factor-alpha promoter and GST-T1 genotype predict skin allergy to chromate in cement workers in Taiwan. *Contact Derm* **57**(5): 309–315.

Watkins SA, Maibach HI. (2009) The hardening phenomenon in irritant contact dermatitis: An interpretative update. *Contact Derm* **60**(3):123–130.

Chapter 5

Mental Health Disorders

Ken Addley[*,†] *and Robert Kerr*[†]

Background

Prior to the emergence of the coronavirus disease 2019 (COVID-19) pandemic in early 2020, mental health and mental health disorders (MHDs) had been one of the most important global public health issues and represented a significant challenge for both employers and employees. At a global level, the pandemic has had a major impact on the mental health of populations in regard to fear, anxiety, depression, post-traumatic stress disorder (PTSD) and suicidal behaviour. A study from China (Wang *et al.*, 2020) indicated that 54% of the survey sample rated the psychological impact of the outbreak as moderate or severe with 29% indicating moderate to severe depressive symptoms and 16% with anxiety. These effects are likely to be more pronounced in those with pre-existing mental health conditions and issues around employment uncertainty and financial concerns will compound the problem (Kinman *et al.*, 2020). It has also impacted on workers across a range of sectors such as transport, retail, cleaning, first responders and

[*] Faculty of Occupational Medicine, Royal College of Physicians of Ireland, Dublin, Ireland.

[†] Department of Management, Leadership & Marketing, Ulster University Business School, Belfast, Northern Ireland, United Kingdom.

Corresponding author: Ken Addley (kenaddley@physicians.ie).

in particular healthcare and long-term care workers (United Nations, 2020) and this will be considered in more detail later in this chapter.

MHDs commonly encountered in the workplace reflect, to an extent, their prevalence in the community from which workforces are drawn. In normal circumstances, the prevalence of non-occupational related MHDs in employees would be expected to be lower than that of the general population due to the healthy worker effect (HWE). The HWE is applied to the difference in morbidity and mortality due to various employment-associated factors that need to be taken into account when comparing the health and mortality experience of workers with that of the general population. In other words, an individual must be relatively healthy compared to the general population in order to be employable in a workforce (Chowdhury, 2017; McMichael, 1976).

It is estimated that a quarter to a third of the European population suffer from an MHD annually with depression and anxiety being the most common. Of interest to public health physicians and indeed employers and their occupational health (OH) professionals, is that only around a half of people will receive professional health support (World Health Organization (WHO), 2018a).

There is a relationship between poor mental health and socioeconomic status whereby poverty, poor working conditions, unemployment and poor education can all contribute to a reduction in well-being and an increased risk of developing an MHD. Other adverse lifestyle factors such as smoking, alcohol abuse, poor diet, obesity and physical inactivity are also associated with MHDs and thereby contribute to other increased non-communicable disease risk such as cardiorespiratory diseases.

The WHO defines mental health (WHO, 2018a) as follows:

- Mental health — a state of well-being in which an individual can realise his or her own potential, cope with the normal stresses of life, work productively and make a contribution to the community.
- MHDs — comprise a broad range of problems, with different symptoms. They are generally characterised by some combination of disturbed thoughts, emotions, behaviour and relationships with others. Examples include, depression; anxiety; bipolar disorders; schizophrenia; adjustment disorders and post-traumatic stress.

Some Key Facts about Mental Health in General

- Around one in 15 people suffer a major depressive episode;
- Around three in 15 people suffer from an anxiety state;
- Depression is twice as common in women;
- In Europe men are five times more likely to commit suicide than women;
- In Europe MHDs account for around 40% of social welfare benefit and disability pensions;
- In 2016, mental health and behavioural disorders represented 6% of total DALYs for all causes globally with major depression representing 2.5% and anxiety 1.08%.

Disability-adjusted life year (DALY) — this is a term used to quantify the burden of disease from the aspect of both mortality and morbidity taking account of standard life expectancy and the incidence/duration/severity of the disease. A DALY for a particular health condition in a population is the sum of the years of life lost due to premature mortality and the years lost due to a disability. One DALY represents one lost year of healthy life and is a measurement of the gap between current health status and that of an ideal health situation where freedom from disease/disability and living to an advance age apply.

Across the world there is variation in the estimated prevalence of MHDs and the associated DALYs — the lowest WHO region is Africa with the highest the Americas (Table 1). MHDs are therefore the leading cause of DALYs in the working age populations of high income countries.

General initiatives to improve and promote better mental health include more investment in mental health services, better training for health professionals in detection and treatment, encouraging community based schemes and offering occupational opportunities (WHO, 2013). Therefore, OH has a key role to play in regard to ensuring that work is "good work" that promotes positive well-being.

Table 1. DALYs for Mental Health Disorders by WHO Region in 2019 (WHO, 2019a)

WHO Region	DALYs (000s) (% of Regional Causes)	
African	18,848	4
Americas	32,673	11
South-East Asia	39,673	6
European	25,476	9
Eastern Mediterranean	15,514	6
Western Pacific	35,951	7
Total (Global)	168,135	7

Mental Health in the Workplace

The WHO Global Strategy on Health, Environment, and Climate Change (WHO, 2019b) identifies workplaces as an essential setting for the prevention of a range of modifiable risks including mental ill health. It is accepted that work/working conditions, is a key social determinant of mental ill health and MHDs are frequently reported by workers globally. The work environment, work organisation and the economic and social context of work creates a psychosocial risk which can lead to a deterioration in both physical and mental health. Good working conditions benefit worker mental health whereas poor working conditions, contribute to or exacerbate the psychosocial status of the individual.

The impact of MHDs on business is significant and in the United Kingdom (UK) in 2018/2019 it has been estimated that 12.8 million working days were lost due to work-related stress, depression or anxiety (Labour Force Survey, 2019). The average prevalence of these conditions across all industries was quoted as 1,380 cases per 100,000 workers. They also accounted for 44% of work-related ill health and 54% of working days lost in that year.

The relationship between work and the causation of MHDs can be complex and any attribution will be a matter of clinical judgement. In a Delphi study, eleven workplace and seven personal factors were

Table 2. Workplace and Personal Factors for Attributing MHDs to Work (Wong *et al.*, 2015)

Workplace Stressors	Personal Factors
High job strain	Previous mental illness
Effort-reward imbalance	Neurotic personality trait
Major trauma at work	Adverse life events
Interpersonal conflict	Adverse social circumstances
Inadequate support	Resilience/coping strategies
Role ambiguity	Family history of mental illness
Person-job mismatch	Secondary gain — financial or otherwise
Organisational injustice	
Organisational culture	
Work scheduling — shifts/long hours	
Job insecurity	

identified that should be considered when attributing mental illness to work (Table 2). In addition, the authors proposed a definition of occupational mental illness — anxiety, depression or both or an adjustment disorder or PTSD which can be reasonably be attributed on a balance of probabilities to workplace stressors rather than to personal factors.

In dealing with MHDs in the workplace a case-management approach that takes account of human resource input, line manager or supervisor context, the employee perspective and their social circumstances is recommended. There should be access to OH services and other multidisciplinary interventions such as counselling, training and rehabilitation. In other words, the "bio-psychosocial" approach is used to acknowledge that the health and well-being of the individual is determined by a combination of biological, psychological and social factors (Black, 2008).

The Challenge of the COVID-19 Pandemic

The emergence of the COVID-19 outbreak has raised several concerns regarding its mental health effect on workers in various sectors including essential workers in transport, retail, cleaning services, first responders and frontline workers, particularly workers in health and long-term care (United Nations, 2020). Many of these workers, and their families, are under exceptional stress, being faced with long hours and extreme workloads, risks of becoming infected and spreading infection to families and communities, concerns about adequacy and availability of PPE, separation from families, loneliness, and physical fatigue. In addition, healthcare and long-term care workers, are faced with difficult moral decisions and witnessing the multiple deaths of patients. Stigmatisation of these workers was also evident in some communities particularly in the early stages of the outbreak (Rajkumar, 2020). It is accepted therefore that healthcare workers (HCWs) have to work in very challenging conditions and are at risk of significant adverse mental health outcomes.

Reports from across the world have highlighted the impact of COVID-19 on mental health among HCWs: In Canada, 47% of health-care workers reported a need for psychological support; in the People's Republic of China, HCWs reported high rates of depression (50%), anxiety (45%), and insomnia (34%); and, in Pakistan, large numbers of health-care workers have reported moderate (42%) to severe (26%) psychological distress (UN, 2020).

Protecting the mental health of HCWs is seen as a priority. The unprecedented nature of the situation is likely to increase the risk of MHDs such as PTSD, depression, other anxiety disorders, substance misuse and suicide (Greenberg, 2020). It has become clear that some individuals including, those with obesity, the immunosuppressed, the presence of chronic medical conditions, Black, Asian and minority ethnic (BAME) background and those who are over 60 are at even higher risk of adverse outcomes and may therefore also be at increased risk of psychological issues. Whilst not a mental health condition, Moral Injury is also recognised as an important consideration and this is defined as psychological distress that results from actions or inactions which violate an individual's moral or ethical code (Greenberg *et al.*, 2020).

According to Greenberg, available evidence suggests that protecting the mental health of HCWs requires consideration of the following key elements:

- Early support and proper preparation of HCWs for the situation and dilemmas they will face;
- Ongoing monitoring by supportive team leaders, access to peer support programmes, psychological therapies and mental health support for those who are seriously or persistently distressed;
- HCWs should have appropriate acknowledgement of the challenging work undertaken and recognition of potential psychological difficulties and support information being provided;
- Staff who do not turn up to work are contacted as their non-attendance may be indicative of poor mental health;
- As normality returns all HCWs should receive "return to normal work" interviews;
- Managers should pay particular attention to HCWs in high-risk groups, such as those with a BAME background, and junior or inexperienced staff who have been working above their expected level of competence;
- Anyone who has been exposed to a potentially traumatic event should be actively monitored, particularly those considered at higher risk of developing mental health problems;
- Given the likelihood that HCWs have been exposed to morally distressing circumstances during the COVID-19 pandemic, most probably repeatedly, managers should help them to make sense of their experiences.

A substantial evidence base supports the notion that health-care managers have a major role in protecting the mental health of their staff as well as in helping those that need additional care and support to access it.

OH professionals also have an important role to play during and after the COVID-19 pandemic. They can provide support to both staff and organisations and give guidance on key issues such safety on the front line and supporting home workers, as well as assisting managers and workers with return to work guidelines either after illness or a period of remote working (Kinman, 2020).

OH services can also assist with ensuring that appropriate occupational hygiene measures such as segregation, ventilation and adequate PPE are being rigorously adhered to. In addition, issues of rehabilitation and redeployment will need to be addressed as will stresses on mental health ranging from adjustment disorders to "burn-out" to PTSD. These conditions are bound to affect many workers who may present symptomatically or through sickness absence or "presenteeism" (defined as workers who are at work but unable to function effectively) (Agius, 2020).

A significant proportion of individuals seem to experience lingering and debilitating symptoms following acute COVID-19 infection typically beyond 12 weeks. This has been termed post-COVID Syndrome or Long Covid and describes the effects of Covid-19 that continues for weeks or months beyond the initial illness. It has been estimated that upwards of 20% of positive patients go on to develop post-COVID Syndrome. Common symptoms include fatigue and sleep disturbance, anxiety and dyspnoea. Clearly this condition will have a major impact on individuals and society post-pandemic (Iqbal *et al.*, 2021).

Case Study 1: COVID-19 — Healthcare Worker Distress

Jane is a 25-year old registered nurse working in a hospital general medical unit which is also assisting in caring for COVID-19 patients. She has been a nurse for three years and enjoyed her job but she feels that the 'horrors', as she describes them, of what she has seen in the pandemic have made her demotivated and now she thinks about changing her career. During her shifts at the height of the pandemic there were multiple deaths on a daily basis and the patients were isolated from their families which made it worse. All of the team on the ward just have to absorb the grief and move on and it's difficult she says.

Jane suffers from constant bad dreams and nightmares which upsets her sleep and she is going into work feeling exhausted and at home she is irritable with her partner and they have constant arguments. She questions herself all the time — did she do the right things at work or could she have done more? She is constantly anxious, tired and irritable. She's expected to be resilient but she says she isn't unbreakable, she is just human and needs to get some help and support or she can't carry on.

Case Study 2: COVID-19 — Healthcare Worker Burnout

Manuel is a 55-year old senior doctor in a hospital medical department. When the pandemic started, he became totally immersed in it and it consumed his whole life. No training he said could have prepared him for what he had to face. Manuel hadn't previously experienced the levels of tiredness he had and said he and everyone on his team was tired 'emotionally, intellectually and, spiritually'.

He admits that he has mild depression and there are locations within his department where he re-experiences memories of difficult cases and decisions he had to deal with. You just go from patient to patient with no time to reflect or process what happened. I worry about what will happen the next day and the life and death decisions I will need to make.

His ordinary day to day life is affected. He is very irritable, easily angered feeling frayed all the time. Sleep is always disturbed with nightmares and flashbacks. He takes no gratitude from the expressions of support from the local community — he's 'not a hero he is just a broken man'.

Both these examples (Case Studies 1 and 2) illustrate how individuals can become overwhelmed and possibly burnt out by what they have to face at work despite being well trained and experienced. The impact of dealing with difficult and challenging situations for prolonged periods takes its toll and manifests itself in poor sleep, nightmares, fatigue, anxiety, and low mood. They show how "moral injury" is present in regard to decision making and that clinical anxiety/depression and some symptoms consistent with PTSD are also evident. The importance of peer support programmes, supervisor support and for severe and persistent distress referral for professional mental health support will be appropriate.

Depression

Depressive disorders are common ranking as the fourth cause of disability globally and increasing in prevalence year on year with currently a lifetime prevalence rate of between 10%–25%. They are more common in women than men and are often not diagnosed and on occasion inadequately treated. Depressive disorders result in significant morbidity and mortality and a significant factor in around 50% of suicides. There are also associations with other conditions including physical such as heart disease and alcohol and substance misuse. The adverse social impact results in dysfunction in families, relationships and legal implication, e.g. drink driving. It also affects work — the ability to get and maintain employment as well as sickness absence and occupational accidents and injuries. The majority of patients with depressive disorders are usually diagnosed at the primary care level and also quite commonly present at OH clinics.

In diagnosing depression, five or more of the core symptoms should be present during the same 2-week period; not regarded as normal for the individual; not secondary to other medical disorders including drug/alcohol misuse or bereavement; and, cause significant distress and/or impairment of social, occupational or general functioning (American Psychiatric Association, 2013). Whilst there may be variation in the clinical presentation including co-existent anxiety and poor memory or concentration, the core symptoms are shown in Box 1.

Box 1. Depressive Disorders — Core Symptoms.

- Depressed mood most of the day, nearly every day, as self-reported or observed by others.
- Diminished interest or pleasure in all or almost all activities most of the day, nearly every day.
- Significant weight loss when not dieting, weight gain or decrease, or increase in appetite nearly every day.
- Insomnia or hypersomnia nearly every day.
- Psychomotor agitation or retardation nearly every day.
- Fatigue or loss of energy nearly every day.
- Feelings of worthlessness or excessive or inappropriate guilt nearly every day.
- Diminished ability to think or concentrate nearly every day.
- Recurrent thoughts of death, recurrent suicidal ideation without a specific plan. In addition, these symptoms cause functional impairment (e.g., social, occupational).
- Are not better explained by substance abuse, medication side effects, or other psychiatric or somatic medical conditions.

Cases can be categorised as mild, moderate or severe depending on the number and type of symptoms present. In DSM V: Mild refers to five core symptoms with minor functional impairment; moderate refers to >5 core symptoms with greater intensity and moderate impairment in functioning; severe refers >5 core symptoms with intense functional impairment; psychotic features such as hallucinations or paranoia may be present (American Psychiatric Association, 2013). Diagnosis in the OH clinic is based on taking a psychiatric history, excluding other causes of the core symptoms and can be aided by the use of standardised questionnaire screening tools such as:

- Hamilton Depression Rating Scale (HAM-D);
- Hospital Anxiety and Depression Scale (HADS);
- Beck Depression Inventory (BDI);
- Patient Health Questionnaire (PHQ9);
- Goldberg Depression and Anxiety Scale.

Depressive episodes can vary in length from 4 to 30 weeks for mild to moderate cases and six months or longer in severe cases. This clearly will have an impact on sickness absence where spells will tend to be lengthy. Positive prognostic factors include acute onset; endogenous depression; early age of onset. Negative indicators include slow onset; neurotic depression; elderly; low self-confidence; co-morbidity and social isolation.

Treatment will usually involve the use of antidepressant medication which is effective in 65–75% of cases. Antidepressants are usually tried for a period of 4 weeks when considering what is adequate (British National Formulary, 2021). Commonly used drugs include selective serotonin reuptake inhibitors (SSRIs) and serotonin/noradrenaline reuptake inhibitors (SNRIs). Medication is usually continued for 6–12 months after improvement and withdrawn gradually monitoring for symptom recurrence. Talking therapies such as Cognitive Behavioural Therapy (CBT) and other psychotherapies may also have a role especially in those where medication is not tolerated. Severe cases may require hospital admission and use of physical therapies such as electro-convulsive therapy.

OH considerations include an awareness that a worker may be depressed and ensuring that they are receiving adequate treatment. The cognitive symptoms associated with depressive episodes and side effects of medication may affect general performance however, particular attention needs to be paid to those working in safety critical jobs. In those cases, robust assessment must be carried out to adequately determine fitness for the specific tasks. As already indicated, attendance at work may be affected due to symptoms such as loss of confidence, low energy, apathy and withdrawal. Getting back to work may include a phased return, involvement of the line manager and re-training and mentoring may be useful depending on the context and length of absence.

Case Study 3: Reactive Depression

John is a 52-year old office worker in a multi-national accounting firm. He has worked for the company for over twenty years during which time the business has been taken over by another firm on two occasions. He spends most of his time carrying out computer activities to the extent that he felt that his life was being dominated by the demands of the computer system rather than the needs of the clients. A lot of time is spent entering details about the various activities connected with client casework — in his view more time than it takes to do the actual accountancy tasks. In addition, he felt that the latest employer wanted to get rid of older staff and gave preference to younger colleagues. He was therefore finding it very difficult to remain focused and cope with his work which resulted in him going absent from work.

John had no previous health problems. He had been married for twenty years when his wife died from breast cancer five years previously after a short illness and that was difficult for him at the time. There were two children who were pursuing their own careers although they were a source of ongoing support for him. As he was absent from work due to sickness, he was referred to occupational health for an assessment.

At assessment, he was quiet and withdrawn. He spoke of the working conditions making him feeling undervalued, demotivated and stressed. Since leaving work there had been some improvement although his sleep remained disturbed and his mood was low at times. He also spoke about the death of his wife and how he hadn't really come to terms with that.

Case study 3 illustrates a very vulnerable man who was trying to cope with demands of his job whilst at the same time feeling undervalued and worthless. He was also trying to deal with the bereavement issues which had been constantly in the background. He was suffering from a reactive depression and was commenced on anti-depressant medication and also referred to the company's external counselling service. When reviewed 6 weeks later, he was feeling much better and was due to return to work the following day. He was going to speak with his supervisor about his job tasks and how he could be supported better. This case highlights how workers can lose their motivation and also how computer systems can dominate people's lives almost like an IT version of a conveyor belt. In addition, people are dealing with issues outside work that when added to in-work pressures can create a situation where coping can be difficult.

Anxiety

Anxiety symptoms are commonly found in the general population and lifetime prevalence is 14.6% — just less than twice that of depression. Comorbidity with other conditions including depression and alcohol/substance misuse is frequent and physical symptoms may be present. There are a number of different types of anxiety including phobic states (panic, social phobia; agoraphobia); generalised anxiety; adjustment disorders; obsessive compulsive disorder (OCD) and PTSD.

In generalised anxiety disorder (GAD), there is excessive worry, feelings of apprehension about everyday events leading to significant distress and functional impairment. Lifetime prevalence is estimated to be around 5.7% with females twice as likely to have the condition compared to men.

Symptoms are related to:

- Autonomic arousal — e.g. fast heart rate, palpitations, sweating, shaking and dry mouth.
- Physical symptoms — e.g. dyspnoea, chest pain, nausea and abdominal pain.
- Mental state — derealisation and depersonalisation. General symptoms such as dizziness, fainting, numbness and tingling.

- Tension — muscle aches and pains, failure to relax, on edge and difficulty swallowing.
- Cognitive — difficulty getting to sleep, poor memory, irritability and excessive worry.

Diagnosis is based on presentation/history and the following questionnaire tools may be helpful:

- Generalised Anxiety Disorder (GAD7);
- Goldberg Depression and Anxiety Scale.

Treatment may include psychological therapies along with a range of anti-anxiolytics, tranquillisers and antidepressants where depression is comorbid.

Case Study 4: Generalised Anxiety

Irene, aged 45, was a Chief Executive Officer of a successful high profile national company and had been in that post for two years. Whilst she had a successful track record in sales and management she was finding it difficult to cope with the challenging demands of the job and she felt just burnt out. Her family doctor had advised her to come out of work and certified her as suffering from stress. As part of their normal procedures, the company HR department asked that Irene be seen by the occupational health physician.

On assessment, Irene appeared anxious and described how she had panic attacks when her heart would race and she would become quite agitated. These occurred when she thought about work, had to deal with e-mails or meet with members of her team or other colleagues. This was a new experience for her as she had previously been an outgoing person with good relationships will her staff and others in work settings. The feelings of anxiety were also impacting on her domestic life as she had become withdrawn, irritable and had lost interest in the family and the things that she normally enjoyed like attending concerts and cooking. In addition, there were financial pressures due to property prices having fallen in the recession.

She was referred for Cognitive Behavioural Therapy and had nine sessions which helped her regain control over her thinking and how she was approaching issues at home and at work. This helped her regain a sense of control in her life that allowed her to better assess and deal with the demands being placed on her. The anxiety and feelings of negativity reduced — allowing a return to work after four sessions with a different perspective. The home life also improved as she was able to resume her hobbies and interests as well as see other problems in a more realistic context.

Even the most successful people can develop problems in coping with demands — not just at work but also at home. The interaction of demands at home and demands at work is also evident. Self-confidence can be lost and negative thoughts can present as inability to make decisions, fear and in some cases panic attacks. Short CBT can be useful to allow people to recognise negative patterns of thoughts or behaviour and to develop new techniques and strategies that allow these to be handled in a rational as opposed to an irrational way. Access to this form of support for employees can be useful for employers to provide.

Case Study 5: Social Phobia

Jason was 32 years old and worked in a back-office telephone call centre for a large public sector organisation. The organisation wanted to set up a customer drop-in centre and Jason was moved to this facility which was open five days a week on a rolling shift basis and involved interacting with customers and dealing with their queries and complaints. At times some of the customers were aggressive and could be verbally abusive. There was a delay in providing training and just before the centre opened staff were given brief instructions.

Jason had always been a reserved and shy person. He lived at home with his parents and apart from at work he had little social responsibility and few friends. He found that he had difficulty talking to people and got confused and forgot what it was he was trying to say. This made him feel humiliated and embarrassed and he got annoyed with himself for being so inadequate. He developed feelings of unworthiness, and severe anticipatory anxiety when going into work. He was unable to sleep and couldn't wait for the weekends to get away from it. He approached his supervisor asking to be moved; however, there were no alternative posts available.

The organisation had an occupational health service and he was seen by the doctor who diagnosed social anxiety and phobia. Jason was advised to contact the external counselling service and Jason gave them a call. He discussed his situation with them and they arranged to see him. He was given cognitive strategies to consider how he was interpreting and dealing with situations. This led to him being part of a group session where he was sharing his views with others under the supervision of the therapist. Eventually Jason was able to feel more comfortable in his role at work and although he still had some anxiety, his thinking about the situations which made him anxious were more manageable and he felt in control of things.

Organisations making changes to how they do their business may have an impact on the health and well-being of their employees. The importance of job training cannot be overstated to ensure that employees have the knowledge and skills to carry out the tasks. Keeping the situation under review and providing a means whereby feedback can be provided is also an important element when new ways of working are introduced. Lastly, selecting the appropriate staff to do particular jobs is also crucial to avoid a mismatch between job tasks and employee characteristics.

Adjustment Disorders

Adjustment disorders are mental health symptoms that occur within a defined timeframe of a particular environmental or psychosocial stressor — 1 month (ICD-10) or 3 months (DSM-V) — and should not last longer than 6 months after the stressor has been removed. In addition, bereavement or grief reactions are excluded. There is usually marked distress and impairment of normal functioning. Symptoms include those of depression; anxiety; emotional upset; and disturbed conduct. Prevalence is estimated to be in the region of 5–20% depending on the setting. Whilst there may be individual predisposition, the condition would not arise in the absence of a triggering event or stressor.

Distinction needs to be made between adjustment disorder and PTSD where in the latter it is likely that the triggering event will be more severe and life threatening. Adjustment disorders are often seen in the workplace where an event, e.g. a disciplinary matter, has triggered a dysfunctional psychological reaction in the worker. Treatment may involve engagement with a talking therapy such as CBT and antidepressants or anxiolytics may be required for cases that are resistant to this approach or symptoms persist. The difficulty is avoiding prolonged sickness absence and promoting an early return to work. In instances where the stressor is work-related, mediation between the employer and the employee may be beneficial as may a mentored return to work programme.

Bereavement Reactions

It is very common for individuals to experience an episode of depressive symptoms following a bereavement (a loss event — usually a death) of a family member or loved one. The context of the situation, the relationship bond, the personality and experience of the person involved will determine the strength or otherwise of the severity and course. Normal bereavement or grief reaction will include the following: disbelief; shock; numbness; guilt; anger; feeling sad; preoccupation with the deceased; low mood; lack of sleep; and weight loss. Normally these will lessen with time and the presence and intensity will be variable. The end point is reaching a point of acceptance. The average duration is around 6 months although cultural differences will play a part. It is generally accepted that the intensity of grief is at its height for the loss of a child, followed by a spouse/partner then a parent. An abnormal reaction will present as very intense or prolonged stages of bereavement with other serious psychological pathology. Generally, in the workplace, bereaved employees are supported by their employer and their co-workers and this is helpful in dealing with the situation. Many organisations allow a period of leave to be taken and some may facilitate access to bereavement counselling for those that may need it. Returning to work may be assisted by going back on a reduced hours basis — a phased return — building up to full time hours within an agreed time period.

Post-traumatic Stress Disorder

This is a condition which occurs after a traumatic event that leads to a combination of severe mental health disturbance along with involuntary re-experiencing of the event; hyper-arousal and startling; and avoidance. PTSD also has a major impact on a person's ability to function in their social interactions and ability to work. Whilst PTSD may be encountered in any worker — there are jobs where it is more likely to a risk, e.g. fire and police services; military; front-line health service workers; and train drivers.

In the DSM V criteria (American Psychiatric Association, 2013) the person involved has to have one or more of the following:

- directly experienced the traumatic event;
- witnessed the traumatic event in person;
- learns that the traumatic event occurred to a close family member or close friend (with the actual or threatened death being either violent or accidental); or,
- experiences first-hand repeated or extreme exposure to aversive details of the traumatic event (not through media, pictures, television or movies unless work-related).

Other diagnostic criteria also include meeting specific stipulations and symptoms from each of four symptom clusters: intrusion, avoidance, negative alterations in cognitions and mood, and alterations in arousal and reactivity. Other criteria concern duration of symptoms; assessment of functioning; and, clarifying that symptoms are not attributable to a substance/alcohol or co-occurring medical condition.

Screening questionnaires available for PTSD include:

- PTSD checklist for DSM-V (PCL-5) (Weathers *et al.*, 2013a);
- Clinician-administered PTSD scale for DSM-5 (CAPS-5) (Weathers *et al.*, 2013b).

Treatments include trauma-focused CBT and eye movement desensitisation and reprocessing (EMDR); medication such as anti-depressants for those who are very distressed, unstable or unable to engage with psychological therapy. In regard to outcome, estimations suggest that 50% will recover within 12 months and 30% will be chronic. Recovery is aided by good social support and the absence of any further traumatic events.

Case Study 6: PTSD

Maria had been a firefighter for six years and had dealt with quite a few serious and dangerous incidents during that time. Recently she found that one incident in particular was playing on her mind — it was the disturbing scene of one of her colleagues, who had gone into a building just in front of her, being killed within metres of her when part of a burning building collapsed on top of him. Maria found that these images were becoming more frequent and the scenes from that night would run repeatedly through her mind and disrupt her focus on work. Sounds and smells she experienced both in work and at home recreated horrific memories. She found herself avoiding socialising with her work colleagues, as this acted as a trigger for the images. At home, her partner was complaining how she was always irritable and bad tempered with problems relaxing and calling out in her sleep which was much more restless than it had been. Sudden or unexpected loud noises made her jump.

Maria was beginning to avoid going home until late, walking at times aimlessly around the neighbourhood where she lived. She had also started to call into a local bar for drinks — something which she rarely did before.

Maria spoke to one of her colleagues who was very supportive and thought she might have PTSD. He recommended that she be referred to the fire service occupational health department where the diagnosis was confirmed. Maria agreed to participate in therapy on a one to one basis with a therapist. She developed an understanding of what was happening and involved her partner in some of the sessions. The therapist discussed the trigger incident and identified the activities, people, sounds, and smells that set off her symptoms. In addition to therapy, medication helped Maria relieve some of their symptoms and decrease the intrusive memories and her levels of anxiety. It also reduced the irritability, improved sleep and she was startling less at loud sounds. After six months her symptoms had dramatically alleviated. She was able to remain at work and carry out a full range of firefighter duties. She also remained under review by occupational health for a further period of six months.

The symptoms of PTSD can be quite intrusive and disabling both mentally and physically. Relationships and normal day-to-day functioning can also be impaired. In addition, often those with PTSD will resort to the misuse of alcohol, illegal substances or prescribed drugs. It is important to be able to feel supported and enter into therapy that suits the individual, e.g. group therapy was not deemed appropriate for this case. Also, other therapy such as EMDR was not required. Organisations that are at high risk for PTSD should have in place policies and procedures to lessen the risk and also to help those who suffer get early treatment and therapy. In many cases, individuals will get control of their symptoms through a combination of therapy, medication, and the support of colleagues, family and friends.

Schizophrenia and Psychosis

Schizophrenia and related psychotic illnesses represent disorders of brain function with characteristic signs and symptoms. These include:

- Hallucinations — either visual or auditory with the latter in the form of hearing negative comments leading to paranoia;
- Delusions — fixed false beliefs unshakeable by logical reasoning which may be persecutory, thought interference or passivity;
- Thought disorder — abnormal flow of thoughts interfering with speech and writing.

These disorders have a severe impact on an individual's quality of life both socially and importantly, occupationally. Schizophrenia affects about one in 100 people with a lifetime risk of between 15 and 19 per 1,000 of the population. It is usually diagnosed in late adolescence or early adulthood. There are effective treatments which can help stabilise symptoms which allow some to lead relatively normal lives. Studies have estimated that the average employment rate in western societies is around 12–39% (Evensen *et al.*, 2016) and so employment, whilst many can struggle to find competitive paid jobs — the possibility of work and remaining in it and in particular in supported work schemes, is seen as a realistic prospect (Drake, 2018).

Case Study 7: Schizophrenia

Brian, now aged 34, was diagnosed at the age of 22 with schizophrenia following graduation from university. From that time, he had been in and out of employment, with several long term-jobs, a work placement and some periods of long-term unemployment. This most recent spell in unemployment led to him receiving help from support groups, which helped him to find his current position. He had not been able to find employment suitable to his university degree and had been working in low skilled and manual roles in the hospitality, leisure and currently as a labourer in a warehouse in a large service industry company. After being employed for six months he had been absent from work for six weeks and when reviewed at occupational health the diagnosis became apparent. He had not disclosed his mental health problems to his employers as he felt it would have resulted in him not being employed and he didn't want them to know. He saw being in work as important to him and he had a fear of losing his job.

Case Study 7 highlights how fear of stigma is an important issue and may lead to the withholding of health information. How relevant the diagnosis is in regard to any tasks undertaken will be part of a risk assessment process. Disability discrimination employment legislation, where it is present, will usually require employers to consider how adjustments or accommodations to jobs might be helpful in providing access to or maintaining people in employment.

Bipolar Disorders

Bipolar disorders are mental health conditions that cause unusual shifts in mood, energy, activity levels and concentration. These were formerly referred to as manic-depressive illness or manic depression, and in severe cases, can impact the ability of the patient to carry out day-to-day tasks. Periods of extreme elation, irritability and energised behaviour (manic or hypomanic episodes) alternate with periods of sadness, indifference, and hopelessness (depressive episodes). Patients often do not have insight into their condition and are unable to recognise the likely harmful or undesirable effects of these mood episodes.

The condition is typically diagnosed during late adolescence or early adulthood; and the symptoms can vary over time. It is a treatable condition, and a prescribed treatment plan can often result in management of symptoms and improvement in quality of life. Treatment is usually lifelong. There are three types of bipolar disorder (National Institute of Mental Health, 2020). Untreated or unstable bipolar disorders can lead to difficulties in both accessing work and also in maintaining it. This highlights the need for those with the condition to seek appropriate care and treatment.

Bipolar I disorder

This is a severe form of bipolar disorder with manic episodes that can last at least seven days, or extreme manic symptoms necessitating immediate hospital care. Depressive episodes, typically of two weeks duration or more usually occur as well. Episodes of depression with mixed features (with depressive symptoms and manic symptoms at the same time) may also present.

Bipolar II disorder

This less severe form of bipolar disorder presents with both depressive episodes and hypomanic episodes, but not full-blown manic episodes typical of Bipolar I Disorder.

Cyclothymic Disorder

Cyclothymic disorder (or cyclothymia) can present as episodes of hypomanic symptoms as well as periods of depressive symptoms lasting for years. The symptoms are less severe, and do not meet the diagnostic requirements for hypomanic or depressive episodes.

Case Study 8: Bipolar Disorder

Lloyd is a 24-year old laboratory technologist who worked for 2 years in his current job. Six months ago, he started to behave unusually with wild mood swings. He was unaware of the disruption caused at work by his altered behaviour.

On some days he would be very excitable and come up with grandiose plans to reorganise work. He would talk incessantly about how his plans would improve the organisation. He would also ignore Standard Operating Procedures and use his own methods for laboratory testing, as he thought the "short-cuts" he took were superior, and that the SOPs were slowing him down in his work. He needed little sleep and seemed to be always jumpy. At work, he bought expensive gifts for his colleagues which were accompanied by effusive notes of thanks and appreciation.

On other days he would be absent from work, and when contacted, was found to be sitting morosely at home and unable to do even simple things. He would talk very slowly, be very forgetful and had trouble concentrating or making decisions.

Lloyd was seen by a doctor, and diagnosed with bipolar disorder. He was treated with medication (Lithium) and showed some improvement initially. However, after a short period, he stopped medication on his own, and defaulted follow-up, resulting in a flare up of his condition. After a few months, he resigned from work to pursue his dreams of being a full-time musician.

Alcohol and Substance Misuse

Those with the greatest likelihood of experiencing alcohol problems in society, tend to be more represented in those of working age. Depending on the culture, high prevalence of alcohol use may mean that workers will present with problems of misuse including acute intoxication and chronic addiction. The typical picture is that of denial and cover-up and often a degree of collusion with co-workers making dealing with the problem very difficult for managers and supervisors. Whilst this section will discuss mainly alcohol problems — substance misuse would follow the same principles.

A review into the impact of drug or alcohol addiction in work (Black, 2016) found that the workplace itself can be a factor in encouraging increased levels of alcohol consumption with evidence of particular risk factors including: long working hours; high physical demand and risk of injury; monotony; tight deadlines; poor supervision and job insecurity.

The impact of alcohol misuse on lost productivity in the UK has been estimated at being over £7.3 billion annually with the cost of workplace hangovers between £1.2 billion and £1.4 billion (Institute of Alcohol Studies, 2019). Other organisational impacts include absenteeism; poor job performance; indiscipline; misconduct; and, increased injuries at work. The potential for serious adverse performance-related consequences are clearly evident in safety critical jobs such as transport, construction and heavy machinery.

Assessment in OH clinics will involve understanding what the issues are in regard to work performance, absence from work and whether there have been any particular incidents. The standard medical approach would be adopted looking for the accepted signs/symptoms of alcohol misuse. Clearly, the assessment should focus on obtaining an accurate picture of the person's drinking behaviour and the use of screening questionnaires may be helpful such as the following:

- CAGE brief screening questionnaire (see Table 3) (Ewing, 1984);
- Alcohol Use Disorders Identification Test (AUDIT) (WHO, 2001);
- Fast Alcohol Screening Test (FAST) (Hodgson *et al.*, 2002).

Table 3. Cage Brief Screening Questionnaire for Identifying At-Risk Drinking or Drugs Use

Each question scores 1 point and a total score of 2 or greater is considered clinically significant and would require further assessment (sensitivity of 93% and a specificity of 76% for the identification of problem drinking). The questions can also be used for drug use by substituting drinking with drug use.
C Have you ever felt you should **C**ut back on your drinking?
A Has anyone ever **A**nnoyed you by criticising your drinking?
G Have you ever felt **G**uilty about your drinking?
E Have you ever had a drink early in the morning as an **E**ye-opener?

Onward referral for assessment and treatment may be required, including use of external counselling services. Prognosis is better if individuals can remain in work and are prepared to admit to having a problem and comply with a programme of recovery. Certain types of safety critical jobs will require high standards of fitness that those with alcohol and drug misuse problems will be unlikely to satisfy. For these jobs routine and unannounced random drug and alcohol testing may be a part of the job contract. These tests may utilise breath, blood, urinary or hair samples.

Many organisations will have an alcohol and substance misuse policy that regards the problem as a combination of health, performance and disciplinary issues. These policies tend to offer support to the employee providing they are compliant. The main reasons why organisations introduce policies to help manage drug and alcohol misuse at work are: to promote safety at work; to support employee health; and because of concerns over deteriorating employee performance.

Commonly used management interventions to help employees with drug and/or alcohol problems include:

- Provision of specialist counselling services;
- Use of disciplinary procedures;
- Random/regular alcohol testing;
- Referral to OH professionals.

Out of those employees that organisations have referred for treatment or supported through rehabilitation, just over 60% remained working for the organisation after successfully managing their problem (Chartered Institute of Personnel and Development, 2007).

Case Study 9: Alcohol Misuse

Michael was 55 years old and worked as general surgeon at his local hospital. He liked his job, felt in control at work but wasn't happy with how he was feeling. Pressures in his personal finances and relationships were having an impact on his ability to cope. There were no apparent issues around his professional or clinical competence.

He presented with poor sleep, morbid thoughts and when he left work in the evenings he felt emotional, drained and negative about his domestic life including the demands of his ex-wife and how he would pay his various bills. He admitted to taking alcohol when he arrived home to steady himself. This had started some years ago as an occasional glass of spirits but had increased to three or four large measures every evening and more at the weekends. This bothered him and made him lethargic, irritable and sad. He knew he should cut down and he was annoyed when one of his children had criticised him for his drinking which made him feel guilty. He also admitted to taking some alcohol in the mornings — although he said this was when he was on holiday and not when he was working. He was clear that he had a problem and wanted help.

He was seen by an addiction psychiatrist who prescribed a short course of chlordiazepoxide to help ease his withdrawal. He was also receiving extended brief intervention therapy with an addiction counsellor. Michael had opted for total abstinence and after a period of two months was feeling better, had remained alcohol free and was still at work. He was able to deal with his finances having sought the help of a financial adviser and was more positively engaged with his family.

Alcohol problems in the workplace can be difficult to detect initially. However, in some cases a crisis will ensue and it becomes obvious that alcohol misuse has been going on for many years. Certain occupations are at a higher risk than others — and there are jobs that carry a safety critical component where alcohol is incompatible with safe working, e.g. airline pilots; train drivers; surgeons. Indeed, in the latter group there will be a fitness to practice issue. Denial is a key feature in alcohol abuse, misuse and dependency. Overcoming this and getting a willingness to admit to a problem is fundamental to a successful treatment outcome. Using a standard assessment approach including, e.g. CAGE or AUDIT screening will be beneficial. Many organisations have an alcohol policy in place to help support and rehabilitate employees who have admitted that they have a problem.

Personality Disorder

Personality is the innate and enduring characteristics of an individual which shapes their attitudes, thoughts and how they behave in response to events. In normal life there will be a variation how these are manifest from individual to individual. When these personality characteristics lead to distress and dysfunction then the diagnosis of personality disorder (PD) is made. There are problems in cognition (thoughts about self and others): Affect (emotional responses) and behaviour (interpersonal relationships, social functioning and impulse control). It will be clear that if these are extreme, intense or inappropriate then difficulties may arise in occupational settings.

PDs are classified by both ICD-10 and DSM-V for example: paranoid; schizoid; dependent; anxious; obsessive; anti-social and histrionic. These are complex issues and the difficulty, except for the extreme cases, is determining what is within the normal range of personality behaviour. Employees may be referred to OH having exhibited what might be referred to as bizarre behaviour at work. It is important to rule out other causes such as alcohol or drug misuse or psychosis. Treatment is difficult and expert advice will usually be required so that a tailored management plan can be compiled. The ability to remain in work is generally determined by the nature of the job, control of the unwanted behaviours and stability of the condition.

Stress at Work

Stress is one of the major contemporary challenges of work with around half of European workers indicating that stress is common in their workplace. In EU workplaces it contributes to almost half of all lost working days. By definition, stress occurs when the demands of the job are excessive and exceed the worker's capacity to cope with them. Among the most frequently mentioned causes of work-related stress are job reorganisation or job insecurity, long working hours, excessive workload, harassment, violence at work, and lack of involvement (EU-OSHA, 2020).

In discussing stress, it is useful to consider the psychosocial work environment which is a collective term for the work-related psychological and social influences on health — either negative or positive. Within this psychosocial work environment there are psychosocial risks which can arise from poor work design, organisation and management, as well as a poor social context of work. These in turn may result in negative psychological, physical and social consequences such as work-related stress, burnout or depression. A positive psychosocial environment enhances good performance and personal development, helping to sustain a worker's well-being (EU-OSHA, 2020). For the organisation, negative effects include poor performance, high absenteeism — which is likely to be lengthy and presenteeism and high rates of accident and injury.

Estimates of the cost to businesses and society are significant and run into billions of euros at a national level. A systematic review of published studies from Europe, Australia and Canada (Hassard *et al.*, 2018) estimated the total cost of work stress to be considerable and ranged from US$221.13 million to $187 billion. In the review, productivity related losses were observed to contribute to the majority of the total cost (between 70% and 90%), with health care and medical costs the remaining 10–30%.

Three influential models of occupational stress have established a relationship between psychosocial working conditions and health:

1. *Demand–control imbalance* — has three main dimensions: psychological demands; decision latitude, comprising two sub-scales, skill utilisation and decision authority; and social support at work from colleagues and supervisor. The combination of high levels of psychological demands and low levels of decision latitude (job strain) may increase the risk of deleterious effects on health, especially mental health. Health risks may also be increased by low levels of support (called iso-strain when combined with job strain) (Karasek, 1979).
2. *Effort–reward imbalance* — includes two dimensions: effort at work, which may be conceptually close to psychological demands, and reward in terms of esteem, job promotion and job security. These have been found, separately or combined as effort–reward imbalance, to be associated with negative mental health outcomes (Siegrist *et al.*, 1986).
3. *Organisational injustice* — refers to an employee's perception of their organisation's behaviours, decisions and actions and how these influence the employees own attitudes and behaviours at work. In other words, it is about perceptions of fairness. These perceptions can be classified into three categories: distributive (the perceived fairness

regarding a person's perceived input versus the reward obtained), procedural (the process followed to arrive at a particular outcome) and interactional (the manner in which information is communicated and the explanation given) (Greenberg, 1987).

Psychosocial Risk Management — The Management Standards

The Management Standards were developed by the UK Health and Safety Executive in 2004 to help reduce the levels of work-related stress reported by British workers (Health and Safety Executive, 2004). The approach uses an Indicator Tool — a freely available 35-item measure of exposure to seven dimensions of the psychosocial work environment that, if not properly managed, can lead to harm to employees. These dimensions include job demands, job control, managerial support, peer support, relationships, role and change. The approach has since its launch been widely used and validated (Health and Safety Executive, 2004; Health and Safety Executive, 2019). The management standards were developed from earlier work using psychosocial risk management assessment which identified a suite of major psychological hazards (Table 4) that are evident in workplaces (Cox, 1993).

The psychosocial domains addressed by the Management Standards are as follows:

Table 4. Ten Categories of Psychosocial Hazard (Adapted from Cox, 1993)

Psychosocial Hazards	Description
Job content	Lack of variety or short work cycles, fragmented or meaningless work, underuse of skills, high uncertainty, continuous exposure to people through work.
Workload and work pace	Work overload or underload, machine pacing, high levels of time pressure, continually subject to deadlines.
Work schedule	Shift working, night shifts, inflexible work schedules, unpredictable hours, long or unsociable hours.
Control	Low participation in decision making, lack of control over workload, pacing, shift working etc.

(*Continued*)

Table 4. (*Continued*)

Psychosocial Hazards	Description
Environment and equipment	Inadequate equipment availability, suitability or maintenance, poor environmental conditions such as lack of space, poor lighting or excessive noise.
Organisational culture and function	Poor communication, low levels of support for problem solving and personal development, lack of definition of, or agreement on, organisational objectives.
Interpersonal relationships at work	Social or physical isolation, poor relationships with superiors, interpersonal conflict, lack of social support.
Role in organisation	Role ambiguity, role conflict and responsibility for people.
Career development	Career stagnation and uncertainty, under-promotion or over-promotion, poor pay, job insecurity, low social value to work.
Home-work interface	Conflicting demands of work and home, low support at home, dual career problems.

1. **Demands** (workload, skills, abilities);
2. **Control** (over pace of work, development opportunities, work patterns);
3. **Support** (feedback and support from managers and between colleagues, employees are aware of support and how to access it);
4. **Relationships** (promotion of positive behaviours, avoiding conflict and dealing with unacceptable behaviour);
5. **Role** (clear and compatible requirements and responsibilities);
6. **Change** (timely consultation and support during organisational change).

The Management Standards adopted a five-step process to help employers identify the main causes of stress and stimulate practical improvements through targeted interventions. The five steps are as follows:

1. Identification of psychosocial hazards.
2. Identification of who might be harmed and how.

3. Evaluation of the risks.
4. Recording of findings.
5. Monitoring and reviewing.

The standards allow organisations to: demonstrate good practice through a step-by-step risk assessment approach; allow assessment of the current situation using pre-existing data, surveys and other techniques; promote active discussion and working in partnership with employees and their representatives; help decide on practical improvements that can be made; help simplify risk assessment for work-related stress by — identifying the main risk factors, helping employers focus on the underlying causes and their prevention, and by providing a yardstick by which organisations can gauge their performance in tackling the key causes of stress.

Case Study 10: Example of a Risk Assessment Approach

A prominent hospital in Dublin set itself the task of identifying and delivering on opportunities to improve employee wellbeing. Financial and operational commitment was secured from senior management through presentations to the Executive Committee. Other employee wellbeing stakeholders were identified and engaged with during this process. These included Occupational Health and Safety Advisors internal and external, union and employee representatives and charity partners. The importance of clear communication for the success of the project was paramount and staff and senior stakeholders were kept updated throughout via a multiplatform "cascade" communication system.

The 'Work Positive Profile,' a risk management tool developed by the Health and Safety Authority (Ireland) and Employee Wellbeing Limited (Wellhub), was chosen to assess potential risk to employee health across work domains such as; demands, control, support, role, relationships (Work Positive^{CI}, 2021). It also reports employee wellbeing levels using the World Health Organisation's WHO-Five Wellbeing Index (WHO-5) and provides benchmark scores for comparison with other Irish organisations. Staff were informed and invited to engage with the audit through various forms of communication in the hospital, such as posters, *emails, flyers at photocopiers. Confidential personal feedback was offered to each person who completed the questionnaire on their own health and well-being and the overall results were presented to the Hospital Executive Committee.*

The 'Work Positive Profile' results were considered within the context of other sources of information on employee wellbeing, including short and long term absence records, health and safety records, and results from previous attitudinal surveys. Employee age, gender, work pattern and occupational grouping were also considered. The 'Work Positive Profile' findings were generally positive and highlighted that peer support was a particular area of strength. However, a few areas of concern were also identified. Focus groups facilitated by an external consultant were used to explore underlying issues and generate suggestions and potential solutions. Focus group findings were presented to the Executive Committee.

The solution: Positive Work Environment Initiative which is a cross-functional team was created to develop, implement, evaluate, and sustain an on-going yearly Quality Improvement Plan designed to improve the health and wellbeing of employees. Survey results were summarised and disseminated to all staff alongside the new Quality Improvement Plan. By year-end a number of planned objectives had been reached including:

- *Mandatory "Dignity at Work" training for all staff members;*
- *A "Staff Recognition Showcase Day" was created to champion positive behaviours and celebrate good practice;*
- *Discussion and agreement of a "Positive Workplace Behaviour Protocol."*
- *Each employee had the opportunity to contribute and comment on a draft protocol created by the Positive Working Environment Group. This represents the behaviours that the staff identified as being most important to embed within the culture of the organisation;*
- *A "Conflict Resolution Pathway" was created and disseminated to all staff;*
- *Management training in conflict coaching was made available to senior managers.*

Staff engagement across the organisation was very high with almost 87% of staff attending training in positive workplace behaviours and contributing to the appropriate workplace behaviour protocol. A follow-up "Work Positive Profile' audit was conducted the following year. The results indicated significant improvements had been made across a number of the work domains. Employee wellbeing levels had dramatically improved and the percentage of employees at risk of anxiety or depression had dropped. Additional questions were inserted into the survey to explore employee interest in potential wellbeing initiatives for the coming year. The results of the follow-up survey, were used to create the next year's Quality Improvement Plan.

Work Engagement and Psychological Well-being

Work engagement is an approach designed to ensure that employees are committed to their organisation's goals and values, motivated to contribute to organisational success and able to enhance their own well-being. It has become increasingly popular over recent years and is considered to be an important predictor of work-related physical and psychological well-being (Green *et al.*, 2017; Oshio *et al.*, 2018; Sakuraya *et al.*, 2017).

It is characterised by high levels of personal energy, mental resilience and persistence in the face of difficulties (vigour and vitality), a sense of work significance, inspiration and enthusiasm (dedication); and being happily immersed in one's work (absorption). Work engagement is positively related to work performance (Bakker *et al.*, 2018), and positively related to job resources (the physical, psychological, social, or organisational resources an individual has to deal with job demands such as having control over one's job) and is negatively associated with sickness absenteeism, burnout and high job demands. Many business organisations worldwide collect employee survey data on work engagement as a key indicator for employee health, well-being and productivity (Bailey *et al.*, 2017).

Individual work engagement is a dynamic concept and so will vary across time and responds to changes within the business and variance in other personal external factors. Maintaining, supporting and monitoring work engagement is important and there are a number of measures with the most common tool the nine item Utrecht Work Engagement Score (UWES-9) (Schaufeli and Bakker, 2004).

Exemplar organisations recognise the importance of good employee mental and physical well-being and how that will benefit worker engagement with the organisation. At the same time, they will be aware of how negative workplace characteristics will have an adverse effect which reduces engagement with the resultant negative consequences that will have for the business and the employee's psychological well-being.

Work Embitterment

Embitterment is common in the community and so is increasingly seen in workplaces and can present in OH settings with distressed individuals who have a chronic obsessive anxiety type condition generated by a perceived sense of injustice, characterised by blame attributed to the assumed perpetrator(s) of the injustice, and a determination to seek redress (Sensky, 2020). Chronic embitterment usually presents with the embittered person perceiving themselves to have been unjustly treated and the injustice has not been satisfactorily resolved (Linden, 2003). The person's distress is usually attributed to a manager and/or the employing organisation.

In some instances, evidence may exist to show the person has been unfairly treated or on the contrary, there may be no supporting evidence at all. Regardless of the evidential nature of the condition, it is appropriate for the OH practitioner to consider how the person is coping, with the injustice itself left for others to deal with (Sensky, 2010). The condition affects the person's ability to function effectively at work and indeed in the severe chronic form they may be absent from work for prolonged periods. In addition, litigation may be instigated by the individual as a means, as they perceive it, of resolving or compensating them for their grievance.

Information about rumination, sleep disturbance, and impact on family and activities of daily living should be sought. All can be adversely impacted when the condition is severe. Assessing the individual for OCD, depression, anxiety and drug and alcohol misuse will also be useful (Sensky *et al.*, 2015). Clinical experience suggests that outcomes vary widely and are difficult to predict, although willingness to engage with interventions may be a useful indicator.

Evidence for effective interventions is lacking although for some CBT may assist as may mediation or restorative justice interventions (Linden *et al.*, 2011). Mindfulness approaches can contribute to reducing rumination and distress with injustice-resolution-focused coaching might also be beneficial.

Types of Interventions

Psychosocial risk interventions can be grouped according to the stages of prevention and their associated targets of change, namely primary-, secondary- and tertiary-level interventions.

Primary-level interventions

Primary-Level Interventions are proactive and aim to prevent exposure to occupational hazards by eliminating or reducing identified risks at source. Examples of primary-level interventions are job redesign, workload management and workforce training that focuses on preventative actions (e.g. Mental Health First Aid).

Case Study 11: Mental Health First Aid (MHFA)

Mental Health First Aid (MHFA) originated in Australia in 2000 and has been defined as: the help provided to a person developing a mental health problem or in a mental health crisis or experiencing the worsening of a mental health problem. The first aid is given until appropriate professional help is received or until the crisis resolves. This concept distinguishes the initial assistance given by a layperson from ongoing carer roles and from professional help (Morgan et al., 2018). This MHFA course is an adaptation of the first aid training model used for physical health emergencies and it covers developing mental health problems (e.g. depression, psychosis, substance misuse problems) and mental health crises (e.g. suicidal, self-injuring, exposure to a traumatic event).Over the past two decades MHFA has been taken into workplace settings globally to provide early interventions to employees experiencing mental ill-health problems in work, or as a consequence of their work.

Reviews have reported positive improvements amongst groups of workers immediately following the training and up to six months after (Booth et al., 2017; Kitchener et al., 2015; Jorm and Ross, 2018). These improvements included increased knowledge, preparedness and confidence to intervene to help others.

The objective is not to create therapists but to equip people with skills to give initial help prior to the instigation of professional help and give confidence in approaching a person in distress. MHFA can be adopted for use in organisations and businesses and is particularly relevant to line managers and supervisors.

Secondary-level interventions

Secondary-level interventions attempt to improve the employee's ability to cope with exposure to occupational stressors, or to reverse, reduce or slow the progression of ill-health caused by exposure. Secondary-level interventions are usually based around individual employee training sessions (e.g. stress management, time management, emotional resilience, work-life balance training).

Case Study 12: Emotional Resilience Training

Emotional resilience is about being able to positively deal with or adapt to an adverse event in life and be able to bounce back into normal emotional functioning and not remain trapped in negative emotions such as irritability, anxiety, aggression and depression (Luthans, 2002).

Emotional resilience is defined as the ability to generate positive emotions and recover quickly from negative emotional experiences and it is an important component of psychological resilience (Southwick, 2012; Wu et al., 2013). It has two basic elements: the ability to generate positive emotions when facing negative emotional stimuli and the ability to recover from negative emotional experiences (Davidson, 2000; Conway and McDonough, 2006).

Emotional resilience is more likely to lead to emotionally directed coping, which is related to the individual's emotional efforts in stressful situations. This adaptive mechanism restores and maintains normal emotional levels in the face of major events. Through interaction between the individual and the environment, adaptation can occur. Emotional resilience has a substantial impact on the individual's mental health and social adaptation.

Tertiary-level interventions

Tertiary-level interventions are reactive in nature and aim to minimise the negative health effects associated with chronic exposure to psychosocial risks. Examples of tertiary-level interventions include Employee Assistance Programmes, return-to-work programmes and other rehabilitative measures that provide psychological support.

Case Study 13: Employee Assistance Programme (EAP)

Many organisations have accepted the need to help their workers deal with personal and professional issues that might impact on their attendance or performance at work. Employee Assistance Programmes (EAPs) have been adapted to fulfil this role of maintaining and improving the effectiveness and health and well-being of employees.

An EAP is therefore designed to assist productivity issue and attendance issues within the workplace, and support employees to identify and resolve personal concerns that may affect job performance. These might include health, stress, emotional, family, relationship or other personal issues as well as financial, alcohol, drug and legal matters (UKEAPA, 2011). In considering an EAP, an employer will want to carry out a risk assessment of needs, what type of service delivery model best fits with the outcome of that process and what components will be required in the schedule of services and at what cost. Occupational health practitioners can play an active role in this process.

Conclusion

MHDs pose a very significant challenge to people both inside and outside of the working environment. The potential is high for adverse consequences to negatively impact on the well-being and functioning of individuals, their families and for those in employment, the businesses and organisations they work for. Greater awareness of the importance of good mental health, access to appropriate services and employment-based strategies to promote good mental health at work is a prerequisite to creating and maintaining healthy and productive workforces.

References

Agius R. (2020) Covid-19 and Health at Work. *Occup Med (Lond)* **70**(5): 349–351.

American Psychiatric Association. (2013) *Diagnostic and statistical manual of mental disorders* (Fifth Edition). Washington DC, American Psychiatric Association.

Bailey C, Madden A, Alfes K, Fletcher L. (2017) The meaning, antecedents and outcomes of employee engagement: A narrative synthesis. *Int J Manag Rev* **19**: 31–53.

Bakker AB, Albrecht S. (2018) Work engagement: Current trends. *Career Dev Int* **23**: 4–11.

Black CM. (2008) *Working for a healthier tomorrow: Dame Carol Black's review of the health of Britain's working age population.* London, The Stationery Office.

Black CM. (2016) *An independent review into the impact on employment outcomes of drug or alcohol addiction, and obesity.* London, Department for Work and Pensions.

British National Formulary. (2021) *Antidepressant drugs.* [Online] Available from: https://bnf.nice.org.uk/treatment-summary/antidepressant-drugs.html. [Accessed on 23 June 2021].

Booth A, Scantlebury A, Hughes-Morley A, Mitchell N, Wright K, Scott W, McDaid C. (2017) Mental health training programmes for non-mental health trained professionals coming into contact with people with mental ill health: A systematic review of effectiveness. *BMC Psychiatry* **17**(1): 196.

Chowdhury R, Shah D, Payal AR. (2017) Healthy worker effect phenomenon: revisited with emphasis on statistical methods – A review. *Indian J Occup Environ Med* **21**(1): 2–8.

Chartered Institute of Personnel and Development. (2007) *Managing drug and alcohol misuse at work.* [Online] Available from: https://www.cipd.co.uk/knowledge/culture/well-being/drug-alcohol-misuse-work-report. [Accessed on 23 May 2021].

Conway AM, McDonough SC. (2006) Emotional resilience in early childhood: Developmental antecedents and relations to behaviour problems. *Ann N Y Acad Sci* **1094**(1): 272–277.

Cox T. (1993) *Stress research and stress management: Putting theory to work.* Subbury, HSE Books

Davidson RJ. (2000) Affective style, psychopathology, and resilience: Brain mechanisms and plasticity. *Am Psychol* **55**(11): 1196–1214.

Drake RE. (2018) Employment and schizophrenia: Three innovative research approaches. *Schizophr Bull* **44**(1): 20–21.

EU-OSHA. (2020) *Psychosocial risks and stress at work.* [Online] Available from: https://osha.europa.eu/en/themes/psychosocial-risks-and-stress [Accessed on 23 May 2021].

Evensen S, Wisløff T, Ullevoldsæter Lystad J, Bull H, Ueland T, Falkum E. (2016) Prevalence, employment rate, and cost of schizophrenia in a high-income welfare society: A population-based study using comprehensive health and welfare registers. *Schizophr Bull* **42**(2): 476–483.

Ewing JA. (1984) Detecting alcoholism. The CAGE questionnaire. *JAMA* **252**(14): 1905–1907.

Green PI. Jr, Finkel EJ, Fitzsimons GM, GinoF. (2017) The energizing nature of work engagement: Toward a new need-based theory of work motivation. *Res Organ Behav* **37**: 1–8.

Greenberg J. (1987) A taxonomy of Organizational Justice Theories. *Acad Man Rev* **12**: 9–22.

Greenberg N. (2020) Mental health of health-care workers in the COVID-19 era. *Nat Rev Nephrol* **16**: 425–426.

Greenberg N, Docherty M, Gnanapragasam S, Wessely S. (2020) Managing mental health challenges faced by healthcare workers during covid-19 pandemic. *BMJ* **368**: m1211.

Hassard J, Teoh K, Visockaite G, Philip Dewe P, Cox, T. (2018) The cost of work-related stress to society: A systematic review. *J Occup Health Psychol* **23**(1): 1–17.

Hodgson R, Alwyn T, John B, Thom B, Smith A. (2002) The FAST Alcohol Screening Test. *Alcohol* **37**(1): 61–66.

Health and Safety Executive. (2004) *The management standards. Health and safety executive*. Sudbury, HSE Books.

Health and Safety Executive. (2019) *Tackling Work-related Stress using the management standards approach: A step-by-step workbook*. Norwich, The Stationary Office.

Institute of Alcohol Studies. (2019) *Alcohol in the workplace*. London, Institute of Alcohol Studies.

Iqbal FM, Lam K, Sounderajah V, Clarke JM, Ashrafian H, Darzi A. (2021) Characteristics and predictors of acute and chronic post-COVID syndrome: A systematic review and meta-analysis. *EClinicalMedicine* **36**: 100899. Available from: doi:10.1016/j.eclinm.2021.100899

Jorm AF, Ross AM. (2018) Guidelines for the public on how to provide mental health first aid: Narrative review. *BJPsych Open* **4**(6): 427–440.

Karasek RA. (1979) Job demands, job decision latitude, and mental strain: Implications for job design. *Admin Sci Q* **24**: 285–308.

Kinman G, Teoh K, Harriss A. (2020) Supporting the well-being of healthcare workers during and after COVID-19. *Occup Med (Lond)* **70**(5): 294–296.

Kitchener BA., Jorm AF, Kelly CM. (2015) *Mental Health First Aid International Manual*. Australia, Mental Health First Aid International.

Labour Force Survey. (2019) *Self-reported work-related ill health and workplace injuries*. [Online] Available from: https://www.hse.gov.uk/statistics/lfs/index.htm. [Accessed on 23 May 2021].

Linden M. (2003) Posttraumatic embitterment disorder. *Psychother Psychosom* **72**: 195–202.

Linden M, Baumann K, Lieberei B, Lorenz C, Rotter M. (2011) Treatment of posttraumatic embitterment disorder with cognitive behaviour therapy based on wisdom psychology and hedonia strategies. *Psychother Psychosom* **80**: 199–205.

Luthans F. (2002) The need for and meaning of positive organizational behaviour. *J Organ Behav* **23**: 695–706.

McMichael AJ. (1976) Standardized mortality ratios and the 'healthy worker effect': Scratching beneath the surface. *Occup Med (Lond)* **18**: 165–168.

Morgan AJ, Ross A, Reavley NJ. (2018) Systematic review and meta-analysis of Mental Health First Aid training: Effects on knowledge, stigma, and helping behaviour. *PLoS One* **13**(5).

National Institute of Mental Health. (2020) *Bipolar disorder*. [Online] Available from: https://www.nimh.nih.gov/health/topics/bipolar-disorder/index.shtml. [Accessed on 23 May 2021].

Oshio T, Inoue A, Tsutsumi A. (2018) Associations among job demands and resources, work engagement, and psychological distress: Fixed-effects model analysis in Japan. *J Occup Health* **60**: 254–262.

Rajkumar RP. (2020). COVID-19 and mental health: A review of the existing literature. *Asian J Psychiatr* **52**: 102066.

Sakuraya A, Shimazu A, Eguchi H, Kamiyama K, Hara Y, Namba K, Kawakami N. (2017) Job crafting, work engagement, and psychological distress among Japanese employees: A cross-sectional study. *Biopsychosoc Med* **11**: 6.

Schaufeli W, Bakker A. (2004) *Utrecht work engagement score (UWES), preliminary manual.* [Online] Available from: https://www.wilmarschaufeli.nl/publications/Schaufeli/Test%20Manuals/Test_manual_UWES_English.pdf. [Accessed on 23 May 2021].

Sensky T. (2010) Chronic embitterment and organisational justice. *Psychother Psychosom* **79**: 65–72.

Sensky T, Salimu R, Ballard J, Pereira D. (2015) Associations of chronic embitterment among NHS staff. *Occup Med* **65**: 431–436.

Sensky T. (2020) Chronic embitterment — its management in occupational health. *Occup Med (Lond)* **70**(6): 389–391.

Siegrist J, Siegrist K, Weber I. (1986) Sociological concepts in the etiology of chronic disease: The case of ischemic heart disease. *Soc Sci Med* **22**: 247–253.

Southwick SM, Charney DS. (2012) The science of resilience: Implications for the prevention and treatment of depression. *Science* **338**(6103): 79–82.

UKEAPA. (2011) *EAPs: A buyer's guide.* Derby, UK Employee Assistance Professionals Association.

United Nations. (2020) *Policy brief: COVID-19 and the need for action on mental health.* [Online] Available from: https://unsdg.un.org/resources/policy-brief-covid-19-and-need-action-mental-health. [Accessed on 23 May 2021].

Wang C, Pan R, Wan X. (2020) Immediate psychological responses and associated factors during the initial stage of the 2019 coronavirus disease (COVID-19) epidemic among the general population in China. *Int J Environ Res Public Health* **17**: 1729.

Weathers FW, Litz BT, Keane TM, Palmieri PA, Marx BP, Schnurr PP. (2013a) *The PTSD checklist for DSM-5 (PCL-5).* Vermont, USA, National Center for PTSD.

Weathers FW, Blake DD, Schnurr PP, Kaloupek DG, Marx BP, Keane TM. (2013b) *The clinician-administered PTSD scale for DSM-5 (CAPS-5).* Vermont, USA, National Center for PTSD.

WHO. (2001) *The alcohol use disorders identification test. Guidelines for use in primary care.* [Online] Available from: https://www.who.int/publications/i/item/audit-the-alcohol-use-disorders-identification-test-guidelines-for-use-in-primary-health-care. [Accessed on 23 May 2021].

WHO. (2013) *Mental health action plan 2013–2020.* [Online] Available from: https://www.who.int/publications/i/item/9789241506021. [Accessed on 23 May 2021].

WHO. (2018a) *Mental Health. Fact sheet on sustainable development goals: Health targets.* [Online] Available from: https://apps.who.int/iris/handle/10665/340847. [Accessed on 23 May 2021].

WHO. (2019a) *Disease burden, 2000–2019.* [Online] Available from: https://www.who.int/data/gho/data/themes/mortality-and-global-health-estimates/global-health-estimates-leading-causes-of-dalys. [Accessed on 23 June 2021].

WHO. (2019b) *Mental health in the workplace.* [Online] Available from: https://www.who.int/teams/mental-health-and-substance-use/mental-health-in-the-workplace. [Accessed on 23 May 2021].

Wong MCG, Poole CMJ, Agius R. (2015) Attribution of mental illness to work: A Delphi study. *Occup Med (Lond)* **65**: 391–397.

Work Positive[CI] (2021). *Work Positive[CI]*. State Claims Agency; Health and Safety Authority; Critical Incident Stress Management Network Ireland. Available from: https://www.workpositive.ie. [Accessed on 02 October 2021].

Wu G, Feder A, Cohen H, Kim JJ, Calderon S, Charney DS, Mathé AA. (2013) Understanding resilience. *Front Behav Neurosci* 7: 10.

Chapter 6

Musculoskeletal Disorders

Karen Walker-Bone[*,†] *and Jane Frølund Thomsen*[‡]

Case Study 1: Handling Frequent Pain Conditions in Strenuous Work Tasks Demands Multifaceted Measures

Several employees of a cigarette manufacturing company were referred to the local department of occupational medicine because they had taken frequent sick leave with pains in their shoulders, arms, hands, and to a lesser extent their backs. Most of the company's 350-strong workforce worked shifts, operating various machines. Two occupational physicians observed the work activities for two full days. They found that employees spent half of a typical workday at the cigarette production and packaging machines. At older machines, the workers lifted boxes weighing 5–6.5 kg on average at a frequency of twice per minute; but some of the machinery had been updated, providing a technical solution that made this unnecessary. The remainder of the day, workers stocked the machines by replacing rolls of paper or cellophane weighing 7–10 kg, and adding materials, such as bundles of

[*] MRC Versus Arthritis Centre for Musculoskeletal Health and Work, University of Southampton, UK.
[†] MRC Lifecourse Epidemiology Centre, University of Southampton, UK.
[‡] Department of Occupational and Environmental Medicine, Bispebjerg and Frederiksberg Hospital, Copenhagen, Denmark.
Corresponding author: Jane Froelund Thomsen (Jane.Froelund.Thomsen@regionh.dk).

cardboard, at an average rate of once per minute. The rolls were typically placed at or above shoulder height. The work pace was high, with a pressure to keep up with strict timelines, although the general working atmosphere was positive and supportive. The physicians concluded that several procedures posed a heightened risk of upper limb disorder, including the repeated lifting of boxes and handling of heavy rolls above shoulder level. They recommended several actions: rotation of workers to reduce the time spent in handling boxes; more frequent breaks; the repositioning of the rolls to a more suitable location; the introduction of lifting gear; and an accelerated programme of machine replacement. For affected employees they proposed temporary measures to avoid the arm-and back-straining tasks.

Commentary

The combination of biomechanical and psychosocial exposures in this production facility is not uncommon. Part of the work was repetitive, forceful, and physically demanding, as well as time-pressured, leading to an increased risk of musculoskeletal disorders; other elements of the job were similar, but because exposure levels were lower the risks were lower. Whether symptoms were caused by occupation or not in any given worker, they made certain work tasks difficult and sometimes impossible to perform. A fundamental principle of case management in such situations is to reduce biomechanical loads and psychosocial stressors through organisational and technical solutions, and other individually-applied measures. This approach can hasten recovery, reduce sickness absence and prevent job loss.

Introduction

Musculoskeletal symptoms are very common in the general population, while some specific pathologies of the musculoskeletal system, such as carpal tunnel syndrome (CTS), epicondylitis, spinal disc prolapse, and osteoarthritis and inflammatory arthritis are not uncommon. It follows that workers with musculoskeletal complaints will often feature in the clinical caseloads seen by occupational health services.

There are three main possibilities in such work-associated cases: their complaints may be caused by their work, or they may be aggravated, or they may be coincidental and neither caused nor worsened by work. Work-related musculoskeletal disorder (WMSD) is an umbrella term, normally intended to cover the first two of these possibilities. In all scenarios, however, symptoms can make work more difficult, impair productivity, and lead to sickness absence, and in this sense any musculoskeletal disorder in a worker can be considered to be "work-related." In all scenarios, occupational health services will have a duty to manage affected workers effectively, while in the first two there will be a further onus to consider prevention.

Older texts applied terminology such as "repetitive strain injury" (RSI), "occupational overuse syndrome" or "cumulative trauma disorder" for some WMSDs. These terms were used inconsistently and ambiguously and implied causation, hampering research and intervention and therefore, have become obsolete. That work can cause or aggravate musculoskeletal symptoms to an important extent is not in dispute, however; it was documented over 300 years ago (Ramazzini, 1713).

This chapter reviews a range of common work-associated musculoskeletal problems, including back and neck pain, and specific and non-specific complaints at the shoulder, elbow, hand and wrist. For each condition we offer a short account of its descriptive epidemiology, relationship to work, and clinical aspects of its diagnosis and case management in the occupational setting. Some illustrative case studies are interspersed to draw out clinical aspects of case assessment and management.

Back Pain

Case Study 2: Inflammatory Low Back Pain

A 24-year old data processor presented with low back pain and stiffness which was worst when he woke in the morning. He rated the pain as at least 7/10 in intensity on waking and this pain was associated with stiffness which went on for 2–3 hours each day. The pain radiated sometimes to the left buttock and sometimes to the right. The pain was easier at the weekends when he was able to cycle and was somewhat eased by taking

Ibuprofen. He reports that he has had the pain on and off since he was 17 years old but it is much worse over the past 6 months. He started working as a data processor 9 months ago after finishing his degree. The work is mostly desk-based and he works in a multi-user office. Physical examination revealed stiffness of lumbar motion with some tenderness of the lumbar spine and sacro-iliac joints. Magnetic Resonance Imaging (MRI) of the spine and sacro-iliac joints revealed inflammatory changes consistent with ankylosing spondylitis. He was found to have HLA B27. Rheumatological treatment with biologic drugs, combined with education and physiotherapy eased the symptoms markedly. In the workplace, an ergonomic assessment was performed to optimise his chair and workstation. He was encouraged to take hourly breaks and moved to a smaller, more private office where he could stand and stretch regularly without attracting attention. Provision was made for him to store his bicycle at work so that he could cycle to and from work and shower on arrival.

Case Study 3: Low Back Pain Aggravated by Sedentary Work

A 42-year old secretary complains of low back pain for the past one year after changing office. The pain is worse towards the end of the day and is localised to the lower portion of the back with no radiation to the lower limbs. The pain improves every day after she leaves the workplace — she has to walk about 0.5 km to get to the bus station and it takes another half an hour of bus travel to get home. Physical examination revealed a non-tender spinal column with good range of movement and no para spinal spasm. Ergonomic assessment revealed that she used a work station which was too high and her office chair had a fixed height with a soft cushion and no lumbar support. A change of office chair to one with an adjustable height, a firmer cushion with a lumbar support addressed the problem of her back pain.

Commentary

Case Study 2 describes typical inflammatory low back pain (features: worse in the morning, eased by exercise, associated with prolonged morning stiffness, alternating buttock pain, not eased by rest), in this case caused by an axial spondyloarthropathy (ankylosing spondylitis)

(Taurog *et al.*, 2016). The symptoms, whilst not caused by work, were aggravated by sedentary work.

Case Study 3 describes typical non-specific low back pain. In both cases, improving the ergonomics of the workplace and advising the individual relieved symptoms (Schonstein *et al.*, 2003).

Epidemiology, Impact and Costs

Musculoskeletal pain is common and epidemiological studies consistently suggest that the most frequently-affected anatomical site is the low back. Most people reporting low back pain will have non-specific low back pain (Maher *et al.*, 2017).

Estimates vary according to the case definition applied, but data from the global burden of disease summaries suggest that around 18% of people report low back pain at any point in time and 30% report low back pain in the past 1-month (Hoy *et al.*, 2012) and that almost everybody will have an episode of low back pain during their lifetime. Low back pain is more common in women than men and in those aged 40–69 years than in other age groups. The prevalence seems to be higher in high-income countries than middle-income or low-income countries, but does not seem to differ according to rurality.

Such is its ubiquity that low back pain is a leading cause of sickness absence, permanent work disability and years lived with disability both in developed and developing countries (Hoy *et al.*, 2014). Importantly, the number of years lived with disability caused by low back pain increased by 54% between 1990 and 2015 and low back pain is now rated as the number one cause of disability globally (Global Burden of Disease 2015 Disease and Injury Incidence and Prevalence Collaborators, 2016). Most people with a new episode of low back pain take relatively little time off work (two-thirds of those absent from work with an episode of low back pain return within a week), but one in five adults develop disabling low back pain and take many days off (10% in excess of 60 days). It has been estimated that in Western countries, low back pain costs 1–2% of gross national product annually with 80–90% of these costs attributable to productivity loss and disability (Hartvigsen *et al.*, 2018).

Evidence has accumulated to suggest that children and adolescents also commonly experience low back pain with rates of prevalence that increase with age (Swain *et al.*, 2014) and that the risk of low back pain in adulthood in substantially increased (possibly as much as two-fold) by experiencing low back pain in childhood.

Risk Factors for Low Back Pain

There is a vast epidemiological literature exploring the risk factors for low back pain, some of which is conflicting. However, there is consistent evidence of a genetic contribution to the risk of developing low back pain (particularly low back pain that is severe or disabling) (Livshits *et al.*, 2011) (estimated contribution between 21% and 67%) (Hartvigsen *et al.*, 2011). Moreover, there is evidence that pain and general ill-health increase the risk of low back pain. For example, a systematic review including eight cohort studies found consistent evidence that those with a previous episode of low back pain are at an increased risk of future episodes (Taylor *et al.*, 2014). Furthermore, people with comorbid painful (e.g. headache) (Vivekanatham *et al.*, 2019) and non-painful physical health conditions (e.g. diabetes) are also at increased risk of new back pain when compared with people without chronic health conditions (risk increased between 60% and 410% from pooled odd ratios) (Ferreira *et al.*, 2013).

There is also growing awareness that low back pain is rarely an isolated symptom and people who report low back pain, when asked, usually report pain at other anatomical sites. In one study, for example, only 16.8% of responders reported single-site pain whilst 53% reported pain at >1 site (Kamaleri *et al.*, 2008). A number of population-based studies have reported that over 50% of those studied reported multi-site pain (Garland, 2012; Blackwell *et al.*, 2014; Patel *et al.*, 2013). In the international CUPID study, people at work in 24 countries across five continents, were considerably more likely to report multi-site pain than single-site pain (Coggon *et al.*, 2013). Whilst most of the earlier literature about low back pain did not include questions about pain at other anatomical sites, there is growing evidence that reporting pain at other anatomical sites increases the risk of development of new low back pain (Yabe *et al.*, 2020), increases the likelihood of sickness absence and work disability caused by the pain (Hallman *et al.*, 2019; Fernandes and Burdorf, 2016), and increases the risk of persistence (Hallman *et al.*, 2019; Beneciuk *et al.*, 2018).

Equally, people who are pain-free but have psychological distress or other mental health conditions are at increased risk of developing low back pain. For example, in one Canadian study, pain-free people with depression had almost a 3-fold increased risk of developing low back pain over two years of follow-up when compared with people without (OR 2 · 9, 95% CI 1 · 2–7 · 0) (Currie and Wang, 2005). These relationships between comorbid health conditions and risk of low back pain are not yet understood but researchers are currently investigating shared genetic (Pinheiro *et al.*, 2018) and environmental risk factors, including for example: obesity (Zhang *et al.*, 2016), low levels of leisure-time physical activity (Shiri and Falah-Hassani, 2017) and cigarette smoking (Shiri *et al.*, 2010).

Workplace factors

Low back pain is somewhat commoner in people who have heavy manual occupations, but there is wide international variation in the prevalence of reported symptoms and the degree to which symptoms cause disability, even among workers apparently undertaking similar work. In the international CUPID study, for example, the 1-month prevalence of disabling low back pain, ascertained identically among nurses from 18 countries, varied from 9.6% to 42.6% (Coggon *et al.*, 2013).

Job type and occupational activity

Given its impact on the working-aged population, there is intense interest in the role of occupational activities in causing the symptom. However, rates of low back pain vary substantially by industry, country, occupation and job title. A range of physical exposures, including heavy lifting, forceful movements, exposure to whole-body vibration, and awkward working postures, probably underlie associations and contribute to a consistently elevated risk of back pain (Andersson, 1992; Bernard *et al.*, 1997; Louw *et al.*, 2007; Garcia *et al.*, 2014). Thus, Bigos and associates found materials handling the most common type, and improper lifting the most frequent cause of back injury in the Boeing Company (Bigos *et al.*, 1986). Klein and associates, using worker's compensation data found that "over exertions," encompassing lifting, pulling, and throwing, produced 72% of compensation claims (Klein *et al.*, 1984). Steffens and colleagues demonstrated an increased risk of incident low back pain amongst workers exposed to: heavy manual work (OR 5.0, 95% CI 3.3–7.4); awkward postures (OR 8.0, 95% CI 5.5–11.8); who were feeling tired (OR 3.7, 95% CI 2.2–6.3) or who were distracted whilst performing a work task (OR 25.5, 95% CI 3.4–184.5) (Steffens *et al.*, 2015). Frequent lifting of objects weighing more than 10 kg, sudden maximal effort that is unexpected, lifting heavy objects held away from the body, and failing to bend at the knees when lifting are other actions associated with increased risks of low back pain (Lee *et al.*, 2001). In one meta-analysis, a summary prevalence odds ratio of 1.98 (95% confidence intervals 1.56–2.50) was found for low back pain in the past 12 months in 24 groups of professional drivers exposed to whole-body vibration when compared with unexposed controls (administrative officers, manual workers and maintenance operators) (Palmer and Bovenzi, 2015), while in a prospective study of professional drivers, new occurrence of low back symptoms could be related to modeled internal forces of vibration acting upon the spine (Bovenzi *et al.*, 2015).

Combinations of adverse physical exposures, like lifting and awkward posture, probably carry even higher risks. In one study (Kelsey *et al.*, 1984), risks of lumbar disc prolapse were elevated in workers who lifted while twisting their body (versus those avoiding lifting in these circumstances), more so when their knees were straight (relative risk (RR) 6.1) than when bent (RR 2.7).

Importantly, workers from manual occupations have significantly greater sickness absence during back pain episodes. They also have higher rates of disability pensioning, some 4.4–6.5-fold higher in one longitudinal survey based on a 10% sample of the Finnish workforce

(Polvinen *et al.*, 2014). Certain occupations (Elders and Burdorf, 2001), particularly truck driving, nursing (Waehrer *et al.*, 2005), firefighting (Walton *et al.*, 2003) and materials-handling jobs, have been reported to have higher rates of disability from back pain.

Despite these findings, there is currently insufficient evidence to suggest that any one occupational activity has a strong causal link with low back pain when the epidemiological evidence is judged against the Bradford-Hill criteria (Kwon *et al.*, 2011). Moreover, the results of population studies tend to suggest that the overall contribution of physical workplace factors to the burden of back pain and its resultant disability are relatively small (of the order of 10–20%).

Workplace psychosocial factors

Occupational psychosocial risk factors for low back pain include job dissatisfaction, poor relationships with colleagues and/or supervisors, job monotony/repetitiveness, high workplace psychological demands, and poor social support at work (Linton, 2000). Significant associations have also been reported for: job strain (Sitthipornvorakul *et al.*, 2011; Janwantanakul *et al.*, 2012); work-family imbalance (OR 1.27, CI 1.15–1.41); exposure to a hostile work environment (or bullying) (OR 1.39, CI 1.25–1.55); job insecurity (OR 1.44, CI 1.24–1.67); and, in younger and female workers, long working hours (Yang *et al.*, 2016). However, as with occupational physical factors, a strong causal link has not yet been established and, in population studies, the overall contribution of adverse psychosocial factors to the burden would appear to be relatively small.

Aetiology

Back pain is a symptom (like dizziness or dysphagia) and not a diagnosis. As with other symptoms, it can have many causes. However, in the majority of cases (at least 85–90%) no specific underlying pathoanatomical cause can be identified. Prior to access to modern imaging techniques, symptoms have been ascribed to pathologies such as: degenerative disc disease, intervertebral disc prolapse, and disc rupture; but imaging studies have shown that such pathology can commonly be detected in the absence of symptoms. Non-specific low back pain is diagnosed in the absence of any other pathoanatomical cause being identified. Current management strategies rely upon a triage-based approach to exclude the rarer pathoanatomical causes and then focus on symptom management and reassurance.

Clinical Presentation

Low back pain can present as: (1) an acute episode or (2) chronic back pain with episodes of acute exacerbation.

In occupationally-related cases, acute onset may follow lifting or pulling activities, and pain may be experienced immediately, often increasing in severity over a few hours. The individual complains of stiffness in the back, and may have an abnormal posture due to muscular spasm. Pain may radiate down one or both legs but does not usually radiate below the knee in non-specific low back pain. More commonly, the onset of back pain is gradual, without any history of a specific injury or precipitating event. Back pain typically comes on when the person sits or stands for some time, when he does lifting or pulling activities, or when working for any length of time in specific postures, e.g. crouching or squatting. The symptoms are typically reduced or relieved by rest (especially over weekends or periods of annual leave). There is often a previous history of intermittent low back pain. There may be referral of pain to the lower limbs but typically not below the knee.

Case Study 4: Non-Specific Low Back Pain

A 45-year old male worker in a sofa factory reports increasing right-sided low back pain which started approximately 3 weeks ago and is gradually increasing in intensity. He rates the intensity as 2/10 when he wakes up in the morning and 7–8/10 when he finishes his shift at work. The pain does not wake him at night but does cause some discomfort down the back of his right thigh as far as the knee when it is at its most intense. He has no neurological symptoms and is otherwise well. Examination reveals some tenderness of the para-vertebral muscles to the right side, and some stiffness of right sided lateral flexion and right sided rotation but straight leg raise elicits no exacerbation and no neurological signs can be found.

At work, he reports that he has been working on a new task for 2–3 months, which involves leaning forward and to the right every 2 minutes to screw a fitting into the sofa frame. He is the only employee completing this task on the factory line. An occupational health review of him working confirms that the occupational task is requiring intense bending and twisting to the right side and then sustaining of this posture, every 2 minutes. It is clear that this new task needs re-design so that the sofa is re-positioned, not the worker. The help of the worker and his line manager is sought to re-design his workstation so that the task can be performed in a neutral posture. 6 weeks later, the worker reports complete resolution of his symptoms and high satisfaction with having been given chance to help develop the solution.

Commentary

This history is very suggestive of non-specific low back pain and the history and examination are reassuring. A clear relationship in terms of time is seen with the new occupational task and symptoms are better before work and worse after work.

Case Study 5: Prolapsed Inter-Vertebral Disc

A 26-year old brick-layer reports a sudden onset of severe low back pain associated with bilateral leg pain. The pain started suddenly when he was bending forward to pour cement. He describes the pain as 10/10 in intensity since it started and he feels nauseated and sweaty with the pain. The leg pain is also severe and associated with numbness of both feet. Assessment reveals that he is in such severe pain that he undresses with difficulty, attempts to undertake a straight leg raise elicit a severe exacerbation of the symptoms down both legs. Saddle anesthesia is demonstrated to light touch and pinprick. He cannot remember when he last emptied his bladder but says that he does not feel he needs to pass urine. Abdominal examination reveals an enlarged bladder.

Commentary

This history is highly suggestive of a large acute central prolapsed inter-vertebral disc (the presentation is not always so dramatic). The greatest concern is that there is bladder motor dysfunction and saddle anesthesia, suggesting significant lower lumbar cord compromise. Therefore, this man should be sent to the Emergency Department for urgent MRI scanning and possibly emergency surgery.

Assessment and Investigation

As work limitation from low back pain is commonplace, occupational physicians will often see patients with back-associated sickness absence. In doing so, they will need to follow modern guidance and think in terms of triage, aiming to identify the few with severe pathology from the many with non-specific low back pain (Palmer and Greenough, 2013).

A thorough history should include the following questions (the answers to which should be recorded):

- What were you doing when the pain first started?
- Did the pain come on suddenly or gradually?
- Where do you feel the pain, and does it affect anywhere else?
- What is the pain like: sharp, dull, heavy, burning?
- Is the pain constant?
- What positions or movements aggravate the pain, or relieve it?
- Do you feel any patches of numbness or pins and needles?
- Have you had any similar attacks before?
- Have you noticed any change in the control of your bladder or bowels?

Characteristically, non-specific low back pain presents at ages 20–55 years, is confined to the lumbosacral area, buttocks and thighs, is mechanical in nature (varying with activity and time) and occurs in a patient who otherwise appears well. From the history, "red flags" which are indicators of possible serious spinal pathology, are shown below (Waddell, 2004):

- Age at onset <20 or >55 years;
- Constant progressive pain;
- Thoracic pain;
- Pain eased by activity and increased by rest (inflammatory back pain);
- Recent acute trauma (e.g. fall or road traffic accident);
- History of previous malignancy;
- History of treatment with oral corticosteroids;
- Likelihood of immunosuppression (HIV, biological therapy, chemotherapy);
- Structural deformity of the spine;
- Features of cauda equina syndrome; and
- A patient who appears systemically unwell (e.g. with weight loss, fever, night sweats).

"Yellow flags" are factors in the history which may be associated with an increased risk of chronicity and are also worth considering:

- How do you rate your own health? (Poor self-rated health increases the risk);
- History of psychological stress and/or depression?
- Disproportionate illness behaviour?
- Job dissatisfaction?
- Are there any ongoing personal problems: alcohol, marital, financial? (poorer prognosis);
- Any adversarial medico-legal proceedings associated with the back pain? (again poorer prognosis).

Examination should focus on the triage elements:

- Is there any visible spinal deformity?
- How is movement of the spine (including thoracic spine rotation) and lumbar spine (lateral flexion and flexion/extension) motion?
- Is there focal tenderness in a vertebral body (can be suggestive of osteoporotic fracture)?
- What happens with a straight leg raise?
- Are there any detectable neurological signs in the lower limbs?

For most patients, investigations including radiography, magnetic resonance imaging, and computed tomography are not indicated and may be harmful (Clinical Standards Advisory Group, 1994). As well as exposing patients to radiation, over-investigation has the downside of misattributing symptoms and focussing attention on physical causes in circumstances where bio-psychosocial management of symptoms may be more effective (Waddell, 2004). However, in the presence of any red flags in the history or examination, appropriate investigation is indicated and referral to orthopaedics or rheumatology may be appropriate.

Treatment

Non-operative

An episode of acute non-specific low back pain that has lasted for less than six weeks should be treated with education, reassurance, analgesics, minimal rest, early mobilisation as pain allows and an early return to work. Patients should be advised that "bed rest is harmful," despite discomfort, it is much better for their recovery if they remain mobile. People should not be given the impression that they need to be 100% pain free to be able to resume their normal activities or their work.

The vast majority of episodes of low back pain are not serious, and most workers are able to follow this advice and return to work within a short time. In some situations, as when work requires exceptional levels of fitness or is very arduous, a return to full normal duties may not be possible in the short-term. Return to work can be facilitated by a period of lighter duties, with restrictions, for example, on repeated bending, stooping and twisting; activities should be modified, both to allow early return and to minimise the risk of prolonged disability (Johnston *et al.*, 2003; Schonstein *et al.*, 2003; Irwin *et al.*, 2007).

Any restriction of duties should subsequently be reviewed, as reports exist of situations in which they were never lifted (Hiebert *et al.*, 2003). A positive approach by employers to the rehabilitation process and availability of lighter work during convalescence will increase the probability of a successful return to work (Johnston *et al.*, 2003; Schonstein *et al.*, 2003; Irwin *et al.*, 2007).

Resolution of acute symptoms can be expected in nine out of 10 patients within 4–6 weeks. The longer a worker stays away from work, the less likely they are to return to the workforce. Workers with back complaints who are away from work for over 6 months have only a 50% chance of ever returning to work. If they are off work for over 1 year, this probability drops to 25% and if they are away for more than 2 years it is almost zero (Schonstein *et al.*, 2003). Thus, workers still absent at the subacute stage (say six weeks) require a review (for red and yellow flags) and should be actively supported towards a rehabilitation programme, perhaps involving appointment of a case manager and a multidisciplinary care package (Van Tulder *et al.*, 2000; Carroll *et al.*, 2010; National Institute for Health and Clinical Excellence, 2009).

Occupational Health workers should be aware of the STarT Back algorithm for the assessment and triage of cases of low back pain. This evidence-based approach has shown cost-effectiveness and clinical effectiveness in primary care in the UK for the triage of acute low back pain (Hill *et al.*, 2011). Application of a freely-available 9-point clinical assessment tool allows separation of primary care patients into groups by risk of chronicity (low-risk, medium-risk, high-risk). Low-risk patients can be effectively treated with a brief advice/education intervention; medium-risk patients receive the same advice/education but also some physiotherapy and high-risk patients receive the same as both groups above but also psychologically-informed physiotherapy to focus on symptoms/function and address obstacles to recovery with a cognitive behavioural approach.

Surgery

Surgery is not required for the vast majority of low back pain patients. Amongst patients with severe radiculopathy and evidence of a lumbar disc prolapse, discectomy (microdiscectomy, endoscopic microdiscectomy, or laminectomy/laminotomy with discectomy) may be offered to patients, aiming to relieve nerve root compression (Jacobs *et al.*, 2011). For severe low back pain caused by degenerative disc disease, spinal fusion has been the principal operative intervention but remains controversial with limited evidence of effectiveness in systematic reviews (Bydon *et al.*, 2014) and an increased risk of disease in adjacent segments post-operatively (Lee and Choi, 2015). Lumbar total disc replacements have been practised since the 1980s but this procedure has been slow to gain popularity amongst spinal surgeons, partly because it is a difficult procedure to bring safely to a department (with logistical, financial and regulatory challenges). However, the evidence suggests that it may be non-inferior to spinal fusion, less expensive and retain lumbar range of motion with the possibility that it is less likely to cause disease at adjacent segments (Beatty, 2018). Unfortunately, there are few data regarding return to work after spinal surgery and surgeons seem to make different recommendations. However, in principle, the operative treatment and post-operative follow-up should be the same in workers as for the general population (Hodges *et al.*, 2001; Irwin *et al.*, 2007), although in some circumstances the rehabilitation period may be longer. Recovery times tend to be poorer in cases involving an industrial accident or a compensation claim (Hodges *et al.*, 2001).

Prevention of Low Back Pain

In an ideal world all back pain would be preventable. In practice, however, since the symptom is almost ubiquitous in most settings, this is an unrealistic goal. At work, the aim should be to reduce the frequency and severity of acute episodes, reduce the contribution that occupational activity makes to exacerbations of back pain and tackle factors that are likely to perpetuate disability.

Better ergonomics and use of mechanical aids to eliminate or limit manual handling (Snook *et al.*, 1978; Bigos *et al.*, 1992; Ijmker *et al.*, 2007), training in manual handling techniques, reorganisation of work schedules to ensure a more even distribution of hazardous tasks between employees (Stobbe, 1996; Zuhosky *et al.*, 2007; Irwin *et al.*, 2007) and job matching all have a role. Changing the height of workbenches, reducing the weight or size of objects being manipulated and altering the position or mechanics of machinery or tools are other measures which can make the workplace more "back-friendly"

(Stobbe, 1996; Schonstein *et al.*, 2003). Where low back pain is linked with professional driving, the magnitude, duration, and pattern of exposure to whole-body vibration can be reduced by, for example, vehicle design with improved cabin seating and suspension, as well as avoidance of rough uneven surfaces, moderation of vehicle speeds to suit road conditions and taking of sufficient rest breaks (Palmer and Bovenzi, 2015).

Whilst it is ethical and best health and safety practice to advocate a preventive package informed by proper risk assessment, underpinned by management systems for monitoring and enforcement, and based on elements such as good training, an induction period, job rotation, rest breaks and task optimisation, it is dispiriting that the evidence from randomised controlled trials for the effectiveness of ergonomic interventions is disappointing. In a recent systematic review, Sundstrup and colleagues found insufficient evidence from the literature to guide current practices in workplace ergonomics to reduce the risk of musculoskeletal disorders amongst employees undertaking physically-demanding work (Sundstrup *et al.*, 2020). Moreover, their review found strong evidence for no benefit of participatory ergonomics, multifaceted interventions, and stress management to reduce the risk. Hearteningly however, they did find evidence that implementing strength training at the workplace can reduce the risk of musculoskeletal disorders, including low back pain (Sundstrup *et al.*, 2020).

A more fundamental issue in preventing back pain and its consequences is that these are not only caused by mechanical factors in the work environment. Thus, while manipulating the physical environment can be very important, it will not necessarily eliminate new back pain episodes. A further issue to consider is that careless interventions carry the inadvertent potential to make some aspects of the problem worse. Theoretically, for example, since personal beliefs appear capable of influencing symptom chronicity and illness behaviour, undue focus on the harms of work could in extremis foster beliefs that worsen prognosis rather than improve it (Coggon, 2005). A more empirical caution is provided by one randomised controlled trial in which a series of ergonomic interventions resulted in higher rates of job dissatisfaction, mental stress and poor co-worker relations in the target group than in the control group (Haukka *et al.*, 2010).

Upper Limb Disorders

Case Study 6: When Psychosocial and Organisational Factors may Influence the Pain Experience

A large department of radiology introduced a new imaging system. The system did not work well. Instead of the doctor dictating the report to a secretary, a speech recognition system was built in. It was slow, demanded many more "clicks" and often the spoken words were not properly understood and therefore the doctor had to keep a constant eye on and correct the text. They used three screens, one for the images they were describing, one for former images for comparison and one for the text. Thus, their work demanded high concentration and precision. At the same time, there had been an increasing number of examinations. As a result, the doctors were unable to manage their workload within the scheduled time and worked constantly 1–2 hours extra every day. They tried to raise the issue at department meetings but felt not heard at all. The tone at the workplace was quite harsh, both top-down and between colleagues. A substantial number of the doctors developed non-specific pain conditions in the neck, shoulders, arms and hands and some suffered from palpitations, fatigue and sleep disturbances because of worries about their work. After improvements of the system with regard to response times and speech recognition, temporary "export" of some of the X-ray descriptions to a telemedical centre, introducing the possibility of choosing suitable keyboards and pointing devices, and the management addressing the psychosocial aspects of the work environment with a dialogue-based approach, conditions improved.

Commentary

The case illustrates the many-faceted problems that sometimes accompany the introduction of new technology. It highlights the focus on not just the ergonomic challenges but also the combination of organisational issues, highly skilled and responsible work and the importance of an open and involving dialogue. In Case Study 6, the operators of the new system developed some typical work-associated upper limb symptoms and disorders. In the following, the more frequently occurring conditions will be addressed.

Neck Pain

Epidemiology and Risk Factors

Neck pain is a very commonly reported and persistent symptom in the general population. In a British population survey involving some 13,000 adults of working age, 34% reported neck pain in the past 12 months, 11% reported symptoms that had interfered with their everyday activities over the period, and 20% had had symptoms in the past week (Palmer *et al.*, 2001). A review of other studies places the prevalence of chronic neck pain at about 14% to 23% (Palmer and Smedley, 2007). This is in line with a more recent Norwegian, population-based study of 12,250 working respondents showing a prevalence of 16.9% with neck/shoulder pain (Sterud *et al.*, 2014). The incidence of cervical disc herniation (CDH) or radiculopathy varies considerably, ranging from 10.7 to 176 per 100.000 person-years, with a peak incidence in the fifth decade and a tendency of an increased risk for females (Wong JJ *et al.*, 2014; Mansfield *et al.*, 2020).

Neck pain shows an increasing trend with age and is more common and more persistent in women (Palacios-Ceña *et al.*, 2021). Other non-occupational associations with chronic neck pain include smoking, low educational level, unemployment, obesity, local injury, pain at other bodily sites and poor mental health (Palmer and Smedley, 2007).

Early studies showed considerable associations between highly repetitive work with a static flexed position of the neck, e.g. in sewing machine operators (Andersen *et al.*, 1993). In a detailed review, "some evidence" was identified on positive relations with neck flexion, forceful use of the arm, arm posture, prolonged sitting, twisting or bending of the trunk, and hand-arm vibration, while noting some limitations in the evidence base (Ariëns *et al.*, 2000). Another review found reasonable evidence that repeated shoulder movements and neck flexion were associated with neck pain with tenderness (Palmer and Smedley, 2007). Likewise, a prospective study of 12,550 respondents in paid work found that neck flexion and lifting in awkward postures were associated with developing moderate to severe neck pain during the three year follow up period, controlled for neck pain at baseline (Sterud *et al.*, 2014). Several occupational risk factors such as static load, whole body vibration, dynamic movements, G-forces or extreme positions have been suggested for cervical disc herniation. However, none of these have been confirmed as causal factors (Zielinska *et al.*, 2021) As with low back pain, psychological and psychosocial factors (high work pressure, monotonous work and low leadership support) are consistently associated with neck and neck/shoulder pain (Sterud *et al.*, 2014; Green *et al.*, 2018)

Clinical Presentation

The most common clinical complaint is pain in the neck with tightness and pain in the shoulders and interscapular region. This has been labeled "postural neck pain," "fibrositis," "tension neck" or in many other ways (Palmer and Smedley, 2007). Patients who have postural neck pain usually have some restriction of neck movement and tenderness in their neck, shoulder or interscapular muscles.

Occasionally, the pain can be radicular in nature; usually radiating down one arm to the fingers following a dermatomal distribution. This is usually associated with numbness. In these cases, there may be nerve root compression due to nerve impingement by osteophytes in the neural foramina or to a cervical disc herniation. Careful neurological examination can help to localise the level of involvement.

Investigation

Laboratory and other tests are generally not recommended. Radiology tends to reveal degenerative changes (e.g. loss of disc height, osteophytosis of vertebral bodies, and osteoarthritis in nearby zygapophyseal joints and other articulating surfaces) in most adults aged over

30 years, whether symptomatic or not (Lawrence, 1969). Nonetheless, radiographs or MRI images of the cervical spine may be informative in cases with evidence of nerve root or spinal cord compression and may then be clinically indicated.

Management

Van Tulder *et al.* (2007) reviewed studies for treatment of neck pain in the workplace setting and found exercise therapy to be most beneficial. This could be supplemented by non-steroidal anti-inflammatory drugs.

Multidisciplinary biopsychosocial rehabilitation has also been advocated, as well as specific exercise programmes involving strength and endurance training, muscle training, stretching, and relaxation (although with limited evidence at present to justify the effort). In case of a cervical disc herniation and persistent symptoms, evaluation by a neurosurgeon may be relevant.

Fortunately, serious underlying causes of neck pain are rare. Therefore, symptomatic relief and advice to remain active appears to be a sensible pragmatic approach, likely in most cases to be followed by an early return to work. It may help in reducing symptoms if frequent change of position (sitting, standing, walking) and pauses with light exercises are possible during the workday.

The Shoulder

Musculoskeletal disorders of the shoulders are important and frequent health problems in the working population, with considerable impact on sickness absence, healthcare seeking and withdrawal from the labour market (Larsson *et al.*, 2007; van Rijn *et al.*, 2010). Prevalence rates in the general population vary considerably, depending on case definitions. In a study from general practice, the incidence of new cases of shoulder pain was 11.2 per 1,000 person–years (Van der Windt *et al.*, 1995).

In the occupational setting, the relevant shoulder disorders are those of a degenerative origin. As an overarching diagnostic term for disorders occupying the subacromial space, the subacromial impingement syndrome includes non-traumatic shoulder disorders such as the rotator cuff syndrome, biceps tendinitis, acromio-clavicular arthrosis, and frozen shoulder (also known as periarthrosis humeroscapularis or adhesive capsulitis) but others also (Michener *et al.*, 2003). It has been difficult to differentiate between these diagnostic entities in epidemiological studies. The rotator cuff syndrome is the most extensively examined disorder and for this entity the evidence for a causal relationship to several occupational factors is substantial. The prevalence in the general population of subacromial impingement syndrome is reported to be 2–8% (Roquelaire *et al.*, 2006). The prevalence of first-time surgery for subacromial impingement syndrome was 1–2 per 1,000 working age people (Svendsen *et al.*, 2012).

Individual risk factors for rotator cuff syndrome include age, low socioeconomic status, shoulder intensive sports, prior shoulder injury and insulin-dependent diabetes mellitus. Gender is not, or only weakly, associated with the syndrome (van der Molen *et al.*, 2017).

Rotator Cuff Syndrome

Definition and clinical picture

The rotator cuff syndrome is a clinical syndrome characterised by shoulder pain originating from the rotator cuff tendons and adjacent bursae. The condition may be due to bursitis, tendinitis and degenerative tendinosis with partial or complete tears of the rotator cuff tendons, especially of the supraspinatus tendon. A suggested mechanism may be impairment of tendon blood flow due to increased intramuscular pressure during work with the arms elevated or carrying heavy loads (Palmerud *et al.*, 2000).

The main complaints are pain localised to the anterolateral upper part of the arm and limitation of shoulder movements due to pain, especially in mid-range of abduction (approximately 60–120 degrees, also known as "painful arc"). The pain may radiate to the hand and fingers and may disturb sleep at night.

Clinically, typical findings are palpation tenderness at the insertion of the supraspinatus tendon on the greater tuberosity of the humerus, anterolateral pain provoked by resisted movements, especially outward rotation and abduction, and a positive impingement test (inward rotation of the upper arm when abducted or flexed to 90 degrees (Hawkins' test)). Passive range of motion is normal, although this may be difficult to assess due to pain. Normal passive outward rotation distinguishes the condition from frozen shoulder. If rotator cuff lesions are severe, muscle weakness may be detected upon resisted abduction and outward rotation, and atrophy of the supraspinatus and infraspinatus muscles may be visible.

X-ray of the shoulder (out-let view) is used to visualise the subacromial space. Ultrasonography and magnetic resonance imaging are used to assess soft tissue changes (partial and especially total supraspinatus tears, tendinitis and bursitis) and dynamic ultrasonography may assess impingement (Lenza *et al.*, 2013).

Differential diagnoses include arthrosis of the shoulder joint and acromioclavicular joint, shoulder instability, cervical nerve root compression and other nerve disorders, referred pain from conditions in the neck and chest, frozen shoulder, bursitis calcarea and non-specific pain conditions in the shoulder-neck regions.

There are no generally agreed diagnostic criteria for the clinical diagnosis. However, many doctors would consider rotator cuff syndrome to be diagnosed in a case with long lasting function-related shoulder pain, a positive impingement test, anterolateral shoulder pain upon resisted shoulder movements, and after exclusion of differential diagnoses.

Occupational risk factors

The prevalence of rotator cuff syndrome has been found to be two to five times higher in occupations involving highly repetitive work, forceful exertions and working with the hands above shoulder height than in comparison groups without these exposures (Linaker and Walker-Bone, 2015). Occupations with an increased prevalence of the syndrome include assembly line workers in food production and fish processing, welders in shipyards, sewing machine operators and slaughter house workers (Van Rijn *et al.*, 2010; van der Molen *et al.*, 2017). The work-relatedness of rotator cuff syndrome has been further supported by studies showing quantitative exposure-response relations, based on objective measures of exposure (Dalboge *et al.*, 2014; Svendsen *et al.*, 2004; Dalbøge *et al.*, 2020) and of diagnostic outcomes, such as MRI-diagnosed alterations in the supraspinatus tendon (Svendsen *et al.*, 2004) or surgery for subacromial impingement syndrome (Svendsen *et al.*, 2013). Among psychosocial factors, high psychosocial job demands have been associated with rotator cuff syndrome (Van Rijn *et al.*, 2010; van der Molen *et al.*, 2017). However, perceived job demands may also reflect high physical workloads (e.g. fast pace of work).

Treatment of the patient in the occupational setting

Case Study 7: Treatment of the Patient in the Occupational Setting

A 40-year old airport baggage handler was responsible for moving suitcases with an average weight of 15 kg, in total around 5 tonnes of baggage per day. Work positions were very awkward owing to the confined spaces of air craft baggage compartments. He had to lift, push and pull the baggage, often with his upper arm flexed or abducted. He had worked in the job for five years. He presented with right shoulder pain during the last six months. Initially, the pain was intermittent and felt at the time of exertion, but gradually it became more chronic to the point where it was aggravated by elevating the arm without lifting loads. Otherwise he felt in good health and had no other symptoms.

The pain was located to the anterolateral part of his right shoulder, and on palpation he was tender on the greater tuberosity of the humerus. He had difficulty abducting his right arm owing to pain, and his pain was aggravated by resistance. The impingement test was positive. The condition was diagnosed as a rotator cuff syndrome. His work conditions were considered to be a likely cause of the disorder, considering his (young) age and no other obvious risk factors or pathology.

He was recommended a period of arm rest with sick leave for a couple of weeks. He was prescribed a nonsteroidal anti-inflammatory drug (NSAID) and was referred to physiotherapy for a shoulder exercise programme. He was further encouraged to contact the occupational health service of his workplace and his superior to ask for help in reducing his arm-straining duties. This was possible for some months and his shoulder symptoms gradually subsided. However, he was finally fired because he would not go back to his old work for fear of recurrence. This was also his doctor's advice.

His doctor notified the body regulating national health and safety to prevent other new cases. There were some meetings and plans were developed for load reduction, but nothing really happened because it was difficult and costly to change the usual baggage handling systems. His doctor also notified his patient to the workers compensation system regarding occupational diseases. The case was recognised as an occupational disease.

Nonsteroidal anti-inflammatory drugs (NSAID) are effective in the treatment of acute shoulder pain. Intra-articular steroid injection has a moderate short term effect on shoulder pain, but this effect is not superior to that of NSAID treatment (Buchbinder *et al.*, 2003). In recent decades, arthroscopic subacromial decompression has increased dramatically as a treatment for rotator cuff-related shoulder disorders (Svendsen *et al.*, 2012). However, randomised controlled follow-up studies have shown that structured training is just as effective as surgery after 12 months (Haahr *et al.*, 2005), 4–8 years (Haahr *et al.*, 2006) and five years (Ketola *et al.*, 2013; Karjalainen *et al.*, 2019). Indications for surgery in subgroups are uncertain (Ketola *et al.*, 2015). Structured exercise treatment, therefore, seems to be the treatment of choice for shoulder impingement syndrome (Ketola *et al.*, 2013).

Rotator cuff syndrome may have a fairly poor prognosis. Recovery is often protracted and may take several years, while some cases become chronic. In a Danish longitudinal study, approximately 10% of cases with surgery became permanently work disabled (Svendsen *et al.*, 2012). Therefore, careful evaluation of work function is important and advice and support is needed in order to maintain a job.

Biceps Tendinitis

Biceps tendinitis often coexists with rotator cuff tendinitis and is considered to be part of the subacromial impingement syndrome. The long biceps tendon may also become impinged between the head of the humerus and the scapular acromial structures. The symptoms are anterior shoulder pain aggravated by resisted elbow flexion and resisted supination of the forearm (Yergason's test). The condition is less frequent than rotator cuff tendinitis. Treatment and management are the same as for rotator cuff syndrome.

Acromio-Clavicular Arthrosis

Arthrosis of the acromio-clavicular joint is often asymptomatic but may cause local shoulder pain and tenderness, especially on adduction of the arm in the cross-over test (hand on opposite shoulder with elbow in shoulder height). Osteophytes from the arthritic joint may cause subacromial impingement. Risk factors are age and shoulder accidents. There is limited evidence that the condition is caused by physical exposure. Diagnosis is based on symptoms and clinical findings, supplemented with radiology if this is necessary for differential diagnosis and treatment.

Frozen Shoulder

Frozen shoulder is a popular term for adhesive capsulitis, also known as periarthrosis humeroscapularis. The condition is caused by capsular fibrosis and is characterised by pain and progressive stiffness with restricted movements in all directions. The condition can be ruled out if outward rotation is normal. The cause of the development of capsular fibrosis is unknown. There is no evidence that the condition is caused by physical exposure. Treatment with intra-articular steroid combined with physiotherapy may improve the condition, but evidence on this is limited (Maund *et al.*, 2012). Workloads should be adjusted to the capacity of the patient.

Pain in the Elbow and Forearm

Lateral and Medial Epicondylitis

Case definition and clinical features

In lateral and medial epicondylitis, the tendons of the extensor and flexor muscles of the wrist are affected. This results in localised pain caused by degeneration or inflammation of the tendons at the lateral and medial epicondyle. The disorder is diagnosed clinically and characterised by pain in the elbow region and tenderness when the epicondyle is palpated and pain elicited when the hand performs a resisted dorsi-flexion (the lateral epicondyle) or palmar flexion (the medial epicondyle) (Harrington *et al.*, 1998; Yoon *et al.*, 2019)

Prevalence and individual risk factors

Men and women are affected equally. Lateral epicondylitis is more common than medial epicondylitis, but the two conditions often co-exist (Shiri *et al.*, 2011). In the general population, the prevalence of the former is 1–4% and that of the latter is 0.3–1.1% (Shiri *et al.*, 2011). In working populations, estimates vary considerably, from 0.3% to 13.5% for lateral epicondylitis and 0.2% to 3.8% for medial epicondylitis. These differences in prevalence arise from use of different case definitions. High prevalence is found if the case definition only includes self-reported pain and tenderness when palpating the epicondyle whereas also demanding pain elicited with resisted flexion reduces the prevalence considerably (Yoon *et al.*, 2019).

Many cases of epicondylitis occur spontaneously without obvious aetiology. The condition is more prevalent in older age groups and most prevalent between 40 and 60 years of age.

Occupational risk factors

As in other upper limb disorders related to work, the prominent factors suspected of causing epicondylitis are repetitive movements of the extensor and the flexor tendons in the wrist and the use of force, alone or in combination, and elbow posture. Several difficulties exist in determining the work-relatedness of lateral and medial epicondylitis, among which exposure definition is the most challenging. Most studies have used self-reported measures of exposure, but these may be biased by the health status of the individual (affected individuals perhaps recalling their exposures more fully or perceiving them to be higher). Recent studies have defined groups not by job title but by the degree of repetition and forcefulness and arm postures in their work.

The most consistent risk factors linked to epicondylitis have been the exertion of force and force in combination with repetitive movements of the wrist (Fan *et al.*, 2014; Haahr and Andersen, 2003a; Herquelot *et al.*, 2013). However, associations have also been found with repetitive bending of the elbow or hand (Descatha *et al.*, 2013; Walker-Bone *et al.*, 2012)

Although the designs and sample sizes of studies have improved over time, there are still considerable challenges in establishing causal associations. Lack of objectivity in assessment of exposures is compounded by reliance on self-reported symptoms, rather than clinical outcomes.

Treatment of the patient in the occupational setting

Case Study 8: The Highly Skilled Worker: Sometimes A Little Extra Is Needed

A 47-year old plasterer had worked for many years in a company making stucco in buildings of preservation value. Work tasks included making plaster casts of existing stuccos, with sizes varying from huge to very small. Part of the work involved smoothing off the edges from the casting. After processing, the casts were fixed in place, usually to the ceilings of buildings. The work tasks were varied, but characterised by varying periods of repetitive movement, frequent lifting of heavy materials, and working with the hands above head height in combination with forceful manoeuvres. He was highly skilled and therefore very valued by his company and colleagues. Without any apparent changes to his working conditions he gradually developed persistent pain in both epicondyles of the dominant right hand. He then had difficulty lifting even light materials, he dropped things and he had rest pain in his elbow. He was diagnosed with lateral and medial epicondylitis and treated with injections of corticosteroids, but these only provided short-term relief. He received exercise training from a physiotherapist, but with no benefit. An occupational physician visited the workshop and evaluated the different kinds of work task. Several activities were identified that were free of forceful handling. Furthermore, because of his wide experience, he was reassigned for a temporary period to help the manager with administrative work and handling customers. At the same time, the municipal job centre established a short-term arrangement whereby a person paid by public benefits helped the plasterer with his job for several hours daily. Gradually his condition improved and his work output normalised.

Commentary

In the presented case, several work tasks were suspected to have caused the man's elbow problem. However, regardless of aetiology, the plasterer had considerable difficulties in performing his job and needed measures to reduce his exposure. At the same time, it was essential for the workshop to find an economically sustainable solution over the longer term. Reduction of exposure was achieved by careful selection of tasks, aided by temporary financial support through a municipal arrangement. Even without this arrangement, recovery might have been achieved because of the reduction in elbow-straining exposures.

Different kinds of treatment for epicondylitis have been tried through the years but according to guidelines from The American College of Occupational Medicine (ACOEM) (Hegmann *et al.*, 2013), there is not one treatment that has proved to have a lasting effect. Benefits from surgical treatment have not been documented. The condition seems to resolve spontaneously, albeit slowly, regardless of the treatment in most cases. More than 80% of new cases are improved or recovered after a year. Individuals with physically straining jobs tend to have a higher risk of not recovering (Haahr and Andersen, 2003b).

Other conditions causing pain in elbow and forearm

Epicondylitis is the commonest and best studied cause of elbow pain. However, various other conditions around the elbow may be work-related. For example, nerve entrapment may occur following external pressure on the ulnar nerve (ulnar neuropathy, also called cubital tunnel syndrome). A recent case-control study of neurophysiologically verified ulnar neuropathy using an expert-based job exposure matrix reported associations with forceful work, with an exposure-response pattern (Svendsen *et al.*, 2012), but this finding has not been confirmed in other well-conducted studies. Another nerve entrapment involving the sensory part of the radial nerve, radial tunnel syndrome, is quite rare. In a large study of computer workers involving clinical examination, only 0.13% were diagnosed with the condition and no risk factors could clearly be identified (Kryger *et al.*, 2003). In the absence of specific evidence, it is suggested that case management should follow the same principles of exposure reduction illustrated above for epicondylitis.

Hand Pain

Carpal Tunnel Syndrome

Case definition and clinical features

CTS is a nerve entrapment of the wrist involving the median nerve where it passes through a narrow tunnel formed by the carpal bones and a tight ligament. The nerve is accompanied by the flexor tendons in this space-limited tunnel. If these tendons become swollen (in tendovaginitis), then compression of the nerve may result, causing characteristic symptoms of numbness and tingling in the thumb, the index and long finger and part of the ring finger. Symptoms are often worse at night. Weakness of the median-innervated muscles of the hand and muscle atrophy, especially of the thenar eminence, may occur and are often seen in advanced stages of disease. The diagnosis is based on a history of characteristic symptoms and a nerve conduction test performed with surface electrodes showing reduced sensory and/or motor conduction of the median nerve across the carpal tunnel.

In the early stages, symptoms may be relieved by splinting (Franklin and Friedman, 2015). Surgery is a simple procedure with a high success rate, provided that cases are correctly identified by proper preceding diagnostic investigations (Middleton and Anakwe, 2014).

Prevalence and individual risk factors

CTS is the commonest of the nerve entrapments, with a prevalence of 1% to 5% in the general population (Atroshi *et al.*, 1999; Bongers *et al.*, 2007). The disorder is more common in women than men (3:1) with a higher prevalence in the age group 45–64 years among men and an increasing prevalence with age among women. In most cases the aetiology is unknown. Hormonal factors (e.g. pregnancy), obesity, wrist fracture, hypothyroidism, diabetes and inflammatory arthropathy have all been associated with CTS (Middleton and Anakwe, 2014).

Occupational risk factors

There is good evidence that forceful exertions at the wrist and hand, especially in combination with repetitive hand movements, and exposures to hand-arm vibration, are risk factors for the development of CTS (Barcenilla *et al.*, 2012; Palmer *et al.*, 2007a; Van Rijn *et al.*, 2009; Newington *et al.*, 2015). Although the condition has been widely studied, it has been difficult to establish exposure-response relationships for these risk factors and threshold limits for safe use are still not clearly defined. However, recent studies have used goniometer measurements representative of jobs and job tasks establishing job (or job task) exposure matrices. In combination with register information on surgery for CTS, exposure-response relationships have been established for repetitiveness and levels of prevention suggested (Heilskov-Hansen *et al.*, 2016; Lund *et al.*, 2019). Wrist posture may also be of some importance although results have been conflicting. Jobs with hand-straining work tasks include meat cutting, fish processing, house painting, laundry work, certain types of manufacturing jobs and jobs where hand-held tools are used, e.g. in construction work (Herbert *et al.*, 2000; Lund *et al.*, 2019). Computer work, however, does not seem to cause CTS (Thomsen *et al.*, 2008; Andersen *et al.*, 2011).

Treatment of the patient in the occupational setting

Prospects for successful return to work after treatment for CTS are good. After an appropriate interval of sick leave, there should be a gradual return to previous work activities. If the job involves hand-straining tasks, then consideration can be given to options for job modification, or further training for another role. There are no strict definitions of hand-straining work and therefore decisions regarding work modifications should be guided by the eventual occurrence of symptoms (Newington *et al.*, 2015). Hand-held powered vibratory tools should not be used in excess of recommended safety limits (Herbert *et al.*, 2000) (e.g. those defined in Europe by legislation on the control of vibration at work). Although these measures make sense a priori, there is no evidence on their effectiveness in preventing the occurrence of CTS, and no evidence on the benefits of ergonomic positioning and ergonomically designed equipment (O'Connor *et al.*, 2012).

Tenosynovitis of the Hand

Case definition and clinical features

Hand pain is a common symptom that can arise from several underlying pathologies. One common cause is inflammation of the tendons and tendon sheaths, often referred to as tenosynovitis (to denote involvement of the synovial sheaths), or as tendinitis, peritendonitis, tendonitis or tendinopathy (the latter implying a primary pathology of degeneration rather than inflammation) (Khan *et al.*, 2002). In the acute phase of the disorder, the clinical picture is characterised by pain in the affected flexor or extensor tendons, swelling, warm and red colour of the skin and crepitation, i.e. a crunching feeling or sound when palpating the oedematous area. If the extensor tendon and tendon sheath of the thumb (first compartment) are involved, the condition is known as de Quervain's tendinitis, and often has a stenosing element (Huisstede *et al.*, 2014).

Prevalence and individual risk factors

Whereas hand pain is common, the clinical condition of tenosynovitis is not. In one British population survey, it was reported to affect about 1% of men and 2% of women (Walker-Bone *et al.*, 2004); in working populations, prevalence and incidences seem a little higher, depending on case definition (da Costa *et al.*, 2015). Tenosynovitis has been associated with diabetes mellitus and rheumatoid arthritis but no other personal risk factors are well recognised.

Occupational risk factors

Some researchers have suggested that studies of tenosynovitis should adopt a uniform approach to case definition, comprising pain on movement localised to the tendon sheaths and reproduced by resisted active movement (Harrington *et al.*, 1998; Sluiter *et al.*, 2001). Frequently, however, studies have used self-reported pain instead. Consequently, quite large differences in prevalence have been reported between the studied populations (da Costa *et al.*, 2015). A further complication in assessing work-relatedness is that exposure evaluation has typically been based on job titles or self-report (Palmer *et al.*, 2007b), rather than objective measurements. However, in one large follow-up study of industrial workers in monotonous employment, exposures were observed by video (Thomsen *et al.*, 2007). Exertion of force seemed to be the main ergonomic risk factor for tendinitis, high levels of repetition also seemed to play a role, but wrist posture did not seem to matter.

Tenosynovitis is reported to be more prevalent among meat cutters, in the fish processing industry, and in workers undertaking industrial sewing tasks and heavy assembly work. However, there have only been a comparatively small number of studies on risks by occupation and surprisingly limited evidence overall that occupational factors cause tendinitis (Palmer *et al.*, 2007b; Stahl *et al.*, 2003). This weak research base can be contrasted with clinical experience, in which cases arise and are often preceded by a period of unusually intensive hand-straining work. Incidents resolve fairly quickly, and this perhaps explains the difficulty in identifying and studying them epidemiologically.

Treatment of the patient in the occupational setting

In the acute phase of inflammation, it is not possible or advisable to continue with hand-straining work — instead, the hand and arm should be rested. Exercise instructions, hand supports and non-steroidal anti-inflammatory drugs are usually recommended, although evidence on the benefits of any specific treatment is limited. Most cases resolve without sequelae, typically with about 10–30 days of lost work (Palmer, 2003). When the acute phase is over the person can resume work gradually. It may be necessary to change work tasks, at least for a period, if symptoms return (Andreu *et al.*, 2011; Huisstede *et al.*, 2014).

Other causes of hand pain

Arthrosis of the joints in the hand, Dupuytren's contracture and trigger finger other than de Quervain's syndrome have also been associated with exposure at work. Of these, osteoarthritis of the hand is fairly common in women in whom it often starts in their 30s and 40s. Continuous joint overload can lead to joint impairment (Solovieva *et al.*, 2005), and a meta-analysis has reported an association between work involving the pinch or hand grip and osteoarthritis of the proximal interphalangeal and first carpometacarpal joints (Hammer *et al.*, 2014). Whether caused by work or not, hand exercises and joint protection, including working splints, may offer some symptomatic relief.

Conclusion

Musculoskeletal disorders are common in the general population and therefore common amongst working-aged adults. Both biomechanical and psychosocial factors at work can cause musculoskeletal disorders, or contribute to worsening the symptoms, and no matter what the cause, people with these conditions need to be accommodated in the workplace. When a worker reports new musculoskeletal symptoms, the focus should be on: (a) identifying any serious underlying pathology ("red flags"); (b) exploring whether work factors are causing the problem or making it worse; and (c) taking measures to minimise long-term disability. Sometimes, it may be necessary to make changes to work design or activities and this may include reduction of physical or psychological strain, increased breaks, rotation of tasks or additional support from co-workers or managers. In general, prolonged sickness absence is unhelpful resulting in reduced confidence and a poorer chance of ever returning to work and, where possible, these conditions should be managed in the workplace taking an empathic and supportive approach.

References

Andersen JH, Fallentin N, Thomsen JF, Mikkelsen S. (2011) Risk factors for neck and upper extremity disorders among computers users and the effect of interventions: An overview of systematic reviews. *PloS one*, **6**(5): e19691.

Andersson G. (1992) Factors important in the genesis and prevention of occupational back pain and disability. *J Manipulative Physiol Ther* **15**: 43–46.

Andreu JL, Oton T, Silva-Fernandez L, Sanz J. (2011) Hand pain other than carpal tunnel syndrome (CTS): The role of occupational factors. *Best Pract Res Clin Rheumatol* **25**: 31–42.

Ariëns GA, van Mechelen W, Bongers PM, Bouter LM, van der Wal G. (2000) Physical risk factors for neck pain. *Scand J Work, Environ Health* **26**(1): 7–19.

Atroshi I, Gummesson C, Johnsson R, Ornstein E, Ranstam J, Rosen I. (1999) Prevalence of carpal tunnel syndrome in a general population. *JAMA* **282**: 153–158.

Barcenilla A, March LM, Chen JS, Sambrook PN. (2012) Carpal tunnel syndrome and its relationship to occupation: A meta-analysis. *Rheumatol* (*Oxford*) **51**: 250–261.

Beatty S. (2018) We need to talk about lumbar total disc replacement. *Int J Spine Surg* **12**: 201–240.

Beneciuk JM, Lentz TA, He Y, Wu SS, George SZ. (2018) Prediction of persistent musculoskeletal pain at 12 months: A secondary analysis of the optimal screening for prediction of referral and outcome (OSPRO) validation cohort study. *Physical Therapy*, **98**(5): 290–301.

Bernard BP. (ed) (1997). *Musculoskeletal disorders and workplace factors. A critical review of epidemiologic evidence for work-related musculoskeletal disorders of the neck, upper extremity, and low back* (*Publication no. 97–141*). Cincinnati, US Department of Health and Human Sciences/ NIOSH.

Bigos SJ, Battié MC, Fisher LD, Hansson TH, Spengler DM, Nachemson AL. (1992) A prospective evaluation of preemployment screening methods for acute industrial back pain. *Spine* **17**(8): 922–926.

Bigos S, Spengler D, Martin N, Zeh J, Fisher L, Nachemson A, Wang MH. (1986) Back injuries in industry: A retrospective study. II. Injury factors. *Spine (Phila Pa 1976)* **11**(3): 246–251.

Blackwell DL, Lucas JW, Clarke TC. (2014) Summary health statistics for U.S. adults: National health interview survey, 2012. *Vital Health Stat 10* (260): 1–161.

Bongers FJ, Schellevis FG, van den Bosch WJ, van der Zee J. (2007) Carpal tunnel syndrome in general practice (1987 and 2001): Incidence and the role of occupational and non-occupational factors. *Br J Gen Pract* **57**(534): 36–39.

Bovenzi M, Schust M, Menzel G, Prodi A, Mauro M. (2015) Relationships of low back outcomes to internal spinal load. *Int Arch Occup Environ Health* **88**: 487–499.

Buchbinder R, Green S, Youd JM. (2003) Corticosteroid injections for shoulder pain. *Cochrane Database Syst Rev* (1): CD004016.

Bydon M, De la Garza-Ramos R, Macki M, Baker A, Gokaslan AK, Bydon A. (2014) Lumbar fusion versus nonoperative management for treatment of discogenic low back pain: A systematic review and meta-analysis of randomized controlled trials. *J Spinal Disord Tech* **27**(5): 297–304.

Carroll C, Rick J, Pilgrim H, Cameron J, Hillage J. (2010) Workplace involvement improves return to work rates among employees with back pain on long-term sick leave: A systematic review of the effectiveness and cost-effectiveness of interventions. *Disability and Rehabilitation* **32**(8): 607–621.

Clinical Standards Advisory Group. (1994) *Epidemiology review: The epidemiology and cost of back pain.* London, HMSO.

Coggon D, Ntani G, Palmer KT, Felli VE, Harari R, Barrero LH, Felknor SA, Gimeno D, Cattrell A, Serra C, Bonzini M, Solidaki E, Merisalu E, Habib RR, Sadeghian F, Masood Kadir M, Warnakulasuriya SS, Matsudaira K, Nyantumbu B, Sim MR, Gray A. (2013) Disabling musculoskeletal pain in working populations: Is it the job, the person, or the culture? *Pain* **154**(6): 856–863.

Coggon D. (2005) Occupational medicine at a turning point. *Occup Environ Med* **62**: 281–283.

da Costa JT, Baptista JS, Vaz M. (2015) Incidence and prevalence of upper-limb work related musculoskeletal disorders: A systematic review. *Work* **51**(4): 635–644.

Currie SR, Wang J. (2005) More data on major depression as an antecedent risk factor for first onset of chronic back pain. *Psychol Med* **35**: 1275–1282.

Dalbøge A, Frost P, Andersen JH, Svendsen SW. (2014) Cumulative occupational shoulder exposures and surgery for subacromial impingement syndrome: A nationwide Danish cohort study. *Occup Environ Med* **71**(11): 750–756.

Dalbøge A, Frost P, Andersen JH, Svendsen SW. (2020) Exposure-response relationships between cumulative occupational shoulder exposures and different diagnoses related to surgery for subacromial impingement syndrome. *Int Arch Occup Environ Health* **93**(3): 375–380.

Descatha A, Dale AM, Jaegers L, Herquelot E, Evanoff B. (2013) Self-reported physical exposure association with medial and lateral epicondylitis incidence in a large longitudinal study. *Occup Environ Med* **70**(9): 670–673.

Elders LA, Burdorf A. (2001) Interrelations of risk factors and low back pain in scaffolders. *Occup Environ Med* **58**: 597–603.

Fan, Z. J., Silverstein, B. A., Bao, S., Bonauto, D. K., Howard, N. L, Smith, C. K. (2014) The association between combination of hand force and forearm posture and incidence of lateral epicondylitis in a working population. *Hum Factors* 56(1): 151–165.

Fernandes, R, Burdorf, A. (2016) Associations of multisite pain with healthcare utilization, sickness absence and restrictions at work. *Int Arch Occup Environ Health* 89(7): 1039–1046.

Ferreira PH, Beckenkamp P, Maher CG, Hopper JL, Ferreira ML. (2013) Nature or nurture in low back pain? Results of a systematic review of studies based on twin samples. *Eur J Pain (Lond)* **17**(7): 957–971.

Franklin GM, Friedman AS. (2015) Work-related carpal tunnel syndrome: Diagnosis and treatment guideline. *Phys Med Rehabil Clin N Am* **26**(3): 523–537.

Garcia JB, Hernandez-Castro JJ, Nunez RG, Pazos MA, Aguirre JO, Jreige A, Delgado W, Serpentegui M, Berenguel M, Cantemir C. (2014) Prevalence of low back pain in Latin America: A systematic literature review. *Pain Physician* **17**(5): 379–391.

Garland EL. (2012) Pain processing in the human nervous system: A selective review of nociceptive and biobehavioral pathways. *Prim Care* **39**: 561–571.

Global Burden of Disease 2015 Disease and Injury Incidence and Prevalence Collaborators. (2016) Global, regional, and national incidence, prevalence, and years lived with disability for 310 diseases and injuries, 1990–2015: A systematic analysis for the global burden of disease study 2015. *Lancet* **388**: 1545–602.5

Green BN, Johnson CD, Haldeman S, Griffith E, Clay MB, Kane EJ, Castellote JM, Rajasekaran S, Smuck M, Hurwitz EL, Randhawa K, Yu H, Nordin M. (2018) A scoping review of biopsychosocial risk factors and co-morbidities for common spinal disorders. *PloS One* **13**(6): e0197987.

Haahr JP, Andersen JH. (2006) Exercises may be as efficient as subacromial decompression in patients with subacromial stage II impingement: 4–8-years' follow-up in a prospective, randomized study. *Scand J Rheumatol* **35**(3): 224–228.

Haahr JP, Østergaard S, Dalsgaard J, Norup K, Frost P, Lausen S, Holm EA, Andersen JH. (2005) Exercises versus arthroscopic decompression in patients with subacromial impingement: A randomised, controlled study in 90 cases with a one year follow up. *Ann Rheum Dis* **64**(5): 760–764.

Haahr JP, Andersen JH. (2003a) Physical and psychosocial risk factors for lateral epicondylitis: A population based case-referent study. *Occup Environ Med* **60**: 322–329.

Haahr JP, Andersen JH. (2003b) Prognostic factors in lateral epicondylitis: A randomized trial with one-year follow-up in 266 new cases treated with minimal occupational intervention or the usual approach in general practice. *Rheumatol* (*Oxford*) **42**: 1216–1225.

Hallman DM, Holtermann A, Björklund M, Gupta N, Nørregaard Rasmussen CD. (2019) Sick leave due to musculoskeletal pain: Determinants of distinct trajectories over 1 year. *Int Arch Occup Environ Health* **92**(8): 1099–1108.

Hartvigsen J., Hancock MJ, Kongsted A, Louw Q, Ferreira ML., Genevay S, Hoy D, Karppinen J, Pransky G, Sieper J, Smeets RJ, Underwood M, Lancet Low Back Pain Series Working Group. (2018) What low back pain is and why we need to pay attention. *Lancet* (*Lond*) **391**(10137): 2356–2367.

Hartvigsen J, Nielsen J, Kyvik KO, Fejer R, Vach W, Iachine I, Leboeuf-Yde C. (2009) Heritability of spinal pain and consequences of spinal pain: A comprehensive genetic epidemiologic analysis using a population-based sample of 15,328 twins ages 20–71 years. *Arthritis Rheumatism* **61**(10): 1343–1351.

Harrington JM, Carter JT, Birrell L, Gompertz D. (1998) Surveillance case definition for work related upper limb pain syndromes. *Occup Environ Med* **55**: 264–271.

Hammer PE, Shiri R, Kryger AI, Kirkeskov L, Bonde JP. (2014) Associations of work activities requiring pinch or hand grip or exposure to hand-arm vibration with finger and wrist osteoarthritis: A meta-analysis. *Scand J Work Environ Health* **40** 133–145.

Haukka E, Pehkonen I, Leino-Arjas P, Viikari-Juntura E, Takala EP, Malmivaara A, Hopsu L, Mutanen P, Ketola R, Virtanen T, Holtari-Leino M, Nykänen J, Stenholm S, Ojajärvi A, Riihimäki H. (2010) Effect of a participatory ergonomics intervention on psychosocial factors at work in a randomised controlled trial. *Occup Environ Med* **67**(3): 170–177.

Hegmann KT, Hoffman HE, Belcourt RM, Byrne K, Glass L, Melhorn JM, Richman J, Zinni P, 3rd, Thiese MS, Ott U, Tokita K, Passey DG, Effiong AC, Robbins RB, Ording JA, American College of Occupational and Environmental Medicine. (2013) ACOEM practice guidelines: elbow disorders. *J Occup Environ Med* **55**(11): 1365–1374.

Heilskov-Hansen T, Mikkelsen S, Svendsen SW, Thygesen LC, Hansson GÅ, Thomsen JF. (2016) Exposure-response relationships between movements and postures of the wrist and carpal tunnel syndrome among male and female house painters: A retrospective cohort study. *Occup Environ Med* **73**(6): 401–408.

Herbert R, Gerr F, Dropkin J. (2000) Clinical evaluation and management of work-related carpal tunnel syndrome. *Am J Ind Med* **37**: 62–74.

Herquelot E, Bodin J, Roquelaure Y, Ha C, Leclerc A, Goldberg M, Zins M, Descatha A. (2013) Work-related risk factors for lateral epicondylitis and other cause of elbow pain in the working population. *Am J Ind Med* 56(4): 400–409.

Hiebert FR, Skovron ML, Nordin M. (2003) Work restrictions and outcome of non-specific low back pain. *Spine* **28**: 722–728.

Hill JC, Whitehurst DG, Lewis M, Bryan S, Dunn KM, Foster NE, Konstantinou K, Main CJ, Mason E, Somerville S, Sowden G, Vohora K, Hay EM. (2011) Comparison of stratified primary care management for low back pain with current best practice (STarT Back): A randomised controlled trial. *Lancet* (*Lond*) **378**(9802): 1560–1571.

Hodges SD, Humphreys SC, Eck JC, Covington LA, Harrom H. (2001) Predicting factors of successful recovery from lumbar spine surgery among workers' compensation patients. *J Am Osteopath Assoc* **101**(2): 78–83.

Hoy D, Bain C, Williams G, March L, Brooks P, Blyth F, Woolf A, Vos T, Buchbinder R. (2012) A systematic review of the global prevalence of low back pain. *Arthritis Rheumatism* **64**(6): 2028–2037.

Hoy D, March L, Brooks P, Blyth F, Woolf A, Bain C, Williams G, Smith E, Vos T, Barendregt J, Murray C, Burstein R, Buchbinder R. (2014) The global burden of low back pain: Estimates from the global burden of disease 2010 study. *Ann Rheum Dis* **73**: 968–974.

Huisstede BM, Coert JH, Friden J, Hoogvliet P. (2014) Consensus on a multidisciplinary treatment guideline for de Quervain disease: Results from the European HANDGUIDE study. *Phys Ther* **94**: 1095–1110.

Ijmker S, Huysmans MA, Blatter BM, van der Beek AJ, van Mechelen W, Bongers PM. (2007) Should office workers spend fewer hours at their computer? A systematic review of the literature. *Occup Environ Med* **64**(4): 211–222.

Irwin RW, Zuhosky JP, Sullivan WJ, Foye PM, Sable AW, Panagos A. (2007) Industrial medicine and acute musculoskeletal rehabilitation. 5. Interventional procedures for work-related lumbar spine conditions. *Arch Phys Med Rehabil* **88**(3 Suppl 1): S22–S28.

Jacobs WC, van Tulder M, Arts M, Rubinstein SM, van Middelkoop M, Ostelo R, Verhagen A, Koes B, Peul WC. (2011) Surgery versus conservative management of sciatica due to a lumbar herniated disc: A systematic review. *Eur Spine J* **20**(4): 513–522.

Janwantanakul P, Sitthipornvorakul E, Paksaichol A. (2012) Risk factors for the onset of nonspecific low back pain in office workers: A systematic review of prospective cohort studies. *J Manipulative Physiol Ther* **35**: 568–577.

Johnston JM, Landsittel DP, Nelson NA, Gardner LI, Wassell JT. (2003) Stressful psychosocial work environment increases risk for back pain among retail material handlers. *Am J Ind Med* 43(2): 179–187.

Kamaleri Y, Natvig B, Ihlebaek CM, Bruusgaard D. (2008) Localized or widespread musculoskeletal pain: Does it matter? *Pain* **138**: 41–46.

Karjalainen TV, Jain NB, Heikkinen J, Johnston RV, Page CM, Buchbinder R. (2019) Surgery for rotator cuff tears. *Cochrane Database Of Syst Rev* **12**(12): CD013502.

Kelsey JL, Githens PB, White AA, 3rd, Holford TR, Walter SD, O'Connor T, Ostfeld AM, Weil U, Southwick WO, Calogero JA. (1984) An epidemiologic study of lifting and twisting on the job and risk for acute prolapsed lumbar intervertebral disc. *J Orthop Res* **2**(1): 61–66.

Ketola S, Lehtinen J, Rousi T, Nissinen M, Huhtala H, Arnala I. (2015) Which patients do not recover from shoulder impingement syndrome, either with operative treatment or with nonoperative treatment? *Acta Orthopaedica* **86**(6): 641–646.

Ketola S, Lehtinen J, Rousi T, Nissinen M, Huhtala H, Konttinen YT, Arnala I. (2013) No evidence of long-term benefits of arthroscopicacromioplasty in the treatment of shoulder impingement syndrome: Five-year results of a randomised controlled trial. *Bone Jt Res* **2**(7): 132–139.

Khan KM, Cook JL, Kannus P, Maffulli N, Bonar SF. (2002) Time to abandon the "tendinitis" myth. *BMJ* **324**: 626–627.

Klein B, Jensen R, Sanderson L. (1984) Assessment of workers' compensation claims for back strains/sprains. *J Occup Med* **26**(6): 443–448.

Kryger AI, Andersen JH, Lassen CF, Brandt LP, Vilstrup I, Overgaard E, Thomsen JF, Mikkelsen S. (2003) Does computer use pose an occupational hazard for forearm pain; from the NUDATA study. *Occup Environ Med* **60**(11): e14.

Kwon BK, Roffey DM, Bishop PB, Dagenais S, Wai EK. (2011) Systematic review: Occupational physical activity and low back pain. *Occup Med (Lond)* **61**(8): 541–548.

Larsson B, Sogaard K, Rosendal L. (2007) Work related neck-shoulder pain: A review on magnitude, risk factors, biochemical characteristics, clinical picture and preventive interventions. *Best Pract Res Clin Rheumatol* **21**(3): 447–463.

Lawrence JS. (1969) Disc degeneration: Its frequency and relationship to symptoms. *Ann Rheum Dis* **28**: 121–138.

Lee P, Helewa A, Goldsmith C, Smythe H, Stitt L. (2001) Low back pain: Prevalence and risk factors in an industrial setting. *J Rheumatol* **28**(2): 346–351.

Lee JC, Choi SW. (2015) Adjacent segment pathology after lumbar spinal fusion. *Asian Spine J* **9**: 807–817.

Lenza M, Buchbinder R, Takwoingi Y, Johnston RV, Hanchard NC, Faloppa F. (2013) Magnetic resonance imaging, magnetic resonance arthrography and ultrasonography for assessing rotator cuff tears in people with shoulder pain for whom surgery is being considered. *Cochrane Database Syst Rev* **2013**(9): CD009020.

Linaker CH, Walker-Bone K. (2015) Shoulder disorders and occupation. *Best Pract Res Clin Rheumatol* **29**(3): 405–423.

Linton SJ. (2000) A review of psychological risk factors in back and neck pain. *Spine* **25**: 1148–1156.

Livshits G, Popham M, Malkin I, Sambrook PN, Macgregor AJ, Spector T, Williams FM. (2011) Lumbar disc degeneration and genetic factors are the main risk factors for low back pain in women: The UK Twin Spine Study. *Ann Rheumat Dis* **70**(10): 1740–1745.

Louw QA, Morris LD, Grimmer-Somers K. (2007) The prevalence of low back pain in Africa: A systematic review. *BMC Musculoskelet Disord* **8**: 105.

Lund CB, Mikkelsen S, Thygesen LC, Hansson GÅ, Thomsen JF. (2019) Movements of the wrist and the risk of carpal tunnel syndrome: A nationwide cohort study using objective exposure measurements. *Occup Environ Med* **76**(8): 519–526.

Maher C, Underwood M, Buchbinder R. (2017) Non-specific low back pain. *Lancet* **389**: 736–747.

Mansfield M, Smith T, Spahr N, Thacker M. (2020) Cervical spine radiculopathy epidemiology: A systematic review. *Musculoskeletal Care* **18**(4): 555–567.

Maund E, Craig D, Suekarran S, Neilson A, Wright K, Brealey S, Dennis L, Goodchild L, Hanchard N, Rangan A, Richardson G, Robertson J, McDaid C. (2012) Management of frozen shoulder: A systematic review and cost-effectiveness analysis. *Health Technol Assess* (*Winchester*) **16**(11): 1–264.

Michener LA, McClure PW, Karduna AR. (2003) Anatomical and biomechanical mechanisms of subacromial impingement syndrome. *Clin Biomech* (*Bristol, Avon*) **18**(5): 369–379.

Middleton SD, Anakwe RE. (2014) Carpal tunnel syndrome. *BMJ* **349**: g6437.

Molano SM, Burdorf A, Elders LA. (2001) Factors associated with medical care-seeking due to low-back pain in scaffolders. *Am J Ind Med* **40**(3): 275–281.

National Institute for Health and Clinical Excellence. (2009) *Managing Long-Term Sickness Absence and Incapacity for Work. NICE public health guidance 19.* London, NICE Publications.

Newington L, Harris E. C, Walker-Bone K. (2015) Carpal tunnel syndrome and work. Best *Pract Res Clin Rheumatol* **29**(3): 440–453.

O'Connor D, Page MJ, Marshall SC, Massy-Westropp N. (2012) Ergonomic positioning or equipment for treating carpal tunnel syndrome. *Cochrane Database Syst Rev* **1**: CD009600.

Palacios-Ceña D, Albaladejo-Vicente R, Hernández-Barrera V, Lima-FlorencioL, Fernández-de-Las-Peñas C, Jimenez-Garcia R, López-de-Andrés A, de Miguel-Diez J, Perez-Farinos N. (2021) Female gender is associated with a higher prevalence of chronic neck pain, chronic low back pain, and migraine: Results of the Spanish National Health Survey, 2017. *Pain Med* (*Malden, Mass.*) **22**(2): 382–395.

Palmer KT, Bovenzi M. (2015) Rheumatic effects of vibration at work. *Best Pract Res Clin Rheumatol* 1–16.

Palmer KT, Greenough C. (2013) Spinal disorders. In: Palmer, K.T., Brown, I, Hobson, J. (eds.), *Fitness for Work* (5th Ed), Oxford, Oxford University Press.

Palmer KT, Smedley J. (2007) The work-relatedness of chronic neck pain with physical findings: A systematic review. *Scand J Work Environ Health* **33**: 165–191.

Palmer KT, Walker-Bone K, Griffin MJ, Syddall H, Pannett B, Coggon D, Cooper C. (2001) Prevalence and occupational associations of neck pain in the British population. *Scand J Work Environ Health* 27(1): 49–56.

Palmer KT. (2003) Regional musculoskeletal conditions: Pain in the forearm, wrist and hand. *Best Pract Res Clin Rheumatol* **17**: 113–135.

Palmer K, Harris EC, Coggon D. (2007a) Carpal tunnel syndrome and its relation to occupation: A systematic literature review. *Occup Med (Lond)* **57**: 57–66.

Palmer KT, Harris EC, Coggon D. (2007b) Compensating occupationally related tenosynovitis and epicondylitis: A literature review. *Occup Med (Lond)* **57**: 67–74.

Palmerud G, Forsman M, Sporrong H, Herberts P, Kadefors R. (2000) Intramuscular pressure of the infra- and supraspinatus muscles in relation to hand load and arm posture. *Eur J Appl Physiol* **83**(2–3): 223–230.

Patel KV, Guralnik JM, Dansie EJ, Turk DC. (2013) Prevalence and impact of pain among older adults in the United States: Findings from the 2011 National Health and Aging Trends Study. *Pain* **154**(12): 2649–2657.

Pinheiro MB, Morosoli JJ, Colodro-Conde L, Ferreira PH, Ordoñana JR. (2018) Genetic and environmental influences to low back pain and symptoms of depression and anxiety: A population-based twin study. *J Psychosom Res* **105**: 92–98.

Polvinen A, Laaksonen M, Gould R, Lahelma E, Martikainen P. (2014) The contribution of major diagnostic causes to socioeconomic differences in disability retirement. *Scand J Work Environ Health* 40(4): 353–360.

Ramazzini B. (1713). *De Morbis Artificum Diatriba*. Venice, Corona.

Roquelaure Y, Ha C, Leclerc A, Touranchet A, Sauteron M, Melchior M, Imbernon E, Goldberg M. (2006) Epidemiologic surveillance of upper-extremity musculoskeletal disorders in the working population. *Arthritis Rheumatism* **55**(5): 765–778.

Schonstein E, Kenny DT, Keating J, Koes BW. (2003) Work conditioning, work hardening and functional restoration for workers with back and neck pain. *Cochrane Database Syst Rev* **1**: CD001822.

Shiri R, Falah-Hassani K. (2017) Does leisure time physical activity protect against low back pain? Systematic review and meta-analysis of 36 prospective cohort studies. *Br J Sports Medicine* **51**(19): 1410–1418.

Shiri R, Karppinen J, Leino-Arjas P, Solovieva S, Viikari-Juntura E. (2010) The association between smoking and low back pain: a meta-analysis. *Am J Med* **123**: 87.

Shiri R, Viikari-Juntura E. (2011) Lateral and medial epicondylitis: Role of occupational factors. *Best Pract Res Clin Rheumatol* **25**: 43–57.

Sitthipornvorakul E, Janwantanakul P, Purepong N, Pensri P, van der Beek AJ. (2011) The association between physical activity and neck and low back pain: A systematic review. *Eur Spine J* **20**: 677–689.

Sluiter JK, Rest KM, Frings-Dresen MH. (2001) Criteria document for evaluating the work-relatedness of upper-extremity musculoskeletal disorders. *Scand J Work Environ Health* **27**(1): 1–102.

Snook S, Campanelli R, Hart J. (1978) A study of three preventive approaches to low back injury. *J Occup Med* **20**(7): 478–481.

Solovieva S, Vehmas T, Riihimaki H, Luoma K, Leino-Arjas P. (2005) Hand use and patterns of joint involvement in osteoarthritis. A comparison of female dentists and teachers. *Rheumatol* **44**: 521–528.

Stahl S, Vida D, Meisner C, Lotter O, Rothenberger J, Schaller HE, Stahl AS. (2013) Systematic review and meta-analysis on the work-related cause of de Quervain tenosynovitis: A critical appraisal of its recognition as an occupational disease. *Plast Reconstr Surg* **132**: 1479–1491.

Steffens D, Ferreira ML, Latimer J, Ferreira PH, Koes BW, Blyth F, Li Q, Maher CG. (2015) What triggers an episode of acute low back pain? A case-crossover study. *Arthritis Care Res* **67**(3): 403–410.

Sterud T, Johannessen HA, Tynes T. (2014) Work-related psychosocial and mechanical risk factors for neck/shoulder pain: A 3-year follow-up study of the general working population in Norway. *Int Arch Occup Environ Health* **87**(5):471–81.

Stobbe T. (1996) Occupational ergonomics and injury prevention. *Occup Med* **11**(3): 531–543.

Sundstrup E, Seeberg KGV, Bengtsen E, Andersen LL. (2020) A systematic review of workplace interventions to rehabilitate musculoskeletal disorders among employees with physical demanding work. *J Occup Rehabil* **30**: 588–612.

Svendsen SW, Bonde JP, Mathiassen SE, Stengaard-Pedersen K, Frich LH. (2004) Work related shoulder disorders: Quantitative exposure-response relations with reference to arm posture. *Occup Environ Med* **61**(10): 844–853.

Svendsen SW, Dalbøge A, Andersen JH, Thomsen JF, Frost P. (2013) Risk of surgery for subacromial impingement syndrome in relation to neck-shoulder complaints and occupational biomechanical exposures: A longitudinal study. *Scand J Work Environ Health* **39**(6): 568–577.

Svendsen SW, Frost P, Jensen LD. (2012) Time trends in surgery for non-traumatic shoulder disorders and postoperative risk of permanent work disability: A nationwide cohort study. *Scand J Rheumatol* **41**(1): 59–65.

Svendsen SW, Gelineck J, Mathiassen SE, Bonde JP, Frich LH, Stengaard-Pedersen K, Egund N. (2004) Work above shoulder level and degenerative alterations of the rotator cuff tendons: A magnetic resonance imaging study. *Arthritis Rheumatism* **50**(10): 3314–3322.

Svendsen SW, Johnsen B, Fuglsang-Frederiksen A, Frost P. (2012) Ulnar neuropathy and ulnar neuropathy-like symptoms in relation to biomechanical exposures assessed by a job exposure matrix: A triple case-referent study. *Occup Environ Med* **69**: 773–780.

Swain MS, Henschke N, Kamper SJ, Gobina I, Ottová-Jordan V, Maher CG. (2014) An international survey of pain in adolescents. *Bmc Public Health* **14**: 447.

Taurog JD, Chhabra A, Colbert RA. (2016) Ankylosing spondylitis and axial spondyloarthritis. *N Engl J Med* **374**: 2563–2574.

Taylor JB, Goode AP, George SZ, Cook CE. (2014) Incidence and risk factors for first-time incident low back pain: A systematic review and meta-analysis. *Spine J NASSJ* **14**(10): 2299–2319.

Thomsen JF, Gerr F, Atroshi I. (2008) Carpal tunnel syndrome and the use of computer mouse and keyboard: A systematic review. *BMC Musculoskelet Disord* **9**: 134.

Thomsen JF, Mikkelsen S, Andersen JH, Fallentin N, Loft IP, Frost P, Kaergaard A, Bonde JP, Overgaard E. (2007) Risk factors for hand-wrist disorders in repetitive work. *Occup Environ Med* **64**(8): 527–533.

van der Molen HF, Foresti C, Daams JG, Frings-Dresen M, Kuijer P. (2017) Work-related risk factors for specific shoulder disorders: A systematic review and meta-analysis. *Occup Environ Med* **74**(10): 745–755.

Van der Windt DA, Koes BW, de Jong BA, Bouter LM. (1995) Shoulder disorders in general practice: Incidence, patient characteristics, and management. *Ann Rheum Dis* **54**(12): 959–964.

van Rijn RM, Huisstede BM, Koes BW, Burdorf A. (2010) Associations between work-related factors and specific disorders of the shoulder — A systematic review of the literature. *Scand J Work Environ Health* **36**(3): 189–201.

Van Rijn RM, Huisstede BM, Koes BW, Burdorf A. (2009) Associations between work-related factors and specific disorders at the elbow: A systematic literature review. *Rheumatology* (*Oxford*) **48**: 528–536.

van Tulder MW, Ostelo R, Vlaeyen JW, Linton SJ, Morley SJ, Assendelft WJ. (2000) Behavioral treatment for chronic low back pain: A systematic review within the framework of the cochrane back review group. *Spine* **25**(20): 2688–2699.

Van Tulder M, Malmivaara A, Koes B. (2007) Repetitive strain injury. *Lancet* **369**: 1815–1822.

Vivekanantham A, Edwin C, Pincus T, Matharu M, Parsons H, Underwood M. (2019) The association between headache and low back pain: A systematic review. *J Headache Pain* **20**(1): 82.

Waddell G. (2004) *The back pain revolution* (2nd Ed). Edinburgh, Churchill Livingstone.

Waehrer G, Leigh J, Miller T. (2005) Costs of occupational injury and illness within the health services sector. *Int J Health Serv* **35**(2): 343–359.

Walker-Bone K, Palmer KT, Reading I, Coggon D, Cooper C. (2004) Prevalence and impact of musculoskeletal disorders of the upper limb in the general population. *Arthritis Rheum* **51**: 642–651.

Walker-Bone K, Palmer KT, Reading I, Coggon D, Cooper C. (2012) Occupation and epicondylitis: A population-based study. *Rheumatology* (*Oxford*) **51**: 305–310.

Walton SM, Conrad KM, Furner SE, Samo DG. (2003) Cause, type, and workers' compensation costs of injury to fire fighters. *Am J Ind Med* 43(4): 454–458.

Wong JJ, Côté P, Quesnele JJ, Stern PJ, Mior SA. (2014) The course and prognostic factors of symptomatic cervical disc herniation with radiculopathy: A systematic review of the literature. *Spine J NASSJ* **14**(8): 1781–1789.

Yoon SK, Thiese MS, Ott U, Kapellusch J, Merryweather A, Wood EM, Ronna BB, Foster J, Drury DL, Hegmann KT. (2019) The role of elbow tender point examination in the diagnosis of lateral epicondylitis. *J Occup Environ Med* **61**(2): 126–131.

Yabe Y, Hagiwara Y, Sekiguchi T, Sugawara Y, Tsuchiya M, Yoshida S, Sogi Y, Yano T, Onoki T, Takahashi T, Iwatsu J, Tsuji I, Itoi E. (2020) Musculoskeletal pain in other body sites is associated with new-onset low back pain: A longitudinal study among survivors of the great East Japan earthquake. *Bmc Musculoskeletal Disorders* **21**(1): 227.

Yang H, Haldeman S, Lu ML, Baker D. (2016) Low back pain prevalence and related workplace psychosocial risk factors: A study using data from the 2010 national health interview survey. *J Manipulative Physiol Ther* **39**: 459–472.

Zhang TT, Liu Z, Liu YL, Zhao JJ, Liu DW, Tian QB. (2018) Obesity as a risk factor for low back pain: A meta-analysis. *Clin Spine Surg* **31**(1): 22–27.

Zielinska N, Podgórski M, Haładaj R, Polguj M, Olewnik Ł. (2021) Risk Factors of Intervertebral Disc Pathology-A Point of View Formerly and Today-A Review. *J Clin Med* **10**(3): 409.

Zuhosky JP, Irwin RW, Sable AW, Sullivan WJ, Panagos A, Foye PM. (2007) Industrial medicine and acute musculoskeletal rehabilitation. 7. Acute industrial musculoskeletal injuries in the aging workforce. *Arch Phys Med Rehabil* **88**(3 Suppl 1): S34–S48.

Chapter 7

Auditory Disorders

Ailin Razali and Krishna Gopal Rampal†*

Introduction

Noise is a major health hazard in the workplace and with industrialisation there has been marked increase in occupational noise. Auditory disorders as a result of exposure to noise, particularly noise-induced hearing loss (NIHL) is a common health problem among workers exposed to loud noise. The damage often goes undetected until it has negatively affected a worker's daily function. Efficient adaptation by the brain often leads to under-estimation of the loudness of sounds one is exposed to. Prevention of NIHL must remain as the mainstay of NIHL management, as there is still no definitive cure to NIHL to date. Knowledge regarding NIHL therefore, should be made known to all stakeholders involved including the workers, employers, engineers, policymakers and especially health professionals.

*Department of ORL-HNS, International Islamic University Malaysia, Kuantan, Malaysia.
†Cyberjaya University College of Medical Sciences (CUCMS), Cyberjaya, Selangor DE, Malaysia.
Corresponding author: Ailin Razali (ailin.razali@gmail.com).

Epidemiology

Recognition that noise exposure could result in hearing loss dates at least to as far back as the 16th century. The classic text *De Morbis Artificum* (Diseases of Workers) (Ramazzini, 1713), was probably where NIHL was first acknowledged in vivid detail when the noisy ambiance of the coppersmiths in Venice was described. Similarly, deafness amongst blacksmiths (Fosbroke, 1831) and boiler makers (Barr, 1886) have been reported as early as the 1800s.

The World Health Organization (WHO) burden of disease study in the year 2000 estimated that 16% of the disabling hearing loss in adults (over 4 million disability-adjusted life years, DALYs) can be attributed to occupational noise and it ranges from 7% to 21% in various sub-regions. Disabling hearing loss is defined as hearing thresholds of frequencies 500, 1,000, 2,000 and 4,000 Hz greater than 40 dBHL. The effects of the exposure to occupational noise are greater for males than females in all sub-regions and higher in the developing regions (Nelson *et al.*, 2005).

A study by Masterson *et al.* in 2013 reported 22 million workers were exposed to hazardous noise and the prevalence of hearing loss to be 18%. Workers in the mining, manufacturing and construction industries needed better engineering controls for noise and better hearing conservation strategies as these were the groups at higher risk for occupationally related hearing loss.

In the United Kingdom, the estimated number of workers with work-related hearing problems was 17,000 (Labour Force Survey — 2017/2018, 2019/2020). There was a total of 1,125 new cases of occupational deafness reported from 2010 to 2019, with only five of the 1,125 cases being female (Health and Safety Executive, 2020). In Norway, of the 3,392 cases of work-related diseases reported to the Norwegian Labour Inspectorate in 2006; 59% (1987) of the cases were due to NIHL (Samant, 2008). A cross-sectional study involving 180 subjects from 356 workers in the welding unit of three automotive parts factories in Thailand found that prevalence of average hearing levels ≥25 dB(A) at 3,000–8,000z varied between 18.3% and 31.7%. Workers with noise exposure levels exceeding 90 dB(A) had a significantly higher prevalence of hearing loss in both ears than those who had noise exposure levels of less than 86 dB(A) (Sriopas *et al.*, 2017).

Prevalence by Industry

Audiometric testing conducted among 64 subjects working in the ship repair production unit in a shipyard company in Surabaya found 52 (81.2%) subjects diagnosed with clinical sensorineural hearing loss with 32 (61.5%) subjects having experienced deafness in both ears. One employee had severe sensorineural hearing loss (1.9%), two of them had moderate-severe hearing loss (3.8%) and 12 had moderate hearing loss (23.1%). The highest proportion, 37 employees (71.2%) had mild sensorineural hearing loss. In the 17 locations, where noise levels were studied in the repair production unit, 12 of them had noise levels above the recommended threshold value (Sincihu *et al.*, 2019).

A cross-sectional study in Nepal involving 124 woodworkers (88 carpenters, 36 sawyers) from 26 workplaces, showed that 31% of carpenters and 44% of sawyers met the criteria for NIHL, with 7% and 17% respectively meeting WHO criteria for hearing impairment. These workers were exposed to noise levels between 71 to 94 dBA in their workplaces (Robinson *et al.*, 2015).

The mean level of noise in 12 locations in the weaving department of a textile factory in Iraq was found to be between 87 and 96 dB. A total of 113 of the 200 workers studied had NIHL with 41 (22%) of the workers having a 4 kHz notch in the audiograms. Complaints among the workers included having hearing difficulty (29.4%), tinnitus (43.5%), ear discomfort (55.4%) and vertigo/dizziness (29.9%). The mean duration of exposure increased with age and ranged from six years in the 31–35 years age group to 24 years in the ≥50 years age group. The prevalence of NIHL also increased with age with 25% in the 31–35 years age group to 100% in the ≥50 years age group (Hameed *et al.*, 2019).

In a study to compare the prevalence of NIHL among 221 iron and steel workers (exposed group) and 107 primary school teachers (control group) in Tanzania, iron and steel workers and primary school teachers were exposed to average noise levels of 92 dB(A) and 79.7 dB(A). The prevalence of hearing loss, defined as hearing threshold levels ≥25 dB hearing loss in either ear at 3,000, 4,000 or 6,000 Hz, was significantly higher (48%) among the exposed group than among the controls (31%) (Nyarubeli *et al.*, 2019). In a study on the prevalence of NIHL in a gold mining company in Tanzania, a total of 246 audiograms obtained from periodic medical examinations were studied. The prevalence of NIHL was 47%, with 12% with poor hearing and 35% with mild hearing impairment. The proportion of NIHL increased with total years of exposure to noise and underground miners were more affected (71%) than open pit miners (28%) (Musiba, 2015). Exercise instructors are also at risk as they are often exposed to levels exceeding 115 dBA during these sessions (Razali, 2020).

The police force is another group with a high prevalence of hearing loss. In a study by Win *et al.* in 2015, NIHL was noted to be prevalent in 37.7% of male police personnel and 23.9% of the female personnel. The authors reported that their findings are similar to those of other studies, e.g. 28% in French police officers, and notably much higher in countries with greater traffic noise pollution with 66.4% in traffic police personnel in Kathmandu City, 81.2% in traffic police in Pune, India, and 84% in traffic police in Jalgaon Urban Centre in India (Win *et al.*, 2015). NIHL was present in 94% of subjects and the severity of NIHL was mild in 26%, moderate in 38% and severe in 36% of the subjects in a study of the incidence of NIHL among 50 police constables conducted in a medical college in Tamil Nadu India (Kanitha *et al.*, 2018). A study of Finnish Air Force pilots found that the hearing of pilots corresponded to approximately 80th percentile and 9–13 dB better than the 50th percentile of industrial workers. The prevalence of hearing loss of more than 20 dB at 1–4 kHz was found to be 4%, 17% and 27% among administrative personnel, flight deck personnel and flight deck engineers in a Nimitz class aircraft carrier (Rovig, 2004). A cross-sectional study at an airport in Malaysia carried out between November 2008 and March 2009 found that the prevalence rate ratio of hearing loss for non-smokers aged 40 years old and younger, smokers aged 40 years old and younger, non-smokers older than 40 years old and smokers older than 40 years old was 1.0, 1.7, 2.8 and 4.6, respectively (Nasir and Rampal, 2012).

In Spain, a prospective study of predictive factors of occupational NIHL among workers exposed to occupational noise in the construction industry; workers with abnormal audiograms were found to have significantly longer noise-exposure duration. A logistic regression model predicted 78.2% individuals with audiometric abnormality indicating the presence of hearing impairment (Peligrin *et al.*, 2015).

Ultrasound and Vibration

Sound and ultrasound emitted by high intensity ultrasonic devices exceeding known hygienic limits for frequencies 10–20 kHz have a negative influence on auditory function. A study of 55 operators exposed to industrial ultrasonic devices of frequencies 0.5–20 kHz showed that while there was no abnormality in the hearing range 0.5–8 kHz, there was an elevation of hearing threshold in the 10–20 kHz range. For comparison, reference hearing levels from 189 non-exposed persons were used (Grzesik, 1983).

Workers exposed to occupational vibration are also often exposed to excessive noise levels. Sympathetic vasoconstriction has been considered to be responsible for vibration white finger (VWF). It has been suggested that vasoconstriction in the cochlear and peripheral blood vessels may be a common mechanism for NIHL and VWF. Along with exposure to noise and aging, the presence of VWF and an elevated diastolic pressure were found to be major factors responsible in generating sensorineural hearing loss in another study of 122 noise exposed forest workers (Pyykko *et al.*, 1987). Vibration and noise may have the effects of combined exposures on the auditory system.

Vestibular Disturbances

NIHL and vestibular disturbances can co-exist. NIHL and balance disturbance with Meniere's-type symptoms appear to be significantly higher in a study of 18 senior army officers exposed to impulse noise for a prolonged period. Endolymphatic hydrops may be the underlying pathophysiologic mechanism in these cases (Ylikoski, 1988a). Simultaneous mechanical damage to both the cochlear and vestibular partitions by intense impulse noise may be responsible for the subclinical disturbance of the vestibular system among subjects with impulse-NIHL (Ylikoski, 1988b).

Ototoxicity

Solvents (particularly mixed organic solvents, styrene and toluene) are commonly established as being ototoxic either on their own or synergistically (with noise). Current exposure limits for solvents, alone and combined with noise and hearing conservation programmes (HCPs) are not adequate to protect the workers against auditory disorders (Sliwinska-Kowalska, 2007). Organic solvents like toluene, styrene, xylene, and ethylbenzene are known not only to cause OHC dysfunction but also impair the central auditory functions (Fuente and McPherson, 2012). This results in difficulty to understand and discriminate speech despite having normal hearing thresholds (Morata and Lemasters, 1995). Tests that assess the functionality of central auditory system such as speech tests (hearing in noise test), dichotic digit test (DDT), random gap detection (RGD) or gap in noise test (GIN) has shown significant differences between solvent-exposed and nonsolvent exposed workers.

Genetic Studies on NIHL

Genetic studies on NIHL appear to associate some genetic mutations with susceptibility to NIHL. However, a review of ten published studies by Zhang in 2010, for the New Zealand's Accident Compensation Corporation reported that genetic markers currently investigated are not strong risk factors for NIHL and hence the implication on the diagnosis and management of NIHL appears to be limited.

Physics of Sound

Noise refers to "sounds unwanted, undesirable and most times damaging and with intensity varying randomly in time." Wanted sounds similarly can also be harmful if exposures are for too long and too loud. The great variation of sound can render the objective description of noise difficult, something one must do in order to quantify, often legally, the exposure of noise. Hence many descriptors of sounds have been proposed in order to quantify them, and they include decibel values, equivalent levels and frequency weighting.

Sound is produced by vibration of an object causing alternate waves of compression and rarefaction. They need to be transmitted through a medium, and they travel best in solids, followed by liquids and air (or gases) respectively. Sound waves become weaker as they move away from the source. These sound waves will evoke the process of hearing when they reach the ear. Sound waves possess various physical characteristics including frequency, amplitude, and complexity, while the psychological perception of their counterparts are termed pitch, intensity and timbre accordingly.

Frequency

Frequency is the number of times the waveform repeats itself per unit time. It is expressed in cycles per second (Hertz, Hz) where 1 Hz = 1 cycle per second. Wavelength is the distance between peaks or troughs of the sound wave. Wavelength is inversely related to frequency.

Amplitude

Amplitude of sound is the magnitude of displacement of the waveform from the equilibrium to the peak or trough. Amplitude gives rise to the loudness, or intensity of a sound. Sound units measured in dB is perceived as intensity or loudness.

Timbre

The complexity of a sound gives it some identifiable characteristics that are known as timbre. This characteristic of sound is a combination of at least five acoustic parameters including spectrum of the stimulus, its waveform, the sound pressure, the frequency location of the spectrum, and the temporal characteristics of the sound; resulting in what is termed as spectral energy. An example of sounds with different timbre would be the middle C note of a piano and that of a guitar.

Sound Measurement

The amplitude of a sound wave is typically expressed in Pascal units (Pa). 0.00002 Pa (or 20 μPa) is generally considered to be the minimum detectable sound level, while the greatest sound pressure level that can be tolerated is 10 million times over. Since it is difficult to cope with this hugely wide range of numbers the logarithmic scale is used to express the ratio of these intensities.

The decibel scale

Sound in general is measured in the decibel sound pressure level scale (dB SPL). All ratio scales have an arbitrary zero, i.e. a reference point, and in the decibel scale the standardised reference point is 20 μPa. The following formula is used to calculate the sound level in decibels (dB SPL):

$$20 \log_{10} (p_1/p_2) \text{ with } p_2 \text{ being the reference point}$$

Thus, a scale of 200,000,000 to 20 has been effectively compressed to one that is of a more manageable range of 140 to 0 dB. Decibels are relative units of measure and thus cannot be added or subtracted arithmetically.

Another important concept to grasp is the relative change in sound pressure. The inverse square law states that, as the distance is doubled from the sound source (or exposure time is halved, for example), the sound pressure will decrease to half its original value. And because of its logarithmic property, a doubling of sound power will lead to a 3-dB rise (and vice versa, halving it will lead to a 3-dB decrease). This explains why decreasing half the exposure time will actually lead to a 3-dB decrease (3 dB exchange rate) instead of the 5-dB exchange rate.

Equivalent sound pressure level

Sound from various noise sources varies during a working day. In an attempt to objectively quantify the worker's exposure to noise; especially for legislation and enforcement purposes, a time-weighted energy average that represents the total sound energy experienced over a given period has been used. Equivalent level or $L_{eq(t)}$ is the average sound energy received during time "t." The popularity of L_{eq} is two-fold: (1) it is possible to compare widely different sound exposures as a total amount of energy exposed, and (2) it uses a 3-dB trading relationship, making it a more accurate analysis of the hazards posed by noise.

Frequency analysis

Frequency analysis is conducted to determine the intensity of sound by individual frequency. This helps in determining noise source for effective engineering controls to be instituted. An octave band analyzer is used to determine the intensity at each of the frequencies.

Frequency weighting

Frequency weighting scales attempt to overcome the frequency variability of sound measurement and analysis equipment. The three weighting most commonly used in commercially available sound level meters are A, C and Z. A reasonable knowledge is useful as using the wrong weighting scale on a sound level meter measurement could render the measurement irrelevant or even non-compliant to the legal requirement.

The frequency-weightages in a nutshell:

i) A-weighting readings resemble the response of the ear to pure tones (most sensitive only from 500 to 4,000 Hz) and only at a relatively low level (i.e. about 40 dB). Noise can be wide-ranging and hence the possibility of damaging levels being filtered out from being measured is very likely. A-weighting is still used mainly because it has been incorporated in most commercially available sound-level meters, and because it has been around for as long as it has (Fletcher and Munson, 1933).

ii) C-weighting is mostly used to measure peak sound pressures in impulsive noise. It documents more of low-frequency sounds on the human ear compared with the A-weighting and is essentially linear or at least flatter in the lower frequency compared to A-weighting.

iii) Z-weighting is a flat frequency response that doesn't filter any or apply any attenuation or weighting to any frequency. This weightage is more often used in octave band analysis and for determining environmental noise.

Types of noise

Sound can be classified as infrasonic (less than 20 Hz), audible (20–20,000 Hz) and ultrasonic (greater than 20,000 Hz). Noise in the frequency range of 250 Hz to 8,000 Hz is particularly important because this is the range where most speech frequencies fall. A representation of this is shown in the diagram below (Fig. 1), marked by the blue-shaded area, termed as "long-term average speech spectrum" (LTASS) or often known as the "speech banana."

The LTASS demarcates where sounds of speech fell within the audiogram. For many languages such as English or Malay, the consonants give meaning, whereas vowels give strength to the words. Hence in the strictest of principles of speech and audiology, each and every frequency within the speech spectrum (most usually from 250 to 8,000 Hz for many languages) is important for deciphering speech.

This is where the methods of averaging a hearing threshold come into conflict with the above concept. A person thus needs to be able to hear all frequencies well, and not just up to 3 kHz as stated by the AAO-AMA classification. Without the ability to hear, for example, the fricatives (such as /sh/, /f/) and plosives (alveolar plosives such as /t/, /d/), a person will have significant difficulty understanding most, if not all of speech. The usual tenet that speech frequency lies

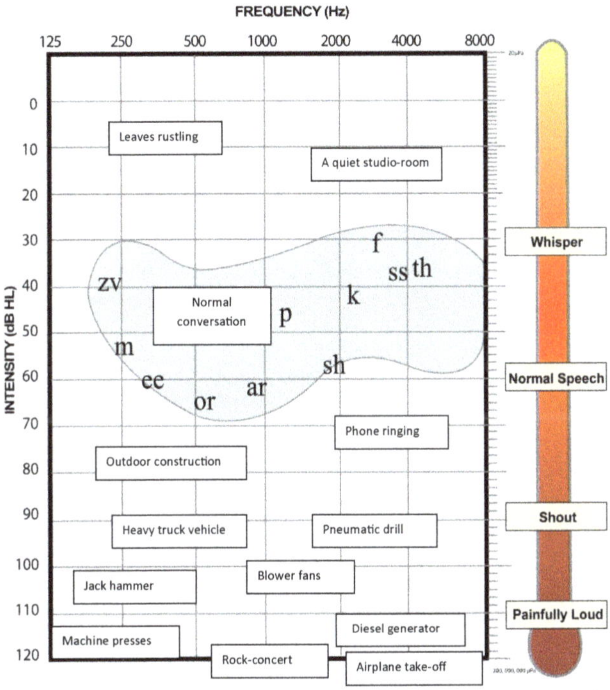

Fig. 1. A diagrammatic representation of everyday sounds in an intensity by frequency graph. The speech spectrum falls into the shaded area.

mostly in the 2,000 Hz region is an anecdote that should not be propagated just to justify the need to come up with an easy and manageable method of classifying hearing impairment.

Generally, there are four types of noise; continuous or steady state, fluctuating, intermittent and impulse noise (Fig. 2). Continuous or steady state noise is sound whose quality and intensity are practically constant over a period of time. It generally varies less than 3 dB. Examples of sources of steady state noise include electrical generators, printing machines and weaving machines.

Fluctuating noise is continuous noise where the intensity of noise varies more than 3 dB.

Intermittent noise is sound whose intensity drops to the ambient level several times. These drops in intensity are for varying periods. An example is using a chain saw to cut logs. Impulse noise or impact noise

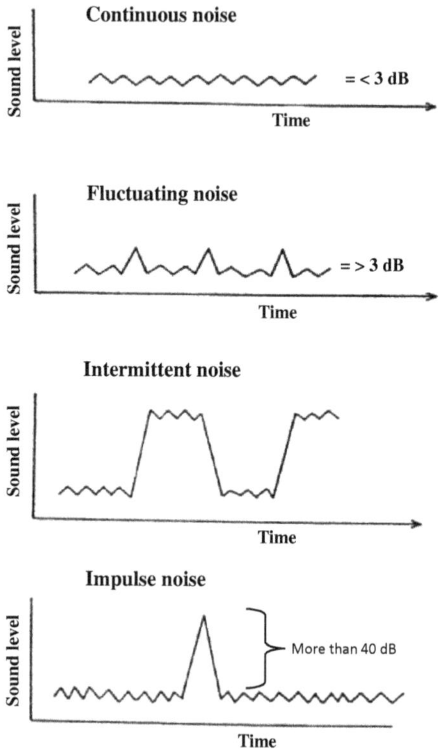

Fig. 2. Types of noise.

is sound with a sudden change of intensity of at least 40 dB. It is of short duration generally less than 0.5 s. Any type of noise can damage the ear, although there are some studies that have proven that high frequency noise is generally more destructive to the hair cells.

Hearing Mechanism

The ear can be divided into the outer, middle and inner ear (Fig. 3). The outer ear is made up of the pinna, the external auditory meatus and canal. It helps conduct sound to the middle ear, amplifies certain frequencies (1–3 kHz) to about 20 dB SPL and bilaterally, is the main player in our ability to localise a distant source of sound. The middle ear is a cavity connected to the outer ear by the tympanic membrane

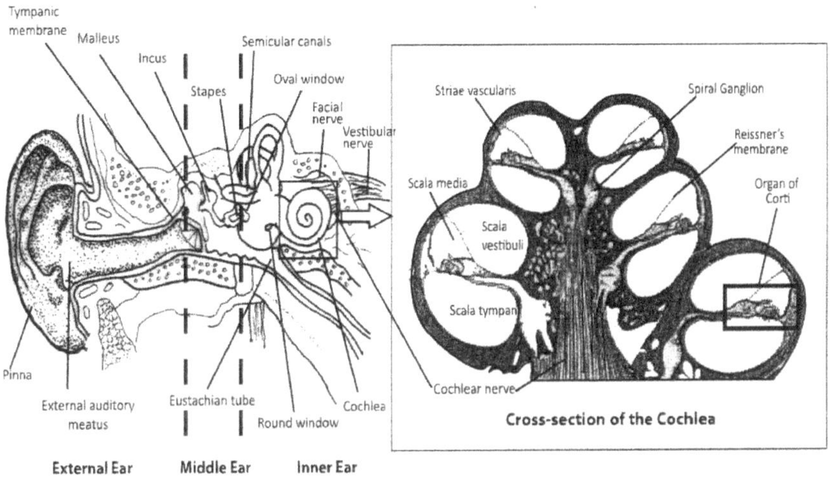

Fig. 3. Diagram of the external, middle and inner ear, with a cross-section view of the cochlea.

and the inner ear by the oval and round windows. It has three bones (ossicular chain) comprising the malleus, incus and stapes. These ossicles conduct sound waves from the external ear to the cochlea. The middle ear's main function is to overcome the impedance of relaying relatively small amount of sound energy from the air onto the fluid medium of the labyrinth while maintaining the same amount of sound energy. The middle ear, via the stapedius muscle, also protects the inner ear from impulsively loud noise.

The cochlea and the semi-circular canals in the inner ear are responsible for hearing and balance respectively. The cochlea, essentially a tube coiled around a central pillar of bone resembles the shape of a snail shell. It is further divided into three chambers (scala vestibuli, media and tympani) by the basilar membrane and the vestibular membrane. All three chambers are filled with fluid that will vibrate when the ossicles in the middle ear passes its energy through the oval window. The organ of Corti (Fig. 4) has about 30,000 hair cells resting on the basilar membrane. The displacement of these hair cells is responsible for triggering the action potential that will then be relayed to the final processing center at the temporal lobe where it will be interpreted as hearing meaningful sounds.

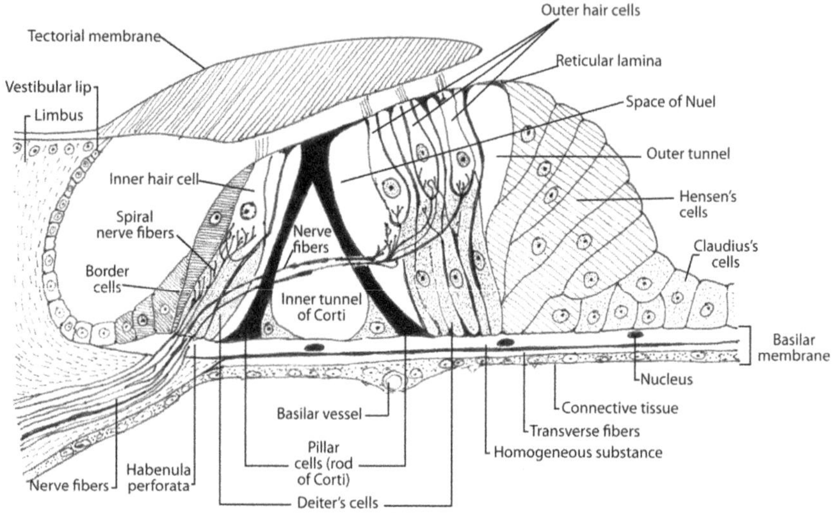

Fig. 4. Organ of Corti.

For physiological purposes, the ear can be divided into the conducting apparatus and the sensorineural apparatus. The conducting apparatus comprises the outer ear, the tympanic membrane, the ossicular chain and labyrinthine fluids. The sensorineural apparatus comprises the organ of Corti in the cochlea, the auditory division of the acoustic nerve and its central connections.

Sound can be transmitted to the inner ear in three modes. The most common route is transmission via the vibrating tympanic membrane by the ossicular chain to the oval window. Sound can be transmitted directly across the middle ear when waves fall on the round window when there is a large perforation in the ear drum. It is also transmitted by bone conduction when sound energy is transmitted to the inner ear through the bones of the skull.

The middle ear serves as a transformer matching acoustic resistance of the air in the outer ear to that of the labyrinthine fluids. Within the cochlea, vibrations in the cochlea fluid are processed such that the frequency, intensity and temporal quality of the sound are transmitted to the auditory nerve and on to the brain. The direction from which the sound originates is assessed by correlating differences between the two sides of the head (differences in loudness and time of reception).

Effects of Noise

The effects of noise can be auditory and non-auditory. Noise can be a nuisance and cause speech interference at 30–80 dBA. It can cause conductive hearing loss if the tympanic membrane is ruptured or the ossicles dislocated caused by loud impulsive noise from an explosion. NIHL occurs from prolonged exposure to noise above 85 dBA. While whole body effects have been noted at intensities of noise greater than 110 dB, NIHL is the most significant problem facing employees in noisy workplaces. The damaging effects of noise depend on overall intensity of noise, total duration of exposure, frequency characteristics of the noise and susceptibility of the individual (Daniel, 2007; Tambs, 2006). A study by Yoon *et al.* (2015) reported that workplaces with high noise exposure were significantly associated with a higher risk of occupational injury. Furthermore, the risk of occupational injury increases with noise exposure level in a dose response relationship (Yoon *et al.*, 2015).

Noise-Induced Hearing Loss

The effects of noise on hearing may be temporary or permanent. The effects are a change in threshold hearing levels and if temporary and reversible following cessation from noise exposure, it is then called temporary threshold shift (TTS). If the loss is irreversible it is a permanent threshold shift (PTS).

TTS is a transitory hearing loss with normal hearing being restored after cessation of noise exposure. The time of recovery from TTS varies. TTS occurs as early as after two min of exposures. The higher the intensity and duration of exposure the higher the TTS. Recovery from TTS begins immediately after cessation of exposure with most of the recovery occurring within 16 h. If loss of hearing due to TTS is less than 30 dB, recovery is usually within 16 h. However, if loss is greater than 50 dB, recovery is only rapid after the first day. In some cases, audiological evoked responses had full recovery only as late as after 30 days.

As TTS usually recovers within 24–48 h, it has not been given much emphasis and hence not much data is available on this issue.

However, a study in a mouse model pointed to the presence of sub-lethal changes to the inner ears that accelerated hearing loss due to aging even though the hearing thresholds were totally restored to normal shortly following the TTS (Kujawa and Liberman, 2006).

NIHL is irreversible permanent sensorineural hearing loss with no recovery on cessation of exposure. The hearing loss typically commences at the 4 kHz frequency and extends to surrounding frequencies with continued exposure. The dip is typically bilateral and symmetrical. Permanent hearing loss may occur without prior onset of TTS.

Case Study 1: Noise-induced Hearing Loss

A 34 year old male has been working in an automotive factory for 14 years with a positive history of hazardous noise exposure. He was examined during the audiometric testing programme that had recently been introduced at his workplace. There was no history of ear discharge, head injury, or any exposure to loud noise outside of his work. Otoscopic examination revealed normal ear canals and intact tympanic membranes bilaterally. Rinne's test was positive and Weber test noted no lateralisation. Pure tone audiometry revealed dips at the 4 kHz region with no air bone gap in both ears (Fig. 5). He was diagnosed as having noise-induced hearing loss based on history of exposure to noise, the dips at the 4 kHz frequency and absence of an air bone gap.

Pathophysiology of noise-induced hearing loss

The basic mechanism involved in NIHL could be broadly classified into mechanically-destructive damage and metabolic stress (Fig. 6).

Mechanical processes

The various mechanical processes that could cause damage to the hair cells as a result of noise exposure include:

1. Violent fluid motion in the cochlea causing the tips of the stereocilia on the outer hair cells (OHCs) to be removed from their

Name: I.C No:

Age: 34 Sex: F /(M) Date: 8/7/2015 Time: 10.00 am

Audiometer: ☑ GSI Audiostar ☐ AC40 ☐ Other: ______ Tester: Ariff

Reliability: Good

AUDIOGRAM

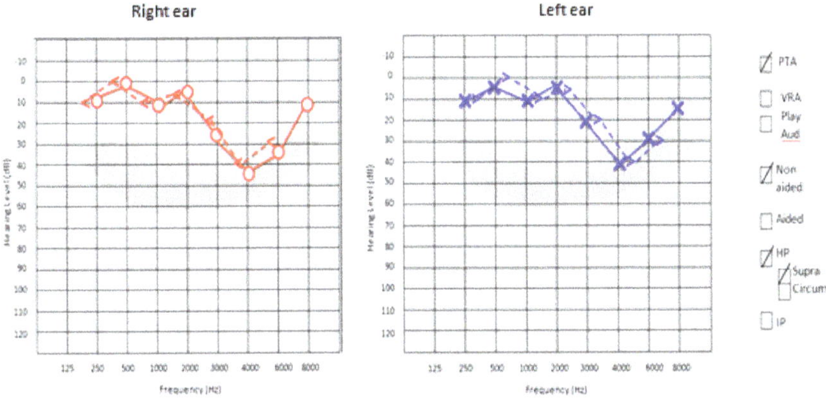

SYMBOLS	LEFT	RIGHT
Air	x	o
Masked Air	▪	▪
Bone	>	<
Masked Bone	]	[
Sound Field Binaural dBSPL		□

Tympanogram					Otoacoustic Emission			Acoustic Reflexes (Screen: 95dB)				
EAR	ECV	SC	MEP	Type	EAR	TEOAE	DPOAE	Ipsi	0.5kHz	1kHz	2kHz	4kHz
RE	1.2	0.2	-5	A	RE			RE				
LE	1.1	0.4	4	A	LE			LE				

Fig. 5. Audiogram of a 34 year old with bilateral NIHL.

points of insertion with the tectorial membrane. In addition, the stereocilia can suffer loss of structural integrity and further reduce its ability to act as mechanoelectrical transducers due to the loss of permeability of protein transduction channels in the surrounding cell membrane.

2. Damage to pillar cells and supporting cells (Deiter's and Hansen's). The loss of these cells will interfere with the local impedance of vibration along the organ of Corti.
3. Damage to the hair cells either directly by detaching the organ of Corti or tearing of the basilar membrane or indirectly from damage of the supporting cells.

4. Rupture of the Reissner's membrane with mixing of the endolymph and perilymph resulting in damage to the hair cells.

The above processes are usually seen when the exposure is to high intensity noise levels and NIHL is of rapid onset.

Metabolic processes

The metabolic processes that could damage to hair cells as a result of noise exposure include:

1. Over stimulation of the OHCs result in excessive mitochondrial activity making them require more energy. The hair cells may then be more susceptible to injury by ischaemia. Vesiculation and vacuolation in the endoplasmic reticulum of the hair cells and swelling of the mitochondria will lead to eventual rupturing of the cell membrane and hair cell loss.
2. Hair cell loss may be due to metabolic exhaustion as a result of disruption of enzyme systems essential for energy production, biosynthesis of protein and ion transport.
3. A significant rise in the intra-cellular calcium levels in the OHCs has been documented. This will lead to cytoskeletal breakdown, membrane defects and DNA damage. The consequences of these damages will be loss of body cell stiffness.
4. Injury to the stria vascularis causes disturbances in Na, K and ATP levels. This results in inhibition of the active transport process and energy utilisation by the sensory cells. The damaged sensory cells create small lesions in the reticular membrane with intermixing of the endolymph and cortilymph with subsequent spread of damage to other sensory cells.
5. Reduction in the cochlear blood flow can occur and this will lead to the increased level of reactive oxygen species (ROS) in the cochlea.
6. Glutamate excitotoxicity will cause swelling and rupturing of the dendritic terminals of the auditory nerve afferent fibres.

The region of the organ of Corti about 8–10 mm from the basal end (tonotopically corresponding to the 4 kHz region of the

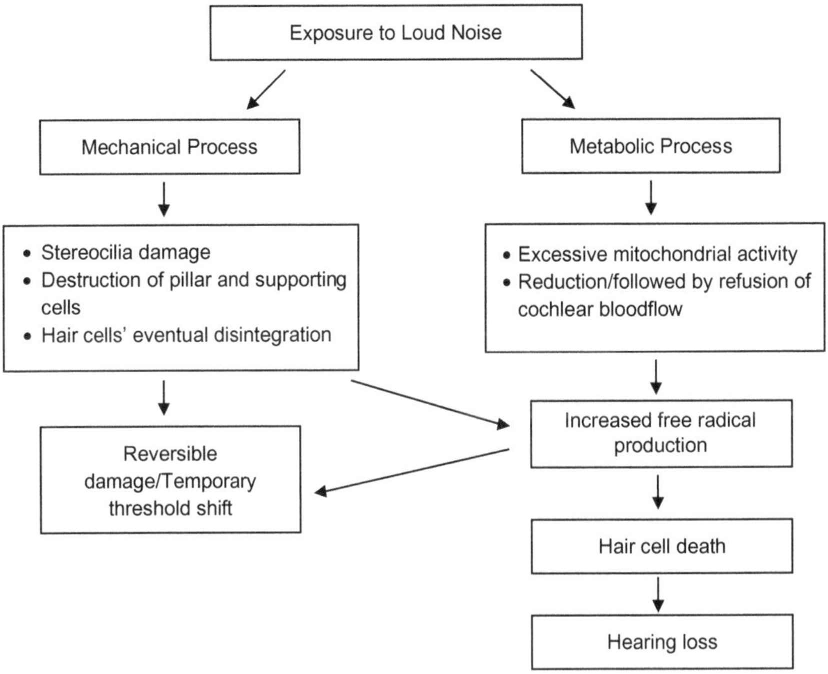

Fig. 6. A flowchart illustrating the pathophysiology of NIHL.

audiogram) is viewed to be uniquely vulnerable to noise. This explains the typical notch around the 4,000 Hz region in NIHL. Several theories have been offered on why NIHL initially involves frequencies surrounding the 4,000 Hz region, and they include:

1. The harmonic amplification theory: The physical structure of the ear canal creates a resonance and amplifies frequencies around this frequency.
2. The absolute sensitivity theory: The ear is most sensitive at the 4,000 Hz region, as evidenced by many established psychoacoustic studies.
3. The biomechanical theory: The energy that is being transferred from the middle ear to the endolymph is greatest as it goes through the first bend of the cochlear. The hair cells located at the first bend are those representing approximately 4 kHz.

4. Middle ear muscle contraction: Chronically intense loud sounds will render the middle ear muscles to contract and reduce only the transmission of low-frequency energy into the cochlea, as opposed to the acute contraction of the muscles which will block the transmission of sound across all the frequencies.

A study to determine the time course of organ of Corti degeneration after noise exposure was conducted in 199 chinchilla cochleae noise exposed animals. The degeneration of hair cells and supporting cells after noise ends was quantitatively demonstrated. The study found OHCs began dying during the exposure and OHC loss slowed down but was still present beyond one month. Inner hair cell loss was delayed until 1–3 weeks postexposure. Outer pillar and inner pillar losses were present at a low level in the acute phase but increased exponentially thereafter. In ears exposed to moderate noise some of these changes in the supporting cells appeared to be reversible while in ears exposed to high-level noise, these changes appeared to indicate impending degeneration (Bohne *et al.*, 2017).

Other Auditory Effects of Noise

Acoustic trauma

Acoustic trauma is usually caused by exposure to sudden loud sounds (illustrated by Case Study 2). Common symptoms include hearing impairment, tinnitus, otalgia, and ear discharge. The likelihood of tympanic membrane perforation in acoustic trauma is higher in ears with current or previous disease, in older workers, in poorly pneumatised middle ear and if the tympanic membrane is perpendicular to the explosion wave (Ritenour *et al.*, 2008).

Case Study 2: Acoustic Trauma with Temporary Threshold Shift

A 31 year old male factory worker was near an explosion at the workplace. He came to the clinic 5 days following the explosion with complaints of hearing loss in both ears and a ringing noise in the left ear.

These complaints began immediately after the explosion. On examination of the ear, there was a small perforation of the tympanic membrane in the right ear and an intact tympanic membrane in the left ear. Pure tone audiometry revealed bilateral severe hearing loss. Tympanometry was flat (type B) in the right ear and normal (type A) in the left ear. His hearing level was monitored regularly and marked improvement in hearing level was noted three weeks later.

Examination two and a-half months later revealed a healed tympanic membrane and normal hearing thresholds bilaterally. He was diagnosed and managed as a case of acoustic trauma with temporary threshold shift.

Tinnitus (ringing noise in the ears) usually presents immediately after noise exposure. It may become permanent on continued exposure. Tinnitus due to noise exposure is usually perceived as high pitched and tonal; the frequency of the tinnitus often reflects the worse frequency of the worker's hearing threshold although tinnitus matching is not an easy task to execute. There is no correlation between the discomfort caused by the tinnitus and audiometric findings. Tinnitus can cause great disability especially if suffered by a young person (Axelsson and Prasher, 2000).

Vertigo can occur after exposure to very extreme noise levels. Temporary vertigo has been described after exposures to the noise of un-silenced jet engines. Temporary or even permanent vertigo can follow firearms explosions. Vertigo is unlikely with ordinary industrial noise exposure. There is associated vestibular involvement only in very severe blast injuries (Tun *et al.*, 2009).

Non-Auditory Effects of Noise

Increased noise levels also produce stress reactions with variations in heart rate, blood pressure, respiration, blood glucose and lipid levels. Increased gastrointestinal motility and peptic ulcers have also been reported (Rahma *et al.*, 2013). Studies have suggested that excessive noise above 55 dBA produces annoyance and a reduction in efficiency. Reported symptoms include chronic fatigue, backache, neck pain, eye-ball discomfort and ear pressure and sleep disturbance (Mahendra and Sridhar, 2008).

Diagnosis of NIHL

The diagnosis of occupational NIHL is based on a history of exposure to noise in the workplace, a clinical examination to exclude other causes of hearing loss and a NIHL audiological profile.

History Taking and Clinical Examination

An occupational history should include detailed, chronological information on current and all previous employment (particularly with respect to noise exposure, including part time jobs held). Information on hobbies and other environmental exposures should also be elicited. The medical history must determine whether the employee has or has had ear disease and whether he has had exposure to ototoxic drugs, e.g. streptomycin. The clinical examination of the ear must exclude the presence of wax, infection and perforation of the tympanic membrane. Vestibular assessment might be necessary in cases where vestibular involvement is suspected.

Case Study 3: Non-occupational Noise Exposure

A steel company established an audiometric programme for its workers for the last 10 years and Mr A, a 35 year old worker in this company has undergone this year's annual audiometric programme. The result showed presence of temporary standard threshold shift (TSTS) and noise induced hearing loss (NIHL) but no hearing impairment yet. After 3 months, the audiogram was reviewed and permanent standard threshold shift (PSTS) was observed. Otoscopic examination revealed normal findings in both ears with no ontological problems or head trauma reported. Tympanometry showed type A (normal) tympanograms in both ears. Mr A did reveal that he had taken up a new hobby for the past 2 years which was playing drums. No hearing protection was worn during these sessions.

A diagnostic pure tone audiometry test was ordered to confirm the type of loss and the result showed sensorineural hearing loss. The audiogram history was reviewed again and noted that this is the first PSTS for the worker for the last 10 years.

He was diagnosed with early sensorineural NIHL with bilateral PSTS and no hearing impairment although the case was determined to be not work related. The Occupational Health Doctor notified the company and ordered a revision of the baseline. The worker was counselled on the need of using hearing protection for his new hobby to prevent developing further deterioration of his hearing.

Pure tone audiometry

Pure tone audiometers have had a long history of use as devices for measuring hearing thresholds (Martin and Stauffer, 1975) and are the current "gold-standard" for assessing hearing thresholds. Pure tone audiometry (PTA) is indispensable both for screening (air conduction) and diagnosis (both air and bone conduction with masking when necessary) of NIHL.

During PTA, pure tones are delivered to the ear through a suitable earphone, the most common being the supra-aural headphones. "Insert ear-phones" can improve the result as it could reduce the incidence of ear-canal collapse and improve interaural attenuation. Circum-aural headphones are occasionally used when the background ambient noise cannot be attenuated, e.g. when a sound-proof room is unavailable. The frequencies tested range from 250 Hz to 8 kHz, at intensities from 20 dB to 120 dB in 5 dB steps. At a minimum, testing at the following frequencies is recommended –0.5, 1, 2, 3, 4, 6 and 8 kHz. A threshold intensity of pure tone is then established, above which the pure tone will be detected and below which it will not. The unit of measurement used is dB HL (decibel hearing level, and not dBA or dB SPL). The response may vary from one testing session to another depending on the skill of the tester, motivation of the worker and the presence of ambient noise. The usual intra-personal variability is 10 dB HL across all frequencies.

PTA testing in the workplace is used to establish the hearing status of employees, identify individuals who are susceptible to noise, monitor hearing loss during the period of employment and as part of a HCP.

Baseline audiometry is usually conducted as part of the pre-employment examination. Periodic audiometry is performed at regular intervals (annually or biannually) to monitor for hearing loss among workers in noisy areas. To obtain a valid audiometric result, the employee should not have been exposed to high noise levels in the past 14 h before baseline audiometry and 12–14 h for periodic audiometry. Audiometers used for PTA must conform to national or international standards and must be calibrated. Background noise levels should be low. Audiometric testing should be carried out and supervised by trained personnel. These requirements have sometimes been incorporated into national health and safety regulations.

Audiological profile of noise-induced hearing loss

The audiologic profile of NIHL is the presence of sensorineural hearing loss, most pronounced in the high frequency region of the audiogram between 3 and 6 kHz. The greatest amount of hearing loss is initially at around the 4 kHz region (4 kHz dip or notch), although this notch could be maximum at anywhere along the 3–6 kHz region. Another important feature is the recovery pattern at the 8 kHz region, hence justifying the 8 kHz inclusion in any hearing test. It is a significant sign of NIHL when seen in individuals with a positive history of noise exposure. The audiometric configuration is bilaterally symmetrical. Continued exposure results in a widening of the 4 kHz notch spreading to adjacent higher and lower frequencies. Higher frequencies of 6 kHz and above are generally affected to a greater extent than frequencies of 2 kHz and below. In very advanced cases the 1 kHz frequency may be affected but rarely to a great extent.

Asymmetrical effects between both ears may result from unequal ear susceptibility, different initial hearing thresholds or specific conditions of work. The audiological profile of advanced NIHL is similar to other high frequency sensorineural hearing loss due to cochlear and supracochlear lesions.

A simple method can be used to classify employees into groups:

1. Where the worsening of hearing thresholds at all frequencies is less than 25 dB HL, the individuals can be deemed to have "normal hearing."

2. Where there is a 25 dB loss or higher at any one frequency individuals are said to have "hearing loss."
3. Where there is a 25 dB loss or higher in the 4 kHz region (including 3 and 6 kHz) plus a recovery pattern at 8 kHz, these individuals are said to have "hearing loss that is suggestive of early NIHL." It would be advisable for the workers who have this to be notified that there are already early changes of NIHL so that appropriate preventive measures can be implemented.
4. Where there is an average loss of 25 dB or more affecting the frequencies 0.5, 1, 2 and 3 kHz with history of noise exposure, it can then be classified as "hearing impairment from NIHL." The worker needs to be notified of his audiological findings and measures such as ensuring that the worker be protected from further exposure to noise, especially for more than 85 dB for >8 h, instituted with engineering and/or administrative controls. The importance of wearing of PPE should be reiterated. Continuing annual audiometry is indicated, and the worker should be sent for further clinical assessment as necessary.
5. Where there is an average increase of 10 dB or more in the frequencies 2, 3 and 4 kHz with a history of noise exposure over time, standard threshold shift (STS) is then said to have been established. The worker needs to be notified, provided with retraining and refitting of hearing protectors and sent for further clinical assessment as necessary.

A decision on whether hearing impairment is due to noise should be made by the medical practitioner only after assessment of the medical and occupational history, considering all sources of exposure to noise, performing an ear examination and reviewing the audiograms.

Fitness to Work

Acceptable hearing level is difficult to define as there is wide individual variation in the degree to which hearing impairment causes hearing disability. Unlike a blind person, an individual with defective hearing has a hidden disability. The hearing-impaired individual should be excluded only in a limited number of jobs where perfect hearing is essential, e.g. radio operators and civil airline pilots. The most appropriate way to judge employability of a hearing-impaired person is to test hearing ability in the intended working environment (a "trade test"). While auditory disorders seldom lead to time off work, the impact is more apparent on efficiency and safety (Kramer *et al.*, 2006). Other auditory disorders that can affect fitness for work include tinnitus, ear discharge, balance disturbances and problems with barometric pressure differences. While the decision on the auditory requirement for fitness for work is usually left to examining medical practitioners, there is guidance on this for specific occupational groups, e.g. firefighters and workers involved in rescue operations and the oil and gas industry.

An off-shore worker for example, would generally need to have an average hearing threshold of not worse than 35 dB in the better ear, without the help of hearing aids. These workers may have difficulty hearing safety warnings and have problems with effective communication in noisy environments. The use of hearing aids is acceptable for existing employees, although care must be taken to ensure that the aids are safe to be used in the rigs/plants.

Interestingly, a review on Auditory Fitness for Duty (AFFD) by Tufts *et al.* (2009) found that audiometric pass-fail and profiling criteria were originally based on medico-legal definitions of handicapping hearing loss and not on fitness-for-duty concerns. The original purpose of pre-employment hearing testing was to safeguard employers against civil claims by ascertaining whether hearing loss was present prior to employment. It was also found that the audiogram often under-predicted the functional performance of individuals with hearing loss as a worker may be able to compensate successfully for hearing loss with experience, skill on the job, familiarity with typical communications, warning signals, and Standard Operating Procedures (SOPs). The forced-whisper test is still utilised by the Federal Highway Administration in the United States for AFFD testing for commercial motor-vehicle operations. Applicants must be able to perceive a forced whispered voice in at least one ear at not less than five feet, with or without use of a hearing aid (Federal Motor Carrier Safety Administration, 2014).

However due to the forced-whisper test having problems with face validity, "inadequate test protocols, calibration, and interpretative criteria" the pure-tone audiogram has largely replaced free-field live-voice tests as the most commonly accepted measure of auditory fitness.

Assessment for Other Auditory Disorders

Tinnitus may be associated with psychological effects including insomnia that may be severe and incapacitating affecting work performance.

Otitis media and otitis externa may affect ability to use ear defenders. Hygiene requirements in the food industry can exclude such cases from working in the preparation or selling of food (Eyears and Hutson, 2019).

Middle ear disease can affect flying and diving. Acute disorientating episodes resulting from vestibular disorders coming on without warning may be a potential danger to employees themselves or to others at work (Eyears and Hutson, 2019). Orientation sense is important in jobs such as diving, driving and flying. This may not be a major concern for those who have warning symptoms, or those who do not work in hazardous areas such as working at heights or handling molten metal, or caustic chemicals.

Hearing Impairment

The American Medical Association (AMA) defines impairment as "a significant deviation, loss, or loss of use of any body structure or body function in an individual with a health condition, disorder, or disease." Some jurisdictions provide compensation for permanent hearing impairment. Permanent impairments have been defined as those that have reached maximum medical improvement (MMI) and are well stabilised and unlikely to change substantially with or without medical treatment (Rondinelli *et al.*, 2008). The term hearing "disability" is now preferred over the term "handicap". Disability is defined as activity limitations and/or participation restrictions in an individual with a health condition, disorder, or disease. Some individuals can be severely disabled by minor impairments and vice versa. Hence the AMA has taken to rating hearing impairments based on hearing thresholds at different frequencies. The Guidelines suggests an average hearing level of 26 dB at 500, 1,000, 2,000 and 3,000 Hz as the onset of hearing impairment.

Hearing impairment can be classified into various categories: normal (not worse than 20 dB HL), mild (20–40 dB HL), moderate (41–70 dB HL), severe (70–90 dB HL) and profound (more than 90 dB HL). "Deafness" is a term that should be avoided as this is a subjective term, and there is no clear cut off point to decide when a person becomes "deaf."

Assessing disability from hearing impairment

While assessment of hearing impairment is based on an individual's hearing, the extent of disability associated with it must take into consideration other work-related factors including the importance of auditory function in the job. Guidelines for total disability compensation due to hearing impairment vary from country to country. They generally require that hearing cannot be restored by hearing aids before benefits are provided. Adjustments for presbycusis are sometimes included when assessing benefits for occupational hearing loss.

Table 1 shows how different organisations assess disability from hearing loss.

Table 1. Methods Calculating Disability from Hearing Impairment*

Organisation or Publication	Frequencies (kHz)	Low Fence	High Fence	Weight Between Ears
*f*AAO-1979	0.5, 1, 2, 3	25	92	5:1
AAOO-1959	1, 2, 3	25	92	5:1
NIOSH-FECA	1, 2, 3	25	92	5:1
Wisconsin State Formula	0.5, 1, 2, 3, 4, 6	35	92	4:1
British Society of Audiology	1, 2, 4	25	92	5:1
The British "Black Book"	1, 2, 3	—		
DHSS	1, 2, 3	40		4:1

Table 1. (*Continued*)

Organisation or Publication	Frequencies (kHz)	Low Fence	High Fence	Weight Between Ears
Compensation for Occupational Injuries and Diseases Act 1993	0.5, 1, 2, 3	25		5:1
Workers Compensation Board, Ontario	0.5, 1, 2, 3	35		5:1
Workers Compensation Board, Quebec	0.5, 1, 2			
Ireland	0.5, 1, 2, 4	20	100	4:1
SOCSO Malaysia	0.5, 1, 2, 3	25	100	5:1

Note: *This table illustrates a lack of concordance in recommendations between organisations.

The use of questionnaires for assessing hearing disability is necessary in spite of its high level of subjectivity (and high variability). Speech test in noise as well as in quiet is deemed more reliable. Commercial and locally validated tests such as the hearing-in-noise-test (HINT) are available and can enable testing using different spoken languages

Prevention of NIHL — Hearing Conservation Programmes

A HCP remains the main approach for minimising the likelihood of hearing loss from exposure to noise in the workplace. It needs to have the commitment and active involvement by both management and employees to ensure the programme is effective and the workers are protected adequately. The most effective approach for controlling noise exposure is through the reduction of noise at source, and if this is not feasible a comprehensive approach comprising risk identification, equipment and job redesign, training and education can be adopted to effectively manage the risk of NIHL and other noise-related health effects.

An effective HCP starts with a thorough noise risk assessment, followed by implementation of noise reduction measures, such as engineering control and administrative control and use of personal hearing protectors if these controls are not sufficient to reduce exposure. Supplementary measures include a yearly pure tone audiometry testing as a secondary preventive measure, informing employees of hazards of noise and imparting appropriate information, instruction and training, and proper record keeping.

Noise Risk Assessment

A HCP should begin with a noise risk assessment (NRA). The need to establish and implement a HCP at a particular workplace depends on the finding of an NRA report. The objective of the assessment would be to identify all employees likely to be exposed to excessive noise. Information regarding specific noise sources and work practices that will help in formulation of new measures to reduce noise as well as to assess the effectiveness of existing control measures will be determined. The NRA would also help in selection of appropriate personal hearing protectors for the workers. Demarcation of hearing protection zone where workers can be "noise-free" could also be done.

Noise Reduction Measures

The measures taken must be based on the findings during noise-risk assessment and must include engineering control, administrative control and personal hearing protectors. The hierarchy of hazard control needs to be followed as much as possible. Engineering control should thus be the most important component of a HCP and other measures are only considered when these are not possible. Engineering noise control methods can be divided into control of noise at source, control of noise propagation and receiver control. Although the initial costs of putting engineering controls in place can be high, it is not a recurrent cost. Complete knowledge of the process is necessary to decide whether noise be controlled at its source or in its path (Figs. 7 and 8).

Measures of controlling noise at source include replacing or substituting equipment with less noisy components, moving the source further from operators, reducing vibration by using absorbing material, and use of silencers for air and gas flow. Measures of noise

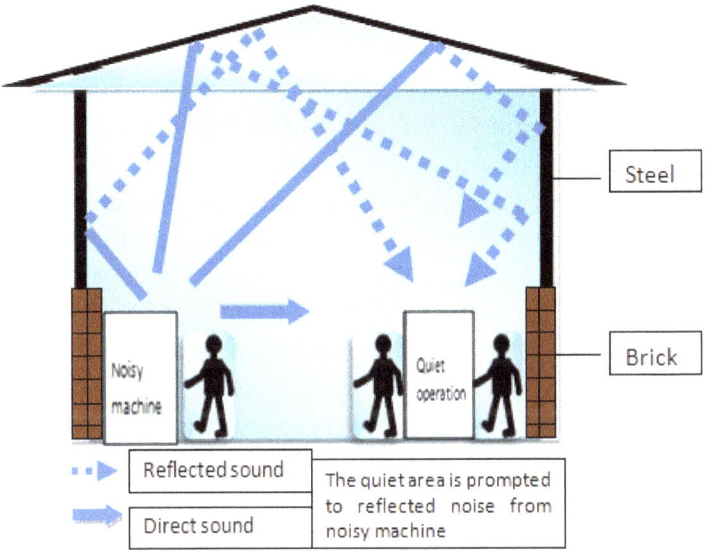

Fig. 7. Area of high noise level.

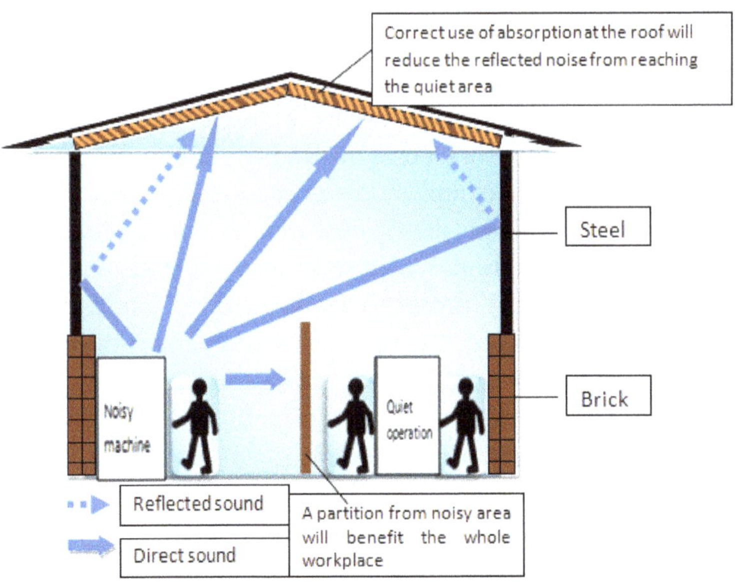

Fig. 8. Area of high noise level with noise control suggestions.

control in the path include acoustical shields, barrier walls, and partial or total enclosures of the noise source. In essence, noise control could involve equipment replacement, equipment relocation, vibration isolation, surface damping, barriers, enclosures, mufflers and source redesign. With appropriate engineering, alterations made within a factory or any workplace, can result in significant reduction in occupational noise (Joy and Middendorf, 2007). For example, recommended engineering noise controls that may be implemented in the South African mines included enclosing noisy places, using correct sound barriers and using curtains and retrofitted noise control packages (Madahana *et al.*, 2020).

Administrative controls reduce individual employee exposures by using the "equal energy principle," which allows a trade-off between noise level and duration of exposure. Under this approach, exposures to noise are allowed if the 8-h time weighted average is kept below the control limits (it also requires compliance with short-term exposure limits). It may also be implemented by switching employees in high noise areas with those in low noise areas after a certain period of time has elapsed. It could also involve scheduling operating times so as to minimise the number of employees exposed to high noise levels. Administrative controls are a poor option for preventing NIHL, because of many reasons including individual differences in susceptibility to noise, and poor compliance with stated schedules for rotation. Also, time-tabling individuals for exposure to a recognised hazard, albeit for a shorter duration, would seem inappropriate.

Hearing protection is meant to supplement the control measures mentioned. Hearing protectors provide an economical means of preventing hearing loss by reducing hazardous exposures to safety levels at the ears of employees (Brady and Hong, 2008). A useful guide in choosing hearing protectors would be to

(1) know how much noise reduction is needed and understand that the noise reduction rating of the hearing protector is laboratory based;
(2) think about the listening situation which includes wearing eye protection, head protection, hands getting dirty and whether the work environment will be very hot or very cold; and

(3) consider comfort and convenience and know that hearing protection works only if worn consistently and correctly every time one is exposed to hazardous noise (Themann, 2020).

Hearing protectors such as ear plugs, ear muffs, molded canal caps, must be made available to all workers exposed to noise levels, especially at or above 85 dB. These should be at no cost to employees, who should be able to select the hearing protectors and be provided training in its use and care. Proper fitting of hearing protectors is important because of the large variation in ear canal diameters and shapes. In some cases, custom-fitted ear plugs may be necessary. The type of hearing protector selected will depend on the attenuation factor (noise reduction rate (NRR) or single noise rating (SNR)) and spectral characteristics of the noise environment that the employees work in. The level of noise attenuation or reduction provided by ear defenders will usually vary from that stated by hearing protection manufacturers to actual field performance. The wearing of double protection (for example ear-muff together with ear plug) is strongly recommended especially when ambient noise levels exceed 100 dBA. Developments in the technology of hearing protectors have produced devices such as head-phones with noise-cancelling technology and wireless connectivity to make vital communication between colleagues working in noisy areas possible.

Audiometric Testing

Audiometry is not a substitute for noise control. However, an audiometric testing programme including baseline, periodic and end-of-employment audiometry are useful as part of a HCP. Adequate training of personnel conducting audiometry, using approved and calibrated audiometers and provision of approved testing booths are essential.

Training and Education

Noise is a well-recognised occupational health problem in most industrialised countries, and employees should be aware of the associated hazards. This may not be so in developing countries. Informing workers of the auditory disorders that can occur from noise exposure is important for the success of a HCP. The "Right to Know" about workplace hazards is gradually but surely being implemented in developing countries.

Record Keeping

Proper record keeping with exposure and hearing status information is crucial for monitoring and medico-legal purposes.

Recent Developments

High-frequency audiometry (8–16 kHz) has been suggested as a tool that can be used to detect early NIHL that has been shown to be present even before the occurrence of hearing loss at the "conventional" frequencies around the 4 kHz region. A study (Singh *et al.*, 2008) has shown that extended high-frequency hearing loss up to 18,000 Hz is noted in workers exposed to noise regardless of their age-group. However, the use of high-frequency audiometry is still very much limited by the reliability and repeatability of these instruments and data regarding this is still limited.

Another tool that could be used for the early detection of NIHL is otoacoustic emission (OAE). OAEs are sounds that are emitted by the OHCs, and there are typically three types of otoacoustic emissions that could be clinically utilised. These are the spontaneous emission, the transient evoked emission (TEOAE) and the distortion product emission (DPOAE). Detection of OAE only takes a few seconds, and as it is an objective test, the patient's full cooperation is not needed. OAEs are also vulnerable to noxious stimuli such as intense noise, ototoxic medication or solvent or hypoxia and tends to be affected much earlier before any change can be detected in pure tone audiometry. However, the use of OAE in HCPs require further evaluation (Shupak *et al.*, 2007) as OAE test also is very sensitive to any conductive elements present in the ear that might be misinterpreted as having NIHL features or abnormal OHCs function. A study of NIHL and OAEs among 241 professional musicians found more intense OAEs with better pure tone hearing thresholds, but as there was large individual differences, its use as an objective test for early detection of NIHL is still yet to be recommended (Jansen *et al.*, 2009).

Several promising developments in the treatment of NIHL have been reported. These include the use of pharmacological agents as antioxidants, magnesium, neurotrophins, vasodilators, neurotrophic factors (NTFs), steroids, calcineurin inhibitors, caspase inhibitors, JNK inhibitors, and Src protein tyrosine kinase (Src-PTK) inhibitors. These have all been shown to be at least partially effective in preventing hair cell death and subsequently hearing loss in animal models (Sakat, 2016).

Conclusion

Auditory disorders in the workplace are common and preventable. Knowledge and awareness of this occupational disease will be essential in encouraging implementation of and compliance with HCPs.

References

Axelsson A, Prasher D. (2000) Tinnitus induced by occupational and leisure noise. *Noise Health* **2**(8): 47–54.

Barr T. (1886) Enquiry into the effects of loud sounds upon the hearing of boilermakers and others who work and noisy surroundings. *Proc Philos Soc Glasgow* **18**: 223–239.

Bohne BA, Kimlinger M, Harding GW. (2017) Time course of organ of corti degeneration after noise exposure. *Hear Res* **344**: 158–169.

Brady J, Hong OS. (2008) Hearing protection: Work climate and hearing protection behaviors in construction workers. *Prof Saf* **51**(11): 18–26.

Daniel E. (2007) Noise and hearing loss: A review. *J Sch Health* 77(5): 225–231.

Eyears J, Hutson K. (2019) Hearing and vestibular disorders. In: Hobson, J., Smedley, J. (eds.), *Chapter 31 in Fitness for Work — The Medical Aspects* (6th Ed), Oxford University Press, pp. 710–725.

Federal Motor Carrier Safety Administration. (2014) *What are the Hearing Requirements for CMV Drivers?*. [Online] Available from: https://www.fmcsa.dot.gov/faq/what-are-hearing-requirements-cmv-drivers. [Accessed on 24 June 2021].

Fletcher H, Munson WA. (1933) Loudness, its definition, measurement and calculation. *J Acoust Soc Am* **5**: 82–108.

Fosbroke J. (1831) Pathology and treatment of deafness. *Lancet* **19**: 645–648.

Fuente A, McPherson B. (2012) *Occupational Chemical-induced Hearing Loss. IntechOpen*. [Online] Available from: https://www.intechopen.com/books/hearing-loss/occupational-chemical-induced-hearing-loss. [Accessed on 24 June 2021].

Grzesik J, Pluta A. (1983) High-frequency hearing risk of operators of industrial ultrasonic devices. *Int Arch Occup Environ Health* **53**(1): 77–88.

Hameed HM, Eleue AH, Hussein FM. (2019) Noise induced hearing loss (NIHL) in Wasit Corporation textile industries. *J Otolaryngol ENT Res* **11**(2): 108–114.

Health and Safety Executive. (2020) *Noise Induced Hearing Loss in Great Britain*. [Online] Available from: https://www.hse.gov.uk/statistics/causdis/deafness/index.htm. [Accessed on 24 June 2021].

Jansen EJM, Hellerman HW, Dreschler WA, De Laat JAPM. (2009) Noise induced hearing loss and other hearing complaints among musicians of symphony orchestras. *Int Arch Occup Environ Health* **83**(2): 153–164.

Joy GJ, Middendorf PJ. (2007) Noise exposure and hearing conservation in U.S. coal mines--a surveillance report. *J Occup Environ Hyg* **4**(1): 26–35.

Kanitha MS, Balasubramanian C, Anandan H. (2018) A Study on noise-induced hearing loss of police constables. *Int J Sci Study* **5**(11): 122–124.

Kramer SE, Kapteyn TS, Houtgast T. (2006) Occupational performance: Comparing normally hearing and hearing-impaired employees using the Amsterdam Checklist for Hearing and Work. *Int J Audiol* **45**(9): 503–512.

Kujawa SG, Liberman MC. (2006) Acceleration of age-related hearing loss by early noise exposure: Evidence of a misspent youth. *J Neurosci* **26**: 2115–2123.

Madahana MC, Nyandoro OT, Moroe NF. (2020) Engineering noise control for mines: Lessons from the world. *South African J Commun Disord* **67**(2): e1–e5.

Mahendra PKV, Sridhar V. (2008) The relationship between noise frequency components and physical, physiological and psychological effects of industrial workers. *Noise Health* **10**(40): 90–98.

Martin FN, Stauffer ML. (1975) A modification of the Tillman-Olsen Method for obtaining the speech reception threshold. *J Speech Hear Disord* **40**(1): 25–28.

Masterson EA, Tak S, Themann CL, Wall DK, Groenewold MR, Deddens JA, Calvert GM. (2013) Prevalence of hearing loss in the United States by industry. *Am J Ind Med* **56**(6): 670–681.

Musiba Z. (2015) The prevalence of noise-induced hearing loss among Tanzanian miners. *Occup Med* **65**(5): 386–390.

Morata TC, Lemasters GK. (1995) Epidemiologic considerations in the evaluation of occupational hearing loss. *Occup Med* **10**(3): 641–656.

Nasir, HM, Rampal, KG. (2012) Hearing loss and contributing factors among airport workers in Malaysia. *Med J Malaysia* **67**(1): 81–86.

Nelson ID, Nelson RY, Concha-Barrientos M, Fingerhut M. (2005) The global burden of occupational noise-induced hearing loss. *Am J Ind Med* **48**(6): 446–458.

Nyarubeli IP, Tungu AM, Bråtveit M, Moen BE. (2019) Occupational noise exposure and hearing loss: A study of knowledge, attitude and practice among Tanzanian iron and steel workers. *Arch Environ Occup Health* **75**(4): 216–225.

Peligrin AC, Canuet L, Rodriguez AA, Morales MP. (2015) Predictive factors of occupational noise-induced hearing loss in Spanish workers: A prospective study. *Noise Health* **17**(78): 343–349.

Pyykko I, Pekkarinen J, Starck J. *(*1987) Sensory-neural hearing loss during combined noise and vibration exposure. *Int Arch Occup Environ Health* **59**: 439–454.

Ramazzini B. (1713) Revised edition 1940. *De Morbis Artificum (Diseases of Workers)*, the Latin text of 1713, revised by WC Wright. Chicago: University of Chicago Press.

Rahma MS, Mustafa BE, Razali A, Shamsuddin N, Althunibat OY. (2013) The correlation between serum leptin and blood pressure after exposure to noise at work. *Noise Health* **15**(67): 375–378.

Razali A, Othman MS, Rahman MS, Misaridin NFI. (2020) Noise exposure and hearing threshold profile among zumba fitness regulars in Kuantan, Pahang, Malaysia. *IIUM Med J Malaysia* **19**(2).

Ritenour AE, Wickley A, Ritenour JS, Kriete BR, Blackbourne LH, Holcomb JB, Wade CE. (2008) Tympanic membrane perforation and hearing loss from blast overpressure in operation enduring freedom and operation Iraqi freedom wounded. *J Trauma* **64**(2): 174–178.

Robinson T, Whittaker J, Acharya A, Singh D, Smith M. (2015) Prevalence of noise-induced hearing loss among woodworkers in Nepal: A pilot study. *Int J Occup Environ Health* **21**(1): 14–22.

Rondinelli RD, Genovese E, Brigham CR. (2008) *Guides to the evaluation of permanent impairment* (6th Ed). [Guideline] American Medical Association, Chicago, Ill.

Rovig G, Bohnker B, Page J. (2004) Hearing health risk in a population of aircraft carrier flight deck personnel. *Mil Med* **169**(6): 429–432.

Samant Y, Parker D, Wergeland E, Wanning A. (2008) The Norwegian Labour Inspectorate's Registry for work-related diseases: Data from 2006. *Int J Occup Environ Health* **14**(4): 272–279.

Sakat MS, Kilic K, Bercin S. (2016) Pharmacological agents used for treatment and prevention in noise-induced hearing loss. *Eur Arch Oto-Rhino-L* **273**(12): 4089–4101.

Shupak A, Tal D, Sharoni Z, Oren M, Ravid A, Pratt H. (2007) Otoacoustic emissions in early noise-induced hearing loss. *Otol Neurotol* **28**(6): 745–752.

Sincihu Y, Steven DM, Taurusia M. (2019) Investigation of noise induced hearing loss at shipyard company, Surabaya. *Indonesian J Occup Saf Health* **8**(3): 321–327.

Singh R, Saxena R, Varshney S. (2008) Early detection of noise induced hearing loss by using ultra high frequency audiometry. *Internet J Otorhinolaryngol* **10**(2).

Śliwinska-Kowalska M. (2007) Exposure to organic solvent mixture and hearing loss: Literature overview. *Int J Occup Med Environ Health* **20**(4): 309–314.

Sriopas A, Chapman RS, Sutammasa S, Siriwong W. (2017) Occupational noise-induced hearing loss in auto part factory workers in welding units in Thailand. *J Occup Health* **59**(1): 55–62.

Tambs K, Hoffman HJ, Borchgrevink HM, Holmen J, Engdahl B. (2006) Hearing loss induced by occupational and impulse noise: Results on threshold shifts by frequencies, age andgender from the Nord-Trøndelag Hearing Loss Study. *Int J Audiol* **45**(5): 309–317.

Themann C. (2020) Choosing the right hearing protector. *Hearing Journal*, Apr 2020,14.

Tufts JB, Vasil KA, Briggs S. (2009) Auditory fitness for duty: A review. *J Am Acad Audiol* **20**(9): 539–557.

Tun C, Hogan A, Fitzharris K. (2009) Hearing and vestibular dysfunction caused by blast injuries and traumatic brain injuries. *Hear Journal* **62**(11): 24–26.

Win KW, Nayake BP, Balalla NBP, Min Z, Lwin MZ, Lai A. (2015) Noise-induced hearing loss in the police force. *Saf Health Work* **6**(2): 134–138.

Ylikoski J. (1988a) Delayed endolymphatic hydrops syndrome after heavy exposure to impulse noise. *Am J Otol* **9**(4): 282–285.

Ylikoski J, Juntunen J, Matikainen E, Ylikoski M, Ojala M. (1988b) Subclinical vestibular pathology in patients with noise induced hearing loss from intense impulse noise. *Acta Otolaryngol (Stckh)* **105**(5–6): 558–63.

Yoon JH, Hong JS, Roh J, Kim CN, Won JU. (2015) Doseresponse relationship between noise exposure and the risk of occupational injury. *Noise Health* **17**(74): 43–47.

Zhang Z. (2010). *Guideline for Diagnosing Occupational Noise-induced Hearing Loss. Epidemiological Review: Some Risk Factors of Hearing Loss.* Research Unit Governance, Policy and Research Accident Compensation Corporation. Part **2**: 30–39.

Chapter 8

Haematological Disorders

Wee Tong Ng and Mark Newson-Smith*[†]

Introduction

Physiology of the Haematological System

Blood cells are derived from multipotent haemopoietic stem cells. These cells self-replicate or differentiate to form committed progenitor cells of the various blood cells lines: erythrocytes, monocytes, neutrophils, eosinophils, basophils, lymphocytes, and platelets. This differentiation is present by the third week of embryonic development, with the presence of primitive nucleated erythrocytes in the yolk sac (Ivanovs *et al.*, 2017).

The healthy adult produces approximately 200 billion red blood cells per day. This process, known as erythropoiesis, occurs within the bone marrow and is mediated by growth factors, such as interleukin 3 (IL-3), and critically, the cytokine erythropoietin. Progenitor cells committed to erythropoiesis divide and differentiate in the bone marrow and are released as reticulocytes into the bloodstream, where they undergo final maturation into erythrocytes (Dzierzak and Philipsen,

*Saw Swee Hock School of Public Health, National University of Singapore, Singapore.

[†]Avon Partnership Occupational Health Services, Avon Partnership Occupational Health Services Centre, Bristol, United Kingdom.

Corresponding author: Mark Newson-Smith (marc.newson-smith@orange.fr).

2013). This process is also regulated by the GATA family of DNA transcription factors, in which mutations and decreased expression has been associated with the development of myelofibrosis (Ling *et al.*, 2018). There has been interest exploring the relationship between chemical agents such as benzene and the development of myeloproliferative conditions. It was suggested that other somatic mutations leading to myelodysplastic syndrome (MDS) had statistical association with benzene exposure but not the other subtypes of myeloproliferative conditions (Gross-Davis *et al.*, 2015). Thus, the lack of diagnostic specificity in studies may affect attribution of myeloproliferative disorders with environmental exposures.

Erythropoietin was discovered in 1977. It is primarily produced by the peri-tubular interstitial cells of the kidneys in response to hypoxia, via an oxygen-sensing mechanism. Secondary sites of production include the liver, spleen, bone marrow, lung, and brain. It modulates the maturation of the erythroblasts into erythrocytes, thus keeping the numbers of mature red blood cells within a narrow homeostatic range (Bhoopalan, Huang and Weiss, 2020). Erythrocytes have a life span of 120 days and the senescent cells are removed by the phagocytic action of reticulo-endothelial cells in the spleen and liver.

There are gender differences in red cell count, and this is attributed to the effect of increased circulating androgens in the male. In males, the normal red cell count is between 4.5 and 6.5×10^{12}/L with haemoglobin of 13.5–18.0g/100 mL. In females, the red cell count is between 4.0 and 5.5×10^{12}/L and haemoglobin of 11.5–16.5g/100 mL.

White cells are formed in the bone marrow and its regulation is less well understood as compared to erythrocytes. Granulocytes can be rapidly mobilised from the bone marrow in response to inflammatory stimulus. Various growth factors in the bone marrow (which includes GM-CSF), promote marrow turnover and its release.

Lymphocytes, on the other hand, mature mainly in the lymphoid tissues, some in the thymus (T-cells) and others (B-cells) in other lymphoid tissues (probably in the Peyer's patches). The prime function of the B-cells is to divide in response to contact with antigens to produce plasma cells which in turn produce antibodies. The T-cells assist the

B-cells in the primary immune response and are also responsible for cell-mediated immunity.

There is little difference in normal white cell values between males and females. The total number of white cells is 4 to 11 × 10^9/L. This is made up of 2.0–7.5 × 10^9/L neutrophils (40–75%), 1.5 to 4.0 × 10^9/L lymphocytes (20–50%), 0.2 to 0.8 × 10^9/L monocytes (2–10%), 0.04 to 0.4 × 10^9/L eosinophils (1–6%) and 0.01 to 0.1 × 10^9/L basophils (<1%).

Occupational Exposures Affecting the Haematological System

Lead (Pb)

Sources of exposure to lead

Lead is a naturally occurring metal that has been used by man since ancient times, where it was used widely as a pigment, a preservative and in the manufacture of alloys such as bronze and pewter. Although it can occur naturally as free lead, it is more often extracted from lead-containing ore such as galena (PbS), anglesite ($PbSO_4$), cerussite ($PbCO_3$) and minimum (Pb_3O_4). The extraction process results in the purified inorganic metal.

In 1853, it was discovered that organic lead (tetra-ethyl lead) could be produced, although it was only in the 1920s that a widespread commercial use was found, as General Motors proposed it as an anti-knock additive to petroleum (Seyferth, 2003). Since then, the environmental impact of leaded emissions has resulted in Europe and the United States of America (USA) legislating out the use of leaded petroleum in cars, although its use remains in certain specialised petroleum compounds, such as leaded aviation fuel. Hence, since the turn of the 21st century, the predominant occupational threat in developed countries has been inorganic lead and its compounds.

Apart from its base metal state, inorganic lead is often used commercially as a compound (oxides, arsenics, sulphurs and chromates). Its ductility, high resistance to corrosion and other properties make it one of the most useful of metals. The largest single use of lead is in the manufacture of lead-acid storage batteries. Lead is also widely used for cathodic protection of the superstructures of ships and bridges, as a component in lead alloys, paint pigments, the production of polyvinyl chloride (PVC) stabilisers, as a glazing agent for earthenware and as a mordant for both cotton dyes and process engraving. This wide application of inorganic lead results in continued exposures to the metal and its compounds in the workplace.

Whilst the ban of leaded petroleum has contributed significantly to the reduction of lead emissions and inhalational risks, large reservoirs still exist worldwide in the environment (soil & dust) from decades of emissions (Tong *et al.*, 2000). Furthermore, emissions from smelting operations (of the lead ore) continue to contribute to this environmental load. In communities where significant industrial pollution exists, anaemia can be a common feature of excessive lead exposure. Furthermore, in many developing countries where secondary lead smelting in small scale enterprises are common, there can be excessive lead exposure. Family members including children are often at risk as they either participate in the smelting or live in proximity as these are usually household enterprises. These issues were reported extensively in the 1970s and 1980s in the U.S.A. However, by 2010, 67% of the world's primary production of lead was in China, with only 8% in North America. The remaining producing countries include Mexico, Peru, India, Russia and Australia (Sullivan, 2015). One notable issue with the shift of production to China has been the lower levels of enforcement with regards to processes, control of emissions and air quality levels in the communities surrounding the smelters. Thus, the consequences of elevated blood levels in children and adults, observed in the lead smelting communities in the U.S.A in the last century, are now being reported in Chinese communities (Zhang, 2012).

Other environmental exposures have also been reported. In 2014, a change in the water source in Flint, Michigan, USA resulted in corrosive leeching of lead from the water pipes into the water supply. As a result, it is estimated that the percentage of children in the city with elevated blood-lead have doubled, from 2.5% in 2013 to 5% in 2015 (Hanna-Attisha *et al.*, 2016).

In 2019, a study was reported from Indonesia, examining the effects of lead on anaemia in children (aged 7–13), in the vicinity of an industrial area conducting lead-acid battery recycling. They reported an increase in the risk of anaemia (OR 3.8), in children exposed to airborne lead concentrations of ≥2 μg/m^3 versus <2 μg/m^3 (Rachmat *et al.*, 2019).

A study from India (Yadav *et al.*, 2020) reported an association between high blood lead levels and antenatal iron deficiency anaemia. As the women with high blood lead levels were housewives with no reported occupational exposure to lead, the study postulated an environmental cause for the elevated blood lead levels.

Anaemia due to lead

- **Inhibition of haem synthesis:** The main mechanism, by which lead causes anaemia in the human body, is via the inhibition of the activities of δ-aminolevulinic dehydratase (δ-ALAD), ferrochelatase and coproporphyrinogen decarboxylase (Chisolm, 1971; Hernberg, 1980). These are critical enzymes in the pathway of haem synthesis, and its reduced synthesis results in decreased haemoglobin production and biochemically detectable anaemia.
- **Promotion of haem breakdown:** The breakdown of haem is catalysed by the enzyme haem oxygenase. The synthesis of this enzyme is regulated by a repressor protein. Lead binds to the -SH group of this repressor protein leading to an increase in haem oxygenase production, which results in increased haem breakdown
- **Decreased life span of erythrocytes:** Lead causes structural and functional changes in the membranes of erythrocytes, which lead to increased osmotic and mechanical fragility and shortened erythrocyte lifespan. The mechanism of action is complex and in vitro studies suggests the involvement of the enzyme P5'N (pyrimidine 5 nucleotidase), inhibition of the Na^+ and K^+ pump as well as reduction in cytochrome oxidative phosphorylation (Sakai *et al.*, 1990). Oxidative damage to erythrocytes, caused by lead, has also been reported to interfere with Ca2+ homeostasis in these cells, leading

to cell distortion and increased fragility (Quintanar-Escorza *et al.*, 2010). There is also some evidence that a decrease in the activity of the P5'N pathway influences Hb levels in workers without manifesting haemolytic anaemia (Kim *et al.*, 2002).

- **Interference with globin chain synthesis:** Lead also inhibits the production of the α and β globin chains, although the effect on the α chain is greater. This may also be a factor in the pathogenesis of lead induced anaemia (White and Harvey, 1972).

Genetic susceptibility

δ-Aminolevulinic dehydratase (δ-ALAD): The ALAD gene is located on chromosome 9q34 (Wetmur, 1986). It codes for the ALAD enzyme which, as shown above, catalyses key steps in haem synthesis. ALAD is expressed in all tissues, with the highest levels in the liver and erythrocytes (Wetmur, 1994). The gene has a polymorphism (ALAD G177C) that gives rise to two alleles, which in turn determines three isozymes, known as ALAD 1-1, ALAD 1-2 and ALAD 2-2 (Battistuzzi, 1981). Studies have focused on trying to determine the susceptibility to lead in the body of the different genotypes. In populations exposed to high lead levels, several studies have found higher levels of blood lead in individuals with ALAD 1-2 and ALAD 2-2, as compared to those with the ALAD 1-1 genotype (Mani *et al.*, 2018; Wetmur *et al.*, 1991; Ziemsen *et al.*, 1986).

Studies that evaluated the bioaccumulation of lead in bone suggest that the ALAD 1-1 genotype sequesters more lead in bone, as compared to ALAD 1-2/2-2 (Fleming *et al.*, 1998). These findings indicated that at high blood lead levels, saturation of binding sites may account for the findings above, whereas in the long term, the ALAD 1-2/2-2 genotype may actually be protective by reducing lead storage in bone. Correlated clinically, in a population exposed to the same level of lead, neuropsychological tests of attention showed better results in the ALAD1-2/2-2 population, suggesting some degree of neuroprotection (Bellinger *et al.*, 1994). It has also been shown that in a lead exposed population, with normal iron levels, the ALAD 1-1 genotype was more likely to be anaemic, further supporting the protective effect of the ALAD1-2/2-2 genotype (Kim *et al.*, 2004). Thus, whilst ALAD 1-2 and ALAD 2-2 may be associated with higher levels of blood lead, the studies also suggest that they may be associated with lower levels of clinical symptoms. This could be due to ALAD 1-2/ 2-2 being more electronegative, binding strongly to red blood cells, and subsequently reducing the availability of lead to target tissues (Mani *et al.*, 2018).

These studies have been done in occupational settings with higher levels of lead exposure. At low and background levels of lead exposure, there is insufficient evidence associating the ALAD polymorphisms with susceptibility to clinical effects of lead. Thus, testing for the ALAD polymorphism in the general population is not warranted at this time (Kelada *et al.*, 2001).

Vitamin D receptor (VDR) gene: Sunlight activates vitamin D in the skin to produce calcitriol. Calcitriol then binds to VDRs in the intestinal walls, which triggers the absorption of calcium from the gut. It has long been postulated that absorption of lead through the gut shares this pathway with calcium. Studies now indicate that genetic polymorphisms of the VDR gene are associated with different levels of lead bioaccumulation in the body (Schwartz *et al.*, 2000).

Diagnosis and management of inorganic lead poisoning

Pre-employment and periodic medical examinations

In many countries, workers exposed to inorganic lead are required to have pre-employment and periodic medical examinations. At pre-employment examinations, baseline haemoglobin and blood lead (PbB) measurements should be determined. Workers with underlying anaemia will require further investigations. Nutritional anaemias and anaemia due to blood loss can be treated. Once treated, these workers can proceed to work in lead environment. However, workers with persistent anaemia like thalassaemia should not work in lead environments.

Periodic medical examinations for workers exposed to lead are required every six months (Centers for Disease Control and Prevention (CDC)/National Institute for Occupational Safety and Health (NIOSH), 2015), where the haemoglobin and blood lead (PbB) measurements should be determined. Although collection of urine for lead measurements may be more convenient and less invasive, urinary samples are prone to contamination during collection, require correction for creatinine clearance and can breakdown during sample transit, resulting in unreliable measurements (Barbosa *et al.*, 2005).

In 2015, CDC/NIOSH designated 5μg/dl as the reference blood level for adults, an elevated blood lead level thus defined as greater than this level. (CDC/NIOSH, 2015) The United States (US) Occupational Safety and Health Administration (OSHA) Lead Standards require workers to be removed from lead exposure when BLLs are equal or greater than 50 μg/dl (construction industry) or 60 μg/dl (general industry) and allow workers to return to work when the BLL is below 40 μg/dl (NIOSH, 2021). Being a cumulative poison, suspension from exposure is not by itself an effective means of preventing the health effects. After a period of suspension, any lowering of PbB is not necessarily a true reflection of the body burden of lead. Suspension merely decreases the rate of increase in body lead burden. It is likely to be effective only if coupled with other preventive measures such as improved engineering controls and safer systems of handling lead at work. Pregnant and lactating females should not be exposed to lead work.

Among workers with a history of high exposure to lead, the erythrocyte activity of δ-ALAD continues to be inhibited out of proportion to the current PbB levels, even after removal from exposure. This is partly due to the high affinity of inorganic lead to the bones. In a steady state, about 90% of the total body burden of lead is present in the bones and teeth. Even with cessation of exposure, bone lead decreases very gradually and continues to leach back into the bloodstream. Bone lead is therefore an important source of 'endogenous exposure' because of its slow turnover and the large storage capacity of the bones (Barry *et al.*, 2019).

However, the routine measurement of erythrocyte activity of δ-ALAD is limited by technical problems. The blood sample must be stored at below 4°C and preferably be measured within 24 hours. For this reason, the measurement of delta-aminolevulinic acid in the urine (ALA-U) is a useful alternative. Due to the inhibition of δ-ALAD of the maturing erythrocytes by lead, the transformation of ALA into porphobilinogen is obstructed. The lowered haem level stimulates the action of ALA synthetase, resulting in an increase in ALA in the serum and urine. However, the correlation between ALA-U and PbB is weaker than that of erythrocyte activity of δ-ALAD.

One of the main goals of regular biological monitoring for lead-exposed workers is to confirm that they are not unduly exposed to high levels of lead in the environment. Where group data shows an increasing trend in average PbB levels, exposures to lead and environmental control measures need to be evaluated and further preventive action taken as necessary. There could be a failure of preventive measures, such as a breakdown of exhaust ventilation or poor housekeeping resulting in higher environmental lead concentrations in the workplace. Poor work practices among workers and improper use of personal protective equipment are further contributing factors to consider.

Health education

Education plays an important role in the mitigation of the negative effects of occupational and environmental lead exposures. Education is commonly targeted at areas where changes in worker habits will make a difference, such as understanding the health effects of lead exposure, avoiding eating with hands and smoking at the work area, good personal hygiene, proper use and maintenance of respirators and preventing secondary exposure to the family and community. In Vietnam, in a community exposed to lead due to battery recycling activities, a combination of low cost engineering interventions and education (three-day workshop and door to door campaign) was able to reduce blood lead levels in the community (Ericson *et al.*, 2018).

Case Study 1: Lead Poisoning in a Child

A mother brought her two-year-old child for a routine checkup with the pediatrician. It was noted that the child had speech and language delay and was small for his age (below the 5th percentile). Initial investigations showed a mild anaemia but little else. On a more thorough history, it was noted that the father worked at a factory that manufactured polyvinyl chloride (PVC) stabilisers. The most common stabilisers are inorganic lead stabilisers. Based on this history, further blood tests were ordered, which showed elevated blood lead levels in the child.

The factory which the father worked at has a policy that work overalls should not be brought home and are laundered by the company. However, the father has a habit of wearing a T-shirt under his overalls, which he wears home each day. He was not careful during the change of clothing and routinely contaminated his T-shirt with lead dust from his overalls. This was subsequently inhaled by his child when he would hold his child before changing out of his work clothes.

Commentary

For workers exposed to powdered lead, it is important that they change out of their work clothing before returning home. Care must be taken at the factory to not mix contaminated overalls with clean clothing. Providing laundry services for contaminated overalls/clothing is a good company policy. Worker's education, in this case, should include elements of personal hygiene, community protection, safe work processes and PPE usage. Compliance to PPE usage will need to be reinforced, for it to be effective.

Use of chelators

Chelating agents are organic compounds capable of binding to metal ions to form a ring structure around the ion called a chelate, the term deriving from the Greek word for claw. The common chelators used for lead poisoning include calcium disodium ethylene diamine tetra acetic acid ($CaNa_2$ EDTA), d-penicillamine (Cupramine) and 2, 3 dimercaptosuccinic acid (DMSA) (Flora, 2014).

$CaNa_2$ EDTA, the most commonly used chelating agent, is not metabolised by the body and following an intravenous injection 50% of it is excreted in an hour and 90% in 7 hours. $CaNa_2$ EDTA only removes extracellular lead and its effectiveness is better when used in combination with dimercaprol (also known as British anti-Lewisite)

(Kim, Kim and Kumar, 2019). Oral EDTA has also been shown to decrease the gastrointestinal absorption of lead. Its role in acute lead poisoning is controversial especially in those with lead encephalopathy. Among patients undergoing EDTA therapy, the encephalopathy symptoms can be increased due to the liberation of bone lead into the blood. Other significant risks of EDTA therapy include renal damage, hypotension and bone marrow depression.

Penicillamine is particularly effective for chelating copper in Wilson's disease and is often used to treat lead intoxication. It has the advantage of oral administration but it interferes with Vitamin B6 metabolism, has the same side effects as penicillin and 10–30% of patients treated with it suffer gastrointestinal problems. Important contraindications for its use are in patients who are allergic to penicillin and those with renal insufficiency (Flora and Pachauri, 2010).

DMSA is very efficient chelator for lead and is effective when given orally. The toxicity of DMSA is low compared to other chelators and its efficiency in chelating a range of heavy metals is very much higher. While its toxicity is relatively low, precautions are necessary for patients with renal or liver impairment, for those with neutropaenia and for those with glucose-6-dehydrogenase deficiency (Blanuša *et al.*, 2005).

A comparison of the effectiveness of EDTA and DMSA in adults with lead poisoning found that both significantly reduced the prevalence of clinical symptoms and the blood lead levels (Sakthithasan *et al.*, 2018). DMSA was considered more effective at reducing blood lead levels while EDTA was more effective in terms of lead mobilisation. It was noted that while treatment with EDTA was more invasive treatment compliance with it was generally much better than with DMSA.

Chelators should be used only in severe lead poisoning with clinical signs and symptoms. 'Prophylactic chelation', that is, the use of chelating agents or related drugs to prevent elevated blood lead or the use of drugs to routinely lower blood lead to predetermined concentrations, is strongly discouraged, and is actually prohibited in certain parts of the world such as in the USA (OSHA, n.d.). Chelation is generally recommended in adults when the blood lead level exceeds 80 μg/dl and those with blood levels between 60 and 80 μg/dl who are showing clinical signs of lead poisoning (Papanikolaou *et al.*, 2005). In children, there is little justification to use chelators when the blood lead is below 45 µg/dl. The main reason for the cautious use of chelators is because of their high nephrotoxicity and the depletion of other essential metals like zinc and iron.

Chelators can be used to aid in the diagnosis of lead poisoning. Following a standard dose of chelator, all the urine excreted over a time period (usually 24 hours) is collected and the lead content estimated. This 'mobilisable' lead content is also a good indicator of the body burden of lead (Hoet *et al.*, 2006).

Methaemoglobinaemia and Oxidative Haemolysis

Work-related methaemoglobinaemia and oxidative haemolysis are caused by several aromatic nitro and amino compounds. Examples include aniline, nitroaniline, toluidine, naphthalene and trinitrotoluene (Bradberry, 2003). These are common in the manufacture of aniline dyestuffs, pesticides, antioxidants in rubber production and explosives. Urea herbicides are also metabolised to aniline-derived products (Watt *et al.*, 2005).

In order for the haemoglobin molecule to carry oxygen molecule effectively, the iron molecule must be in the reduced state (ferrohaemoglobin). When the oxygen is released, the iron molecule is oxidised into the ferric state (ferric haemoglobin or methaemoglobin). The normal individual has less than 1% of methaemoglobin because of effective reduction of methaemoglobin into ferro-haemoglobin via NADH cytochrome b5 reductase.

Methaemoglobin also increases the oxygen affinity to the remaining haem groups of the haemoglobin tetramer resulting in decreasing oxygen delivery to the tissues. Furthermore, the haemoglobin can be denatured and precipitated as Heinz bodies. The presence of Heinz bodies alters the membrane stability of the red blood cells resulting in haemolysis.

Apart from exposure to exogenous oxidative chemicals, inborn structural abnormalities of the haemoglobin as well as decrease in the reduction capabilities from metabolic abnormalities like G6PD (Glucose-6-phosphate dehydrogenase) deficiency cause workers to be more susceptible to oxidative damage. During an acute haemolytic episode, older erythrocytes tend to be destroyed and are replaced by young red cells and reticulocytes. These reticulocytes will have normal G6PD levels and any screening for G6PD activity immediately after an acute haemolytic episode is useless. Workers should therefore be screened for G6PD deficiency at pre-employment if its prevalence is high in the community.

Acute exposure to agents causing methaemoglobinaemia and haemolytic anaemia is usually associated with spills and improper usage. With mild exposure, the worker presents with asymptomatic peripheral cyanosis (i.e. blueness of the nail beds). With more severe exposure, central cyanosis may be present and the patient may complain of breathlessness, headache and fatigue. Freshly drawn blood appears to be dark maroon-brown and does not become red with exposure to air. When the methaemoglobin level is more than 50%, the patient may be disorientated and comatose. Laboratory investigations will reveal hypoxia and subsequently anaemia and haemolysis.

Naphthalene can cross the placenta, and maternal exposure can result in the newborn infant having signs and symptoms of naphthalene toxicity (Molloy *et al.*, 2004; Sahni *et al.*, 2019). Therefore, extra care must be taken to prevent pregnant women from exposure to naphthalene and other similar oxidative chemicals.

Treatment of acute exposure includes rapid recognition and removal of the causal agent. All casualties should be given high-flow oxygen. Central cyanosis not improving with oxygen is useful in diagnosing methaemoglobinaemia and high-flow oxygen will maximise the oxygen carriage by any ferrous haem that remains (Bradberry, 2003). Methylene blue should be administered with care. Methylene blue acts as a cofactor with NADPH to reduce the methaemoglobin to ferro haemoglobin. NADPH is derived from the hexose monophosphate shunt and requires G6PD. Methylene blue in itself has oxidative potential and may precipitate a haemolytic crisis in patients with G6PD deficiency. Hence, methylene blue should only be administered in patients without G6PD deficiency.

Methylene blue is given intravenously as a 1% solution (dose: 1–2 mg/kg) over three to five minutes and will generally significantly reduce the methaemoglobin levels in under an hour (Wright *et al.*,

1999). If the patient responds, the dose could be repeated at hourly intervals. If the patient does not respond, methylene blue administration should be stopped, as the patient may be G6PD deficient. Supportive therapy should be used instead. These patients should be screened for G6PD deficiency 1–2 months after the poisoning episode because during a haemolytic episode, older red blood cells are destroyed and replaced by immature cells. Among patients with G6PD deficiency, the level of the enzyme is normal in these cells.

Ascorbic acid has been recommended as it is also able to reduce methaemoglobin into ferro haemoglobin and does not causes problems in patients with G6PD deficiency (Chikezie and Ekechukwu, 2016). However, the rate of reduction is very slow and it may potentiate renal toxicity.

Workers exposed to oxidative agents should be screened for G6PD deficiency. Biological monitoring would include the end-of-shift measurement of methaemoglobin levels (to be kept below 5%), reticulocyte count and appropriate metabolites (e.g. urinary p-aminophenol for aniline; p-nitrophenol and p-aminophenol for nitrobenzene).

Haemolysis from heavy metals

Arsenic and arsine

Arsenic is often present as a contaminant in metal ore or products. In the presence of hydrogen ions, it reacts to form a volatile, colourless and non-irritating gas, arsine (AsH_3). The gas is much heavier than air and has a garlicky smell. It is easily inhaled and absorbed, as it does not irritate the respiratory tract. Exposure situations include the smelting of metals like zinc and among cleaners of acid storage tanks. Antimony is also present with arsenic and under the same conditions, stibine is also produced. The toxicity of stibine is similar to that of arsine. Arsine gas is also used extensively today in the growth and preparation of crystals and conducting devices in the semiconductor industry.

The mechanism responsible for arsine induced haemolysis is not well understood. However, it is recognised that the presence of oxyhaemoglobin is a necessary component to the overall mechanism as conversion of oxyhaemoglobin to carboxyhaemoglobin prevents the haemolysis of erythrocytes (Rael *et al.*, 2000).

About 20% of all acute arsine poisoning is fatal. Exposure to 250ppm causes death within minutes. Levels of 25–50ppm for more than 30 minutes is also fatal (Pakulska and Czeczak, 2006). At lower concentrations, haemolysis develops after a latent period whose length is inversely proportional to the extent of exposure. Patients are often alarmed by the painless haemoglobin and seek medical attention for it. Associated signs and symptoms include nausea and vomiting, abdominal cramps, headache, malaise, tachycardia, tachypnea and hypotension. Subsequently, acute renal failure may follow.

Anaemia is not present initially. The plasma free haemoglobin is high and the blood appears brownish red from the presence of methaemalbumin (oxidised haemoglobin bound to albumin). Peripheral blood film will show schistocytosis (red cell fragmentation), poikilocytosis, basophilic stippling and polychromatosia. When the haematocrit starts to fall, reticulocytosis increases. The level of unconjugated bilirubin is also raised. Renal function is affected from obstruction by renal tubular haemoglobin casts as well as direct toxicity of arsine on the renal tubular and interstitial cells. Levels of arsenic in the blood and urine are useful indicators for exposure rather than an indication for therapy.

Case Study 2: Arsine Poisoning

A 55 year old male who worked for a company detoxifying water presented with a history of same day low back pain radiating into his groin, both legs and towards his shoulders, which was followed a couple of hours later by gross haematuria (Pullen-James and Woods, 2006). During the patient workup he became hypotensive and it was felt he had sepsis which was supported by the complete blood count results. Overnight his condition deteriorated, his white blood cell went up, his haemoglobin dropped from 11.2– 8.8 mg/dl, and his urine became black. On further questioning the patient stated that his current work involved removing arsenic from water using an acid preparation and while standing above water he was detoxifying he noticed a garlic like smell. Shortly after this information was given two of his co-workers presented with haematuria. Blood and urine samples for arsenic were taken from the first worker which were both elevated. His treatment included an exchange transfusion and dialysis. His co-workers were found to have milder arsine poisoning and did not require the same level of treatment.

Initial therapy includes the management of shock and adequate renal perfusion. Exchange transfusion is required if the free haemoglobin level exceeds 500µg/100ml. Repeated exchange transfusion may be necessary. If renal failure develop, haemodialysis may be indicated. All patients must be monitored closely for further haemolysis and deterioration of renal function (Pullen-James and Woods, 2006). While chelators are used for arsenic poisoning, they are not effective for arsine poisoning (Agency for Toxic Substances and Disease Registry (ATSDR), 2014). Survivors of acute arsine poisoning should be followed up yearly for residual renal impairment.

Lead induced haemolysis

The main effect of inorganic lead is the inhibition of haem synthesis. However, in very high exposure situations, as in the use of a blow-torch on leaded materials, severe acute intravascular haemolysis may occur. It is believed that the inhibition of pyrimidine-5' nucleotidase by lead is similar to the hereditary deficiency of the enzyme. In the hereditary condition, there is accumulation of pyrimidine containing nucleotides within the red blood cells. These nucleotides are believed to compete with adenine nucleotides in binding to active sites of kinases in the glycolytic pathways and affect the membrane stability of the red blood cells (Zanella *et al.*, 2006). In the anaemia associated with chronic lead poisoning one factor is believed to be increased cell membrane fragility resulting in a decreased cell life span. The mechanism for this is not clear but it is associated with inhibition in the activity of sodium and potassium dependent ATPase's (Sharma *et al.*, 2014).

Aplastic Anaemia due to Occupational Exposure

Bone marrow damage is uncommon in industry and only a small percentage of aplastic anaemias are due to environmental and occupational causes. The most common occupational causes are benzene and irradiation.

Benzene

In the past, high benzene exposure has led to toxic aplastic anaemia. There were even cases of fatal aplastic anaemias from exposures exceeding 100ppm. To note, 2019 NIOSH and OSHA occupational exposure limits (8 hour TWA) are 0.1ppm and 1ppm respectively (NIOSH, 2019).

At lower levels of exposure, the changes depend on which type of cell suffer the brunt of the injury. There is however great variation in susceptibility and the evidence of toxicity may appear weeks or years later. There have been reports of cases developing several years after exposure has ceased.

Anaemia is often the first effect to be noted followed by leukopaenia, thrombocytopaenia and finally pancytopaenia. The bone marrow may show evidence of a cellularity with fatty tissue replacement to islands of hyper cellularity without evidence of new cells in the peripheral blood.

Aplastic anaemia due to acute benzene exposure has a better prognosis than idiopathic aplastic anaemia (La Dou and Harrison, 2014). When the patients are removed from exposure, as much as 40% of them may completely recover. However, if hypo cellularity persists for more than 4 to 6 months, recovery is not likely. Those who develop aplastic anaemia after exposure has ceased are also unlikely to recover and may form part of a pre leukaemic syndrome. Bone marrow transplantation and immunosuppressive therapy are the current mainstays of treatment.

Petrochemical industries and petroleum refineries are the main sources of benzene exposure. It is also used in the manufacture of plastics, synthetic fibers and synthetic rubber. In laboratories, benzene is often used for extraction of organic substances. Though the concentration of benzene in industrial solvents (like toluene and xylene) is low, exposure to benzene may be high because of the large volume of industrial solvents used and if the work is carried out in confined spaces.

Biological effect monitoring of benzene-exposed workers includes the haemoglobin level, full blood count and peripheral blood film. End of shift urinary trans-trans-muconic acid (tt-MA) and urinary S-phenylmercapturic acid (SPMA) are the current biomarkers of choice for biological monitoring of benzene-exposed workers. Tt-MA levels can be increased by the consumption of food containing sorbic acid and consequently at lower levels of benzene exposure it is a less reliable marker than SPMA (Hoet *et al.*, 2009; Carrieri *et al.*, 2018). Workers should be followed up periodically for delayed onset of toxicity.

Ionising radiation

Haemopoietic cells are highly radiosensitive. Significant suppression of the haematopoietic system can occur after acute high doses of ionising radiation and is referred to as the haematopoietic syndrome. The full syndrome usually occurs at doses between 0.7 and 10 Gy although mild symptoms can occur at doses as low as 0.3 Gy. Platelets and leucocyte levels will be maximally depressed in 3 to 5 weeks. Aplasia of lymphoid tissues is also common with depression of the immune response. The main causes of death are from fatal haemorrhage and infection. The LD50 is about 2.5 to 5 Gy (Centers for Disease Control and Prevention (CDC), 2018). The most important long term effect is leukaemia.

Exposure situations can be either from acute high dose exposure in nuclear accidents or long term low level exposure as in the practice of radiology. Radiology is used to evaluate the quality of welded joints in various industrial setting.

Case Study 3: Ionising Radiation

A 31 year old male worker presented with a history of anorexia, mild dizziness and generalised weakness over several days. He had been employed as a non-destructive testing worker for 5 years, utilising beams of gamma radiation to carry out radiographic testing (Ahn et al., 2018). The technique is used to test the structure and integrity of a variety of machinery, equipment and structures (e.g. welded joints and metal castings) (International Atomic Energy Agency,1999). His radiation dose measured by a thermoluminescent dosimeter (TLD) for the month before he presented in was 120 mSv. A chromosome aberration test showed an estimated exposure of 1191 mSV, nearly ten times the dose recorded on the TLD.

On presentation the worker was clinically anaemic with a pulse rate of 104 beats per minute. A bleeding tendency along with bruising was found around the venous injection areas and blood testing showed a severe pancytopaenia. The white blood cell count (WBC) was 1360 cells/mm3 (normal range 4000–10800), the absolute neutrophil count (ANC) was 500 cells/mm3 (normal range 1500–8000), the absolute lymphocyte count (ALC) was 680 cells/mm3 (normal range 1500–4000), the absolute monocyte count (AMC) was 179 cells/mm3 (normal range 200–1000), the haemoglobin level was 14.7 g/dL (normal range 12–18), and the platelet levels were 14 × 103/mm3 (normal range 130–450). The worker was prohibited from further work with ionising radiation and was given packed red blood cells along with concentrated platelets. The treatment was repeated 12 days later and around 10 weeks later he was given a further dose of packed RBCs. Over the 13 month follow up period his pancytopaenia slowly improved (Fig. 1) shows the changes in WBC, ANC, ALC and AMC) although the levels did not return to those at his pre-placement examination.

Work-Related Haematological Malignancies

Leukaemias

Ionising radiation, benzene, ethylene oxide and antineoplastic drugs have been shown definitively to cause leukaemia. Other causal

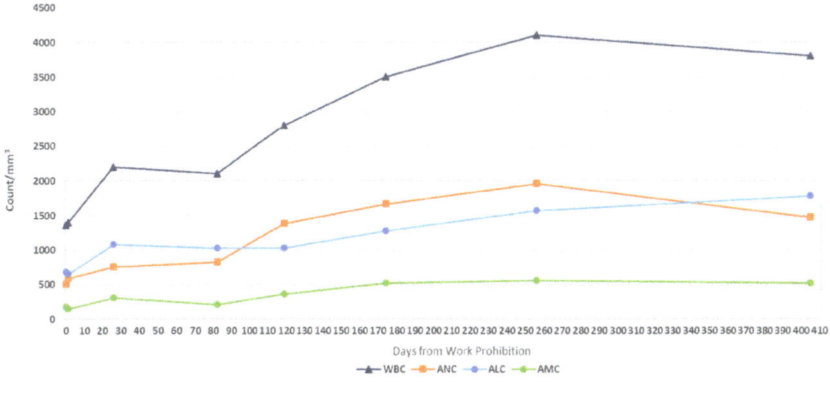

Fig. 1. Blood parameters (white blood cells (WBC), ANC, ALC and AMC) from case of acute radiation syndrome following work prohibition (Ahn *et al.*, 2018).

associations not conclusively established include employment in agricultural work, exposure to formaldehyde and exposure to low frequency electromagnetic radiation. Further description of occupational leukaemia's will be found in the chapter on occupational cancers.

Case Study 4: Leukaemia

The case involves a 43 year old shoemaker who for 6 years prior to presentation was employed in a small workshop where glues with high levels of benzene were routinely utilised (Aksoy et al., 1972). Two years after starting the work he was found to have a pancytopaenia and was diagnosed as having aplastic anaemia due to chronic benzene poisoning. He responded to two months of treatment however continued to undertake his work as a shoemaker.

Four years later the worker presented with fever and ecchymoses having stopped working as a shoemaker some 6 months previously. Ejection systolic murmurs were noted over both the mitral and pulmonary areas and no evidence of lymphadenopathy or hepatosplenomegaly was found. Blood tests showed an RBC of 2.66 million/mm^2 (normal range 4.7–6.1), a haemoglobin of 6.1 gm% (normal range 13.5–17.5), a WCC of 500 (normal range 4000–11000), and myeloblasts at 22% (normally absent). A bone marrow smear was hypercellular with a myeloblast level of 73%, a promyelocyte level of 2%, a myelocyte level of 0% metamyelocyte level of 2% and band forms at 1%.

A diagnosis of Acute Myeloblastic Leukaemia (AML) was made and he was commenced on a course of chemotherapy. Testing after 5 months of treatment showed that he was in remission and he remained so for one year following the start of treatment. He then developed ascites and was admitted to hospital. Testing showed hepatocellular damage possibly related to one of the chemotherapeutic agents he had been given. Just over two weeks later he later died as a result of severe oesophageal bleeding.

Multiple Myeloma

Multiple myeloma is a clonal differentiated B cell neoplasm. Its incidence appears to be on the rise and this has aroused the concern that it may be associated with environmental or occupational factors. Many epidemiological studies have shown an association with agriculture work, benzene exposure, high dose radiation, pesticides and petroleum products. These are however inconclusive (Perrotta *et al.*, 2013)

Conclusion

Occupational exposure to a wide range of chemical agents can cause haematological conditions ranging from anaemia to cancers. The main physical agent found in the workplace that adversely impacts on the haematological system is ionising radiation. Where employees are engaged in activities that may expose them to such agents it is imperative that appropriate risk assessment and risk management regimes are effectively implemented. Appropriate exposure assessment is key and the process may involve health surveillance, biological monitoring and biological effect monitoring.

Management of haematological conditions resulting from exposure to chemical and physical agents in the workplace will depend on nature of the causal agent and resultant health condition. Lead poisonoing, for example, in severe cases can be managed with the use of chelating agents to remove lead from the body. On the other hand, blood cell cancers are treated with the usual management regimes for the condition which are not dependent on the causal factor.

References

Agency for Toxic Substances and Disease Registry (ATSDR). (2014) *Medical management guidelines for arsine.* [Online] Available from: https://wwwn.cdc.gov/TSP/MMG/MMGDetails.aspx?mmgid=1199&toxid=278. [Accessed on 26 April 2021].

Ahn JS, Moon JD, Kang W, Lim H-M, Cho S, Lim D-Y, Park WJ. (2018) Acute radiation syndrome in a non-destructive testing worker: A case report. *Ann Occup Environ Med* **30**: 1–5.

Aksoy M, Dinçol K, Erdhem Ş, Dinçol G. (1972) Acute leukemia due to chronic exposure to benzene. *Am J Med* **52**: 160–166.

Barbosa F, Jr, Tanus-Santos JE, Gerlach RF, Parsons PJ. (2005) A critical review of biomarkers used for monitoring human exposure to lead:

Advantages, limitations, and future needs. *Environ Health Perspect* **113**(12): 1669–1674.

Barry V, Todd AC, Steenland K. (2019) Bone lead associations with blood lead, kidney function and blood pressure among US, lead-exposed workers in a surveillance programme. *Occup Environ Med* **76**(5): 349–354.

Battistuzzi G, Petrucci R, Silvagni L, Urbani FR, Caiola S. (1981) delta-Aminolevulinate dehydrase: A new genetic polymorphism in man. *Ann Hum Genet* **45**(3): 223–229.

Bellinger D, Hu H, Titlebaum L, Needleman HL. (1994) Attentional correlates of dentin and bone lead levels in adolescents. *Arch Environ Health* **49**(2): 98–105.

Bhoopalan SV, Huang LJ, Weiss MJ. (2020) Erythropoietin regulation of red blood cell production: From bench to bedside and back. *F1000 Research* **9**: F1000 Faculty Rev-1153.

Blanuša M, Varnai V, Piasek M, Kostial K. (2005) Chelators as antidotes of metal toxicity: Therapeutic and experimental aspects. *Curr Med Chem* **12**: 2771–2794.

Bradberry S. (2003) Occupational methemoglobinaemia. Mechanisms of production, features, diagnosis and management including the use of Methylene Blue. *Toxicol Rev* **22**(1): 13–27.

Carrieri M, Spatari G, Tranfo G, Sapienza D, Sacapellato ML, Bartolucci GB, Manno M. (2018) Biological monitoring of low level exposure to benzene in an oil refinery: Effect of modulating factors. *Toxicol Lett* **298**: 70–75.

Centers for Disease Control and Prevention (CDC)/National Institute for Occupational Safety and Health (NIOSH). (2015) *Reference Blood Lead Levels (BLL) for Adults in the U.S.* [Online] Available from: www.cdc.gov/niosh/topics/ables/pdfs/Reference%20Blood%20Levels%20for%20Adults-2015-12-18_508.pdf. [Accessed on 25 April 2021].

Centers for Disease Control and Prevention (CDC). (2018) *Acute radiation syndrome. A factsheet for clinicians.* [Online] Available from: https://www.cdc.gov/nceh/radiation/emergencies/arsphysicianfactsheet.htm. [Accessed on 26 April 2021].

Chikezie PC, Ekechukwu CU. (2016) Acute patho-toxicological indicators of methemoglobinemia. *J Acute Dis* **5**(3): 179–184.

Chisolm JJ. (1971) Lead poisoning. *Sci Am* **224**(2): 15–23.

Dzierzak E, Philipsen S. (2013) Erythropoiesis: Development and differentiation. *Cold Spring Harb Perspect Med* **3**(4): a011601.

Ericson B, Duong TT, Keith J, Nguyen TC, Havens D, Daniell W, Karr CJ, Ngoc Hai D, Van Tung L, Thi Nhi Ha T, Wilson B, Hanrahan D, Croteau G, Patrick Taylor M. (2018) Improving human health outcomes with a low-cost intervention to reduce exposures from lead acid battery recycling: Dong Mai, Vietnam. *Environ Res* **161**: 181–187.

Fleming DE, Chettle DR, Wetmur JG, Desnick RJ, Robin JP, Boulay D, Richard NS, Gordon CL, Webber CE. (1998) Effect of the delta-aminolevulinate dehydratase polymorphism on the accumulation of lead in bone and blood in lead smelter workers. *Environ Res* 77(1): 49–61.

Flora S, Pachauri V. (2010) Chelation in metal intoxication. *Int J Environ Res Public Health* 7: 2745–2788.

Flora S. (2014) Toxic metals: Health effects and therapeutic measures. *J Biomed Ther Sci* **1**(1): 46–64.

Gross-Davis CA, Heavner K, Frank AL, Newschaffer C, Klotz J, Santella RM, Burstyn I. (2015) The role of genotypes that modify the toxicity of chemical mutagens in the risk for myeloproliferative neoplasms. *Int J Environ Res Public Health* **12**(3): 2465–2485.

Hanna-Attisha M, LaChance J, Sadler RC, Champney Schnepp A. (2016) Elevated blood lead levels in children associated with the flint drinking water crisis: A spatial analysis of risk and public health response. *Am J Public Health* **106**(2): 283–290.

Hernberg S. (1980) Biochemical and clinical effects and responses as indicated by blood lead concentration. In: Singhal, R.L., Thomas, J.A. (eds.), *Lead toxicity*. Baltimore, Urban and Schwarzenberg.

Hoet P, Buchet J, Decerf L, Lavalleye B, Haufroid V, Lison D. (2006) Clinical evaluation of a lead mobilization test using the chelating agent dimercaptosuccinic acid. *Clin Chem* **52**(1): 88–96.

Hoet P, De Smedt E, Ferrari M, Imbriani M, Maestri L, Negri S, De Wilde P, Lison D, Haufroid V. (2009) Evaluation of urinary biomarkers of exposure to benzene: Correlation with blood benzene and influence of confounding factors. *Int Arch Occup Environ Health* **82**(8): 985–995.

International Atomic Energy Agency. (1999) *Radiation protection and safety in industrial radiography*. Vienna: International Atomic Energy Agency. Safety Reports Series No. 13.

Ivanovs A, Rybtsov S, Ng ES, Stanley EG, Elefanty AG, Medvinsky A. (2017) Human haematopoietic stem cell development: From the embryo to the dish. *Development* **144**(13): 2323–2337.

Kelada SN, Shelton E, Kaufmann RB, Khoury MJ. (2001) Delta-aminolevulinic acid dehydratase genotype and lead toxicity: A HuGE review. *Am J Epidemiol* **154**(1): 1–13.

Kim HS, Lee SS, Lee GS, Hwangbo Y, Ahn KD, Lee BK. (2004) The protective effect of delta-aminolevulinic acid dehydratase 1-2 and 2-2 isozymes against blood lead with higher hematologic parameters. *Environ Health Perspect* **112**(5): 538–541.

Kim J-J, Kim Y-S, Kumar V. (2019) Heavy metal toxicity: An update of chelating therapeutic strategies. *J Trace Elem Med Biol* **54**: 226–231.

Kim Y, Yoo CI, Lee CR, Lee JH, Lee H, Kim SR, Chang SH, Lee WJ, Hwang CH, Lee YH. (2002) Evaluation of activity of erythrocyte pyrimidine 5′-nucleotidase (P5N) in lead exposed workers: With focus on the effect on hemoglobin. *Ind Health* **40**(1): 23–27.

La Dou J, Harrison R. (ed.) (2014) *Current Occupational and Environmental Medicine* (5th Ed). New York, McGraw-Hill.

Ling T, Crispino JD, Zingariello M, Martelli F, Migliaccio AR. (2018) GATA1 insufficiencies in primary myelofibrosis and other hematopoietic disorders: Consequences for therapy. *Expert Rev Hematol* **11**(3): 169–184.

Mani MS, Kunnathully V, Rao C, Kabekkodu SP, Joshi MB, D'Souza HS. (2018) Modifying effects of δ-Aminolevulinate dehydratase polymorphism on blood lead levels and ALAD activity. *Toxicol Lett* **295**: 351–356.

Molloy EJ, Doctor BA, Reed MD, Walsh MC. (2004) Perinatal toxicity of domestic naphthalene exposure. *J Perinatol* **24**(12): 792–793.

NIOSH. (2019) *NIOSH Pocket Guide to Chemical Hazards*. [Online] Available from: https://www.cdc.gov/niosh/npg/npgd0049.html. [Accessed on 26 April 2021].

NIOSH. (2021) *Adult Blood Lead Epidemiology and Surveillance (ABLES)*. [Online] Available from: https://www.cdc.gov/niosh/topics/ables/description.html. [Accessed on 26 Apr 2021].

OSHA. (n.d.) *Regulations (Standards-29 CFR, 1910.1025 App B)*. [Online] Available from: https://www.osha.gov/pls/oshaweb/owadisp.show_document?p_table=STANDARDS&p_id=10032. [Accessed on 25 April 2021].

Pakulska D, Czerczak S. (2006) Hazardous effects of arsine: A short review. *Int J Occup Med Environ Health* **19**(1): 36–44.

Papanikolaou N, Hatzidaki E, Belivanis Tzanakakis G, Tsatsakis A. (2005) Lead toxicity update. A brief review. *Med Sci Monit* **11**(10): 329–336.

Perrotta C, Kleefeld S, Staines A, Tewari P, De Roos AJ, Baris D, Birmann B, Chiu B, Cozen W, Becker N, Foretova L, Maynadie M, Nieters A, de Sanjose S, Miligi L, Costantini AS, Purdue M, Spinelli J, Cocco P. (2013) Multiple myeloma and occupation: A pooled analysis by the International Multiple Myeloma Consortium. *Cancer Epidemiol* **37**: 300–305.

Pullen-James S, Woods S. (2006). Occupational arsine gas exposure. *J Natl Med Assoc* **98**(12): 1198–2001.

Quintanar-Escorza MA, González-Martínez MT, del Pilar IO, Calderón-Salinas JV. (2010) Oxidative damage increases intracellular free calcium [Ca2+]i concentration in human erythrocytes incubated with lead. *Toxicol in Vitro* **24**(5): 1338–1346.

Rachmat B, Kusnoputranto H, Inswiari. (2019) Anemia in children due to airborne lead exposure of used lead acid battery recycling area in Jabodetabek, Indonesia. *Indian J Public Health Res Develop* **10**(11): 1856–1861.

Rael LT, Ayala-Fierro F, Carter DE. (2000) The effects of sulfur, thiol, and thiol inhibitor compounds on arsine-induced toxicity in the human erythrocyte membrane. *Toxicol Sci* **55**: 468–477.

Sahni M, Vibert Y, Bhandari V, Menkiti O. (2019) Newborn infant with mothball toxicity due to maternal ingestion. *Pediatrics* **143**(6): e20183619

Sakai T, Araki T, Ushio K. (1990) Accumulation of erythrocyte nucleotides and their pattern in lead workers. *Arch Env Health* **45**: 273–277.

Sakthithasan K, Lévy P, Poupon J, Garnier R. (2018) A comparative study of edetate calcium disodium and dimercaptosuccinic acid in the treatment of lead poisoning in adults. *Clin Toxicol* **56**(11): 1142–1149.

Schwartz BS, Stewart WF, Kelsey KT, Simon D, Park S, Links JM, Todd AC. (2000) Associations of tibial lead levels with BsmI polymorphisms in the vitamin D receptor in former organolead manufacturing workers. *Environ Health Perspect* **108**(3): 199–203.

Seyferth D. (2003) The rise and fall of tetraethyllead. *Organometallics* **22**: 5154–5178.

Sharma B, Singh S, Siddiqi NJ. (2014) Biomedical implications of heavy metals induced imbalances in redox systems. *BioMed Res Int* **2014**: 640754.

Sullivan M. (2015) Reducing lead in air and preventing childhood exposure near lead smelters: Learning from the U.S. experience. *New Solut* **25**(1): 78–101.

Tong S, von Schirnding YE, Prapamontol T. (2000) Environmental lead exposure: A public health problem of global dimensions. *Bull World Health Organ* **78**(9): 1068–1077.

Watt BE, Proudfoot AT, Bradberry SM, Vale JA. (2005) Poisoning due to urea herbicides. *Toxicol Rev* **24**(3): 161–166.

Wetmur JG, Bishop DF, Cantelmo C. (1986) Human -δ-aminolevulinate dehydratase: Nucleotide sequence of a full-length cDNA clone. *Proc Natl Acad Sci U.S.A.* **83**: 7703–7707.

Wetmur JG, Lehnert G, Desnick RJ. (1991) The δ-aminolevulinate dehydratase polymorphism: Higher blood lead levels in lead workers and environmentally exposed children with the 1-2 and 2-2 isozymes. *Environ Res* **56**: 109–19.

Wetmur JG. (1994) Influence of the common human δ-aminolevulinate dehydratase polymorphism on lead body burden. *Environ Health Perspect* **102**(3): 215–219.

White JM, Harvey DR. (1972) Defective synthesis of and globin chains in lead poisoning. *Nature* **236**(5341): 71–73.

Wright RO, Lewander WJ, Woolf AD. (1999) Methemoglobinemia: Etiology, pharmacology, and clinical management. *Ann Emerg Med* **34**(5): 646–656.

Yadav G, Chambial S, Agrawal N, Gothwal M, Kathuria P, Singh P, Sharma P, Sharma PP. (2020) Blood lead levels in antenatal women and its association with iron deficiency anemia and adverse pregnancy outcomes. *J Fam Med Prim Care* **9**(6): 3106–3111.

Zanella A, Bianchi P, Fermo E, Valentini G. (2006) Hereditary pyrimidine 5′-nucleotidase deficiency: From genetics to clinical manifestations. *British J Hematol* **133**(2): 113–123.

Zhang X, Yang L, Li Y, Li H, Wang W, Ye B. (2012) Impacts of lead/zinc mining and smelting on the environment and human health in China. *Environ Monit Assess* **184**(4): 2261–2273.

Ziemsen B, Angerer J, Lehnert G, Benkmann HG, Goedde HW. (1986) Polymorphism of delta-aminolevulinic acid dehydratase in lead-exposed workers. *Int Arch Occup Environ Health* **58**(3): 245–247.

Chapter 9

Neurological Disorders

Ian Brown and Arjune Sen*†

Introduction

Neurological disorders are an important cause of disability globally. The morbidity is often more significant than the mortality with 6% of the European Union (EU) population suffering a longstanding neurological disorder. Neurological and psychiatric disorders account for 1.4% of all deaths and represent 28% of all lives lived with disability (Menken, 2002). Neurological disorders may therfore have long lasting, perhaps lifelong, effects something that becomes more evident when looking at the prevalence of some common neurological disorders and comparing this with their incidence. Table 1 compares the incidence and prevalence rate for common neurological conditions in the EU.

Neurological disorders can have a significant effect on the ability of an employee to undertake their employment, especially as many neurological conditions are chronic. The incidence of epilepsy is more than ten times lower than the prevalence (Table 1), indicating that

* NHS England and the General Medical Council, Oxford Epilepsy Research Group, Nuffield Department of Clinical Neurology, Oxford University and Oxford University Hospitals, United Kingdom.

† Oxford Epilepsy Research Group, Nuffield Department of Clinical Neurosciences, National Institute of Health Research Biomedical Research Centre, John Radcliffe Hospital, Oxford, United Kingdom.

Table 1. Neurological Disease Rate (Per 100,000 Population)

	Incidence	Prevalence
Epilepsy	40	500
Bell's palsy	20	2
Multiple sclerosis	2	50
Motor neurone disease	1	5
Huntington's chorea	0.5	6

Source: Modified from Weatherall DJ, Ledingham JGG, and Warrell DA (eds.) (1966) *Oxford Textbook of Medicine* (3rd Ed). with the kind permission of Oxford University Press.

the the disorder can be treated, but rarely resolves completely. An occupational physican (OP), should therefore consider the patient's perspective and how the disorder affects function. This "phenomenological" approach was succintly stated by Sir Robert Platt, the President of the Royal College of Physicians of London (from 1957 to 1962), who wrote *"The art of medicine remains the art of identifying the patient's problem — which is something more than merely diagnosing the disease."* Nothing could be more pertinent to the practice of occupational medicine, but the OP has an additional task in appreciating the possibility of an occupational cause and removing the employee from further potential causative exposure. This is a vital responsibility in this medical specialty as such action may protect other employees similarly exposed.

The following groups of symptoms and signs should be considered when making an assessment of a patient with a neurological disorder: memory, cognition, mood, judgment, disinhibition, sensation, and motor function. Some symptoms may well be transient such as loss of conciousness, headache and disturbance of memory and these will usually recover.

The main considerations during the assessment are; severity, progression, prognosis, and removal or separation from further (causative) exposure, especially if occupational factors are deemed to be the cause.

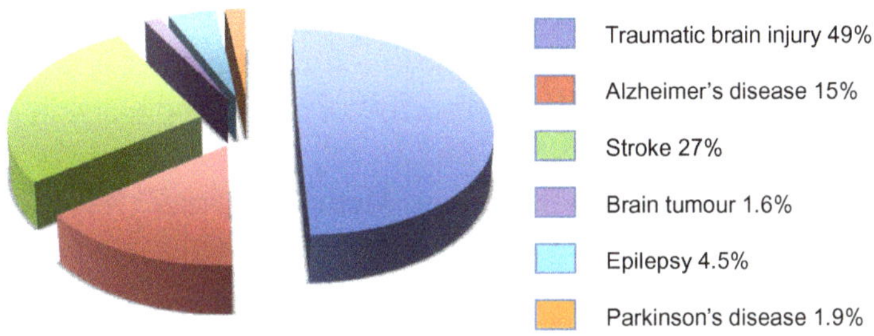

Fig. 1. Brain disorders in the United States of America (Kim and Kang, 2010).

Neurological brain disorders, (central nervous system) that have an effect on occupation and employment are illustrated in the pie chart as shown in Fig. 1.

The effects of the different conditions are predominantly related to brain function and the central nervous system. Stroke (27%), Alzheimers disease (15%) and epilepsy (4.5%) are less commonly caused by work although they may have a devastating effect on employment. This is in contrast to "traumatic brain injury" (TBI) which is significantly causal to impairments at work in almost 50% of the total. A global systematic review (Li *et al.*, 2016) indicated that the majority of traumatic brain injuries were caused by motor vehicle accidents and falls, with a significant number directly associated with work. In our view there was probably a much greater component associated with work, as driving is often a part of the working day and falls from heights may also be work related.

Peripheral nervous system disorders may also compromise work, and the most common is a peripheral neuropathy. This might relate to a wider neurological or systemic disorder, be it idiopathic or be occupationally caused.

The clinician needs to decide on whether a neurological disorder is compromising the central, peripheral or autonomic nervous system or perhaps all three components through a neurodegenerative process (Kim and Kang, 2010). An alternative is to use a dual approach combined assessment considering the aetiological agent and which part of the nervous system is affected.

The examining doctor can initially consider employment generically, but needs to be aware of possible occupational exposures and if such exposure is a possible cause of the neurological disorder. Regardless, the impact of neurological disease on employment is an important responsibility of the OP (irrespective of cause) and below is a brief synopsis of the responsibilities. Considerably more detail can be found in the book "Fitness for Work — The Medical Aspects" (Hobson and Smedley, 2019).

The Impact of Neurological Disease on Employment

As well as the potential of developing neurological illness as a consequence of workplace exposure, neurological conditions can have an impact on an employee's interface and function in the workplace itself. The reasons for this can be principally divided into deficits in motor or other specific functions (e.g. cognitive difficulties) or the impact of episodic conditions on the ability to work. While not all neurological conditions can be covered, the basic approach can be appreciated by evaluation of salient examples in the next few sections.

Disorders of Motor/Sensory Function

Many neurological conditions can affect sensorimotor function be that peripheral (e.g. peripheral neuropathy) or central (e.g. multiple sclerosis or stroke). The OP will need to assess whether the patient can continue to perform the main tasks of their employment. There will need to be assessments, for example, as to ability to control heavy machinery or perform delicate procedures. Moreover, certain occupations require fine dexterity and the impact on employees in these professions will be felt earlier in the disease process than jobs in which motor control is less critical.

Similarly, conditions that cause cerebellar or posterior column dysfunction may result in ataxia and balance difficulties and these symptoms too will be noticed earlier in certain professions (e.g. ballet dancers or professional athletes). In presenting with ataxia, OPs should be aware of potentially reversible contributory factors including alcohol which, of course, may impact work beyond the balance difficulties with which the patient presents.

In all patients, appropriate adaptations should be made to enable employees to continue in their role with, for example, appropriate occupational therapy assessment and input.

Disorders of Cognitive Function

Neurodegenerative conditions (for example Alzheimer's disease, Parkinson's disease, Motor Neurone disease) are principally diseases of older age by which time patients may have left the workplace. There are, though, cases of early-onset Alzheimer's disease, for example, and OPs need to be alert to signs suggesting cognitive or memory impairment. Such changes may initially be quite insidious, with colleagues noting that the affected employee cannot keep up with his/her peers, is less engaged in meetings or, possibly, is exhibiting frank memory difficulties or unusual behaviours. In such cases specialist neurological and neuropsychological advice should be sought.

However, as well as neurodegenerative diseases, many other neurological conditions that affect the central nervous system may also have elements of cognitive difficulty. Notable examples include multiple sclerosis and epilepsy (which is discussed in detail below). Again an awareness of these associations is important and prompt neuropsychometric appraisal should be recommended in patients who begin to exhibit memory or other cognitive difficulties.

Neurological Disorders Characterised by Episodic Symptoms

One of the most common causes of missed days at work is headache and of the primary headache disorders, migraine is by far the most common. Patients with disabling migraine on more than two occasions per month should be referred to their primary care physician or a neurologist for consideration of prophylactic therapy. Current general advice can be accessed through the British Association for the Study of Headaches (BASH, 2021) and the Migraine Trust (Migraine Trust, 2021).

Migraine can associate with focal neurological deficits, but its gradual evolution means that, beyond needing time away from work, headache will not necessarily come to the attention of OPs. In sharp contrast, epilepsy is a condition that will frequently require discussion and is of sufficient prevalence to be considered in its own right.

One in twenty patients will experience a single seizure and even an isolated event can have a significant impact at work. Epilepsy, which affects around 50 million people worldwide, is diagnosed after a patient has experienced two unprovoked seizures or has had a single seizure and there are factors that predict a higher than average risk of seizure recurrence (e.g. positive family history, abnormalities on magnetic resonance imaging (MRI) and/or electroencephalogram). Patients should be advised to exercise due caution so that were they to have a further event the chance of injury to the patient or others is minimised. However, many occupations carry very specific risks were a patient to have a seizure in the workplace such as construction workers, electricians, lifeguards, pilots, cooks and all jobs requiring use of power tools.

Moreover, even a single seizure will result in a restriction on driving. The OP should be familiar with relevant local driving guidelines. In the United Kingdom (UK), a single seizure, with no factors predicting higher than average risk of recurrence, results in a 6-month restriction from driving. In people who have had more than one seizure, or in whom there is considered to be a higher than average risk of seizure recurrence, individuals are required to be free of all seizures for a period of at least 12 months. Special dispensations may apply to those who experience only seizures from sleep or those in whom seizures do not impair awareness or ability to act. More stringent restrictions apply to the UK Group II vehicles (heavy goods, large goods and passenger carrier vehicles) where a single seizure results in a 5-year restriction on driving and people with epilepsy must be free of all events for 10 years before applying to the licensing authority for restoration of their Group II Licence.

Many people drive for their work and many more drive to and from their workplace. Employers should make necessary arrangements to accommodate the driving restrictions. For example, employers may be able to delegate patients to desk duties and arrange for other employees to bring the affected individual to and from work during the period when they cannot drive. There may also be opportunities for the patient to claim relevant government sponsored travel discounts.

In all cases, the OP and employers should work to reduce potential provoking factors for further seizures. Modern light emitting diode (LED) computer screens are unlikely to trigger photosensitive epilepsy owing to no flicker or a very high flicker rate. However, if necessary, appropriate screens can be purchased or screen-guards put in place over the patient's screen. Perhaps most importantly, people with epilepsy should try to avoid, or at least limit, shift-work as the disruption to sleep patterns can lower the seizure threshold. Shift-work is very much part of modern employment, but employers should strive to make the necessary adjustments. As well as in factory work, shifts are prevalent in other occupations, notably in the health and emergency services. Rosters should account for a person's epilepsy and wherever possible the affected employee should be rostered to work daytime shifts to enable adequate sleep overnight. In addition, as with many neurological conditions, epilepsy can associate with cognitive and psychological co-morbidities. For example, approximately one third of people with epilepsy will experience depression. Adequate assessment and treatment of the psychological health of all patients with neurological conditions is fundamental to improving attendance and outcomes in the workplace.

Disorders of Pain Perception

There has evolved an increasing interest in the problem of chronic pain, its management and its effect on an individual's work and enjoyment of life. Conservatively, one in 10 individuals globally suffer with chronic pain and in the UK, at least one third of the population suffers with chronic pain, which is the second most common cause of sickness absence (Dueñas *et al.*, 2016). The source of such pain may well be musculoskeletal or neuropathic but the pathway is always to the thalamus within the brain from which further interpretation/analysis is undertaken, such that the site of the pain is considered (somatosensory cortex), what might have caused the pain (the frontal cortex) and how it should be perceived and understood (the limbic system). Pain is perhaps not traditionally considered a neurological disorder, but the chronicity and disability it causes certainly is and we discuss this briefly below.

The treatment of chronic pain has often been questionable with numerous different approaches that have often not given optimal results and were also not evidence based. The difficulty often arises when the fear of suffering pain becomes "conditioned" in the amygdala, (a part of the limbic system), leading to "fear conditioning" and activity avoidance. In the majority of cases the pain is no longer a warning that activities (possibly work) need to cease. Professor John D. Loeser, Director of the Washington Multidisciplinary Pain Centre, has been credited as the first person to use the multidiciplinary biopsychosocial model in association with chronic pain treatment. This involves case management using the expertise of a physician or specialist nurse with an interest in chronic pain, a clinical psychologist, a physiotherapist and an occupational therapist. Opiates should be avoided. Other medications have been found to be helpful, but the treatment will probably fail without the input of a multidiciplinary team.

Case Study 1: Management of Chronic Pain

Mr. M, an Iraq war veteran is admitted to the hospital for intractable pain in his left arm. He suffered an acute crush injury two years ago while in combat. He has had multiple operations to repair damage but still suffers from chronic unrelenting pain. He clearly states that if the surgeon does not agree to amputate his arm, he has purchased a gun and is planning to commit suicide.

A comprehensive biopsychosocial treatment approach was designed that integrated cognitive behavioural therapy, physiotherapy, relaxation techniques, engagement of his family, and a serotonin-noradrenaline reuptake inhibitor. Over the next 6 months Mr. M noted a substantial improvement in his pain and functional status. Enabling the multidiciplinary biopsychosocial approach Mr M understood the scientific reasons for his chronic pain and behaviour and this allowed him to decatastrophise his thoughts and re-engage with his life — Perhaps even a life saved?

Trauma

Head injury is a major cause of neurological injury at workplaces. Almost 50% of all brain disorders in the USA are attributable to TBI, many due to road traffic accidents. TBI is a major cause of death and severe disability with a million hospital admissions per annum throughout the EU (European Brain Injury Society, 2021). Around 80,000 patients are left with permanent neurological disabilities in the USA annually (Ghajar, 2000). More than 25% of all journeys that resulted in a road traffic accident (RTA) in the UK are reported as work related (including commuting, 10%), and the actual number is probably much higher than this (72% are classified in the category "unknown" (Department for Transport, 2015).

Head injuries at work may be caused by many factors other than driving. Workplace regulations in most countries require the wearing of a protective hard hat. In the USA, around 7,300 occupational TBI deaths occurred between 2003 and 2008. The leading cause was motor vehicle incidents (31%) this was closely followed by falls (29%). The main industry implicated was construction (Tiesman *et al.*, 2011). After a serious head injury it is often many months before the individual can return to work following intensive neurorehabilitation. In very severe cases, survival may lead to such significant brain damage that the worker may never be able to work again.

The Glasgow Coma Scale can predict prognosis reasonably reliably and is an external measure of brain function, especially to verbal commands or physical stimuli (Table 2).

The scale is from 3 to 15 and scores of 8 or below may herald future complications that could significantly affect work potential. Of particular concern will be the possibility of developing epilepsy, disturbances of memory and mood and disorders of voluntary movement.

The OP should play a leading role in considering every aspect of the disability and recommend reasonable adjustments and modification at the workplace. Epilepsy is a special category. Typically (but not necessarily), a head injury would need to be penetrating with tears

Table 2. Glasgow Coma Scale

Component	Description	Score
Best eye response (E)	Spontaneous-open with blinking at baseline	4
	Opens to verbal command, speech or shout	3
	Opens to pain, not applied to face	2
	None	1
Best verbal response (V)	Oriented	5
	Confused conversation, but able to answer questions	4
	Inappropriate responses, words discernible	3
	Incomprehensible speech	2
	None	1
Best motor response (M)	Obeys commands for movement	6
	Purposeful movement to painful stimulus	5
	Withdraws from pain	4
	Abnormal(spastic) flexion, decorticate posture	3
	Extensor (rigid) response, decerebrate posture	2
	None	1

in the dura or significant intra-cerebral bleeding to cause epilepsy. Known toxic causes are gross overexposure to chlorinated hydrocarbons and ingestion of organochlorine insecticides. Lead encephalopathy can also, but rarely, cause convulsions in children (Brown and Prevett, 2019). If epilepsy does result, then anti-seizure medication may reduce or abort attacks. Choice of anti-seizure medication must always be individualised to ensure that it has the least effect on cognition, mood, reaction time and drowsiness.

Case Study 2: Epilepsy and Driving

A 35 year-old female UK university researcher attends a hospital epilepsy clinic because of long standing thought disturbances where she suddenly feels unfamiliar with her environment and faces and colors become distorted. There are no motor problems. The events occur in clusters and may happen many times in one day or there may only be a single event in several weeks. She currently drives her motor vehicle on university business and also uses the car to take her three children to school. After a number of investigations a diagnosis of focal seizures was made. She is started on an anti-seizure medication, but this made her drowsy and did not abort the disturbances.

Clinicians need to give the patient advice about driving which is an essential part of the patient's job. She reports to the university occupational health service and the OP discusses the case with the neurologist and car driving licensing authority. She was allowed to continue to drive as changes in UK Class 1 motor vehicle driving regulations will allow an individual with epilepsy to continue to drive if the events they suffer do not in any way impair consciousness or their ability to control the motor vehicle. Different countries and jurisdictions, though, have different regulations and guidelines. Patients must always be informed fully of the existing national driving regulations and adhere to these at all times. Failure to do so may well be dangerous and will invalidate their insurance cover.

Aetiological Agents

About 40% of chemicals in the workplace are known to affect the nervous system and about 30% of occupational standards are based on behavioural or neurological endpoints (Lucchini *et al.*, 2005). Much of our knowledge of the effects of neurotoxicants on workers' health comes from epidemiological studies. These studies are important because they provide evidence of the effects of long-term exposure to many neurotoxicants.

Metals

Arsenic

Exposure to arsenic can occur in different settings. In Singapore, for example, the commonest exposures to arsenic were from the production of electronics components and wood preservation industries (Chia *et al.*, 1993a). Although the electronics industry had the most number of workers, their exposure is usually very low. The exposure is confined to the manufacture of electronic wafers where arsenic is used to enhance electrical conductivity. This process is enclosed although exposure is possible during maintenance (LaDou, 1990).

Arsenic exposure was once potentially high in wood preservation plants with dust generated during the pouring and mixing of dry wood preservatives chemicals, athough no dust is generated in those using the paste form of wood preservative, skin contact is unavoidable during the release of treated wood from the pressurised tanks (Ho *et al.*, 1982). At the end of 2003, the United States wood treatment industry stopped using arsenic for wood preservation and it has been replaced with the less toxic mix of copper and a quaternary ammonium compound and arsenic has slowly been phased out globally.

High levels of arsenic can though, be found in drinking water for both natural and anthropogenic sources. Workers occupationally exposed to arsenic and residents in areas with high arsenic content in drinking water, can be at higher risk for the development of adverse effects and arsenic has become a worrying contaminant of ground water in several countries, especially Bangladesh (Uddin and Huda, 2011).

Other exposures to arsenic include manufacture of glass (used to remove bubbles from molten glass), alloy manufacture, manufacture and use of antifouling paints, taxidermy (arsenic trioxide) and pottery (arsenic trichloride). In many museums that conserve and exhibit biological specimens for display, arsenic was often found as a preservative and continued to be used until around 1970, but its use is waning because of toxicity. Museum conservators though should always be aware of the exposure risk and use personal protective equipment when handling and restoring early specimens.

The carcinogenic properties of this metal are well known but it can also cause a peripheral neuropathy which is not a common feature of acute arsenic poisoning. Arsenic is thought to damage the peripheral nerves by reacting with the thiol groups of proteins, especially enzymes. In chronic arsenic exposure, the typical neurological manifestation is a combined sensory and motor polyneuropathy (Heyman *et al.*, 1956; Feldman *et al.*, 1979) with paresthesia and

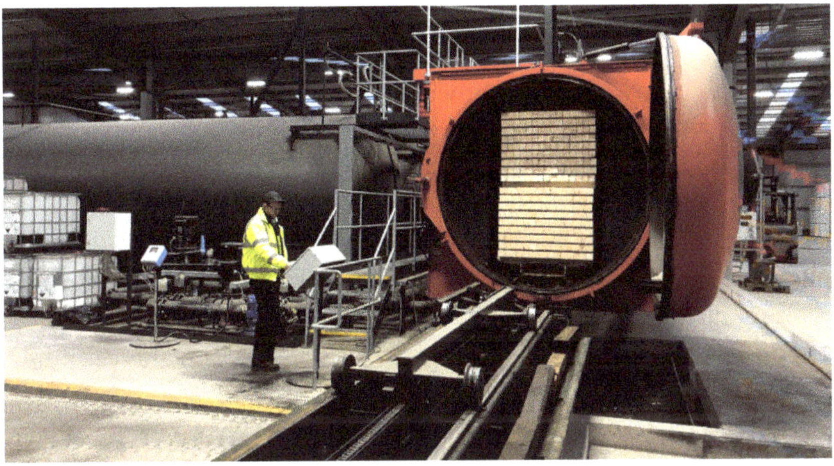

Fig. 2. Wood being placed into a pressurised tank for treatment with preservatives. (Reproduced with the kind permission of James Jones Ltd and the Timber Decking and Cladding Association.)

painful hyperesthesia often being the initial presenting symptoms. Sensory deficits are more prominent and motor defects appear initially in the distal parts of the lower limbs with wasting of the extensor muscles of the feet and toes. Involvement of the upper limbs is less common and central nervous system effects are rare. Exposure to arsenic is also associated with mucosal irritation, a desquamating rash, myalgia and white transverse Mees lines in the fingernails (Ropper *et al.*, 2019). Chronic occupational exposure at levels above the air concentration of 10 $\mu g/m^3$ can cause increased neurological symptoms and dose-related abnormalities of visual evoked potential, nerve conduction studies and electroencephalography (Halatek *et al.*, 2009).

Lead

Lead is still a major global toxicological problem. The Institute for Health Metrics and Evaluation (IHME) estimated that in 2017, lead exposure accounted for 1.06 million deaths and, more significantly, 24.4 million years of healthy life lost (disability-adjusted life years (DALYs)) worldwide due to long-term effects on health. The highest burden was in low- and middle-income countries. IHME also estimated that in 2016, lead exposure accounted for 63.2% of the global burden of idiopathic developmental intellectual disability, 10.3% of the global burden of hypertensive heart disease, 5.6% of the global burden of the ischaemic heart disease and 6.2% of the global burden of stroke (IHME, 2019).

Common industries where workers can be exposed to lead include smelters, factories producing fabricated metal products and the telecommunications, electronics, plastics, and storage battery industries. Exposure once occured in printing, (type setting), but most printing now is digital. Lead though is still used in the manufacture and use of antifouling paints, manufacture and use of glazes for China porcelain, enamels, glazed tiles and lead soldering.

Organic lead exposure is mainly confined to its use as an anti-knock agent. This application is now becoming obsolete with current international environmental legislation in most countries.

Lead can damage both the central and peripheral nervous systems. Lead exerts its toxic effects by its ability to substitute for other polyvalent cations, particularly divalent cations, such as calcium [Ca^{2+}] and zinc [Zn^{2+}] and the inhibition of enzymes that contain sulphydryl (–SH) functional groups. The earliest symptoms of exposure are fatigue, lethargy, and drowsiness often disturbing the employee's work and social life. Lead poisoning may present as an encephalopathy acutely and a nerve palsy more chronically. Acute encephalopathy, characterised by delusion, delirium and hallucination, is rare and is associated with very high exposure, usually to organic lead. Radial nerve palsy, presenting as "wrist-drop", is now an uncommon complication of lead poisoning. Typical significant poisoning in adults with metallic or inorganic lead presents with abdominal colic, anaemia and muscle weakness. Motor effects predominate over sensory symptoms. The abdominal discomfort is often associated with abnormalities of intestinal movement and may reflect autonomic dysfunction. The patient may regrettably therefore end up in an acute surgical ward awaiting an exploratory laparotomy if the doctor does not take a detailed history and discovers the possibility of lead exposure.

Neurobehavioural changes, consistent with a mild toxic encephalopathy, have been reported in lead workers. These consist of sleep

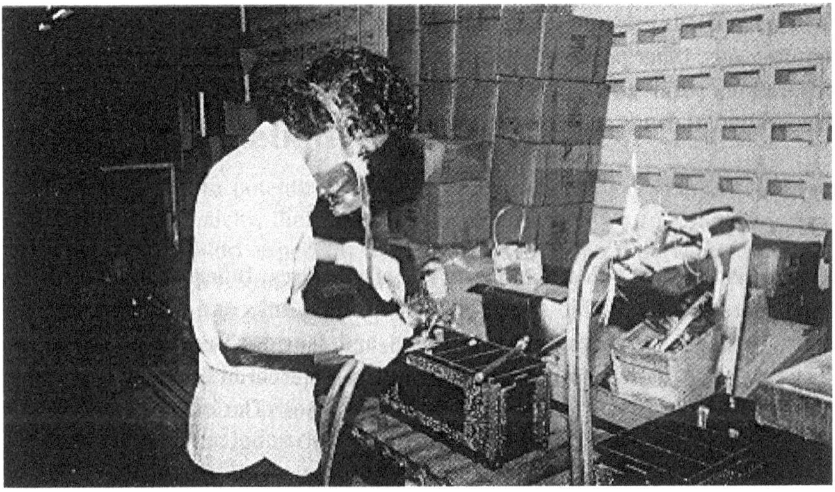

Fig. 3. Burning of lead ingot to join the connectors in the assembly of storage batteries.

difficulties, headaches, fatigue, difficulty in learning new material and adjusting to new situations. Neurobehavioural testing will show elevated mood disorders, deficits in memory and impairment of visuomotor performance. Chia *et al.* (1997) and Schwartz *et al.* (2005) reported that cumulative exposure to lead affects performance on neurobehavioural tests in adults, especially perceptual and motor skills, and long-term cognitive effects.

Studies on occupational lead exposure have shown that neurotoxic effects can begin at blood lead levels around 18 μg/dL (Murata *et al.*, 2009). Severe neurological defects have been reported for blood lead (BPb) concentrations of 100 to 200 μg/100mL (Nordberg, 1976). Radial palsy can develop if BPb levels exceed 120 μg/mL. There is no evidence in adults of peripheral neuropathy below BPb levels of 40 μg/mL (Jeyaratnam *et al.*, 1985; Chia *et al.*, 1996).

Manganese

Manganese is used in the manufacture of dry cell batteries, animal feed, matches and fireworks and in the iron and steel industry. Exposure typically occurs in mining, ferroalloy production, smelting, welding, refining and milling of manganese compounds. A study conducted by Gan *et al.* (1988) reported that the highest manganese exposure was in manganese mills. Other studies indicate highest levels in mining and ferroalloy production (IEH/IOM, 2004).

Although manganese is relatively non-toxic to the adult human and an essential trace element, high exposure to manganese will cause acute behavioural manifestations and manganese miners were reported to develop irritability, nervousness and emotional lability. Some experienced visual and auditory hallucination and compulsive, repetitive behaviours. Exposure for at least 2–3 years to airborne manganese concentrations above 1 mg/m^3 (World Health Organization, 1981) is believed to be sufficient for the development of neurologic abnormalities. There does though appear to be a marked individual susceptibility (Emara *et al.*, 1971).

Chronic excessive manganese exposure may lead to poisoning of the central nervous system called "manganism." The first description of "manganism" was published by Couper in 1837 (Couper, 1837) only 20 years after the first description of the "shaking palsy" by Sir James Parkinson (Parkinson, 2002). Manganism involves a degenerative change of the basal ganglia producing extrapyramidal symptoms similar to Parkinsonism. At the early stage, it presents with asthenia, somnolence, muscular tenderness, irritability and apathy. Later, it involves disorders of gait, dysarthria, mask-like facies, tremor and dysdiadochokinesis (Chandra *et al.*, 1974). Following chronic exposure to manganese air levels above 200 $\mu g/m^3$, early signs of motor function impairment can be shown by neurobehavioural tests (Lucchini *et al.*, 1999; Lucchini *et al.*, 2009) and MRI (Chang *et al.*, 2009). Prolonged exposure to lower levels may be responsible for Parkinsonism symptoms, as shown in manganese exposed welders (Racette *et al.*, 2001; Racette *et al.*, 2005). Chronic exposure to the manganese-containing fungicide, maneb can also cause Parkinsonism symptoms.

Case Study 3: Manganese Poisoning

A 50 year-old woman had been exposed to manganese for 21 years (1963–1984) in the course of her work in the manganese mills. The patient had suffered from palpitations and tremors since 1968 and was initially thought to have hyperthyroidism. In 1980, she developed headache, giddiness, palpitation, salivation, failing memory, lower limb myalgia, myasthenia, intermittent muscular spasms and numbness in the arms and legs. Physical examination at that time showed her hands, tongue and eyelids to be tremulous with rigidity or hypertonicity of muscles and a positive finger-nose test. Following consideration of her occupational history and the extent of exposure to manganese at work, the patient was subsequently diagnosed with chronic mild manganese poisoning by the occupational diseases diagnosis group (Ky et al., 1992).

Mercury

Mercury is used as a flowing cathode in chlor-alkali plants producing chlorine, hydrogen and sodium hydroxide by brine electrolysis (the Castner–Kellner process). The mercury is kept under brine or water during normal operations but mercury exposure can occur during maintenance and refitting when the electrolysing chambers are drained off exposing the mercury. Mercury is also used to recover gold by amalgamation in an extraction heating process that can cause occupational exposure and contamination of air, soil, rivers and lakes. Mercury was used for the felting of the wool when hat making and was depicted in the "Mad Hatter" in Lewis Carol's "Alice in Wonderland." This practice is now rarely undertaken and the mercury has been replaced by hydrogen peroxide which was much safer to use in felting.

Workers in the small-scale gold-mining sector are thought to use mercury more than in any other small industry especially in many regions across Africa, Asia and South America (Swain *et al.*, 2007). In the laboratory, elemental mercury is used as a pressure medium in instruments for carrying out pressure, volume and temperature measurement.

Other possible sources of exposure to mercury include amalgam preparation in dentistry (although less common nowadays with the availability of newer non-mercury dental materials), production of thermometers and neon lights, paint and pigment manufacture, and in the pharmaceutical industry (preparation of drugs and disinfectants).

Tremor is the characteristic sign of inorganic mercury poisoning. A fine tremor involving the eyelids, lips, tongue and fingers can progress to a very coarse tremor. Handwriting may become irregular, shaky and illegible. A mixed peripheral neuropathy can also occur, though this is uncommon (Vroom *et al.*, 1972). The neurological signs are thought to be due to the oxidation of elemental mercury to the divalent ionic form which binds to thiol groups of proteins in the nervous system. Also, selenium containing enzymes are permanently inhibited and this causes oxidative damage to the nervous system (Carvalho *et al.*, 2008). Mercury's irreversible inhibition of selenium-dependent enzymes (Spiller, 2017) may inactivate *S*-adenosyl-methionine, which is necessary for catecholamine catabolism by catechol-*O*-methyl transferase. Due to this inability to degrade catecholamines (e.g. adrenaline), a person suffering from mercury poisoning may therefore experience profuse sweating, tachycardia, increased salivation, hypertension and of course the tremor described above.

Inorganic mercury can also cause the behavioural changes referred to as "erethism." It is characterised by nervousness, insomnia, loss of memory, irritability and excessive shyness. Erethism is now uncommon as it is usually associated with very high levels of mercury exposure. However, low-level exposure to mercury vapors can cause concentration difficulties and mild impairment of cognitive functions (Piikivi and Hanninen, 1977). Alterations in visual fields, contrast sensitivity and color discrimination have been detected in workers exposed to low levels of mercury vapor (average urinary mercury of 22.3 µg/g creatinine) (Barboni *et al.*, 2009). Neuroendocrine changes (increased serum prolactin) and motor coordination imbalance were observed in workers from chloroalkali plants and the production of thermometers and neon lamps, with average urinary mercury levels of 8.3 µg/g creatinine (Lucchini *et al.*, 2003). Organic mercury (often methyl mercury) is usually ingested accidently and through environmental contamination or incidents. Mercury in this form is very easily absorbed via the gut and causes cerebellar ataxia, dysarthria and constriction of the visual fields due to damage of the visual cortex.

Organic Solvents

Organic solvents are typically colorless liquids with a distinct smell and a low boiling point, hence they evaporate easily. Common uses of organic solvents are in dry cleaning (tetrachloroethylene), as paint thinners, (toluene and turpentine), as nail polish removers, (acetone, methyl acetate, ethyl acetate), as spot stain removers, (hexane, petrol ether), and in perfumes, (ethanol). They are also used in printing inks and surface coatings as diluents for paints, spreading preparations for papers and fabrics and for extracting oils, fats and other substances from different materials.

Toluene is probably the most extensively reported organic solvent for causing toxic encephalopathy especially among solvent abusers (King, 1981). It is widely used as a paint, lacquer and ink diluent.

Shoe making, leather and glove industries were among the most frequently reported sources of peripheral neuropathy from organic solvents (Spencer *et al.*, 1980). The main solvents responsible were n-hexane, methyl n-butyl ketone and carbon disulphide. Most of the cases occurred in subjects who work in small, poorly ventilated rooms (Gilioli, 1983).

Case Study 4: Chronic Toxic Encephalopathy from Organic Solvents

A 55-year old man was seen at a medical clinic on many occasions for the previous few months for giddiness. He was well before going to work and only developed giddiness after beginning his work. Physical examinations were normal on all these occasions. He was referred to the Occupational Health Clinic and his occupational history revealed that this patient had been working as a fitter in a shipyard for the last 15 years. Each day he had to use considerable amounts of degreasing agents to clean the ship's engine. Over the last few months, he had started to develop giddiness especially after degreasing in enclosed spaces. Further investigations were conducted and revealed that his symptoms were suggestive of early chronic toxic encephalopathy due to organic solvent exposure.

It was only in the late twentieth century that experimental, clinical and epidemiological studies confirmed that exposure to organic solvents can result in neurobehavioural effects as well as causing a peripheral neuropathy (Hänninen, 1985; Johnson, 1987).

As a generalisation, the more lipophilic the solvent the more potent are its central nervous system depressant characteristics. Behavioural methods have frequently been used to study the effects of exposure to organic solvents. Today, the pre-narcotic effects from acute solvent exposures are now widely accepted as are the more chronic CNS effects from long-term low-level exposures (Iregren, 1996). Exposure to mixtures of solvents can cause deficits of attention and cognitive processing speed (Meyer-Baron *et al.*, 2008). Long term exposure leads, in some workers, to the development of chronic solvent induced encephalopathy (CSE) a non-progressive disease in which deterioration ceases when the employee is withdrawn from further exposure. Cerebral impairment has been localised to the fronto-striato-thalamic networks (Visser *et al.*, 2008) and at a neurobiochemical level organic solvents have been found to alter the function of a variety of ligand gated ion channels (Beckstead *et al.*, 2000) and increase neurodopamine transmission within the mesolimbic reward pathway (Reigel *et al.*, 2004).

In general, acute exposure to high concentrations of organic solvents causes confusion, dizziness, headache, poor concentration, motor incoordination and other related symptoms. Most of these symptoms are reversible if the exposure concentrations are modest but residual deficits may persist. The behavioural effects of solvents associated with chronic exposure can be divided into three levels of increasing severity (Johnson, 1987). The first involves mood changes — easy fatigability, decreased reactivity to environmental stimuli and some degree of mental confusion. Neurobehavioural tests are usually normal but symptoms of depression, irritability, fatigability and confusion are present. The second level is represented by a mild toxic encephalopathy that includes features of mood disorder together with impaired cognitive function. Sleep disorders and memory impairments are also common. The third level is chronic dementia and represents the least common and advanced form of CNS effects. The prognosis for phase 1 is good. Workers can fully recover if they are quickly removed from the excessive solvent exposure.

The prognosis for phase 2 depends on its severity. In the early stages of phase 2, recovery is complete. However, if removal from exposure does not happen in early phase 2, recovery may be impaired. The third stage of the disease is not reversible. However, removal from exposure would still be recommended as this will prevent the further deterioration of the disease (Chia, 1998).

Long and medium term exposure to organic solvents containing carbon disulphide, n-hexane, 2-hexanone and methyl n-butyl ketone are well known to cause mixed peripheral neuropathies (Baker *et al.*, 1985). These solvents cause a distal axonopathy. Carbon disulphide is directly toxic by reacting with protein amino groups (Graham *et al.*, 1995), whereas n-hexane, 2-hexanone and methyl n-butyl ketone toxicity is dependent on the production of the neurotoxic γ-diketone metabolite, 2,5-hexanedione.

Heavy solvent exposure is therefore associated with a number of adverse effects including mild cognitive impairment, hearing loss, and sub-clinical colour vision deficits. Whether these agents are risk factors for neurodegenerative diseases is less clear although dementia has been demonstrated in chronic high-level unprotected exposure. Solvents are important agents in the workplace and occupational physicians should continue to urge employers and the self-employed to adopt appropriate control measures to minimise solvent exposures and protect the health of the employees.

Case Study 5: Peripheral Neuropathy from n-Hexane

A 40 year-old female production worker from an electronic factory complained of numbness of her hands. She had been diagnosed with diabetes 10 years earlier and her blood glucose was well controlled with oral hypoglycaemic agents. She was initially diagnosed by her physician with a peripheral neuropathy secondary to diabetes mellitus.

In a follow-up appointment for her diabetes, it was found that she used solvents to clean electronic components and the solvent contained n-hexane as a contaminant. She was therefore then suspected to have developed a solvent induced periphery neuropathy caused by the n-hexane exposure. After the contaminated solvent was replaced, she recovered completely and did not experience any further dyasesthesia of the hands.

Pesticides

The Food and Agriculture Organization (FAO, 2003) defines a pesticide as any substance or mixture of substances intended to prevent, destroy or control any pest. This includes vectors of human or animal disease, unwanted species of plants or animals causing harm during or otherwise interfering with the production, processing, storage, transport, or marketing of food, agricultural commodities, wood and wood products, or animal feedstuffs. It also includes chemicals that may be administered to animals for the control of insects, arachnids, or other pests in or on their bodies. According to their use, pesticides can be classified into seven main categories: insecticides, fungicides, herbicides, acaricides, molluscicides, rodenticides and nematicides (depending on the target organism).

Approximately 90% of all pesticides are used for commercial crop protection with the remainder for building material pest control, horticulture, and home and garden purposes. Those who are usually exposed are employees who prepare and/or apply pesticides as part of their job, although the general and bystander public may sometimes also be affected following inadvertent exposure, especially by spray drift. Common work exposure situations usually involve agricultural workers and horticultural workers. In horticulture, occupational exposure to the pesticide occurs predominantly during the dilution of the concentrate with water and in the spraying of the mixture. Workers involved in the formulation and manufacture of pesticides and packers who perform "repackaging" of pesticides are also exposed. These operations are often undertaken in warehouses or cottage industries with little or no preventive measures adopted. Although regulation in the EU is stringent with clear guidelines on exposure prevention, the policing of these regulations can be patchy.

Insecticides have a common mode of action on the nervous system neuro-biochemistry shared by most living organisms including insects and humans. It is often only the dose that renders insecticides less toxic to humans, as insects have a smaller body mass and weight. Generally these chemicals interfere with the membrane transportation of sodium, potassium, calcium and/or chloride ions (Ecobichon, 2001). The effects of pesticides on the nervous system may be due to their acute toxicity as in the case of most insecticides or they may possibly contribute to chronic disorders such as Parkinson's disease and chronic fatigue syndrome although clear associations have not been unequivocally proven. There have, though been a number of reports and studies associating mixed pesticide exposure with Parkinsonian symptoms. More specifically, they include agricultural workers exposed primarily to organochlorine pesticides (Elbaz *et al.*, 2009). Use of the non-selective bypyridyl herbicide paraquat, chlorophenoxy herbicides and the insecticide and acaricide, permethrin, (synthetic pyrethroid) have also been associated with Parkinsonism in farmers (Tanner *et al.*, 2009). The strength of the association with the organochlorine and chlorophenoxy group was greatest (Elbaz *et al.*, 2009).

Organochlorine Compounds

The commonest organochlorine pesticides used are dichlorodiphenyltrichloroethane (DDT), chlordecone (Kepone), aldrin, dieldrin, endosulfan and lindane. Significant overexposure to organochlorine insecticides is one of the few causes of non-medicinal chemically-induced convulsions. These chemicals are being used once again as a more persistent and long lasting chemical control of disease carrying insects, although there are still environmental and food contamination concerns about their effects on the environment and the food chain as they are lipophilic and will persist in human and animal fat.

Organochlorines have a primary neuro-biochemical effect which causes repetitive discharges of neurones and both acute or subacute intoxication produces a picture of generalised nervous system excitability; apprehension, excitability, dizziness, headache, disorientation, confusion, weakness, paresthesia, muscle twitching, tremor, convulsions and coma. This is an example of hyper-responsiveness and the postulated mechanism at the level of the neuronal membrane is change in permeability to potassium ions, reducing potassium transport across the membrane. There is also an effect on sodium channel closure and inhibition of ATPase, which will interfere with repolarisation (Matsumura, 1985; Brown *et al.*, 2010).

Organophosphorus Compounds and Carbamates

Organophosphorus and carbamate poisoning is a major public health problem in developing countries, resulting in significant morbidity and mortality. Although the actual incidence of organophosphate poisoning is difficult to establish due to challenges of collecting data for surveillance, it is estimated to cause 250,000 to 350,000 deaths per year globally (Pershin *et al.*, 2014) which is about 10% of all global poisoning episodes.

Organophosphorus insecticides and carbamates are both cholinesterase inhibitors. They are used most commonly in agriculture and are probably the most frequent cause of chemically-related neurological disease among agricultural workers especially from developing countries. Dithiocarbamates like Maneb and Mancozeb are also widely used as fungicides and have also been shown to cause neurotoxic effects in workers and they also contain manganese which can also be toxic.

Acute poisoning by these chemicals is caused by inhibition of the acetylcholinesterase enzyme (which can be measured in whole blood to assess exposure to organophosphates). Symptoms and signs described are both muscarinic, (miosis, salivation, vomiting, diarrhea, bronchial hypersecretion) and nicotinic (muscular fasciculation, tremor, muscular cramps, paralysis) in addition to central nervous system effects (impaired consciousness, convulsions, coma). Significant acute symptomatic exposure will result in effects on the peripheral nervous system. The inhibition of acetylcholinesterase is virtually permanent with organophosphorus compounds (enzyme phosphorylation) but reversible with carbamates (enzyme carbamylation).

Following the acute cholinergic symptoms with organophosphates, an intermediate syndrome may occur in 1–4 days and last between 5 and 18 days. The major effects are muscular weakness of all muscle groups and this is a life threatening condition as breathing can be compromised. This may be followed by a delayed polyneuropathy after an interval of 2–3 weeks. Organophosphorus pesticide induced delayed polyneuropathy (OPIDP) is characterised by a "second" motor neurone flaccidity which is followed in some cases by a long term spasticity, hypertonicity, hyperreflexia and clonus indicative of damage to the pyramidal tract and a Wallerian "dying back" of large diameter axons (Brown *et al.*, 2010). Evidence of long-term central nervous system effects in humans (sheep dippers "flu" or "the chronic (fatigue) syndrome from low dose chronic exposure to organophosphates" is contradictory and current evidence does not fully support the existence of clinically significant neuropsychological effects, neuropsychiatric abnormalities or peripheral nerve dysfunction (Costa *et al.*, 2008).

Case Study 6: Cholinesterase Monitoring in a Worker Exposed to Organophosphorus

*An employee on an organophosphorus manufacturing plant was subject to regular cholinesterase monitoring as a practical method of biological effect monitoring and the occupational physician (OP) received the following graphical result on a temporal run chart (Control limit: 7.86053; Upper control limit: 12.72; lower control limit: 3.0011. I*True Depression).*

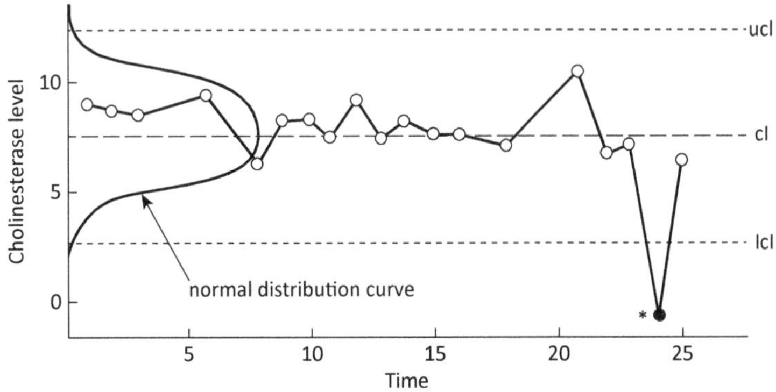

The cholinesterase level has become depressed in this individual by more than two standard deviations from the individual's mean and this

is therefore a significant escalation of exposure. The employee was symptomatic with clinical features consistent with cholinergic effects. The OP immediately withdrew the employee from further exposure and the levels improved over the next few weeks. The OP's next responsibility was to thoroughly investigate how the exposure occurred, and to recommend suitable preventive measures to reduce the likelihood of similar effects re-occurring in this employee or other co-workers.

The above graph is reproduced with the kind permission of Wiley Global Permissions, originally in chapter 19 (author Ian Brown) of Occupational Health — Risk Assessment and Management (1999), editors Sadhra and Rampal (Blackwell Science Ltd).

Impact of COVID-19 on Neurological Illness and Occupational Health

The COVID-19 (SARS-COV2) pandemic has wrought untold misery on the world since first emerging in Wuhan, China in 2019 (Wu *et al.*, 2020). Although a highly infectious and devastating illness, COVID-19 seems to not be a particularly neuro-tropic virus with, for example, far less propensity to result in acute seizures than SARS or MERS, (Kuroda, 2021). The previously reported increase in Guillan Barre Syndrome seems to not be substantiated (Keddie *et al.*, 2021). COVID-19 can, though, result in thromboembolic disease including stroke (Tan *et al.*, 2020), with all of the attendant complications that can result for future work. It may also lead to "long COVID" and profound difficulties through fatigue, sleep problems, low mood, anxiety and persistent dyspnoea (Huang *et al.*, 2021). Also, COVID has had immense impact on health care workers, many of whom report exhaustion and significant mental health illness as a consequence of working through the pandemic, often with limited or no personal protective equipment.

COVID-19 infection has also been found to have both psychiatric sequelae and psychiatric antecedents (Taquet *et al.*, 2021). Survivors have an increased rate of new onset psychiatric disorders, and prior psychiatric disorders are associated with a 65% higher risk of COVID-19 infection.

In terms of neurological illness, COVID-19 is likely to have far greater indirect than direct impact. The vast redeployment of healthcare workers and resources in already stretched systems, means that routine care is substantially delayed. Operations for back pain, carpal tunnel syndrome as well as epilepsy surgery, deep brain stimulation and even some neuro-oncology procedures have all been delayed. The consequences of this and the lost work capacity that inevitably follows have yet to be quanitified. At the time of writing, the UK Government are considering prioritising cases according to whether procedures will enable people to return to work rather than time on a waiting list. This perhaps reflects the desperate need to return to economic productivity as vaccination programmes, hopefully, help quell the COVID storm.

Clinical Investigation of Neurotoxicity from Possible Occupational Exposure

There are many problems in trying to establish a direct cause-effect relationship when examining workers exposed to potentially neurotoxic agents who demonstrate signs and symptoms of neurotoxicity (especially those related to central nervous system effects).

The nervous system responds to neurotoxic substances in many ways. The actual mechanism responsible for neurotoxic effects is still unclear for many substances. Furthermore, little information is generally available about the possible neurotoxic properties of many chemicals. Only a small number of the estimated 60,000 chemicals in the workplace have been evaluated for neurotoxic effects. However, around 2000 new chemicals are being introduced into industries each year (US Department of Health and Human Services, 2021). For chemicals with known neurotoxic properties there is considerable uncertainty about the level and duration of exposure required to produce neurotoxic effects.

In addition, workers are generally exposed to a mixture of chemicals. For example, pesticides often have a solvent carrier and therefore, it is can be very difficult to isolate the effects of a single chemical. To complicate matters further, the "multi-hit" theory makes the CNS particularly susceptible to cumulative exposure via multiple agents compared to a single exposure (Lucchini and Zimmerman, 2009; Cory-Slechta, 2005).

Very few symptoms or signs of neurological impairment are specific for a particular chemical. It may be difficult to differentiate occupational from other (non-occupational) causes of neurological dysfunction. For example, symptom reporting may not be very useful in the diagnosis of chronic solvent-induced encephalopathy which needs further objective evaluation with specific neuropsychological testing (Bast-Pettersen, 2009).

In order to establish that the presenting problem is one that is related to or caused by work exposure, a detailed occupational history is essential. This should be followed by environmental assessment and monitoring (where feasible) to determine the types of agents and level of exposure. Biological monitoring of the employee and other workers may also give a better picture of the body burden to the exposed substance.

How to Distinguish Between an Occupational and a Non-Occupational Disease

Occupational history

In general, the symptomatology of a non-occupational neurological disorder cannot easily be differentiated from that of an occupational related disease; apart from a suggestive exposure history. This is where a comprehensive and detailed occupational history becomes particularly important in helping to distinguish an occupational disease from one that is not work-related. The following is a suggested checklist for taking a comprehensive occupational history (Box 1).

Subjective symptoms questionnaire

Recording of subjective complaints using a standardised questionnaire is important to provide a consistent information base for all patients with neurotoxic exposure. Symptom reports are usually the first manifestation of the disease before any detectable neurological or psychological testing. Subtle changes could be detected, especially if the standardised questionnaire is used periodically for workers. Box 2 shows a sample of one such questionnaire (Johnson, 1987).

Box 1. Occupational History.

Presenting Illness Enquiry:

- Are your symptoms associated with work? i.e. do the symptoms improve during vacations or weekends? Identify patterns suggesting either improvement or exacerbation on withdrawal from exposure.
- Do any other workers have similar symptoms? Identifying others who may also have been affected can lead to further enquiries that clarify the individual patient's problem.
- Are you currently exposed to any metals, solvents, pesticides or other chemicals? Think of the possible neurotoxic agents; remember that there are many substances with possible effects on the nervous system that we may not be aware of.
- Who else did you see regarding the problems?
- This is a valuable way of getting further information from others who may have seen the patient at an earlier phase of the disease, e.g. behavioural changes.

Work History:

- List in chronological order all employment undertaken with dates of engagement and leaving. Describe a typical workday and job duties. Ascertain the degree and duration of exposure to possible neurotoxic substances.
- Was protective equipment issued? If so, did you use it? How frequently did you use it? Consider if protection was given to workers and whether the protection was adequate. Also check if respirators or other airway protection used are the appropriate types.
- Is ventilation in your workplace adequate? Obtain a general impression of adequacy and type of ventilation by air movement and odors.
- Was a pre-employment examination performed? What about periodic medical examinations? Important information could be obtained regarding baseline results and trends of results if these examinations were conducted.
- Besides your regular work, do you have another job? If so please list additional jobs. Some significant exposures may not be due to the regular job but occur during a part-time job outside normal working hours.
- Ask about abnormal circumstances at the workplace. Has there been any increase in workload recently? Was there a breakdown/shutdown? Have there been any changes to the production line or introduction of new chemicals? Identify possible outbreaks or clusters of a neurological condition at the workplace.

Box 2. Symptom Questionnaire.

Chronic Symptoms:

Below is a list of questions concerning symptoms you may have had. Circle the appropriate number if you have been experiencing the symptoms in the past month. If you have experienced the symptom, please indicate in the space provided. ((1) Not at all; (2) A little; (3) Moderately; (4) Quite a bit; (5) Extremely)

- Are you tired more easily the than expected for the amount of activity you do?
- Have you felt lightheaded or dizzy?
- Have you had difficulty concentrating?
- Have you been confused or disoriented?
- Have you had trouble remembering things?
- Have your relatives noticed that you have trouble remembering things?
- Have you had to make notes to remember things?
- Have you found it hard to understand the meaning of newspaper, magazines and books you have read?
- Have you felt irritable?
- Have you felt depressed?
- Have you had heart palpitations even when not exerting yourself?
- Have you had a seizure? ((1) No; (2) Yes; (3) More than one seizure)
- Have you been sleeping more often than is usual for you?
- Have you had difficulty falling asleep?
- Have you been bothered by incoordination or loss of balance?
- Have you had any loss of muscle strength in your legs or feet?
- Have you had any loss of muscle strength in your arms or hands?
- Have you had difficulty moving your fingers or grasping things?
- Have you had numbness or tingling in your fingers lasting more than a day?
- Have you had numbness or tingling in your toes lasting more than a day?
- Have you had headaches at least once a week?
- Have you had difficulty driving home from work because you felt dizzy or tired, even though you slept enough?
- Have you felt 'high' from the chemical you smell at work?
- Have you had a lower tolerance for alcohol (takes less to get drunk)

Box 2. (*Continued*)

Acute Symptoms During the Workday:
During the last month that you have worked, have you noticed that you felt or experienced any of the following symptoms during the workday:

- Headaches
- Tired
- Lightheaded or 'high'
- Difficulty concentrating
- Confusion
- Difficulty remembering things
- Irritable
- Incoordination
- Loss of muscle strength

If you have answered yes to any of the symptoms above, do these symptoms come on when you are using a specific substance? Please explain.

If the patient has answered "yes" to a specific symptom, further information should be sought if the symptoms associate with using a specific substance or undertaking a particular job.

Clinical history and examination

Other than a general history and clinical physical examination of the various systems, specific emphasis should be placed on the nervous system. The neurological examination should include examination of the cranial nerves, strength, co-ordination, sensation, gait and tendon reflexes (Baker *et al.*, 1987). Particular emphasis should be placed on a careful assessment of higher cortical function and mental state examination as suggested above. At our clinic in Oxford we often assess higher cortical function using the Addenbrooke's Cognitive Examination (ACE), which was developed by Hodges and Larner (2017) and is now designated ACEIII (Bruno and Schurmann Vignaga, 2019). This is an extended cognitive screening technique, originally designed to detect dementia and differentiate Alzheimer dementia from frontotemporal dementia. It was also developed to overcome the neuropsychological omissions present in the Mini Mental State Examination

(MMSE). The aim of ACE was to be a screening technique that evaluates the principal cognitive functions and grants free access to health professionals. In this way, ACE turns into a relatively brief cognitive screening tool, which takes 15–20 minutes to administer and is useful in the detection of dementia syndromes regardless of aetiology. If the ACEIII is suggestive of impairment, more detailed testing can be undertaken as described below.

Peripheral nerve function

Peripheral neuropathies are common and increase with age. Around 50% are idiopathic and of all the possible causes, of which there are many, only a few are occupational. The simple mnemonic below will act as a useful memory aid when considering the possible causes of a peripheral neuropathy ("A CHEAP DRUG LIST"):

- **A** — alcohol
- **C** — Collagenosis and cobalamin
- **H** — Hereditary
- **E** — Endocrine, (not diabetes)
- **A** — Amyloid
- **P** — Porphyria
- **D** — Diabetes melitus
- **R** — Relapsing (chronic inflammatory)
- **U** — Uraemia
- **G** — Guillian-Barre syndrome
- **L** — Lead
- **I** — Iatrogenic, e.g. vincristine
- **S** — Sarcoidosis
- **T** — Tumours

This is a comprehensive generic list containing many relatively common non-occupational causes, and includes only one occupational cause (lead). Other occupational causes are exposure to n-hexane, vibration, and acrylamide.

Early symptoms of peripheral nerve dysfunction are numbness or tingling of the extremities, usually starting in the lower limbs then the upper limbs. Sensory nerves innervating the feet are longer than those innervating the hands and many toxins cause length-dependent neuropathy. If exposure persists, weakness (again distal more than proximal) may accompany the sensory symptoms. Examination may reveal diminished vibration or pain sensation and bilaterally reduced or absent ankle reflexes. Atrophy and muscular fasciculation may develop later.

Central nervous system

Acute exposure to high concentrations of a neurotoxic substance generally results in a non-specific narcotic effect. The toxic substance is usually easy to identify because of the acute onset of symptoms when the exposure occurs.

Chronic low-level exposure is much more difficult to relate to central nervous system dysfunction because of the lack of specific symptoms, the lack (in many instances) of objective methods for assessment, biases introduced by compensation and a possible "healthy worker effect." The most common presenting symptoms are difficulty with concentration and memory. Verbal reasoning, remote and recent memory, complex concept formation and dexterity may also be affected (Baker *et al.*, 1987b). In addition, patients may report headache, light-headedness, vertigo, blurred vision, poor co-ordination, tremor and weakness of the extremities. The more severely affected patients can complain of difficulties with attention and organisational ability together with general depression, irritability and fatigue.

It must be stressed that patients who have been exposed to a central neurotoxin (e.g. solvents) may complain of cognitive dysfunction without any other physical signs. A standard neurobehavioural test battery is therefore an important adjunctive examination tool.

Diagnostic and Laboratory Tests

Tests of exposure

Environmental monitoring

Environmental monitoring is used to assess the types of chemical and exposure levels at the work site. Wherever possible, personal monitoring of the workers should be carried out rather than a collection of static area samples. This is especially so for workers who have to move around the workplace and are not stationed at a particular work process. It is best to consult an industrial hygienist for the environmental monitoring, however, in certain factories the safety officer or engineer may be able to undertake the monitoring if they have been trained. Knowledge of the types of chemicals that the workers are exposed to and the exposure levels are very useful data that a physician will need to obtain.

Biological monitoring

Biological monitoring or biological effect monitoring is complementary to environmental monitoring. Where biological monitoring techniques are available, these provide information on body burden (internal exposure) that reflects the balance between uptake, biotransformation and excretion in contrast to environmental monitoring that measures airborne concentration in the workplace or breathing zone.

Biological monitoring is especially useful where skin absorption or inadvertent ingestion could be a significant route of exposure. Where it is difficult to measure the actual chemical or metabolite in the body or urine, biological effect monitoring can act as a surrogate for the body burden, i.e. cholinesterase levels following organophosphorus exposure (see above).

Skin exposure to solvents is especially common among painters, degreasers and printers (Chia *et al.*, 1993b). It is a common practice for these workers to use solvents to clean paint, ink or oil stains from their skin (Chia *et al.*, 1987). Oral ingestion of metal dust can also be a significant factor especially in some cultural practices. For example, oral ingestion of lead through the eating of food with hands contaminated by lead compounds among Malay workers in Singapore could be a possible cause for higher mean blood levels than the mean blood levels of their Chinese counterparts (Chia *et al.*, 1991). For chronic effects, the current biological monitoring results may not be reflective of past exposure and it would, therefore, be more useful to look at serial results of biological markers rather than a single result.

Biological monitoring for some of the heavy metals is well established. Blood lead and manganese are useful measures of body burden. This is similarly true for the urinary levels of mercury, arsenic and manganese. Measures of red blood cell or plasma cholinesterase activity are useful in determining the acute effects of organophosphate exposure ("biological effect monitoring"). There are, however, a limited number of biological monitoring techniques applicable to solvents. Examples of solvents that have a biological exposure index (BEI) include carbon disulphide, dimethylformamide (DMF), n-hexane, methanol, methyl chloroform, methyl ethyl ketone (MEK), perchloroethylene, styrene, toluene, trichloroethylene, xylenes (ACGIH, 2020). Even for the limited solvents with BEIs the facilities for analysis of these substances or their metabolites are only available in certain specialist laboratories around the world. Table 3 shows biomarkers for monitoring exposure to some known neurotoxic chemicals.

Table 3. Biomarkers for Monitoring Exposure to Some Neurotoxic Chemicals (ACGIH, 2020)

Chemical Agents	Biological Fluid	Value	Remarks/ Sampling Time
Metals			
Arsenic, elemental and soluble inorganic compounds	Urine	35 μg As/L	End of work week
Inorganic Lead	Blood	200 μg/L	Not critical
Mercury Total inorganic mercury	Urine	20 μg/g creatinine	Prior to shift
Solvents			
Carbon disulphide	Urine(2-thiothiazolidine-4-carboxylic acid)	0.5mg/g creatinine	End of shift
Methanol	Urine	15 mg/L	End of shift
Methyl Ethyl Ketone	Urine	2 mg/L	End of shift
Toluene	Urine (Hippuric acid)	0.03mg/L	End of shift
	Blood	0.02mg/L	Prior to last shift of workweek

Tests to Confirm Clinical Findings or to Detect Subclinical Effects

Neurophysiological and neuro-radiological tests

Electroencephalogram

An electroencephalogram (EEG) records the (cortical) electrical activity of the brain through application of small electrodes to the scalp. In recent years, imaging studies have somewhat supplanted it as a method for localising anatomical pathology. However, EEG remains a useful pathophysiological tool, detecting abnormal cerebral function that cannot be visualised radiographically or magnetically. Thus, the use of EEG is more appropriate in the evaluation of transient states (e.g. seizures), evolving conditions (e.g. encephalitis) and global disorders (e.g. dementia).

Studies of significant EEG findings among workers exposed to solvents are equivocal. Seppalainen (1973) reported that abnormalities were more frequent among patients with mild solvent poisoning. The abnormalities were usually slow wave abnormalities, one-third focal and about two-thirds diffuse or generalised. However, no increase in the frequency of abnormal EEGs was found among industrial or car painters exposed to solvents at about 30% of the hygiene limits in comparison to reference groups of manual workers without solvent exposure (Seppalainen *et al.*, 1973; Elofsson *et al.*, 1980). A more recent study (Keski-Säntti *et al.*, 2008) looked at quantitative EEGs and found that the power of the frontal theta band was increased in the solvent exposed group, but the findings in this study did not reach statistical significance. Theta oscillations in the frontal areas of the brain indicate significant activity in memory maintenance and this may be worthy of further exploration.

EEGs of patients who have been intoxicated by toluene may show diffuse or focal slow or sharp wave complexes (Aminoff, 2012). In general, EEG may be useful in detecting encephalopathy processes, but the findings are non-specific and it cannot confirm that an abnormality is due to an occupational related disease.

Electromyography/Nerve Conduction Studies

Peripheral neurophysiological assesments, which include motor and sensory nerve conduction studies (NCS) and needle electrode examination of muscles (EMG), are valuable and sensitive. It can recognise and distinguish abnormalities of the anterior horn cell, dorsal sensory ganglion cells, nerve roots, peripheral nerve, neuromuscular junction, muscle membrane and muscle fibre.

EMG/NCS is a sensitive and useful method of identifying and diagnosing patients with a mild toxic neuropathy. The prominent feature of neuropathy caused by various solvents is the distal slowing of both motor and or sensory conduction velocities (depending on the causative agent) (Allen *et al.*, 1975; Cianchetti *et al.*, 1976). EMG/NCS has also showed neurogenic abnormalities in patients with n-hexane polyneuropathy (Sobue *et al.*, 1978).

Owing to its sensitivity, the examiner must be cautious of over interpretation of EMG/NCS results. A study at the Mayo Clinic found that up to a third of unselected patients with an EMG diagnosis of polyneuropathy had minor or subclinical disease thought not to warrant intervention by the clinician (Thomas and Dale, 1981; Aminoff, 2012). To avoid problems of over interpretation, EMG should be a focused and restricted examination with specific questions asked:

- Does the worker have a polyneuropathy detectable by NCS/EMG?
- Is this polyneuropathy due to agent exposure or is it due to some concomitant disease?

Computerised Tomography and Magnetic Resonance Imaging

Computed Tomography (CT) is not very useful as a diagnostic tool for toxic encephalopathy. Orbaek *et al.* (1987) studied 32 patients with chronic toxic encephalopathy due to occupational exposure to organic solvents. They concluded that chronic toxic encephalopathy induced by solvents revealed no evidence of brain atrophy on CT, despite poor psychometric test performance.

MRI is one of several technological advances that have occurred in recent years. MRI uses a magnetic field and radio frequency waves (not radiation). It is non-invasive and is based on the principle of imaging of the hydrogen proton (Gilman, 1992). The intensity of images in a certain region of CNS is given by the "proton spin-lattice relaxation time" (T_1), a measure of the rate at which the protons (hydrogen nuclei) return to thermal equilibrium after being disturbed in a magnetic field. The T_1 rate, and consequently the contrast in brain MRI, is influenced by water and fat content and by the presence of paramagnetic ions, such as manganese, iron and copper. Manganese accumulates selectively in the globus pallidus of the basal ganglia and can be visualised by brain MRI. A semi-quantitative method to compute a Pallidal Index can be used to assess manganese deposition in the brain and has been found to be predictive of neurobehavioural alterations in welders (Chang *et al.*, 2009). MRI is also very useful for examining the brain pathology that follows long term solvent exposure, especially to toluene. Continued toluene use or abuse leads to severe irreversible cognitive impairment, which is an important clue for diagnosis in adolescents and young adults, because this population is not usually affected by dementia, and toluene abuse is widespread in a proportion this population. Alterations depicted on images include diffuse periventricular white matter lesions that are hyperintense.

Neurobehavioural tests

A variety of neurobehavioural methods are available for evaluating effects on the nervous system in working populations exposed to chemical and physical agents. However, these methods have important limitations. Standardisation of techniques has often been variable. Various factors can influence test performance and mask the impact of exposure. In addition, specific abnormal neurobehavioural results often cannot be related to specific neuropathological processes or disease conditions.

The selection of the neurobehavioural tests will depend on the settings and purposes under which testing is performed and the kind of trained persons suitable for performing the tests in different situations. Anger (2003) gives an excellent critical exploration of neurobehavioural tests and systems and is worth consulting before embarking on a test programme.

World Health Organization Neurobehavioural Core Test Battery

At the clinic level, prospective surveillance programmes could be developed for monitoring workers exposed to neurotoxic agents and a short standardised neurobehavioural test would be useful. A suggested test battery is the World Health Organization Neurobehavioural Core Test Battery (NCTB). The complete set of tests is given in Table 4. The details of this test battery are described by Anger (2003) as well as many related test systems and their limitations. This test battery was reconsidered in 2014 with some minor amendments (Anger, 2014).

Factors influencing test performance

Test scores are influenced by many factors other than exposure to toxicants. These factors can confound the interpretation of the results if they are not recognised and controlled for in testing. Generally, these factors can be classified as: patient factors, examiner factors and environmental factors.

Table 4. World Health Organization Neurobehavioural Core Test Battery

Test	Functional domain tested
Profile of mood states	Affect
Simple reaction time	Attention/response speed
Digit span	Auditory memory and working memory
Santa Ana dexterity test	Manual dexterity
Digit symbol	Perceptual-motor speed
Benton visual retention	Visual perception/memory
Aiming (pursuit aiming II)	Motor steadiness

Patient factors to be considered include age, sex, education, socio-economic status, health and drug history, circadian rhythms, fatigue and motivation. Examiners should preferably be from the same culture and be able to speak fluently in the subject's native language. Examiners must interact with all subjects in a consistent and standardised manner. Environmental factors which could affect the tests include lighting, noise, temperature and humidity. Anger (2003) suggests the following planning regime:

1. The primary factor guiding test selection is the chemical to which the population is exposed
2. Computer based test systems are preferred for standardisation and to avoid bias
3. Include supplemental test of motivation, standardised measures of physical and psychological symptoms and intellectual or educational level
4. Administer test to a sample from the target population to identify problems and develop an accurate measure of statistical power, considering multiple comparisons
5. Select a comparison population as similar to exposed participants as possible
6. Collect information on sex, age, education, (years and cultural or ethnic group for data analysis, at a minimum.

Interpretation of the results

One major problem in the interpretation of test results is the lack of baseline data of the worker's performance prior to exposure to toxicants. The non-specific nature of the toxicant in question, and the variability of the worker performance create problems in interpretation. Efforts should be made to obtain the baseline data wherever possible. As with neurophysiological tests, serial results are more often more meaningful and important than a single test for individual diagnosis.

Other tests

A worker with a neurological disorder with an appropriate history may not be suffering from a work related disease. To further elucidate the pathological processes additional haematological and biochemical tests may also be necessary.

Assessment of Clinical Status

Pre-Employment Examinations

As in any pre-employment examination certain general principles apply: Is the worker fit for the particular job for which he is seeking employment? What are the baseline examinations and investigations that should be conducted?

To answer these questions with sufficient confidence the attending physician must know the job requirements and the possible hazards. What is the working environment? What is the work process? What are the work tools? (Noise and vibration also need to be considered). Does the job expose the worker to any substances that may cause the individual to be more susceptible to developing ill-health? The physician would also need to know the likely agents that the worker may be exposed to and the likely target organs of those toxins. Based on this knowledge, the appropriate tests may be conducted to obtain appropriate baseline results. Wherever possible, the relevant biological monitoring markers (Table 3) should be measured to determine the pre-exposure levels.

In addition, workers who are exposed to organic solvents could be given a subjective symptoms questionnaire (Box 2) and a standard neurobehavioural test (Table 4). These questionnaires and tests become very useful during the periodic medical examination to evaluate early cases of toxic encephalopathy.

Workers with certain medical conditions/complications may be more susceptible to neurotoxic substances at the workplace. Extra caution must be taken in deciding if such individuals are fit for employment. When in doubt, it is always good practice to consult and discuss the worker's medical condition with specialists in that particular field.

Periodic Examinations

The objective of periodic examinations is the detection of early cases, subclinical effects or excessive absorption of the exposed substances.

The frequency of the examination is dependent on the degree of exposure to the hazard.

History taking and clinical examination should be specific to the hazard concerned. It is good practice to study the relationship of the results over different medical examination periods (see cholinesterase trends in Case Study 6). Rising trends in the result should alert the physician to the likelihood of excessive absorption or early effects of the agent. Appropriate interventions should then be carried out, the simplest is removal from exposure. Therefore, if the workers' biological monitoring results exceed the permissible values, they should be transferred to another area where there is no exposure to the hazard. Similarly, this would apply to workers who develop symptoms and or signs of neurological or behavioural dysfunction.

Fitness to Return to Work

Whether a worker is fit to return to work (with possible further exposure to the neurotoxic agent) will depend on the cause of the exclusion. If it is due to excessive absorption, e.g. high blood lead levels, then when the blood lead levels return to the permissible level (and there is no other contraindication) the worker can return to the former job.

In a situation where a worker develops a peripheral neuropathy due to a neurotoxic substance and subsequently recovers, re-exposure to the causative agent should be prohibited. Of course many neurological conditions are unrelated to the work environment but may impair an employee's work ability or make the work environment less safe. There are many common neurological conditions that may well occur in the working lifetime and will need careful assessment by the OP to ensure that appropriate adjustment and job modification have been undertaken and the employee is safe and will not impair the safety of others. Perhaps the most common neurological conditions are the effect of head injury, epilepsy (that may be related to head injury), stroke and the more chronic and insidious effects of neurodegerative disorders such as multiple sclerosis, Parkinson's disease and Motor Neurone disorders.

Conclusion

As has been discussed, the potential impact of the working environment on neurological health is enormous. Similarly, many chronic neurological conditions can affect the ability of the patient to function appropriately in a given employment. The responsibility of the OP is to maximise the employment potential for any given patient, while also ensuring safety of that employee and others. As well as being aware of possible work related reversible factors, it is also important to appreciate the significant co-morbidities that may associate with neurological disease. In particular, patients with neurological conditions are prone to cognitive and psychological difficulties, irrespective of the underlying disorder. There may also be significant psychosocial impact beyond the confines of work itself, for example being unable to drive. A holistic approach which addresses all these aspects and close liaison with the patient's primary care physician and neurologist should help to improve outcomes.

References

ACGIH. (2020) *Threshold Limit Values for Chemical Substances and Physical Agents and Biological Exposure Indices.* Cincinnati, ACGIH

Allen N, Mendell JR, Billmaier DJ, Fontaine RE, O'Neill J. (1975) Toxic polyneuropathy due to methyl n-butyl ketone. An industrial outbreak. *Arch Neurol* **32**: 209–218.

Aminoff MJ. (2012) *Aminoff's Electrodiagnosis in Clinical Neurology* (6th Ed). Philadelphia, Pennsylvania, Elsevier Saunders.

Anger WK. (2003). Neurobehavioral tests and systems to assess neurotoxic exposures in the workplace and community. *Occup Environ Med* **60**: 531–538.

Anger WK. (2014) Reconsideration of the WHO NCTB strategy and test selection. *Neurotoxicology* **45**: 224–231.

BASH. (2021) *British Association for the Study of Headache.* [Online] Available from: https://www.bash.org.uk/. [Accessed on 17 May 2021].

Baker EL, Smith TJ, Landrigan PJ. (1985) The neurotoxicity of industrial solvents: A review of the literature. *Am J Ind Med* **8**: 207–217.

Baker EL, Seppalainen AM. (1987) Human aspect of solvent neurobehavioral effects. *Neurotoxicology* 7(4), 43–56.

Barboni MT, Feitosa-Santana C, Zachi EC, Lago M, Teixeira RA, Taub A, da Costa MF, de Lima Silveira LC, Ventura DF. (2009) Preliminary findings on the effects of occupational exposure to mercury vapor below safety levels on visual and neuropsychological functions. *J Occup Environ Med* **51**(12): 1403–1412.

Bast-Pettersen R. (2009) The neuropsychological diagnosis of chronic solvent induced encephalopathy (CSE) — a reanalysis of neuropsychological test results in a group of CSE patients diagnosed 20 years ago, based on comparisons with matched controls. *Neurotoxicology* **30**(6): 1195–1201.

Beckstead MJ, Weiner JL, Eger EI, 2nd, Gong DH, Mihic SJ. (2000) Glycine and gamma-aminobutyric acid(A) receptor function is enhanced by inhaled drugs of abuse. *Mol Pharmacol* **57**(6): 1199–1205.

Brown I, Chiordini A, Somaruga C. (2010) Pesticides and other Agrochemicals. In: Baxter, P.J., Aw, T., Cockcroft, A., Durrington, P., Harrington, J. M. (eds.), Hunter's diseases of occupations. Boca Raton, Florida, United States, CRC Press.

Brown I, Prevett M. (2019) Epilepsy. In: Hobson, J., Smedley, J. (eds.), Fitness for work (6th Ed), Oxford, United Kingdom, Oxford University Press.

Bruno D, Schurmann Vignaga S. (2019). Addenbrooke's cognitive examination III in the diagnosis of dementia: A critical review. *Neuropsychiatric Dis Treat* **15**: 441–447. Published online 2019 Feb 15. doi: 10.2147/NDT.S151253, PMCID:

Carvalho CML, Hashemy SI, Lu J, Holmgren A. (2008) Inhibition of the human thioredoxin system: A molecular mechanism of mercury toxicity. *J Biol Chem* **283**(18): 11913–11923.

Chandra SV, Seth PK, Mankeshwar JK. (1974) Manganese poisoning: Clinical and biochemical observation. *Environ Res* 7: 374–380.

Chang Y, Kim Y, Woo ST, Song HJ, Kim SH, Lee H, Kwon YJ, Ahn JH, Park SJ, Chung IS, Jeong KS. (2009) High signal intensity on magnetic resonance imaging is a better predictor of neurobehavioral performances than blood manganese in asymptomatic welders. *Neurotoxicology* **30**(4): 555–563.

Chia SE. (1998) Exposure to solvents and behavioral effects (Editorial). *Singapore Med J* **39**: 191–192.

Chia SE, Chia HP, Ong CN, Jeyaratnam J. (1997) Cumulative blood lead levels and neurobehavioral test performance. *Neurotoxicology* **18**: 793–804.

Chia SE, Chia KS, Ong CN. (1991) Ethnic differences in blood lead concentration among workers in a battery manufacturing factory. *Ann Acad Med Singapore* **20**(6): 758–761.

Chia SE, Chia KS, Chia HP, Ong CN, Jeyaratnam J. (1996) Three-year follow-up of serial nerve conduction among lead-exposed workers. *Scand J Work Environ Health* **22**: 374–380.

Chia SE, Ong CN, Phoon WH, Tan KT, Jeyaratnam J. (1993a) Neurobehavioral effects on workers in a video-tape manufacturing factory in Singapore. *Neurotoxicology* **14**(1): 51–56.

Chia SE, Phoon WH, Lee HS, Tan KT, Jeyaratnam J. (1993b) Exposure to neurotoxic metals among workers in Singapore: An overview. *Occup Med* **43**(1): 18–22.

Chia SE, Tan KT, Kwok SF. (1987) A study on the health hazard of toluene in the polythene printing industry in Singapore. *Ann Acad Med Singapore* **16**(2): 294–299.

Cory-Slechta DA. (2005) Studying toxicants as single chemicals: Does this strategy adequately identify neurotoxic risk? *Neurotoxicology* **26**(4): 491–510.

Costa LG, Giordano G, Guizzetti M, Vitalone A. (2008) Neurotoxicity of pesticides: A brief review. *Front Biosci* **13**: 1240–1249.

Couper J. (1837) On the effects of black oxide of manganese when inhaled into the lungs. Br *Ann Med Pharmacol* **1**: 41–42.

Cianchetti C, Abbritti G, Perticoni G, Siracusa A, Curradi F. (1976) Toxic polyneuropathy of shoe-industry workers. A study of 122 cases. *J Neurol Neurosurg Psychiatry* **39**(12): 1151–1161.

Dueñas M, Begoña O, Salazar A, Mico JA, Failde I. (2016) A review of chronic pain impact on patients, their social environment and the health care system. *J Pain Res* **9**: 457–467. Available from: doi: 10.2147/JPR.S105892.

Ecobichon DJ. (2001) Toxic effects of pesticides. In: Klaassen, C.D. (ed.), *Casarett and Doull's toxicology. The basic science of poisons* (6th Ed). New York, McGraw-Hill, pp. 763–810.

Elbaz A, Clavel J, Rathouz PJ, Moisan F, Galanaud JP, Delemotte B, Alpérovitch A, Tzourio C. (2009) Professional exposure to pesticides and Parkinson's disease. *Ann Neurol* **66**(4): 494–504.

Elofsson SA, Gamberale F, Hindmarsh T, Iregren A, Isaksson A, Johnsson I, Knave B, Lydahl E, Mindus P, Persson HE, Philipson B, Steby M, Struwe G, Söderman E, Wennberg A, Widén L. (1980) Exposure to organic solvents. A cross-sectional epidemiologic investigation on occupationally exposed care and industrial spray painters with special reference to the nervous system. Scand *J Work Environ Health* **6**(4): 239–273.

Emara AM, El-Ghawabi SH, Madkour OI, El-Samra GH. (1971) Chronic manganese poisoning in the dry battery industry. *Br J Ind Med* **28**: 78–82.

European Brain Injury Society. (2004) *European Brain Injury Society.* [Online] Available from: https://ebissociety.org/. [Accessed on 17 May 2021].

Food and Agriculture Organization. (2003) *International Code of Conduct on the Distribution and Use of Pesticides. FAO, Rome.* [Online] Available from: http://www.fao.org/3/y4544e/y4544e00.htm.

Feldman RG, Niles CA, Kelly-Hayes M, Sax DS, Dixon WJ, Thompson DJ, Landau E. (1979) Peripheral neuropathy in arsenic smelter workers. *Neurology* **29**: 939.

Gan SL, Tan KT, Kwok SF. (1988) Biological threshold limit values for manganese dust exposure. *Singapore Med J* **29**: 563–568.

Ghajar J. (2000) Traumatic brain injury. *Lancet* **356**: 923–929.

Gilioli, R. (ed.) (1983) *Neurobehavioral Methods in Occupational Health.* Oxford, Pergamon Press.

Gilman S. (1992) Advances in neurology. *New Engl J Med* **326**(24): 1608–1616.

Graham DG, Amarnath V, Valentine WM, Pyle SJ, Anthony DC. (1995) Pathogenetic studies of hexane and carbon disulfide neurotoxicity. *Crit Rev Toxicol* **25**(2): 91–112. Available from: https://doi.org/10.3109/10408449509021609.

Halatek T, Sinczuk-Walczak H, Rabieh S, Wasowicz W. (2009) Association between occupational exposure to arsenic and neurological, respiratory and renal effects. *Toxicol Appl Pharmacol* **239**(2): 193–199.

Hänninen H. (1985) Twenty-five years of behavioral toxicology within occupational medicine: A personal account. *Am J Ind Med* 7(1): 19–30.

Heyman A, Pfeiffer JB, Willet RW, Taylor HM. (1956) Peripheral neuropathy caused by arsenical intoxication. *New Engl J Med* **254**: 401.

Ho SF, Phoon WH, Tan KT, Kwok SF. (1982) Study on the usage and health hazards of arsenic in wood preservation plants. *Proc 10th Asian Conf Occup Health* **2**: 563–568.

Hobson J, Smedley J. (2019) *Fitness for Work — The Medical Aspects* (6th Ed). Oxford, United Kingdom, Oxford University Press.

Hodges JR, Larner AJ. (2017) *Cognitive Screening Instruments: A practical Approach* (2nd Ed). Berlin, Springer.

Huang C, Huang L, Wang Y, Li X, Ren L, Gu X, Kang L, Guo L, Liu M, Zhou X, Luo J, Huang Z, Tu S, Zhao Y, Chen L, Xu D, Li Y, Li C, Peng L, Li Y, Cao B. (2021) 6-month consequences of COVID-19 in patients discharged from hospital: A cohort study. *Lancet* (*Lond*) **397**(10270): 220–232.

Institute for Environment and Health/Institute of Occupational Medicine Occupational (IEH/IOM). (2004) *Exposure Limits: Criteria Document for Manganese and Inorganic Manganese Compounds* (Web Report W17), Leicester, UK, MRC Institute for Environment and Health. [Online] Available from: http://www.iehconsulting.co.uk/IEH_Consulting/IEHCPubs/HumExpRiskAssess/w17.pdf.

IHME. (2017) GBD compare. [Online] Available from: https://vizhub.healthdata.org/gbd-compare/. [Accessed on 17 May 2021].

Iregren A. (1996) Behavioral methods and organic solvents: Questions and consequences. *Environ Health Perspect* **104**(2): 361–366.

Jeyaratnam J, Devathasan G, Ong CN, Phoon WO, Wong PK. (1985) Neurophysiological studies on workers exposed to lead. *Br J Ind Med* **42**: 173–177.

Johnson BL. (1987) *Prevention of Neurotoxic Illness in Working Populations.* New York, John Wiley and Sons.

Keddie S, Pakpoor J, Mousele C, Pipis M, Machado PM, Foster M, Record CJ, Keh R, Fehmi J, Paterson RW, Bharambe V, Clayton LM, Allen C, Price O, Wall J, Kiss-Csenki A, Rathnasabapathi DP, Geraldes R, Yermakova T, King-Robson J, Lunn MP. (2021) Epidemiological and cohort study finds no association between COVID-19 and Guillain-Barré syndrome. *Brain* **144**(2): 682–693.

Keski-Säntti P, Kovala T, Holm A, Hyvärinen HK, Sainio M. (2008) Quantitative EEG in occupational chronic solvent encephalopathy. *Hum Exp Toxicol* **27**(4): 315–320.

King M. (1983) Long term neuropsychological effects of solvent abuse. In: Cherry, N, Waldron, H.A. (eds.), *The neuropsychological effects of solvent exposure.* Colt Foundation, Havant, Hampshire, pp. 75–84.

Kim EA, Kang SK. (2010). Occupational neurological disorders in Korea. *J Korean Med Sci* **25**, 26–35

King MD, Day RE, Oliver JS, Lush M, Watson JM. (1981) Solvent encephalopathy. *Br Med J* (*Clinical Research Ed.*) **283**(6292): 663–665.

Kuroda N. (2021) Epilepsy and COVID-19: Updated evidence and narrative review. *Epilepsy Behav* **116**: 107785.

Ky S, Deng HS, Xie PY, Hu W. (1992) A report of two cases of chronic serious manganese poisoning treated with sodium para-amino salicylic acid. *Br J Ind Med* **49**: 66–69.

LaDou J. (1990) Health issues in the micro-electronics industry. *J Occup Med Singapore* **2**: 9–22.

Li M, Zhao Z, Yu G, Zhang J. (2016) Epidemiology of traumatic brain injury over the World: A Systematic Review. *Austin Neurol Neurosci* **1**(2): 1007.

Lucchini R, Apostoli P, Perrone C, Placidi D, Albini E, Migliorati P, Mergler D, Sassine MP, Palmi S, Alessio L. (1999) Long-term exposure to "low levels" of manganese oxides and neurofunctional changes in ferroalloy workers. *Neurotoxicology* **20**(2–3): 287–297.

Lucchini R, Calza S, Camerino D, Carta P, Decarli A, Parrinello G, Soleo L, Zefferino R, Alessio L. (2003) Application of a latent variable model for a multicentre study on early effects due to mercury exposure. *Neurotoxicology* **24**(4–5): 605–616.

Lucchini R, Benedetti L, Albini E, Alessio L. (2005) Neurobehavioral science in hazard identification and risk assessment of neurotoxic agents – What are the needs for further development? *Int Arch Occup Environ Health* **78**: 427–437.

Lucchini R, Zimmerman N. (2009) Lifetime cumulative exposure as a threat for neurodegeneration: Need for prevention strategies on a global scale. *Neurotoxicology* **30**: 1144–1148.

Lucchini RG, Martin CJ, Doney BC. (2009) From manganism to manganese-induced parkinsonism: A conceptual model based on the evolution of exposure. *Neuro Mol Med* **11**(4): 311–321.

Matsumura F. (1985) Toxicology of insecticides. New York, Plenum Press.

Menken M. (2002) Demystifying neurology. *BMJ* **324**(7352): 1469–1470. Available from: https://doi.org/10.1136/bmj.324.7352.1469.

Meyer-Baron M, Blaszkewicz M, Henke H, Knapp G, Muttray A, Schäper M, van Thriel C. (2008) The impact of solvent mixtures on neurobehavioral performance: Conclusions from epidemiological data. *Neurotoxicology* **29**(3): 349–360.

Migraine Trust. (2021) *The Migraine Trust*. [Online] Available from: https://www.migrainetrust.org/. [Accessed on 17 May 2021].

Murata K, Iwata T, Dakeishi M, Karita K. (2009) Lead toxicity: Does the critical level of lead resulting in adverse effects differ between adults and children? *J Occup Health* **51**(1): 1–12.

Nordberg GF. (1976) Effects and dose-response relationships of toxic metals. A report from an international meeting. *Scand J Work Environ Health* **2**(1): 37–43.

Orbaek P, Lindgren M, Olivecrona H, Haeger-Aronsen B. (1987) Computed tomography and psychometric test performance in patients with solvent induced chronic toxic encephalopathy and healthy controls. *Br J Ind Med* **44**(3): 175–179.

Parkinson J. (2002). Neuropsychiatric classics: James Parkinson: An essay on the shaking palsy. *J Neuropsych Clin Neurosc* **14**: 223–236.

Peshin SS, Srivastava A, Halder N, Gupta YK. (2014) Pesticide poisoning trend analysis of 13 years: A retrospective study based on telephone calls at the National Poisons Information Centre, All India Institute of Medical Sciences, New Delhi. *J Forensic Leg Med* **22**: 57–61.

Piikivi LT, Hanninen H. (1977) Psychological performance and long-term exposure to mercury vapors. In: Hernberg, S, Kahn, H. (eds.), *Proceedings from effects of early action of toxic substances on the organism.* Helsinki, Tallinn, Institute Experimental and Clinical Medicine of the Ministry of Health, pp. 165–169.

Reigel AC, Ali SF, Torinese S, French ED. (2004) Repeated exposure to the abused inhalant toluene alters levels of neurotransmitters and generates peroxynitrite in nigrostriatal and mesolimbic nuclei in rat. *Ann NY Acad Sci* **1025**: 543–551.

Uddin R, Huda NH. (2011) Arsenic poisoning in bangladesh. *Oman Med J* **26**(3): 207. Available from: https://doi.org/10.5001/omj.2011.51.

Department of Transport. (2015) Reported road casualties. Great Britain: 2014 Annual report. [Online] Available from: https://assets.publishing.service.gov.uk/government/uploads/system/uploads/attachment_data/file/467465/rrcgb-2014.pdf. [Accessed on 17 May 2021].

Racette BA, McGee-Minnich L, Moerlein SM, Mink JW, Videen TO, Perlmutter JS. (2001) Welding-related parkinsonism: Clinical features, treatment, and pathophysiology. *Neurology* **56**(1): 8–13. Available from: https://doi.org/10.1212/wnl.56.1.8.

Racette BA, Tabbal SD, Jennings D, Good L, Perlmutter JS, Evanoff B. (2005) Prevalence of parkinsonism and relationship to exposure in a large sample of Alabama welders. *Neurology* **64**(2): 230–235. Available from: https://doi.org/10.1212/01.WNL.0000149511.19487.44.

Ropper A, Samuels M, Klein J. (2019) *Adams and Victor's Principles of Neurology* (11th Ed). New York, McGraw-Hill Medical.

Schwartz BS, Lee BK, Bandeen-Roche K, Stewart W, Bolla K, Links J, Weaver V, Todd A. (2005) Occupational lead exposure and longitudinal decline in neurobehavioral test scores. *Epidemiology* **16**(1):106–113. Available from: doi: 10.1097/01.ede.0000147109.62324.51.

Seppalainen AM, Lindstrom K, Martelin T. (1980) Neurophysiological and psychological picture of solvent poisoning. *Am J Ind Med* **1**: 31–42.

Seppalainen AM. (1973) Neurotoxic effects of industrial solvents. Electroencephalogr Clin *Neurophysiol* **34**: 702–703.

Spencer PS, Schaumburg HH, Sabri MI, Veronesi B. (1980) The enlarging view of hexacarbon neurotoxicity. *Crit Rev Toxicol* 7(4): 279–356. Available from: https://doi.org/10.3109/10408448009037489.

Spiller HA. (2017) Rethinking Mercury: The role of selenium in the pathophysiology of mercury toxicity. *Clin Toxicol* **56**(5): 1–14.

Sobue I, Iida M, Yamamura Y, Takayanagui T. (1978) N-hexane polineuropathy. *Int J Neurol* **11**(4): 317–330.

Swain EB, Jakus PM, Rice G, Lupi F, Maxson PA, Penn JMP, Spiegel SJ, Vaiga MM. (2007) Socio economic consequences of mercury use and pollution. *Ambio* **36**: 45–61.

Tan YK, Goh C, Leow A, Tambyah PA, Ang A, Yap ES, Tu TM, Sharma VK, Yeo L, Chan B, Tan B. (2020) COVID-19 and ischemic stroke: A systematic review and meta-summary of the literature. *J Thromb Thrombolys* **50**(3): 587–595.

Tanner CM, Ross GW, Jewell SA, Hauser RA, Jankovic J, Factor SA, Bressman S, Deligtisch A, Marras C, Lyons KE, Bhudhikanok GS, Roucoux DF, Meng C, Abbott RD, Langston JW. (2009) Occupation and risk of Parkinsonism: A multi-centre case-control study. *Arch Neurol* **66**(9): 1106–1113.

Taquet M, Luciano S, Geddes JR, Harrison PJ. (2021) Bidirectional associations between COVID-19 and psychiatric disorder: Retrospective cohort studies of 62 354 COVID-19 cases in the USA. Lancet. *Psychiat* **8**(2): 130–140.

Thomas JE, Dale AJD. (eds.) (1981) Clinical examinations in neurology. Philadelphia, WB Saunders.

Tiesman HM, Konda S, Bell JL. (2011) The epidemiology of fatal occupational traumatic brain injury in the U.S. *Am J Prev Med* **41**(1): 61–67. Available from: https://doi.org/10.1016/j.amepre.2011.03.007.

US Department of Health and Human Services. (2021) National Toxicology Program. [Online] Available from: https://ntp.niehs.nih.gov/. [Accessed on 17 May 2021].

Visser I, Lavini C, Booij J, Reneman L, Majoie C, de Boer AG, Wekking EM, de Joode EA, van der Laan G, van Dijk FJ, Schene AH, Den Heeten GJ. (2008) Cerebral impairment in chronic solvent-induced encephalopathy. *Ann Neurol* **63**(5): 572–580.

Vroom FQ, Greer M. (1972) Mercury vapor intoxication. *Brain* **95**: 305–318.

World Health Organization. (1981) Manganese. Environmental Health Criteria 17. [Online] Available from: https://apps.who.int/iris/rest/bitstreams/1312025/retrieve. [Accessed on 17 May 2021].

Wu F, Zhao S, Yu B, Chen YM, Wang W, Song ZG, Hu Y, Tao ZW, Tian JH, Pei YY, Yuan ML, Zhang YL, Dai FH, Liu Y, Wang QM, Zheng JJ, Xu L, Holmes EC, Zhang YZ. (2020) A new coronavirus associated with human respiratory disease in China. *Nature* **579**(7798): 265–269.

Chapter 10

Occupational Infections

Li Yang Hsu, Wee Hoe Gan† and David Koh‡*

Introduction

Occupational infections are diseases caused by pathogenic microorganisms that are associated with work activity. The infections are varied, and most are not confined to occupational situations alone. To be labelled as an occupational infection, that occupational setting or activity must predispose the worker to a higher risk of exposure to the microorganism, with a recognised increased risk of infection and disease (Aw *et al.*, 2017).

The control of any occupational infection requires a detailed knowledge of its epidemiology, clinical features, reservoir, mode of transmission, incubation period and communicable period. To prevent and control infection, measures are necessary to eliminate the source of infection and the route of transmission. Susceptible workers can be offered protection with immunisation, if a vaccine exists, or

* Saw Swee Hock School of Public Health, National University of Singapore, Singapore.
† Department of Occupational and Environmental Medicine, Singapore General Hospital; Changi Aviation Medicine Centre, Changi General Hospital; and Duke-NUS Medical School, National University of Singapore, Singapore.
‡ PAPRSB Institute of Health Sciences, Universiti Brunei Darussalam, Brunei Darussalam *and* Saw Swee Hock School of Public Health and Yong Loo Lin School of Medicine, National University of Singapore, Singapore.
Corresponding author: Wee Hoe Gan (gan.wee.hoe@singhealth.com.sg).

with available post-exposure prophylaxis (PEP), following a known exposure.

Occupational infections can be classified in several ways, such as by mode of transmission (e.g. blood-borne, vector-borne, contact, droplet, airborne), by aetiological agent (e.g. viruses, bacteria, rickettsia, fungi), and by occupational groups at risk (e.g. healthcare workers (HCWs), farmers, forestry workers, vets, zoo staff).

This chapter will cover selected common occupational infections categorised by mode of transmission.

Blood-Borne Infections

In spite of work control processes and the development of devices with sharps injury protection features, occupational infections transmitted through sharps injuries and contact with body fluids remain a major concern for HCWs. The United States (US) Centers for Disease Control and Prevention (CDC) reported that approximately 385,000 needlestick and other sharps injuries affected hospital-based HCWs each year (CDC, 2021a). Nurses and doctors are most commonly affected, often during suturing and other intraoperative procedures, administering injections, and drawing blood (International Safety Center, 2019; Leong *et al.*, 2019).

In addition to patient-to-HCW transmission of blood-borne infections, HCW-to-patient transmission of blood-borne viruses is also an occupational concern in certain settings. "Exposure-prone procedures (EPPs)" are those "where the worker's gloved hands may be in contact with sharp instruments, needle tips or sharp tissues inside a patient's open body cavity, wound or confined anatomical space, where the hands or fingertips may not be completely visible at all times" (Public Health England, 2017). Three conditions must be fulfilled for the transmission of a blood-borne infection from an infected HCW to a patient during an EPP, namely the HCW must sustain an injury or have a condition that allows for exposure; the HCW's blood must come into contact with a patient's wound, traumatised tissue, mucous membranes or similar portal of entry; and the HCW must be sufficiently viraemic (Ogunremi *et al.*, 2019).

The use of sharps cannot be avoided in healthcare and other industries such as those providing tattooing services. Preventing occupational blood-borne infections is therefore essential and of considerable public health importance. The World Health Organization (WHO) lists the prevention of sharps injuries as its first of five World Patient Safety Day 2020–2021 Goals (WHO, 2020a). The approach of "standard precautions" has been advocated, where all blood, tissues, and some body fluids are treated as a potential source of infection and additional infection prevention measures such as the use of appropriate personal protective equipment (PPE), safe injection practices and hand hygiene are applied to all patients, regardless of the knowledge of their infection status (Occupational Safety and Health Administration, 2021). Engineering (e.g. self-sheathing needles) and work practice controls (e.g. not recapping needles, containerisation through discarding sharps immediately after use) are effective in reducing the incidence of such occupational injuries.

While different diseases such as malaria and haemorrhagic fever may be transmitted through contaminated sharps, the most important blood-borne infections in the occupational setting are Hepatitis B, Hepatitis C and human immunodeficiency virus (HIV).

Human Immunodeficiency Virus

HIV is the retrovirus that causes acquired immune deficiency syndrome (AIDS). The main modes of spread are sexual contact, injecting drug use and mother-to-infant vertical transmission, with only a small proportion of cases acquired from occupational transmission. The US CDC reported 58 confirmed cases of occupational transmission of HIV to HCWs up to December 2013, and with only one case reported since 1999 (CDC, 2019). The risk of HIV infection through needlestick injury ranges from 0.03% to 0.3%, determined by factors such as the depth of penetration, volume of contaminated blood inoculated, hollow needle injuries, and possibly the viral load of the source (Wyzgowski *et al.*, 2016). The risk of transmission is approximately 0.09% after mucous membrane exposure to infected blood or body fluids (Kuhar *et al.*, 2013).

The British Association for Sexual Health and HIV (BASHH) guidelines recommend that PEP should be routinely offered following an occupational exposure from a source known to be HIV positive, if the HIV viral load is detectable or unknown (BASHH, 2021). PEP is generally not recommended if the HIV status of the source is unknown, or if the source is known to be HIV positive but with undetectable HIV viral load (<200 copies/mL) (Expert Advisory Group on AIDS, 2013).

The early initiation of PEP is important. The rule-of-thumb is as soon as possible, ideally within 2 h of exposure and no later than 72 h. Treatment is usually with three or more antiretroviral drugs comprising a combination of nucleoside reverse transcriptase inhibitors, integrase inhibitors, protease inhibitors and non-nucleoside reverse transcriptase inhibitors for a duration of 4 weeks. The HCW should also have follow-up evaluations at regular intervals to review the health status and for repeat HIV screening tests. Nwaiwu *et al.* (2017) followed up 266 HCWs who were exposed to HIV-contaminated body fluids, of whom 21.1% of them received PEP. The seroconversion rate was 0%, supporting PEP as an effective exposure management strategy.

Given that most occupational exposures do not result in HIV transmission, and balancing against the potential side effects of antiretroviral drugs, the decision to start or not to start PEP is not always a straightforward one. For example, while PEP is generally not recommended when the source has undetectable HIV viral load, the psychological stress experienced by the affected HCW cannot be dismissed and may be a dominant factor to initiate and continue PEP (Aribou *et al.*, 2020).

In the United Kingdom (UK), pre-employment HIV testing is required for HCWs who perform EPPs (Public Health England, 2020a). This policy is designed to maintain public confidence in health services and reduce the need for look-back patient notification exercises. HCWs can decline to be tested, in which case they would not be cleared for EPP work. With the availability of highly active combination antiretroviral therapy (cART), viral suppression in treated HCWs can now be effectively maintained. Those who are on effective cART and have a viral load of <200 copies/ml, or are demonstrated to be an "elite controller" (a person living with HIV who is not receiving cART and is capable of immunologically suppressing viraemia, i.e. maintaining the viral load below the limits of assay detection for at least 12 months, based on at least three separate viral load measurements) may perform EPPs. In addition, these HCWs must be entered in a central confidential register, subject to viral load testing every 3 months, and be under the joint supervision of a consultant occupational physician and the primary treatment physician. The US adopts similar guidelines for HCWs living with HIV performing EPPs, who need to agree to take advice from an oversight panel on recommended practices to minimise the risk of exposure events (Henderson *et al.*, 2020). The guidelines further stipulate that there is no justification for, nor benefit gained from, the routine notification of patients managed by this group of HCWs who are already under the guidance of the oversight panel.

Hepatitis B

The hepatitis B virus (HBV) is a small virus belonging to the hepadnavirus family of DNA viruses. It has an outer lipoprotein coat, which is detectable as hepatitis B surface antigen (HBsAg) and an internal hepatitis B core antigen (HBcAg). Hepatitis B e antigen (HBeAg) is a marker of high infectivity, although a subset of HBeAg negative patients may have a high viral load. HBV is transmitted through sexual contact, injecting drug use, from mother to infant and through contact with infected blood and body fluids. Following infection, complete clearance of the virus is possible or a chronic carrier state can develop. The carrier state manifests as the persistence of HBsAg and/or HBeAg. Carriers have an increased lifetime risk of chronic liver disease, cirrhosis, hepatocellular carcinoma and can transmit the infection to others.

Occupational infection of HCWs with HBV has declined, especially in countries where hepatitis B vaccination is incorporated as part of the national immunisation schedule. A systematic review published by Danzmann *et al.* (2013) revealed 27 large nosocomial HBV outbreaks affecting 212 patients. There was even a reported outbreak cluster where a surgeon infected 19 patients with HBV. The risk of acquiring HBV infection from a needlestick injury from a highly infectious HBeAg positive source is 22–31%, and seroconversion will occur in 23–37% of the exposed individuals (Schillie *et al.*, 2013).

Recombinant DNA vaccines against HBV infection are both effective and confer prolonged protection even after anti-HBs antibodies have waned. The standard vaccination schedule is a 3-dose series at 0, 1 and 6 months. If the vaccine series is interrupted after the first or second dose, the next dose should be administered as soon as possible. The second and third doses should be at least 8 weeks apart. For those who did not receive primary hepatitis B vaccination in childhood, an accelerated schedule may be implemented for occupational groups at higher risk, such as phlebotomists and HCWs performing EPPs. This accelerated schedule requires the vaccine to be given at 0, 1, and 2 months and for those who are at continued risk, a fourth dose can be given at 12 months for maximum, long-term protection. Anamnestic responses to HBsAg following challenge occur even years after vaccination, suggesting the role of immune memory in long-term protection (Damme, 2016).

In HCWs, anti-HBs titers should be checked 1–2 months after the primary course of vaccination. Individual workers should be informed of their result so that they know if they are protected and advised on what to do if they are subsequently exposed. Anti-HBs levels of 10m IU/mL or more are accepted as protective. In general, immunocompetent persons who have demonstrated immunological response to the primary vaccination series do not need booster vaccinations in the future. This is supported by a 30-year prospective study by Bruce *et al.* (2016), which found no significant breakthrough infections in the those vaccinated. Of the cohort, 51% of the vaccinees still retained detectable anti-HBs antibodies 30 years after vaccination.

Individuals who do not respond to the primary course of hepatitis B vaccination should be evaluated to exclude chronic hepatitis B infection, if not already done so. They should be given an additional dose of hepatitis B vaccine. Averhoff *et al.* (1998) showed that 47% of HCWs without serologic response after a primary vaccination series developed vaccine-induced seroprotection after one additional vaccine dose. If there is still no protective antibody level detected, these individuals should receive two more vaccine doses. Cumulatively, approximately 69% of HCWs in Averhoff's study demonstrated detectable anti-HBs antibodies after the second vaccine series. If available, a different brand of hepatitis B vaccine may be administered for the second series.

A hepatitis B vaccine non-responder is a person who does not develop protective anti-HBs antibodies after completing two full vaccine series. Older age, obesity and other chronic diseases may be factors that affect serologic response to vaccination. Vaccine non-responders should be counselled about their risk of infection if they come into contact with infected blood and body fluids in the course of their work. Those cleared to conduct EPPs should undergo annual testing for serological signs of HBV infection (Henderson *et al.*, 2020). They will require Hepatitis B immune globulin (HBIG) (0.06 mL/kg) administered via intramuscular injection for PEP. The first dose of HBIG should be administered as soon as possible after exposure, with the second dose one month later.

WHO estimates that 257 million persons are living with chronic HBV infection in 2015 (WHO, 2020b). Individuals living with blood-borne diseases, including HBV, continue to form part of the workforce including in occupations carrying the risk of disease transmission to others. HCW-to-patient transmission of HBV was more prevalent in the 1990s and earlier. However, the incidence has since declined substantially due to screening; the practice of standard and additional precautions, especially during the performance of EPPs; and the promulgation of professional guidelines on the occupational restrictions of HCWs living with HBV (Lewis *et al.*, 2015).

In general, HCWs living with HBV should be restricted from performing EPPs if the hepatitis B viral load (HBV DNA) is at or above 200 IU/mL (Public Health England, 2020a). They may be cleared for EPPs if two hepatitis B viral load (HBV DNA) samples taken no less than 4 weeks apart show a viral load result below 200 IU/ml. In the UK, this group of HCWs need to be registered in a central confidential register. They should also be subjected to annual and post-exposure testing for HBV viral load as long as they continue to perform EPPs (Henderson *et al.*, 2020).

Hepatitis C

The development of direct-acting antivirals (DAAs) has resulted in effective treatment regimens of persons with chronic hepatitis C virus (HCV) infections. DAAs target specific points in the viral life cycle and are classified by their mechanisms of action, namely NS3/4A protease inhibitors, NS5A inhibitors, NS5B nucleoside polymerase inhibitors and NS5B non-nucleoside polymerase inhibitors. Current therapeutic regimes are generally associated with high sustained virologic response (SVR) rates exceeding 90%, where HCV RNA is not detectable on blood test 24 weeks after the completion of the antiviral therapy. DAAs are associated with improved clinical outcomes with a reduction in the risk of liver cirrhosis, decompensation, and liver-related and all-cause mortality (Jacobson *et al.*, 2017). Persons who achieved SVR are generally considered cured of the infection and the rates of late relapse are very low (Smith-Palmer *et al.*, 2015).

The risk of occupational HCV infection through exposure to infected blood from needlestick or sharps injuries is estimated to be 0.2% (CDC, 2020a). The risk of transmission from mucous membrane exposure is extremely low. Medical and laboratory staff, and HCWs who perform EPPs are at higher risk of occupational infection (Westermann *et al.*, 2015).

New HCWs should be offered screening for hepatitis C with HCV antibody, though being HCV positive or declining the screening test will generally not affect the employment of HCWs not performing EPPs. A positive screening test should be followed up with a HCV RNA test.

Given the low risk of HCV transmission through EPPs from a HCW whose HCV status is unknown, the UK Advisory Group on Hepatitis does not recommend routine hepatitis C screening for HCWs already conducting EPPs unless they are aware of possible exposure (Public Health England, 2020a). HCWs with active HCV infection should be restricted from performing EPPs and treated, until they have achieved SVR. Both the UK (Public Health England, 2020a) and US (Henderson *et al.*, 2020) guidelines accept undetectable HCV RNA at 12 weeks upon completion of treatment as acceptable for consideration to reinstate EPP privileges.

PEP for HCV exposure is currently not recommended. From a theoretical viewpoint, PEP would be effective if it can prevent the cellular entry of HCV. However, the pathogenesis of early HCV infection is not well understood. In addition, the DAAs target post-cellular entry processes and will presumably not be effective in preventing hepatocyte entry. Given the low incidence of HCV transmission in the occupational setting and the availability of highly efficacious and safe DAAs for HCV treatment, PEP is assessed not be to cost effective (Naggie *et al.*, 2017).

Case Study 1: Needlestick Injury in a Pregnant Dentist

A dentist who is at 14 weeks of gestation is performing a root canal procedure on her 28-year-old male patient. After injecting the local anaesthetic and as she was withdrawing the needle-and-syringe ensemble from the oral cavity, the used needle accidentally punctured her left index finger. The needle had penetrated her surgical gloves and resulted in a puncture wound with bleeding.

Following an exposure to a used sharp or needle with a penetrating wound, the wound should be washed liberally with soap and water and free bleeding should be encouraged. For splash injuries to mucous membranes including conjunctivae, the area should be irrigated and contact lenses removed. The injury should be reported promptly.

All HCWs should have immediate, 24-hour access to an expert service including a designated doctor. Such a service is best delivered by an Occupational Health Department but out-of-hours cover may be provided by the Emergency Department. The affected HCW should be assessed for the risk of transmission of HIV, HBV and HCV and the need for post-exposure management. The risk assessment is based on the type of body fluid involved and the route and severity of the exposure. Injuries from sharp objects that result in a breach of the skin barrier and exposure of mucous membranes (including the eye) are significant injuries. Most body fluids pose a risk of transmission. The exceptions are urine, vomit, faecal matter and saliva unless visibly bloodstained. Saliva in the context of dentistry is considered blood stained. Transmission has been reported following bites from HBV-infected persons (Lohiya et al., 2013).

As a routine, the designated doctor or member of the clinical team (not the exposed worker) should approach the source patient (if known) and obtain informed consent, after pre-test discussion, to test for anti-HIV, HBsAg and HCV RNA. Testing of source patients should be completed timely because it has a bearing on the risk assessment of the occupational injury and where relevant, the decision on PEP for the affected HCW.

If the affected HCW is pregnant, dolutegravir (an integrase inhibitor) should be avoided in the HIV PEP regimen as it has been associated with an increased risk of neural tube defects in infants (Kuhar et al., 2013). The combination of elvitegravir, cobicistat, emtricitabine and tenofovir should also be avoided because of reduced drug levels during pregnancy. Due to the risk of HIV transmission through breast milk, women who are breastfeeding may wish to consider temporary discontinuation until after the follow-up period and she has been cleared of HIV infection.

To protect against occupational HBV transmission, an unvaccinated HCW should receive one dose of HBIG and the first dose of hepatitis B vaccine as soon as possible after exposure. Both HBIG and hepatitis B vaccine are not contraindicated in pregnant or lactating women. As anti-HBs may be detectable up to six months after administration, it may be necessary to defer anti-HBs testing to later than the standard 1–2 months after the last vaccine dose, in order to ascertain that the serological response is from hepatitis B vaccination (Schillie S et al., 2013).

Zoonoses

Zoonotic infections are caused by microbes that normally infect animals, but are transmitted to humans who come into contact with these microbes either via direct contact with the animals that harbour them, or indirectly through the environment, contaminated food and water, as well as vectors such as mosquitoes and ticks that bite both humans and animals (CDC, 2017a). Certain occupations such as farming, veterinary practice, forestry, foraging and zookeeping have an increased risk of zoonotic infections because of higher animal contact. A significant proportion of these microbes are able to transmit between humans, resulting in outbreaks. Those microbes that have successfully made the transition towards being a human pathogen and which are stably maintained in the human population (i.e. HIV, SARS-CoV-2, influenza) are discussed elsewhere in this chapter.

Because the list of occupational zoonotic infections is extensive and there is no internationally agreed priority list given the diversity of occupations and zoonoses in different countries, the infections discussed below were selected from a comparison of several major publications and reports focusing on zoonoses in different parts of the world (CDC, 2017b; Hidajat and de Vocht, 2020; Vonesch *et al.*, 2019).

Anthrax

Anthrax affects humans primarily as an occupational infection although this aspect has been overshadowed by its potential role as a biological weapon (D'Amelio *et al.*, 2015). It is the name given to the disease caused by *Bacillus anthracis*, an aerobic, gram-positive, sporulating bacterium which is endemic in the soil of the tropics (WHO, 2012). The spores may remain dormant for decades and are present in soil and animal hides, horn, bones and bone meal. In tropical and subtropical regions worldwide, occupations such as farming, meat processing and veterinarians are at higher risk of anthrax, although the disease is now very rare in high and middle-income countries because of animal and human vaccination programmes (Chambers *et al.*, 2021). Human anthrax occurs in three distinct forms based on the mode of transmission.

Cutaneous anthrax is the most common (about 95% of all cases), and occurs 1–5 days following introduction of spores into the skin. Skin lesions begin as papules that progress after a week into relatively painless characteristic black eschars with regional lymphadenitis if untreated. The majority of cases resolve, although disseminated disease can develop in approximately 20% of those infected, with a high fatality rate (Chambers *et al.*, 2021).

Gastrointestinal anthrax occurs following consumption of spores, with clinical presentations that run the range from asymptomatic to gastrointestinal bleeding and septicaemia.

Inhalational anthrax leads to the most fatal outcomes, with an incubation period of up to 10 days followed by initial influenza-like symptoms. Rapid progression to septic shock and haemorrhagic mediastinitis may occur, with fatality rates that exceed 50% (Chambers *et al.*, 2021). This is also termed "woolsorter's disease" after a recognition of the increased risk in workers exposed to the spores present in untreated wool. Cleaning, preparation, and treatment of wool and hides originating from endemic areas before export has helped to reduce the incidence of anthrax.

Cutaneous anthrax is diagnosed clinically. As with other forms of anthrax, laboratory confirmation by bacterial cultures, serology or PCR where available can be sought. Treatment includes supportive care and antibiotics. There is no human-to-human transmission of anthrax, hence no special infection prevention measures are necessary in the healthcare setting.

Brucellosis

Brucellosis is a Gram-negative bacterial disease that affects a wide range of animals worldwide. Four *Brucella* species cause virtually all known human infections — *Brucella mellitensis* (which is the most common and also the most virulent), *B. abortus*, *B. suis*, and *B. canis.* The first is found in sheep and goats, whereas the latter three have cattle, pigs and dogs, respectively as primary host animals (CDC, 2021b).

The bacterium is transmitted to humans via close contact with livestock, consumption of unpasteurised dairy products or eating undercooked meat. It may rarely spread between humans via contaminated aerosols, blood transfusions, or transplacentally from mother to fetus (Corbel *et al.*, 2006). The occupational groups at greatest risk of brucellosis are animal breeders, abattoir workers, veterinarians, laboratory workers and hunters, usually exposed via direct contact with animal fluids or non-compliance with biosafety standards in the case of laboratory workers (Pereira *et al.*, 2020).

The incubation period is highly variable, ranging from a week to 2 months (Hayoun *et al.*, 2020). The initial presentation is non-specific, resembling influenza, although myalgia and fever are usually predominant. If untreated, a complex of rising and falling fevers, night sweats, anorexia, myalgia, arthralgia and weakness may occur, giving rise to the term "undulant fever." Any part of the body may be involved, including the heart valve (resulting in endocarditis), sacroiliac joints, and the brain. In infected pregnant women, spontaneous abortion, foetal death, preterm delivery and rarely congenital malformations have been described (Vilchez *et al.*, 2015).

Brucellosis can be diagnosed via cultures of blood, although more commonly via serological tests. Prolonged antibiotic treatment with doxycycline combined with other drugs such as rifampicin and aminoglycosides remain the mainstay of therapeutic management. Prevention is primarily via elimination of infection in animals via vaccination of livestock or culling of infected animals. Where that is not feasible, food safety measures, occupational hygiene and raising awareness are necessary (Corbel *et al.*, 2006; Hayoun *et al.*, 2020). Laboratory staff need to be informed if they are receiving clinical samples from patients with suspected brucellosis.

Hepatitis E

Once thought to be a human pathogen endemic in low- and middle-income countries (LMICs) in Asia and Africa, the hepatitis E virus (HEV) is now understood to have a broad host range that includes pigs, camels, bats, bears and minks (Vonesch *et al.*, 2019; Kenney, 2019). Genotypes 1–4 are associated with human disease, with swine — including pigs in the commercial pork industry and wild boars — being the principal reservoir for HEV-3 and -4 (De Schryver *et al.*, 2015). Although non-occupational faecal-oral transmission remains the most common mode of HEV spread among humans, a recent systematic review showed that working with pigs, in hospitals, or in forestry in non-endemic countries was associated with higher risks of HEV seropositivity (Wilhelm *et al.*, 2020).

The majority of HEV human infections are asymptomatic, with <5% developing symptoms of acute hepatitis with elevated liver enzymes and jaundice. A rare few develop extra-hepatic manifestations including neurological injuries (European Association for the Study of the Liver, 2017). Progression to liver failure is rare, and virtually all infections are self-limiting. No specific treatment exists. While a vaccine has been licensed in China (Hecolin®), it is not available elsewhere in the world (WHO, 2020c).

Nipah Virus

Nipah virus was discovered in an outbreak in Malaysia in 1998 that affected 283 persons and caused 109 deaths (Chua, 2003). Amongst the occupational groups affected were pig farmers, abattoir workers (also reported in neighbouring Singapore), pork vendors, and HCWs. The causative agent is a paramyxovirus, with transmission following contact with pigs and/or infected individuals. Fruit bats are the natural host of the virus. The presenting clinical features of infection include fever, headache, dizziness, vomiting, reduced consciousness, non-productive cough, myalgia, and focal neurological signs. Laboratory investigations show thrombocytopaenia and raised serum aminotransferases in about a third of cases (Goh *et al.*, 2000).

Public health measures taken to limit the spread of the outbreak included restricting the movement of pigs and destroying affected herds. The epidemic peaked and cases declined towards the end of 1999. Reports of re-emergence of the infection in countries such as Bangladesh (Islam *et al.*, 2016) have not been associated with occupational exposures in the community, although nosocomial transmission to healthcare staff has been reported, likely through close contact and respiratory droplets (Sazzad *et al.*, 2013).

Leptospirosis

Leptospirosis is caused by members of the slow-growing mobile spirochetes *Leptospira* spp. that are present worldwide. *Leptospira interrogans* is the species most commonly associated with human disease; others include *L. borpetersenii*, *L. santarosai*, and *L. noguchii* (Teo *et al.*, 2018). Multiple animal species act as both maintenance and incidental hosts of *Leptospira* spp., although rats are probably the most important maintenance hosts in the urban setting, shedding the bacteria through urine and infecting humans as well as other animals via contact with the contaminated environment. People in occupations with increased risk of direct or indirect contact with rodent urine are at increased risk of leptospirosis. These include sewage workers, garbage collectors, agricultural workers, and manual labourers (Mwachui *et al.*, 2015; Barragan *et al.*, 2017).

The incubation period is 10 days on average (range of 2–26 days). Fever, chills, myalgia, red eyes, fatigue, and loss of appetite are common clinical symptoms at presentation. Clinical course is varied, with most cases being asymptomatic or mild, while rarely the disease can worsen dramatically with the onset of jaundice, kidney failure and respiratory failure — the eponymous Weil's disease (Teo *et al.*, 2018). Diagnosis can be challenging, as cultures and commonly available serological tests are less sensitive. Treatment with antibiotics such as ceftriaxone or doxycycline is unnecessary except for severe disease. Preventive measures include risk communication and health education, with the use of protective clothing and footwear for those at risk, as well as chemoprophylaxis with doxycycline (CDC, 2020b). Vaccines are available only in a few countries such as France and Cuba.

Livestock-associated MRSA

Methicillin-resistant *Staphylococcus aureus* (MRSA) is one of the most common and best-known antibiotic-resistant bacteria worldwide (Hsu *et al.*, 2005; Aires-de-Sousa, 2017). Its importance is due to the large number of infections caused by the organism, as well as its resistance to all but the newest beta-lactam antibiotics, rendering treatment far more challenging. Originally believed to be a primary human commensal, it was first isolated in UK hospitals in 1960, before reports of community infections unassociated with healthcare contact arose in the 1980s. In the early 1970s, MRSA causing bovine mastitis in Belgium was isolated, but the issue of livestock-associated MRSA really came to prominence in the early 2000s with the association of MRSA infections and pig farming in the Netherlands (Voss *et al.*, 2005). Subsequent research revealed specific clonal lineages of MRSA that are able to infect both animals and humans, several of which are present in livestock worldwide (Aires-de-Sousa, 2017). Unsurprisingly, livestock workers — particularly those in the porcine industry — and veterinarians are at highest risk of livestock-associated MRSA infections (Chen and Wu, 2020), although person-to-person transmission via contact can occur with livestock-associated MRSA and hospital outbreaks are well described (Sieber *et al.*, 2019).

MRSA can cause a wide range of infections, but most commonly skin and soft tissue infections. Such infections can be treated with a variety of antibiotics, although not the commonly prescribed beta-lactam antibiotics. Prevention in the agricultural setting largely involves improving hygienic farming practices and reducing the use of antibiotics in livestock (Speksnijder *et al.*, 2015).

Lyme Disease

This is caused by the spirochete *Borrelia burgdorferi*, and named after the area in the United States where a cluster of cases was first reported in 1997. Most cases occur in the US although it is also present the Europe, especially the Scandinavian countries, Germany, Austria and Slovenia (Shapiro and Auwaerter, 2002). Deer and rodents are the natural hosts, and humans are infected from bites by ixodid ticks, which are the vectors for the disease. Outdoor workers such as forestry workers, hunters and foragers are at increased risk of Lyme disease (Richard and Oppliger, 2015).

Clinical manifestations are generally divided into early localised disease, early disseminated disease and late disease. Early localised disease is characterised by erythema migrans, a single ovoid rash observed up to a month after an infected tick bite (Shapiro and Auwaerter, 2002). Even if untreated, the lesion will disappear within 4 weeks. Early disseminated disease presents in a variety of ways, including multiple erythema migrans accompanied by fever and fatigue, aseptic meningitis with or without neuritis, or carditis with varying degrees of heart block. Late Lyme disease typically manifests as arthritis affecting large weight-bearing joints, although rarely chronic encephalomyelitis can occur. Post-infectious sequelae are present in up to 10% of patients, presenting as chronic fatigue syndrome.

Laboratory diagnosis is challenging as cultures are often impossible, and serological tests have varying sensitivities and specificities (Branda and Steere, 2021). Treatment depends on manifestations of disease, although antibiotics such as penicillin, cephalosporins and tetracyclines are often effective, except for post-infectious sequelae. Minimising risk for infection in endemic areas include education and training for workers, use of insect repellents and insecticides, and personal protective measures when working at sites with leaf litter and bushes (National Institute for Occupational Safety and Health, 2017).

Orf

This zoonotic infection is often included in chapters on occupational infections because of its odd sounding name rather than the severity of the infection. Orf is a self-limiting localised blister lesion usually on the hands caused by a parapox virus. It affects communities involved in farming sheep and goats. A third of Welsh farmers responding to a questionnaire reported having ever suffered from orf (Buchan, 1996). Twenty percent of the 251 respondents reported more than one previous episode. The infection was also common amongst family members. Complications reported include a rash and blisters on the face, body or mouth.

Q Fever

Q fever (the "Q" stands for "query," labelled at a time when the cause was unknown) is a worldwide zoonosis caused by a spore-forming rickettsia, *Coxiella burnetti*. The microbe has a broad host range, but the most common animal reservoirs through which humans are infected are cattle, sheep and goats (Anderson *et al.*, 2013). It is transmitted by droplets containing the excreta or fluids of infected animals, particularly during birthing, and other forms of transmission are rare. Therefore, farm workers, veterinarians and abattoir workers are most at risk.

Acute Q fever typically presents as a relatively benign, non-specific febrile illness 2–3 weeks post-exposure, with symptoms persisting for weeks if untreated. It can however be asymptomatic or rarely, present as severe pneumonia. Chronic Q fever is rare, manifesting months to years after acute infection. The most common presentation is endocarditis (inflammation of the heart valves); rarely osteoarticular infection, chronic hepatitis or pulmonary disease may develop.

The organism is challenging to culture and diagnosis is often made by serological testing or less commonly, by PCR in early stages of disease. The antibiotic doxycycline is used in the treatment of acute Q fever, but a combination of doxycycline and hydroxychloroquine is required for several months for chronic Q fever. A vaccine (Q-Vax) is available for humans at risk of infection but not widely licensed.

Vector-Borne Occupational Infections

These are infections transmitted by insect vectors and affect workers in occupations that expose them to the risk of such insect bites (Aw and Harrison, 1998). These occupations include forestry workers and those working in rural areas.

Malaria

Malaria is an endemic infection in many tropical areas in Asia, Africa and South America. It is caused by different strains of *Plasmodia* (e.g. *falciparum, vivax, ovale* and *malaria*), and is transmitted by the bite of Anopheles mosquitoes. These vectors breed in pools of stagnant water. *Plasmodium falciparum* causes cerebral malaria, and a severe haemolysis, which can present as "blackwater fever," which describes the resulting haemoglobinuria causing the urine to have a characteristic dark discolouration. Malaria also presents as hepatomegaly and splenomegaly. Malaria is diagnosed by identifying the malaria parasite in red blood cells from a thick blood film stained with Giemsa's stain.

There were an estimated 229 million malaria cases in 2019 in 87 malaria endemic countries. Twenty-nine countries, mostly in Africa, accounted for 95% of malaria cases globally. Malaria deaths have reduced steadily over the period 2000–2019, from 736,000 in the year 2000 to 409,000 in 2019. About 95% of malaria deaths globally were in 31 countries. Nigeria (23%), the Democratic Republic of the Congo (11%), the United Republic of Tanzania (5%), Mozambique (4%), Niger (4%) and Burkina Faso (4%) accounted for about 51% of all malaria deaths globally in 2019 (WHO, 2020d).

Workers from temperate areas sent to rural and forested areas in the tropics appear to be particularly susceptible, and are advised to take malaria chemoprophylaxis before, during and after their return from working in such areas. Up-to-date advice on the need for malaria prophylaxis when travelling to different countries is available from national and international websites (Chiodini *et al.*, 2021; WHO, 2021).

Simian malaria is a zoonotic disease caused by *Plasmodium knowlesi* infection. The common natural reservoir of the parasite is the macaque monkey and the vector is the *Anopheles* mosquito. Human cases of *P. knowlesi* infection has been reported in all South East Asian countries in the last decade, and it is currently the most common type of malaria seen in countries such as Malaysia and Brunei. *Plasmodium knowlesi* malaria can be an occupationally acquired infection that is seen among persons who work in jungles. Between 2007 and 2017, 73 cases of *P. knowlesi* infection were notified and confirmed to the Ministry of Health in Brunei. Of these, 15 cases (21%) were documented as work-related, and 28 other cases (38%) were classified as probably related to work (due to incomplete history). The occupations of those with probable and confirmed work related infections were border patrol officers, Armed Forces and security personnel, Department of Forestry officers, boatmen (Case Study 2) and forestry researchers. (Koh *et al.*, 2019).

Case Study 2: Simian Malaria in a Boatman

A 37-year-old male longboat operator's job was to transport visitors upriver to a university forestry field research centre located in the deep jungle (Fig. 1). Macaques were frequently seen along the riverbanks.

He presented to the clinic with complaints of fever for seven days, associated with headache and body ache. He was ferrying passengers to the research centre prior to the onset of his symptoms.

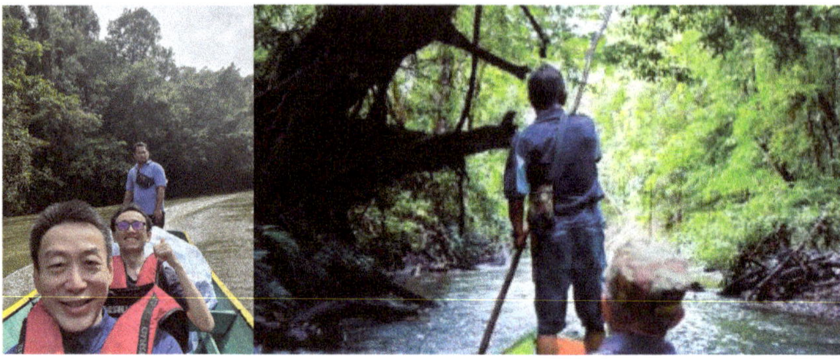

Fig. 1. Longboat operator working in deep jungle areas.

On examination, he was found to be febrile (39.1 degree Celsius), with stable vital signs. Laboratory results showed anaemia, moderate thrombocytopaenia, deranged liver function test results and increased creatinine levels. Dengue and Chikungunya viral screens were negative, with P knowlesi seen in a blood film examination.

In Singapore, the first reported locally acquired human *P. knowlesi* infection in 2007 was a soldier who trained in a forested area where long tailed macaques were frequently encountered. Subsequent disease surveillance detected four additional cases in 2007 and another in 2008. All occurred among military personnel who had undergone training in forested areas (Wong *et al.*, 2011).

The risk of this zoonotic infection extends to tourists and overseas visitors who have to travel to the jungle in the course of their work. It can be minimised with the recommended use of chemoprophylaxis for those going on duty into the jungles, application of mosquito/insect repellents, and use of repellent impregnated uniforms and bed nets in jungle camp sites.

Occupational Infections Spread Mainly by Aerosols or Droplet Infection

Tuberculosis

Tuberculosis (TB) is an infection of the lungs and/or other organs, due to *Mycobacterium tuberculosis* (MTB). TB is typically spread by inhalation of droplets from an infectious case and this depends on the presence of cough and MTB in the sputum together with the proximity and duration of contact. Droplet aerosols may also be generated in healthcare settings during autopsies, bronchoscopy and intubation. Only about 5% of those who are infected develop clinically apparent primary disease. In most, the primary TB focus heals spontaneously but MTB may survive within the lesion, giving rise to latent TB infection (LTBI). This latent form may reactivate later in life and this has important implications for global TB control. The lifetime risk of reactivation is usually estimated at 5–15% (Kiazyk and Ball, 2017) and depends on age, chronic disease and immuno-suppression particularly HIV/AIDS.

The incidence of active clinical TB varies greatly between countries and within countries. The highest rates are seen in South Asia and Sub-Saharan Africa. Risk factors for TB are exposure to MTB and immunosuppression and these particularly affect immigrants and travelers from high incidence countries, the elderly, close contacts of infectious cases, those living in poor housing conditions and those with poor health and nutrition because of homelessness, drug abuse or alcoholism.

Before 2001, the tuberculin skin test (TST) was the only practical and commercially available immunologic test for *Mycobacterium tuberculosis.* However, blood tests that measure T-cell interferon-gamma release in response to unique TB antigens are now widely used. These tests are known collectively as interferon-gamma release assays (IGRAs). There are currently two interferon gamma release assays commercially available: QuantiFERON-TB Gold In tube (QIAGEN, Germany) and T.Spot.TB (Oxford Immunotec, UK). The sensitivity of IGRA is comparable to TST whilst the specificity is consistently greater than TST in all groups. A higher level of concordance between IGRA and TST was observed in non-BCG vaccinated populations than in those who were BCG vaccinated. To date, there is no conclusive evidence on the cost-effectiveness of adopting a single modality (either TST or IGRA) vis-à-vis a sequential dual modality (TST/IGRA) in screening risk groups for LTBI, such as HCWs and recent arrivals (e.g. workers) from high TB incidence countries. Some studies comparing the use of single TST test against single IGRA test suggest that the higher initial cost of an IGRA screening test is offset by the lower post-screening costs arising from additional medical consultations, imaging investigations with chest X-ray, and chemoprevention (Nienhaus *et al.*, 2011; Sousa *et al.*, 2021). However, many factors affect cost-effective analyses and the most appropriate screening test for any setting, such as the background population prevalence of LTBI, and the sensitivity, specificity and prevailing cost of these tests (Auguste *et al.*, 2016).

Cross sectional studies of LTBI prevalence using IGRA have been reported among HCWs in South Korea and China. Among 1,655 HCWs in a 740-bed general hospital in South Korea who were surveyed, 271 persons tested positive and the prevalence of LTBI was 16% (95% CI; 15–18%) (Yeon *et al.*, 2018). About a third (33.9%) of 487 HCWs working in 31 TB-designated hospitals in southeastern China who underwent LTBI testing were found to be positive for LTBI (Chen *et al.*, 2019).

TB has important occupational health dimensions. HCWs including mortuary staff have twice the expected incidence of TB, allowing for age, sex and ethnic factors (Meredith *et al.*, 1996). There may also be an excess TB risk in other occupations such as prison staff although studies that show this are subject to reporting bias and confounding factors such as country of birth and social, economic and lifestyle factors (Seidler *et al.*, 2005). TB incidents in institutions and other community settings are an increasingly problem. For example, in England in 2019, 7.7% (274) people of working age diagnosed with TB were HCWs (Public Health England, 2020b). Typical scenarios include a patient who is admitted to hospital with TB but not appropriately isolated leading to potential exposure of other patients, or a HCW recruited from a high TB incidence country who later develops TB and exposes his/her patients to TB. A retrospective review by Chia *et al.* (2020) of 32 TB exposure events involving 881 HCWs showed a 2.5% Quantiferon conversion rate on follow-up over 8 weeks post-TB exposure.

HCWs, particularly those working in low and middle income countries (LMICs) with high TB incidence, are at increased risk of LTBI and TB disease. A systematic review of the prevalence and incidence of LTBI in HCWs in LMICs and associated factors (Apriani *et al.*, 2019) included 85 studies (32,630 subjects) from 26 LMICs. The prevalence of a positive TST was 14–98% (mean 49%); and the prevalence of a positive IGRA was 9–86% (mean 39%). Countries with TB incidence of ≥300 per 100,000 had the highest prevalence (TST: pooled estimate 55%, 95% CI 41–69%; IGRA: pooled estimate 56%, 95% CI 39–73%). Annual incidence estimated from the TST was 1–38% (mean 17%); while the annual incidence estimated from the IGRA was 10–30% (mean 18%). The prevalence and incidence of a positive test was associated with years of work, work location, TB contact and job category.

Most countries implement pre-employment screening for HCWs because of the public health implications of infectious TB in a HCW. Evidence-based guidelines for managing the occupational health aspects of TB have been published (National Institute for Health and Care Excellence, 2019). HCWs who will have contact with patients or clinical specimens should be screened for LTBI before employment. Screening should comprise a health questionnaire and documentary evidence of BCG status, TST or IGRA in the preceding 5 years. If documentary evidence is not available, or is negative, then a TST or IGRA test should be carried out. An IGRA test is preferred in screening employees from high TB prevalence countries. Those who are TST/IGRA positive are evaluated clinically and may be offered a course of LTBI treatment to prevent later re-activation of disease.

HCWs and laboratory staff who have contact with patients and/or clinical materials are more likely than the general population to be exposed to MTB. In certain countries with low TB incidence such as the UK, unvaccinated, TST/IGRA-negative individuals aged 16–35 who are at occupational risk of TB exposure are recommended to receive BCG (UK National Health Service, 2019). These include veterinary and other staff such as abattoir workers who handle animal species known to be susceptible to TB, such as simians; prison staff working directly with prisoners; staff of care homes for elderly people; and staff of hostels for homeless people and facilities accommodating refugees and asylum seekers. There is limited evidence that the BCG vaccine is effective for adults older than 35 years old.

Case Study 3: Healthcare Worker with Tuberculosis

A healthcare assistant (HCA) attends the employee health clinic with a seven-month history of cough, sputum, weight loss and night sweats. She has acid-fast bacilli in her sputum and changes on her chest X-ray typical of pulmonary tuberculosis. Originally from Zimbabwe, she has been working in local health services for five years. She was initially employed by a neighboring hospital where she underwent pre-employment screening. She then left to work in a community nursing home. To supplement her income, through a staffing agency, she works extra shifts in local hospitals.

This HCA should be seen urgently by the local TB service so that treatment can be initiated under the supervision of a respiratory specialist with TB experience. He/she should be mindful of the possibility of drug resistant TB and the possibility of HIV co-infection. She should be isolated at home until deemed no longer infectious and her close household contacts should be identified for screening according to best practice.

Her patients and work colleagues have been exposed to a TB infection risk. An incident meeting should be convened involving the local occupational health services, public health authorities, the TB service and managers of the healthcare premises where she has worked. A risk assessment should be made based on: the degree and duration of infectivity; what patients she has cared for; the nature of the care provided and the care environment; and whether any of the patients are unusually susceptible to infection because of age, immunosuppression and other susceptible factors. A similar risk assessment should be made for her work colleagues. Patients and staff who are deemed to have been exposed for long enough to be equivalent to *household contacts* or if they are particularly susceptible to infection should be managed as equivalent to household contacts and should be traced, screened and if deemed necessary, offered testing for TB. Tracing and testing contacts with lesser degrees of exposure is not generally beneficial; however, the exposure should be documented in the contact's clinical notes and his/her medical attendant should be informed. The contact should receive information on symptoms of TB and advised to seek medical consultation if necessary.

When the HCW was recruited from overseas and first employed in the health services, she would have undergone TB screening appropriate for a newly employed HCW. Because she had documentary evidence of having had BCG in the past, no testing was carried out. However, she should have been screened to the higher standard advised for new entrants from high-incidence settings (Henderson and Howard, 2017). New employees who are from countries of high TB incidence should have a chest X-ray and a TST/IGRA test. The HCW was symptomatic for several months before she sought medical attention.

Reminders of the symptoms of TB, and the need for prompt reporting should be sent annually to staff who may be exposed to TB. When a staff member moves jobs, documentary evidence of the results of past screening should be reviewed. If this is not available, then re-screening should be carried out. The same standards for pre-employment checks should apply to providers of temporary staff. Health clearance appropriate to a HCW's duties should be verified before the individual undertakes any clinical work. This also applies to agency staff. Agencies should be responsible for supplying staff who are fit to practice but the managers of the healthcare setting in which the temporary workers are based should satisfy themselves that the staff they receive have the necessary clearance.

Rubella

Rubella infection in a pregnant woman can result in congenital abnormalities in the newborn. These abnormalities may vary in severity, but are in any case preventable by ensuring that all pregnant women are immune to rubella. Rubella vaccination or infection in childhood will confer immunity. However, where this has not occurred, an additional preventive procedure is to ensure that all HCWs, regardless of sex, are immunised against rubella (Public Health England, 2013). This will further reduce the likelihood of HCWs transmitting the infection to non-immune pregnant women through contact in the occupational setting.

At pre-employment assessment of both male and female health care staff, hospital occupational health services can check whether there is a past history of rubella infection. If there has not been previous infection, or if there is uncertainty regarding this, then the presence of rubella antibodies can be checked. In the absence of rubella antibodies, the individual should be immunised and this recorded in the occupational health records.

Legionnaire's Disease

Legionnaire's disease is caused by *Legionella pneumophila*, and is spread by inhalation of aerosols (UK Health and Safety Executive, 2021). The organism was first identified in 1976 after a number of attendees at an American Legion convention at the Bellevue Stratford hotel in Philadelphia became ill with a "flu"-like illness. Clinical features included high fever, chills, cough, headache, and mental confusion. Some patients developed diarrhea, vomiting and delirium. There were a number of fatalities (the case fatality rate is around 10%), and epidemiological and laboratory investigation led to isolation of the causative organism, *Legionella pneumophila*. Occupational groups or members of the public can be affected. Elderly male smokers with pre-existing respiratory illness or other serious illness appear to be more susceptible to Legionella infection.

While the organism is ubiquitous, it has been responsible for outbreaks associated with hot water and air-conditioning systems in large buildings such as office blocks, hotels, and hospitals. Well-publicised outbreaks include those linked to hospital cooling towers in the UK, the BBC building in London, and an aquarium in Melbourne, Australia. Prevention of outbreaks is by ensuring that the temperature of water supplied to hospitals and large buildings are maintained at temperatures below 20°C or above 60°C. At these temperature extremes, the organism is unable to flourish (WHO, 2007). For delivery of hot water to users, the temperature at delivery should be reduced to prevent scalding. Refrigerated food display units with humidifiers have been identified as a source of Legionella causing two deaths from Legionnaire's disease (Comm Dis Surv Centre, 2000). Preventive measures include proper maintenance of these machines with antibacterial treatment and regular testing of the ultraviolet lamps, which are part of these units.

Emerging Coronaviruses

Three novel coronaviruses have emerged over the past two decades as important viral pathogens causing severe respiratory illness in humans. The severe acute respiratory syndrome coronavirus (SARS-CoV) first appeared in late 2002 in Guangdong province, China (Hui and Zumla, 2019); the Middle East respiratory syndrome coronavirus (MERS-CoV) first emerged in Saudi Arabia in 2012 (Chan *et al.*, 2015); and the cause of the COVID-19 pandemic — SARS-CoV-2 — in late 2019 in Wuhan, China (Zhu *et al.*, 2020).

All three viruses are believed to be of animal origin — specifically bats (Jelinek *et al.*, 2021). Dromedaries are the main animal reservoir for MERS-CoV, which has been identified in camel herds in several countries in the Middle East, Africa and South Asia (Chan *et al.*, 2015). The intermediate hosts of the other two viruses are less certain, although SARS-CoV had been isolated from civet cats in China, where these animals were considered a delicacy (Hui *et al.*, 2019).

Human-to-human spread via respiratory droplets has been well documented with all three coronaviruses, with large super-spreading events that are more in keeping with airborne spread seen rarely with SARS-CoV (Yu *et al.*, 2004) and more frequently with SARS-CoV-2 (Morawska and Cao, 2020).

The relatively short-lived SARS epidemic took place between November 2002 and July 2003, with an estimated 8,437 cases and 813 deaths across 32 countries and territories (Hui *et al.*, 2019), after which it has not re-emerged.

MERS has an even higher case-fatality rate exceeding 30%, with 2,584 laboratory-confirmed cases and 886 known deaths in 27 countries as of May 2021 (World Health Organisation Regional Office for the Eastern Mediterranean, 2021). Although MERS-CoV spreads far less efficiently than the other two coronaviruses, recurrent occupational and recreational infections and small outbreaks have occurred owing to its widespread distribution in camel herds. The largest outbreak of MERS-CoV occurred in 2015 in South Korea, with 186 laboratory-confirmed cases and 38 deaths (Korea Centers for Disease Control and Prevention, 2015).

The COVID-19 pandemic is still ongoing at the time of writing, with almost 194 million confirmed cases and over four million deaths worldwide as of July 2021. Although the case-fatality rate is the lowest of all three coronaviruses, its greater efficacy at transmission has resulted in the highest number of deaths and ongoing sustained human-to-human spread.

HCWs are a major high-risk group for infection by these emerging coronaviruses. HCWs have accounted for over 10% of MERS and SARS cases worldwide, with a lower proportion in SARS-CoV-2 owing to its greater transmissibility in the community. Besides HCWs, other occupational groups such as social, transport, education and other essential workers are at higher risk of COVID-19 (SAGE EMG — Transmission Group, *2021*).

Persons infected by any of the three coronaviruses typically present with fever and respiratory symptoms, although SARS and MERS are more likely to be associated severe lower respiratory tract involvement, whereas a significant proportion of COVID-19 infections are asymptomatic, although still infectious to others (Wilmes *et al.*, 2021). A significant proportion — ranging from between 20% and 70% depending on study — of symptomatic COVID-19 patients continue to have symptoms for at least six months post-recovery from the acute illness, most commonly fatigue, muscle weakness and sleeping difficulties (Crook *et al.*, 2021). This ill-defined condition has been termed post-acute COVID-19 syndrome or long COVID (Crook *et al.*, 2021).

Whereas there is neither specific treatment nor vaccine for SARS and MERS, the intense concentration of public and private scientific resources on COVID-19 has resulted in the identification of a number of therapeutic options for severe COVID-19, including dexamethasone and tocilizumab, the latter being a monoclonal antibody targeting interleukin-6 receptor originally used for rheumatoid arthritis (Infectious Diseases Society of America, 2021). A large number of vaccines have been developed against COVID-19, with the largest global vaccination campaign against a disease in progress at the time of writing.

General principles for prevention and control, such as early detection and isolation of cases are essential in preventing spread of illness. The main infection prevention and control measures are aerosol (wearing a surgical or N95 mask within 1m of patients) and contact precautions (wearing gown and gloves on entering patients' rooms and removing them on leaving). Patients infected with any of the emerging coronaviruses should ideally be placed in negative pressure rooms or in rooms where room exhaust is filtered through high-efficiency particulate air filters. Airborne precautions with at least six air changes per hour should be applied in treatment rooms when performing aerosol-generating procedures (ISARIC PHE, 2017). HCWs are also on the priority list for vaccination against COVID-19 worldwide.

Other Respiratory Viruses

Many other respiratory viruses can present with a syndrome of severe respiratory illness including influenza viruses, respiratory syncytial virus and human metapneumovirus. In recent years, influenza viruses have circulated in seasonal (H3N2, H1N1) and avian (including H5N1) forms. In April 2009, "Swine flu" caused by a new strain of influenza A, *Pandemic (H1N1) 2009* emerged. Since then, there have been more reports of human infections with influenza A viruses normally found in swine (now known as "variant viruses"), likely due to a combination of improved diagnostics, enhanced surveillance and possibly a true increase in swine-to-human transmission (CDC, 2012). Workers who raise or work with pigs, and pork producers are at risk. Preventive measures against occupational infection include vaccinating pigs for swine influenza, practicing hand hygiene before and after exposure to the animals, and avoiding close contact with animals that appear ill. In addition, these workers should be vaccinated against seasonal influenza. While this will not protect against variant virus infection, vaccination is nonetheless important to reduce the risk of transmission of seasonal influenza between workers, from humans to pigs, and decrease the likelihood of co-infection of workers with human and variant influenza viruses.

When pandemic influenza is widespread in a community, there is a risk of spread from patient to HCW and from HCW to patient within the healthcare environment. The former carries the greater risk usually as a result of an unprotected HCW undertaking aerosol generating procedures on an infected patient. Spread in both the healthcare setting and the community can also occur through fomite transmission. The practice of regular hand hygiene, masking, and remaining at home when unwell with acute respiratory symptoms are simple measures that can limit transmission. An ecological study by Wei *et al.* (2020) found an association between an increase in the proportion of HCW vaccinated with seasonal influenza vaccine and the reduction in nosocomial influenza incidence in a tertiary inpatient setting, suggestive a protective effect.

General principles for prevention and control, such as early detection and isolation of cases are essential in preventing spread of illness. In a recent incident, an imported case of MERS remained undiagnosed for 9 days in South Korea, leading to the largest outbreak of MERS outside the Middle East, with 188 secondary infections (Fu and Wang, 2016). While the exact transmission mechanism for MERS is not well understood, the adoption of standard, contact and airborne precautions is recommended for HCW protection. Source control may also be implemented by placing a surgical mask on the suspect or infected patient, as tolerated.

With the emergence of the COVID-19 pandemic in 2020, the PPE for HCWs managing patients with influenza-like illness has generally been enhanced to include gowns, gloves, eye protection (goggles or face shield), and respiratory protection equivalent to a fit-tested National Institute for Occupational Safety and Health (NIOSH)-certified disposable N95 filtering face-piece respirator (Public Health England, 2020c). Patients should be placed in negative pressure rooms or in rooms in which room exhaust is filtered through high-efficiency particulate air filters. Airborne precautions with at least six air changes per hour should be applied in treatment rooms when performing aerosol-generating procedures.

Table 1. Other Examples of Occupational Infections

Occupations at Risk	Mode of Transmission	Disease	Organism
Laboratory staff and other health care workers	Needle stick injuries	Malaria Syphilis	*Plasmodium spp* *Treponema pallidum*
Clinical staff and other health care workers	Droplet infection and contact with infected material	Haemorrhagic fever	Marburg virus, Ebola virus
Bird breeders	Aerosols Droplet infection from chickens	Psittacosis/ ornithosis Conjunctivitis	*Chlamydia psittaci* Newcastle virus
Farmers	Close contact/ Droplet infection	Meningitis	*Streptococcus suis*
Hairdressers	Close contact	Ringworm	*Microsporum audouini*
Gardeners	Injury from thorny plants	Sporotrichosis	*Sporothrix schenckii*

Conclusion

There are many other infections that affect occupational groups. Some are rare and exotic (as those acquired by laboratory workers); and others are common with a clear link between infection and work activity (Collins *et al.*, 1997). Table 1 provides further examples of occupational infections, the causative agents, and the mode of transmission.

In the individual case where an occupational infection is suspected, it is important to take an adequate occupational history. If feasible, a workplace visit to assess the system of work can help confirm the likelihood of the infection being acquired through workplace factors. A high index of suspicion will ensure that occupational infections are not missed. If an occupational source is not recognised, there will be a continuing risk to other workers in the same work area, and the affected individual may be at risk of re-infection on return to work, especially if immunity following the initial infection does not occur.

References

Aires-de-Sousa M. (2017) Methicillin-resistant *Staphylococcus Aureus* among animals: Current overview. *Clin Microbiol Infect* **23**(6): 373–380.

Anderson A, Bijlmer H, Fournier PE, Graves S, Hartzell J, Kersh GJ, Limonard G, Marrie TJ, Massung RF, McQuiston JH, Nicholson WL, Paddock CD, Sexton DJ. (2013) Diagnosis and management of Q fever — United States, 2013: Recommendations from CDC and the Q Fever Working Group. *MMWR Recomm Rep* **62**(RR-03): 1–30.

Apriani L, McAllister S, Sharples K, Alisjahbana B, Ruslami R, Hill PC, Menzies D. (2019) Latent tuberculosis infection in healthcare workers in low- and middle-income countries: An updated systematic review. *Eur Respir J* **53**(4): 1801789.

Aribou ZM, Wijaya L, Gan WH. (2020) To offer or not to offer: A conundrum on ascertaining whether post-exposure prophylaxis is indicated in occupational exposure of HIV. *Health Sci Rep* **3**(2): e152.

Auguste P, Tsertsvadze A, Pink J, Court R, Seedat F, Gurung T, Freeman K, Taylor-Phillips S, Walker C, Madan J, Kandala NB, Clarke A, Sutcliffe P. (2016) Accurate diagnosis of latent tuberculosis in children, people who are immunocompromised or at risk from immunosuppression and recent arrivals from countries with a high incidence of tuberculosis: Systematic review and economic evaluation. *Health Technol Assess* **20**(38): 1–678.

Averhoff F, Mahoney F, Coleman P, Schatz G, Hurwitz E, Margolis H. (1998) Immunogenicity of hepatitis B vaccines. Implications for persons at occupational risk of hepatitis B virus infection. *Am J Prev Med* **15**(1): 1–8.

Aw TC, Harrison J. (1998). Exposure-based Hazards: Biological. In: Herzstein, J.A, Fleming, LE, Bunn, W.B. (eds.), *International occupational and environmental medicine*. St Louis, Michigan, Mosby.

Aw TC, Blair I, Babcock HM. (2017) Occupational infections. *Infect Dis* 647–655.e1.

Barragan V, Olivas S, Keim P, Pearson T. (2017) Critical knowledge gaps in our understanding of environmental cycling and transmission of *Leptospira spp. Appl Environ Microbiol* **83**(19): e01190–17.

BASHH. (2021) *UK Guideline for the use of HIV post-exposure Prophylaxis 2021*. [Online] Available from: https://www.bashhguidelines.org/media/1269/pep-2021.pdf. [Accessed on 15 July 2021].

Branda JA, Steere, AC. (2021) Laboratory diagnosis of lyme borreliosis. *Clin Microbiol Rev* **34**(2): e00018–19.

Bruce MG, Bruden D, Hurlburt D, Zanis C, Thompson G, Rea L, Toomey M, Townshend-Bulson L, Rudolph K, Bulkow L, Spradling PR, Baum R, Hennessy T, McMahon BJ. (2016) Antibody levels and protection after hepatitis B vaccine: Results of a 30-year follow-up study and response to a booster dose. *J Infect Dis* **214**(1): 16–22.

Buchan J. (1996) Characteristics of orf in a farming community in mid-Wales. *Brit Med J* **313**(7051): 203–205.

CDC. (2012) *Swine Influenza (Influenza in Swine)*. [Online] Available from: https://www.cdc.gov/flu/swineflu/influenza-in-swine.htm. [Accessed on 1 August 2021].

CDC. (2017a) *Zoonotic Diseases*. [Online] Available from: https://www.cdc.gov/onehealth/basics/zoonotic-diseases.html. [Accessed on 17 April 2021].

CDC. (2017b) *Prioritizing Zoonotic Diseases for Multisectoral, One Health Collaboration in the United States*. [Online] Available from: https://www.cdc.gov/onehealth/pdfs/us-ohzdp-report-508.pdf. [Accessed on 17 April 2021].

CDC. (2019) *HIV and Occupational Exposure*. [Online] Available from: https://www.cdc.gov/hiv/workplace/healthcareworkers.html. [Accessed on 15 July 2021].

CDC. (2020a) *Hepatitis C Questions and Answers for Health Professionals*. [Online] Available from: https://www.cdc.gov/hepatitis/hcv/hcvfaq.htm#f1. [Accessed on 18 July 2021].

CDC. (2020b) *CDC Yellow Book 2020: Health Information for International travel*. New York, Oxford University Press.

CDC. (2021a) *Sharps Safety for Healthcare Settings*. [Online] Available from: https://www.cdc.gov/sharpssafety/index.html. [Accessed on 11 July 2021].

CDC. (2021b) *Brucellosis*. [Online] Available from: https://www.cdc.gov/brucellosis/index.html. [Accessed on 17 April 2021].

Chambers J, Yarrarapu SNS, Mathai JK. (2021) *Anthrax infection*. [Online] Florida, StatPearls Publishing. [Online] Available from: https://www.ncbi.nlm.nih.gov/books/NBK535379/#article-19041.s4.

Chen C, Wu F. (2020) Livestock-associated methicillin-resistant Staphylococcus aureus (LA-MRSA) colonization and infection among livestock workers and veterinarians: A systematic review and meta-analysis. *Occup Envirron Med* oemed-2020-106418.

Chan JF, Lau SK, To KK, Cheng VC, Woo PC, Yuen KY. (2015) Middle East respiratory syndrome coronavirus: another zoonotic betacoronavirus causing SARS-like disease. *Clin Microbiol Rev* **28**(2): 465–522.

Chen B, Hua G, Wang X, Wang F, Peng Y, Ge E, Upshur R, Dai R, Wei X, Jiang J. (2019) Prevalence and determinants of latent tuberculosis infection among frontline tuberculosis healthcare workers in southeastern China: A multilevel analysis by individuals and health facilities. *Int J Infect Dis* **79**: 26–33.

Chia SZG, How KBM, Chlebicki MP, Ling ML, Gan WH. (2020) A retrospective review of tuberculosis exposure among health care workers in a tertiary hospital. *Am J Infect Control* **48**(6): 650–655.

Chiodini PL, Patel D, Goodyer L, Ranson H. (2021) *Guidelines for Malaria Prevention in Travellers from the United Kingdom, 2021.* [Online] Available from: https://www.gov.uk/government/publications/malaria-prevention-guidelines-for-travellers-from-the-uk. [Accessed on 29 July 2021].

Chua KB. (2003) Nipah virus outbreak in Malaysia. *J Clin Virol* **26**(3): 265–275.

Collins CH, Aw TC, Grange JM. (1997) *Microbial diseases of occupations, sports and recreations.* Oxford, Butterworth-Heinemann.

Comm Dis Surv Centre. (2000) Legionella from guests of Welsh hotel indistinguishable from humidifier isolates. *Commun Dis Rep CDR Wkly* **10**(16): 141.

Corbel MJ, Elberg SS, Cosivi O. (eds). (2006) *Brucellosis in humans and animals.* [Online] Available from: https://www.who.int/csr/resources/publications/Brucellosis.pdf. [Accessed on 17 April 2021].

Crook H, Raza S, Nowell J, Young M, Edison P. (2021) Long covid-mechanisms, risk factors, and management. *BMJ* **374**: n1648.

D'Amelio E, Gentile B, Lista F, D'Amelio R. (2015) Historical evolution of human anthrax from occupational disease to potentially global threat as bioweapon. *Environ Int* **85**: 133–146.

Damme PV. (2016) Long-term protection after hepatitis B vaccine. *J Infect Dis* **214**(1): 1–3.

Danzmann L, Gastmeier P, Schwab F, Vonberg RP. (2013) Health care workers causing large nosocomial outbreaks: A systematic review. *BMC Infect Dis* **13**: 98.

De Schryver A, De Schrijver K, Francois G, Hambach R, van Sprundel M, Tabibi R, Colosio C. (2015) Hepatitis E virus infection: An emerging occupational risk? *Occup Med (Lond)* **65**(8): 667–672.

Expert Advisory Group on AIDS. (2013) *Updated Recommendation for HIV Post-exposure Prophylaxis (PEP) Following Occupational Exposure to a Source with Undetectable HIV viral Load.* [Online] Available from:

https://assets.publishing.service.gov.uk/government/uploads/system/uploads/attachment_data/file/275060/EAGA_advice_on_PEP_after_exposure_to_UD_source_Dec13.pdf. [Accessed on 15 July 2021].

European Association for the Study of the Liver. (2017) EASL clinical practice guidelines on hepatitis E virus. *J Hepatol* **68**(6): 1256–1271.

Fu C, Wang S. (2016) Nosocomial infection control in healthcare settings: Protection against emerging infectious diseases. *Infect Dis Poverty* **5**(1): 30.

Goh KJ, Tan CT, Chew NK, Tan PSK, Kamarulzaman A, Sarji SA, Wong KT, Adbullah BJJ, Chua KB, Lam SK. (2000) Clinical features of Nipah virus encephalitis among pig farmers in Malaysia. *New Engl J Med* **342**(17): 1229–1235.

Hayoun MA, Muco E, Shorman M. (2020) *Brucellosis.* [Online] Florida, StatPearls Publishing. Available from: https://www.ncbi.nlm.nih.gov/books/NBK441831/. [Accessed on 17 April 2021].

Henderson DK, Dembry LM, Sifri CD, Palmore TN, Dellinger EP, Yokoe DS, Grady C, Heller T, Weber D, Rio CD, Fishman NO, Deloney VM, Lundstrom T, Babcock HM. (2020) Management of healthcare personnel living with hepatitis B, hepatitis C, or human immunodeficiency virus in US healthcare institutions. *Infect Control Hosp Epidemiol* 1–9.

Henderson M, Howard SJ. (2017) Screening for latent tuberculosis in UK health care workers. *Occup Med (Lond)* **67**(8): 641–643.

Hidajat M, de Vocht F. (2020) Occupational zoonoses potential in Southeast Asia. *Occup Med (Lond)* **70**(5): 323–326.

Hsu LY, Wijaya L, Tan BH. (2005) Management of healthcare-associated methicillin-resistant *Staphylococcus aureus. Expert Rev Anti Infect Ther* **3**(6): 893–905.

Hui DSC, Zumla A. (2019) Severe Acute Respiratory Syndrome: Historical, epidemiological, and clinical features. *Infect Dis Clin North Am* **33**(4): 869–889.

Infectious Diseases Society of America. (2021) *IDSA guidelines on the treatment and management of patients with COVID-19.* [Online] Available from: https://www.idsociety.org/practice-guideline/covid-19-guideline-treatment-and-management/. [Accessed on 29 July 2021].

ISARIC PHE. (2017) *Treatment of MERS-CoV: Information for Clinicians. Clinical Decision-making Support for Treatment of MERS-CoV patients.* [Online] Available from: https://assets.publishing.service.gov.uk/government/uploads/system/uploads/attachment_data/file/638628/MERS_CoV_guidance_for_clinicians.pdf. [Accessed on 29 July 2021].

International Safety Center. (2019) *EPINet Report for Needlestick and Sharp Object Injuries.* [Online] Available from: https://internationalsafetycenter.org/wp-content/uploads/2020/06/2019-EPInet-Needlestick-Sharps-Summary.pdf. [Accessed on 11 July 2021].

Islam MS, Sazzad HM, Satter SM, Sultana S, Hossain MJ, Hasan M, Rahman M, Campbell S, Cannon DL, Ströher U, Daszak P, Luby SP, Gurley ES. (2016) Nipah virus transmission from bats to humans associated with drinking traditional liquor made from date palm sap, Bangladesh, 2011–2014. *Emerg Infect Dis* **22**(4): 664–670.

Jacobson IM, Lim JK, Fried MW. (2017) American Gastroenterological Association Institute Clinical Practice Update-Expert Review: Care of patients who have achieved a sustained virologic response after antiviral therapy for chronic hepatitis C infection. *Gastroenterology* **152**(6): 1578–1587.

Jelinek HF, Mousa M, Alefishat E, Osman W, Spence I, Bu D, Feng SF, Byrd J, Magni PA, Sahibzada S, Tay GK, Alsafar HS. (2021) Evolution, ecology, and zoonotic transmission of betacoronaviruses: A review. *Front Vet Sci* **8**: 644414.

Kenney SP. (2019) The current host range of Hepatitis E viruses. *Viruses* **11**(5): 452.

Kiazyk S, Ball TB. (2017) Latent tuberculosis infection: An overview. *Can Commun Dis Rep* **43**(3–4): 62–66.

Koh GJN, Ismail PK, Koh D. (2019) Occupationally acquired *Plasmodium Knowlesi* malaria in Brunei Darussalam. *Saf Health Work* **10**(1): 122–124.

Korea Centers for Disease Control and Prevention. (2015) Middle East respiratory syndrome coronavirus outbreak in Republic of Korea, 2015. *Osong Public Health Res Perspect* **6**(4): 269–278.

Kuhar DT, Henderson DK, Struble KA, Heneine W, Thomas V, Cheever LW, Gomaa A, Panlilio AL, US Public Health Service Working Group. (2013) Updated US Public Health Service guidelines for the management of occupational exposures to human immunodeficiency virus and recommendations for postexposure prophylaxis. *Infect Control Hosp Epidemiol* **34**(9): 875–892.

Leong XYA, Yee FZY, Leong YY, Tan SG, Amin IBM, Ling ML, Tay SM. (2019) Incidence and analysis of sharps injuries and splash exposures in a tertiary hospital in Southeast Asia: A ten-year review. *Singapore Med J* **60**(12): 631–636.

Lewis JD, Enfield KB, Sifri CD. (2015) Hepatitis B in healthcare workers: Transmission events and guidance for management. *World J Hepatol* 7(3): 488–497.

Lohiya GS, Tan-Figueroa L, Lohiya S, Lohiya S. (2013) Human bites: Bloodborne pathogen risk and postexposure follow-up algorithm. *J Natl Med Assoc* **105**(1): 92–95.

Meredith S, Watson JM, Citron KM, Cockcroft A, Darbyshire JH. (1996) Are healthcare workers in England and Wales at increased risk of tuberculosis? *BMJ* **313**(7056): 522–525.

Morawska L, Cao J. (2020) Airborne transmission of SARS-CoV-2: The world should face the reality. *Environ Int* **139**: 105730.

Mwachui MA, Crump L, Hartskeerl R, Zinsstag J, Hattendorf J. (2015) Environmental and behavioural determinants of leptospirosis transmission: A systematic review. *PLoS Negl Trop Dis* **9**(9): e0003843.

Naggie S, Holland DP, Sulkowski MS, Thomas DL. (2017) Hepatitis C virus postexposure prophylaxis in the healthcare worker: Why direct-acting antivirals don't change a thing. *Clin Infect Dis* **64**(1): 92–99.

National Institute for Health and Care Excellence. (2019) *Tuberculosis NICE guideline [NG33]*. [Online] Available from: https://www.nice.org.uk/guidance/ng33. [Accessed on 29 July 2021].

National Institute for Occupational Safety and Health. (2017) *Lyme disease*. [Online] Available from: https://www.cdc.gov/niosh/topics/lyme/recommendations.html. [Accessed on 17 April 2021].

Nienhaus A, Schablon A, Costa JT, Diel R. (2011) Systematic review of cost and cost-effectiveness of different TB-screening strategies. *BMC Health Serv Res* **11**: 247.

Nwaiwu CA, Egro FM, Smith S, Harper JD, Spiess AM. (2017) Seroconversion rate among health care workers exposed to HIV-contaminated body fluids: The University of Pittsburgh 13-year experience. *Am J Infect Control* **45**(8): 896–900.

Ogunremi T, Defalco K, Johnston BL, Vearncombe M, Joffe AM, Cleghorn B, Cividino M, Wong DK, Mazzulli T, Wong J, Isinger MA, Robert Y, Boucoiran I, Dunn K, Henry B. (2019) Preventing transmission of blood-borne viruses from infected healthcare workers to patients: Summary of a new Canadian Guideline. *Can Commun Dis Rep* **45**(12): 317–322.

Occupational Safety and Health Administration. (2021) *Worker Protections Against Occupational Exposure to Infectious Diseases*. [Online] Available from: https://www.osha.gov/bloodborne-pathogens/worker-protections. [Accessed on 15 July 2021].

Pereira CR, de Almeida JVFC, de Oliveira IRC, de Oliveira LF, Pereira LJ, Zangeronimo MG, Lage AP, Dorneles EMS. (2020) Occupational exposure to *Brucella spp.*: A systematic review and meta-analysis. *PLoS Negl Trop Dis* **14**(5): e0008164.

Public Health England. (2013) *Rubella: The Green Book Chapter 28.* [Online] Available from: https://assets.publishing.service.gov.uk/government/uploads/system/uploads/attachment_data/file/148498/Green-Book-Chapter-28-v2_0.pdf. [Accessed on 1 August 2021].

Public Health England. (2017) *Emergency Healthcare Workers, Exposure Prone Procedures (EPPs) and the Exposure Prone Environment: Advice from the United Kingdom Advisory Panel for Healthcare Workers Infected with Bloodborne Viruses (UKAP).* Available from: https://fphc.rcsed.ac.uk/media/2237/ukap_emergency_healthcare_workers_epps_and_exposure_prone_environment_published.pdf. [Accessed on 12 July 2021].

Public Health England. (2020a) *Integrated Guidance on Health Clearance and the Management of HCWs Living with BBVs (Hepatitis B, Hepatitis C and HIV): August 2020.* [Online] Available from: https://www.gov.uk/government/publications/bbvs-in-healthcare-workers-health-clearance-and-management. [Accessed on 17 July 2021].

Public Health England. (2020b) *Tuberculosis in England. 2020 Report (Presenting Data to End of 2019).* [Online] Available from: https://assets.publishing.service.gov.uk/government/uploads/system/uploads/attachment_data/file/943356/TB_Annual_Report_2020.pdf. [Accessed on 1 August 2021].

Public Health England. (2020c) *Guidelines for PHE Health Protection Teams on the Management of Outbreaks of Influenza-like Illness (ILI) in Care Homes.* [Online] Available from: https://assets.publishing.service.gov.uk/government/uploads/system/uploads/attachment_data/file/932991/Guidelines_for_the_management_of_outbreaks_of_influenza-like_illness_in_care_homes_05_11_2020.pdf. [Accessed on 1 August 2021].

Richard S, Oppliger A. (2015) Zoonotic occupational diseases in forestry workers — Lyme borreliosis, tularemia and leptospirosis in Europe. *Ann Agric Environ Med* **22**(1): 43–50.

SAGE EMG — Transmission Group. (2021) *COVID-19 Risk by Occupation and Workplace.* [Online] Available from: https://assets.publishing.service.gov.uk/government/uploads/system/uploads/attachment_data/file/965094/s1100-covid-19-risk-by-occupation-workplace.pdf. [Accessed on 29 July 2021].

Sazzad HMS, Hossain MJ, Gurley ES, Ameen KMH, Parveen S, Islam MS, Faruque LI, Podder G, Banu SS, Lo MK, Rollin PE, Rota PA, Daszak P, Rahman M, Luby SP. (2013) Nipah virus infection outbreak with nosocomial and corpse-to-human transmission, Bangladesh. *Emerg Infect Dis* **19**(2): 210–217.

Schillie S, Murphy TV, Sawyer M, Ly K, Hughes E, Jiles R, de Perio MA, Reilly M, Byrd K, Ward JW, Centers for Disease Control and Prevention (CDC). (2013) CDC guidance for evaluating health-care personnel for hepatitis B virus protection and for administering postexposure management. *MMWR Recomm Rep* **62**(RR-10): 1–19.

Seidler A, Nienhaus A, Diel R. (2005) Review of epidemiological studies on the occupational risk of tuberculosis in low-incidence areas. *Respiration* **72**(4): 431–436.

Shapiro ED, Auwaerter P. (2002) *Borrelia Burgdorferi (Lyme Disease)*. [Online] Available from: http://www.antimicrobe.org/new/b84.asp#t2. [Accessed on 17 April 2021].

Sieber RN, Larsen AR, Urth TR, Iversen S, Moller CH, Skov RL, Larsen J, Stegger M. (2019) Genome investigations show host adaptation and transmission of LA-MRSA CC398 from pigs into Danish healthcare institutions. *Sci Rep* **9**(1): 18655.

Smith-Palmer J, Cerri K, Valentine W. (2015) Achieving sustained virologic response in hepatitis C: A systematic review of the clinical, economic and quality of life benefits. *BMC Infect Dis* **15**: 19.

Sousa S, Rocha D, Silva JC, Ribeiro AI, Goncalves G, Almeida A, Correia AM, Duarte R, Carvalho C. (2021) Comparing the cost-effectiveness of two screening strategies for latent tuberculosis infection in Portugal. *Pulmonology* S2531-0437(21)00091-X.

Speksnijder DC, Mevius DJ, Bruschke CJM, Wagenaar JA. (2015) Reduction of veterinary antimicrobial use in the Netherlands. The Dutch success model. *Zoonoses Public Health* **62**(Suppl 1): 79–87.

UK Health and Safety Executive. (2021) *What is Legionnaires' Disease?* [Online] Available from: https://www.hse.gov.uk/legionnaires/what-is.htm. [Accessed on 29 July 2021].

UK National Health Service. (2019) *Who Should have the BCG (TB) Vaccine?* [Online] Available from: https://www.nhs.uk/conditions/vaccinations/when-is-bcg-tb-vaccine-needed/. [Accessed on 1 August 2021].

Teo AKJ, Bramley A, Sa'at ZAA, Fernandez CJ, Chng WC, Tan BZ, Hsu LY, Pang J, Ooi SP. (2018) A review of leptospirosis epidemiology, transmission and risk factors. *Epidemiol News Bull Q* **44**: 111–117.

Vilchez G, Espinoza M, D'Onadio G, Saona P, Gotuzzo E. (2015) Brucellosis in pregnancy: Clinical aspects and obstetric outcomes. *Int J Infect Dis* **38**: 95–100.

Vonesch N, Binazzi A, Bonafede M, Melis P, Ruggieri A, Iavicoli S, Tomao P. (2019) Emerging zoonotic viral infections of occupational health importance. *Pathog Dis* 77(2): ftz018.

Voss A, Loeffen F, Bakker J, Klaassen C, Wulf M. (2005) Methicillin-resistant *Staphylococcus aureus* in pig farming. *Emerg Infect Dis* **11**(12): 1965–1966.

Wei WE, Fook-Chong S, Chen WK, Chlebicki MP, Gan WH. (2020) The impact of healthcare worker influenza vaccination on nosocomial influenza in a tertiary hospital: An ecological study. *BMC Health Serv Res* **20**(1): 636.

Westermann C, Peters C, Lisiak B, Lamberti M, Nienhaus A. (2015) The prevalence of hepatitis C among healthcare workers: A systematic review and meta-analysis. *Occup Environ Med* **72**(12): 880–888.

Wilhelm B, Waddell L, Greig J, Young I. (2020) A systematic review and meta-analysis of predictors of human hepatitis E virus exposure in non-endemic countries. *Zoonoses Public Health* **67**(4): 391–406.

WHO. (2007) *Legionella and the Prevention of Legionellosis.* [Online] Available from: https://www.who.int/water_sanitation_health/emerging/legionella.pdf. [Accessed on 1 August 2021].

WHO. (2012) *Research Priorities for Zoonoses and Marginalized Infections.* [Online] Available from: https://apps.who.int/iris/bitstream/handle/10665/75350/WHO_TRS_971_eng.pdf. [Accessed on 17 April 2021].

WHO. (2020a) *World Patient Safety Day 2020–2021 goals.* [Online] Available from: https://www.who.int/campaigns/world-patient-safety-day/sign-up-for-wpsd-2020-2021-goals. [Accessed on 15 July 2021].

WHO. (2020b) *Hepatitis B.* [Online] Available from: https://www.who.int/news-room/fact-sheets/detail/hepatitis-b. [Accessed on 18 July 2021].

WHO. (2020c) *Hepatitis C.* [Online] Available from: https://www.who.int/news-room/fact-sheets/detail/hepatitis-e. [Accessed on 17 April 2021].

WHO. (2020d) *World Malaria Report 2020: 20 Years of Global Progress and Challenges.* [Online] Available from: https://www.mmv.org/sites/default/files/uploads/docs/publications/World_Malaria_Report_2020.pdf. [Accessed on 29 July 2021].

WHO. (2021) *WHO guidelines for Malaria.* [Online] Available from: https://www.who.int/teams/global-malaria-programme/guidelines-for-malaria [Accessed on 29 July 2021].

World Health Organization Regional Office for the Eastern Mediterranean. (2021) *Middle East respiratory syndrome.* [Online] Available from: http://www.emro.who.int/health-topics/mers-cov/mers-outbreaks.html. [Accessed on 29 July 2021].

Wilmes P, Zimmer J, Schulz J, Glod F, Veiber L, Mombaerts L, Rodrigues B, Aalto A, Pastore J, Snoeck CJ, Ollert M, Fagherazzi G, Mossong J, Goncalves J, Skupin A, Nehrbass U. (2021) SARS-CoV-2 transmission risk from asymptomatic carriers: Results from a mass screening programme in Luxembourg. *Lancet Reg Health Eur* **4**: 100056.

Wong PSJ, Tan CH, Lee V, Li MZI, Lee KS, Lee PJ, Singh B, Ng LC. (2011) Molecular epidemiological investigation of *Plasmodium knowlesi* in humans and macaques in Singapore. *Vector-borne Zoonotic Dis* **11**(2): 131–135.

Wyzgowski P, Rosiek A, Grzela T, Leksowski K. (2016) Occupational HIV risk for health care workers: Risk factor and the risk of infection in the course of professional activities. *Ther Clin Risk Manag* **12**: 989–994.

Yeon JH, Seong H, Hur H, Park Y, Kim YA, Park YS, Han CH, Lee SM, Seo JH, Kang JG. (2018) Prevalence and risk factors of latent tuberculosis among Korean healthcare workers using whole-blood interferon-γ release assay. *Sci Rep* **8**(1): 10113.

Yu IT, Li Y, Wong TW, Tam W, Chan AT, Lee JH, Leung DY, Ho T. (2004) Evidence of airborne transmission of the severe acute respiratory syndrome virus. *N Engl J Med* **350**: 1731–1739.

Zhu N, Zhang D, Wang W, Li X, Yang B, Song J, Zhao X, Huang B, Shi W, Lu R, Niu P, Zhan F, Ma X, Wang D, Xu W, Wu G, Gao GF, Tan W, China Novel Coronavirus Investigating and Research Team. (2020) A novel coronavirus from patients with pneumonia in China, 2019. *N Engl J Med* **382**(8): 727–733.

Chapter 11

Renal Disorders

*Huw Rees**, *Doris T. Chan*†, *and Steve Riley*‡

Introduction

Kidney disease is a general term used to describe a broad range of clinical conditions that disrupt the structure and function of the kidney. The various clinical presentations can be attributed to a multitude of underlying causes, as well as, numerous renal and extra-renal pathological processes. Occupational and environmental exposures are important aetiological agents. This chapter provides an overview of kidney disease, followed by examples of recognised agents encountered in workplaces that can cause renal tract damage.

Overview of Kidney Disease

Definition and Classification of Kidney Disease

The international organisation Kidney Disease: Improving Global Outcomes (KDIGO) developed standardised definitions and

* College of Biomedical and Life Sciences, Cardiff University School of Medicine, Cardiff. South Wales Fire & Rescue Service, Llantrisant *and* Powys teaching Health Board, Bronllys, United Kingdom.
† Department of Renal Medicine, Sir Charles Gairdner Hospital, Nedlands, Australia.
‡ College of Biomedical and Life Sciences, Cardiff University School of Medicine, Cardiff, United Kingdom.
Corresponding author: Huw Rees (ReesHG1@cardiff.ac.uk).

Table 1. Definition and Staging of AKI (Khwaja, 2012)

AKI is defined as any of the following:

- Increase in SCr by ≥0.3 mg/dL (≥26.5 μmol/L) within 48 h; or
- Increase in SCr to ≥1.5 times baseline, which is known or presumed to have occurred within the prior 7 days; or
- Urine volume <0.5 mL/kg/h for 6 h.

Stage	Creatinine	Urine Output
1	1.5–1.9 times baseline OR ≥0.3 mg/dL (≥26.5 μmol/L) increase	<0.5 mL/kg/h for 6–12 h
2	2.0–2.9 times baseline	<0.5 mL/kg/h for ≥12 h
3	3.0 times baseline OR Increase in SCr to ≥4.0 mg/dL (≥353.6 μmol/L) OR Initiation of kidney replacement therapy OR, In patients <18 years, decrease in eGFR to <35 mL/min per 1.73 m^2	<0.3 mL/kg/h for ≥24 h OR Anuria for ≥12 h

classification systems for the different types of kidney disease based on the duration and severity of kidney impairment (Levey *et al.*, 2020b). Acute kidney injury (AKI) is defined as the abrupt decline in kidney function or glomerular filtration rate (GFR), within 48 h to 7 days, which may or may not be accompanied by loss of urine output (Table 1). Chronic kidney disease (CKD) is defined as the presence of kidney damage or gradual loss of kidney function for at least 3 months regardless of the underlying cause and sub-classified for presence of albuminuria (Fig. 1). Finally, the term acute kidney disease (AKD) was coined to define kidney damage or GFR <60 mL/min/1.73 m^2 which persists between 7 and 90 days from the onset kidney injury, without classification for severity. Loss of kidney function or GFR is estimated using serum creatinine (SCr)-based equations while structural abnormalities are identified through examination of urine and imaging of the renal tract.

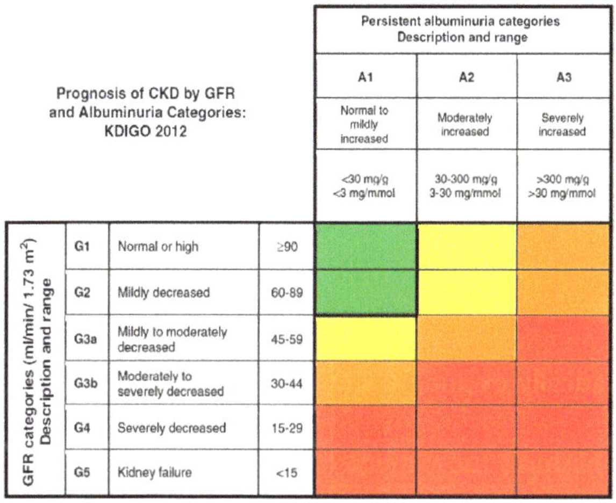

Green: low risk (if no other markers of kidney disease, no CKD); Yellow: moderately increased risk; Orange: high risk; Red, very high risk.

Fig. 1. Stages of CKD by GFR and albuminuria category (Levey *et al.*, 2011).

Standardisation in the definition and classification of kidney disease has provided a common language to allow for improved communication and awareness of kidney disease and its risk factors, enabled more accurate determination of the epidemiology of the various types of kidney disease, and facilitated the development of strategies for disease prevention, management and development of clinical practice guidelines to improve patient outcomes (Levey and Levin, 2017)

An important limitation of the AKI and CKD staging systems include the lack of consideration for the underlying aetiology or pathological diagnosis which may have important implications for disease progression and prognosis (Hall and Himmelfarb, 2017). In CKD, the absence of age-, gender- and race-related thresholds for GFR has the potential to mislabel otherwise stable and asymptomatic patients who may not require further evaluation or intervention. Both SCr and GFR are insensitive markers of kidney function and injury. Significant kidney disease may be present with little change in SCr or GFR due to adaptive changes in the glomeruli to maintain kidney function. GFR estimates are also inaccurate in non-steady state which is of particular importance when evaluating patients with AKI (Levey *et al.*, 2020a)

History Taking and Examination in Renal Disease

It is important to consider the clinical context within which the renal assessment is being made. When an abnormal SCr is identified the clinician should consider any previous records to distinguish between AKI, acute on CKD and CKD. The absence of a prior raised SCr does not automatically exclude CKD but should prompt the exclusion of an AKI.

In establishing the patient history the presence of co-morbidity provides an important indicator of potential kidney disease. Obtaining a thorough occupational history is equally important in order to identify and prevent toxic exposure which may further contribute to kidney impairment (see Occupational Renal Disease later in this chapter). Diabetes mellitus, cardiovascular disease, alongside other chronic disease are risk factors for the presence of both AKI and CKD. A history of diarrhea, vomiting, heart failure and sepsis all hint towards reduced kidney perfusion and likely pre-renal insult. There should be a high index of suspicion for a post-renal or obstructive cause in those with a known prior history of renal calculi, prostatomegaly or intraabdominal malignancy. Symptoms that relate to potential kidney dysfunction include difficulties in micturition (poor urine flow, frequency or dysuria), the observation of visible haematuria, or pain related to the renal angle or lumbar region. Whilst non-specific, the presence of peripheral edema, new onset shortness of breath or rash could also indicate kidney problems. It is important to consider medication use, either prescribed or over the counter, as many drugs can have nephrotoxic effects, e.g. renin–angiotensin receptor blockers, non-steroidal anti-inflammatory drugs (NSAIDs) or cyclooxygenase-2 (COX-2) inhibitors.

The examination should seek to establish direct evidence of kidney problems and its causes. Hypertension is a common cause and consequence of CKD, and its presence, particularly in the younger age groups should lead to a formal evaluation of kidney function. On the other hand, hypotension in the right clinical context would support a pre-renal cause for kidney injury. Abdominal examination should seek to identify palpable kidneys that may be the result of polycystic kidney disease, the presence of a renal bruit that might indicate renal vascular disease or an enlarged bladder indicating bladder outflow obstruction. The examination of the prostate, in men, is an important consideration should there be any concerns about bladder outflow obstruction.

Figure 2 highlights important clinical considerations when assessing a patient with abnormal kidney function. Following this flow chart will guide the generalist through some of the diagnostic considerations and help in discussions with specialist teams during referral (Fig. 2).

Assessment of Kidney Function

Serum creatinine

SCr is the most commonly used marker to estimate renal function given that it is principally excreted through the kidneys by filtration and has minimal tubular reabsorption. It is the ideal marker for serial monitoring of kidney function given its low cost, convenience (single blood sample) and wide availability. However, its accuracy is affected by factors that affect muscle mass such as age, gender, race, consumption of red meat and degree of renal impairment.

Equations to estimate glomerular filtration rate

Whereas direct measurement of GFR is cumbersome, the availability of traceable SCr assays and SCr-based equations to better estimate GFR (eGFR) have allowed for routine reporting of eGFR in most laboratories around the world. The 2009 Chronic Kidney Disease Epidemiology Collaboration (CKD-EPI) creatinine equation has now overtaken the 4-variable Modification of Diet in Renal Disease study (MDRD) equation as the preferred method for calculating eGFR in North America, Europe and Australia (Levey *et al.*, 2020a). However, it is important to note that these equations may still be unreliable in those at extremes of age and body weight, in those with excess dietary

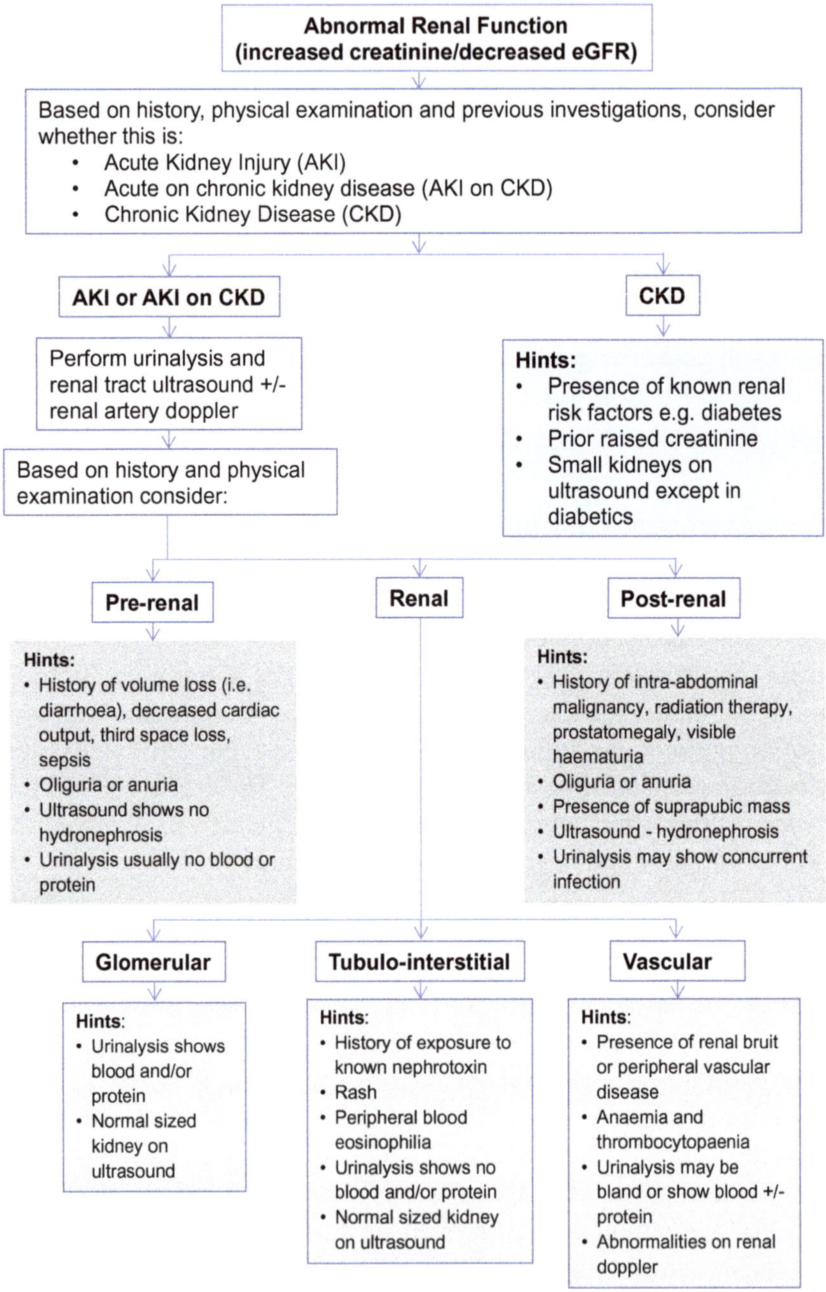

Fig. 2. Assessment of the patient with abnormal kidney function.

intake of creatinine or creatine, in the presence of muscle diseases or atrophy, and in some ethnic groups. Furthermore, neither equation has been validated in patients with AKI. In some, confirmatory testing utilising eGFR based on serum cystatin ($eGFR_{cys}$) or the combination of SCr and cystatin ($eGFR_{cr\text{-}cys}$) or formal measurement of GFR using exogenous filtration marker may be considered (Levey *et al.*, 2020a).

Clinical Syndromes

Patients with kidney disease are often asymptomatic and the diagnosis is largely dependent on measurement of GFR using SCr, examination of the urine or kidney imaging. However, there are a few clinical syndromes which should alert towards the presence of an underlying intrinsic kidney disease (Table 2).

Table 2. Clinical Syndromes and Examples of Primary Renal Pathological Diagnoses

Clinical Syndrome	Primary Renal Pathological Diagnoses
Asymptomatic haematuria	IgA nephropathy Thin basement membrane disease Alport's syndrome Polycystic kidney disease Henoch Schonlein purpura
Asymptomatic proteinuria	Membranous nephropathy Focal segmental glomerulosclerosis Laminopathies
Nephrotic syndrome	Minimal change disease Membranous nephropathy Focal segmental glomerulosclerosis Laminopathies
Acute nephritis	Post-infectious glomerulonephritis Mesangiocapillary/membranoproliferative glomerulonephritis
Rapidly progressive glomerulonephritis	ANCA positive associated vasculitis Anti-glomerular basement membrane disease
Chronic glomerulonephritis	Any of the primary renal pathological diagnoses

Haematuria

Haematuria, defined as the presence of red blood cells (RBC) in the urine, can either be visible (gross or macroscopic haematuria) or detected only by urine dipstick or microscopy (micro-haematuria). Given the high false positive and negative rates associated with urine dipsticks, urine microscopy is required to confirm the diagnosis of micro-haematuria and exclude spurious causes which do not require further investigation (Table 3). However, it is important to recognise haematuria (visible and non-visible) in the presentation of renal tract cancer, depending on age and risk factors, and the timely investigation of true haematuria through referral via local urological guidelines. Micro-haematuria is formally defined as the presence of more than 3 RBC per high powered field (HPF) in two or more properly collected urine samples, and in the absence of an obvious benign cause (Sharp *et al.*, 2013).

Micro-haematuria is often asymptomatic and is usually detected as part of routine medical examination such as pre-employment medicals. Patients with asymptomatic haematuria may require a renal biopsy to obtain a histological diagnosis if associated with abnormal or worsening renal function and/or significant proteinuria.

Proteinuria and nephrotic syndrome

The glomerular basement membrane of the kidney is an effective barrier to the appearance of large molecular proteins such as albumin and other proteins into the urine. It is injury to this filtration barrier and its associated structures that lead to the presence of an abnormal

Table 3. Some Causes of Spurious Haematuria

Benign Causes of Haematuria	Causes of "Red Urine"
Recent exercise	Haemoglobinuria (false + dipstick)
Menses	Myoglobinuria (false + dipstick)
Sexual activity	Foods: beetroot, rhubarb, carrots, blackberries
Recent instrumentation	Medications: rifampicin, isoniazid, methyldopa, senna, povidone iodine others
	Porphyria
	Factitious

Table 4. Classification of Proteinuria

	Albumin: Creatinine in mg/g (mg/mmol)	Protein: Creatinine Ratio mg/g (mg/mmol)
Normal	<30 (<3.5)	<150 (<15)
Microalbuminuria	30–300 (3.5–35)	—
Macroalbuminuria or macroproteinuria	>300 (>30)	>450 (>45)
Nephrotic range proteinuria	—	>3,000 (>300)

Notes: To convert mg/g to mg/mmol, multiply by 0.113.
To convert mg/mmol to g/day, divide by 100.

amount of protein in the urine. Proteinuria is often used interchangeably with albuminuria, particularly in diabetic kidney disease, given that albumin is the predominant protein in the blood. Proteinuria is typically classified based on the amount of albumin or protein found in the urine as measured preferably in a spot urine sample (albumin creatinine ratio or protein creatinine ratio) or alternatively using a 24-h urine sample (Table 4).

Nephrotic syndrome is characterised by the presence of heavy proteinuria, defined as >3.0 g of protein excretion per day, peripheral edema and hypoalbuminaemia (serum albumin of <30 g/L or <3.0 g/dL). Other associated features include hypertension, hyperlipidaemia and lipiduria. All patients with nephrotic range proteinuria or nephrotic syndrome require further assessment and referral to a nephrologist regardless of kidney function. Diabetic kidney disease is the most common secondary cause of nephrotic syndrome in adults. Amongst the primary glomerulonephritis, the commonest cause of nephrotic syndrome in adults are membranous nephropathy (recent evidence shows an association with the presence of anti-phospholipase A2R antibody) and focal segmental glomerulosclerosis, followed by minimal change nephropathy.

Acute nephritis and rapidly progressive glomerulonephritis

Acute nephritis is characterised by acute onset oliguria with impaired kidney function and passing of dark or "coca-cola" colored urine. This is usually associated with edema, hypertension and presence of haematuria and proteinuria on urinalysis. On the other hand, rapidly progressive glomerulonephritis (RPGN) is used to describe haemoproteinuria that is associated with a rapid decline in GFR over days to months. Systemic symptoms may be present but are often subtle. Both acute nephritis and RPGN are medical emergencies which require immediate nephrology referral for further assessment given that delay in initiation of therapy can lead to irreversible kidney injury.

Chronic glomerulonephritis

Patients with chronic glomerulonephritis are often asymptomatic and may only come to attention due to hypertension. Diagnosis is often based on the presence of advanced stage CKD, persistent haematuria and or proteinuria, and small kidney size on imaging.

Clinical Consequence of Renal Disease

There is increasing recognition that both AKI and CKD have immediate and long-term adverse consequences not only for the affected individual but also on the healthcare system. AKI has been associated with significant increase in patient mortality, duration of hospitalisation and cost (Ikizler *et al.*, 2021). CKD is associated with a markedly increased risk of cardiovascular disease (CVD)-related morbidity and mortality and is still considered as the “highest risk group” for CVD that contributes significantly to global morbidity and mortality (GBD Chronic Kidney Disease Collaboration, 2020). Complications of CKD which include hypertension, anaemia, malnutrition, bone disease, neuropathy and decline in overall functional status begins when GFR falls below 60 mL/min/1.73 m^2 and this worsens progressively with decline in renal function. Recently, there is growing recognition that AKI and CKD form part of a continuum rather than distinct clinical syndromes with shared risk factors and outcomes (Duff and Murray, 2020). This highlights the need for a coordinated multidisciplinary approach to the early identification and initiation of appropriate management for both syndromes to reduce disease progression and improve patient outcome.

Occupational Renal Disease

The kidneys have a very high blood flow, are the principal excretory organs in the body, and have a smaller but significant metabolic and storage functions. Because of this they have high exposures to environmental toxins leading to acute cortical injury, CKD and stage 5 kidney failure.

Case Study 1: A Worker With Chronic Kidney Disease

Mr. A is a 45 year old electrician/maintenance craftsman working for a municipal authority in the United Kingdom (UK).

In 2009, he is diagnosed with hypertension, and treated by his General Practitioner. In 2014 he presents with fatigue, has a serum creatinine estimation and is diagnosed with chronic kidney disease. The precise cause is not clear. He is referred to an occupational health department by his manager. He is treated with four different anti-hypertensive drugs, and his blood pressure is well controlled, without any postural hypotension. His nephrologist has told him that he will probably have to start dialysis treatment within the next 12 months. He might be eligible to receive a kidney transplant "in a few years' time."

Mr. A complains of tiredness and finds difficulty coping with the prospect of having dialysis treatment. However, he does not want to retire because he does not have many years' pension contributions. Neither does he want to see the counsellor attached to the occupational health department.

Over the next two years he takes several weeks' sickness absence each year with a variety of symptoms, and this takes him over his employer's policy threshold for management action. His occupational physician advises the manager that he probably falls within the remit of the UK 2010 Equality Act (Office for Disability Issues, 2015), and that "reasonable adjustments" should be made to accommodate him in work. His manager discounts some of his sickness absence. Mr. A is given regular appointments at the Occupational Health Department, but attends only sporadically.

Mr. A's kidney function deteriorates, in 2017 an arterio-venous fistula is created and he starts haemodialysis. He needs dialysis three times a week, with each session lasting about four hours at a hospital 30 km from his home. This means that his shift pattern has to be altered to accommodate the treatment. The renal unit offers him a dialysis machine at home, that would save hours of travelling time but he declines, because he does not want the responsibility of complex equipment in his home. He is also offered peritoneal dialysis comprising either four 30-minute exchanges each day or an automated system to run overnight, but he lacks the confidence to proceed with this.

He complains of tiredness, but insists that he is able to carry out all his duties. He continues to take several weeks' sickness absence each year with ill-defined symptoms. On one occasion he takes two weeks sick leave after being admitted to the local district general hospital with fluid overload — it emerged that he typically drank three pints of beer, several nights a week. He complains that he is under pressure from his manager to take less sick leave.

In the following years, his sickness absence record improves, but his work output remains low.

Efficient occupational health management is often a long-term process of negotiation between the occupational clinician, the employee and the manager. This should be informed by local health and safety legislation, equality legislation, and ethical considerations such as beneficence and patient autonomy. It is possible that a small commercial company would not have been able to afford the adjustments given to Mr. A.

Chemicals Toxic to the Kidneys

A number of industrial materials cause AKI related to the level of exposure. For example, arsenic (As) causes acute tubular necrosis and bladder cancer, while arsine (AsH_3) gas causes acute tubular necrosis as a direct effect, but also secondary to haemolysis and haemoglobinuria. Such materials are toxic to multiple organ systems (Table 5).

There is sometimes a clear association between disease and occupational exposure; for example AKI following arsine exposure, or CKD in workers with very high body burdens of heavy metals that are readily estimated. However, very often the cause of stage 5 kidney

Table 5. Toxic Effects of Arsenic (Agency for Toxic Substances & Disease Registry, 2007)

Acute Effects	Chronic Effects
GI tract inflammation/ corrosion following ingestion	Skin pigmentation, keratosis and squamous cell carcinoma
Circulatory collapse	Peripheral neuritis
Acute renal tubular necrosis	Fatty cardiac degeneration and conduction defects
	Skin, lung and bladder cancer

failure cannot be identified (Warrell *et al.*, 2010; Jameson *et al.*, 2018). Several factors make epidemiological studies difficult. Renal toxicants do not usually produce unique histological changes, most occupational renal toxicity has a long latent period, and there may be multiple confounders, e.g. several different toxic exposures, hypertension and diabetes mellitus (Schnellmann, 2019) In developing countries, exposure may occur via both occupational and non-occupational routes. For example mercury from eating sea-food, and cadmium from arable crops (Ufelle and Barchowsy, 2019) For the most part, surveillance data on the prevalence of acute occupational kidney injury and chronic occupational kidney disease are not available. Case reports in the modern medical literature are rare, but are probably under-reported from developing and middle-income countries.

Kidney disease nomenclature is complex. Table 6 summarises the histo-pathological changes and clinical syndromes following different occupational insults.

Filtration of high molecular weight protein (principally albumin) and loss from the glomerulus into Bowman's capsule is normally very limited, but following glomerular damage, albuminuria occurs. Similarly, the proximal tubule normally reabsorbs most low-molecular weight proteins, but following damage, these are lost, along-with enzymuria from the brush border (Schnellmann, 2019). AKI is identified by measuring SCr, and identifying reduced urine output. Occupational epidemiological studies typically employ more sensitive markers of AKI such as micro-proteinuria (β2-microglobulin, alpha-1 microglobulin, or retinol binding protein) and enzymuria (N-acetyl-β-D-glucosaminidase, gamma glutamyl transpeptidase,

Table 6. Occupational Renal Insults (Warrell *et al.*, 2010; Jameson *et al.*, 2018; Schnellmann, 2019)

Toxic Insult	Histo-Pathological Change	Clinical Syndrome
Heavy metals Mercuric chloride Arsenic Arsine (haemoglobinuria) Carbon tetrachloride Toluene Venoms Dehydration (pre-renal failure) Heat stroke Trauma (myoglobinuria)	Acute tubular necrosis	AKI CKD
Lead Cadmium	Proximal tubular damage, Chronic Tubulo-interstitial nephritis	CKD CKD
Mercury	Membranous Glomerulonephropathy	CKD
Hydrocarbons	Anti-glomerular basement membrane disease	Rapidly progressing glomerulonephritis AKI CKD

or alkaline phosphatase). They are principally used as research tools, and while toxicity causing micro-proteinuria and enzymuria is clearly undesirable, there is a lack of robust longitudinal studies demonstrating that micro-proteinuria or enzymuria progress to CKD (De Broe *et al.*, 2010; Byber *et al.*, 2016; Scientific Committee on Occupational Exposure Limits (SCOEL), 2017)

The rest of this section will describe the principal industrial substances associated with chronic occupational renal disease.The chapter will only briefly describe their other toxic effects. Other substances with renal effects, such as bismuth, silver, copper sulfate, and uranium will not be discussed (Murunga and Zawada, 2007).

In general, only limited treatment is available for the conditions described, and primary prevention using the hierarchy of control is essential (National Institute for Occupational Safety and Health (NIOSH), 2015).

Lead and Compounds

Exposures and prevalence of disease

Inorganic lead compounds are widely used in industry because of their density, anticorrosive properties, malleability and colour (Tables 7 and 8)

The People's Republic of China is currently the principal producer and user of lead in the world (International Lead Association, 2020). In developing countries, substantial occupational exposure occurs from activities such as smelting, recycling lead from batteries and craft industries like the manufacture of fishing weights, fire-arm bullets and

Table 7. Industrial Exposure to Inorganic Lead Compounds

Use	Mode of Exposure
Metallic lead and alloys	Smelting Recycling plants
Lead acid batteries	Manufacture
PVC plastic stabilisers	Manufacture
Lead pigments	Pottery manufacture
Lead painted steel structures Lead sheathed cabling	Demolition and scrap work
Bullets	Manufacture and firing ranges

Table 8. Estimated World Lead Usage (International Lead Association, 2020)

Year	Total Usage
2002	6.67 million tonnes
2012	10.54 million tonnes

traditional cosmetics. Waste from old industrial sites also causes high exposures. In lower-income socio-economic groups, occupational and non-occupational exposures often over-lap (Meyer *et al.*, 2008; Ye and Wong, 2006; United Nations Environment Programme (UNEP), 2010b; International Lead Association, 2020; Agency for Toxic Substances and Disease Registry, 2020).

In developed countries lead production and usage is declining. In the United States for example, lead levels in general populations have fallen substantially in recent decades, reflecting reductions in both occupational and non-occupational exposure (Centers for Disease Control & Prevention, 2020). Reports of occupational toxicity in the recent literature are rare (Kaneko *et al.*, 2020; Zhang *et al.*, 2016). However, Zhang *et al.* (2010) estimated that between 1990 and 2005, most Chinese work-places exceeded Occupational Exposure Standards for Lead. Despite the emergence of occupational health services in the People's Republic of China, national surveillance data on occupational lead toxicity is not published. It is calcuated that in 2017 lead caused 1.06 million deaths world-wide, largely from cardiovascular conditions. The highest rates were in low and middle income countries (World Health Organization (WHO), 2020a).

The threshold of exposure at which lead causes CKD is not clear, and evidence from studies in general populations and lead workers give apparently conflicting results. Large cross-sectional studies of general populations suggest that relatively low blood lead levels (e.g. <5–10 μg/100 mL of blood) may be a risk factor (Agency for Toxic Substances and Disease Registry, 2020; Ekong *et al.*, 2006). Because of persistent lead storage in the body, these observations may be confounded by high historical exposures, and similar evidence from prospective studies are only available from small population samples.

In contrast, large prospective cohort studies of lead workers with mean blood lead levels of 19.6 μg/100 mL (Gwini *et al.*, 2012) and 44.3 μg/100 mL (McElvenny *et al.*, 2015) showed little increased mortality from renal diseases. But these studies may have been confounded by the healthy worker effect (Hu *et al.*, 2007).

The bulk of both occupational and non-occupational exposure probably results from ingestion and inhalation of lead dust. Inhalation is more important when there are high levels of airborne fume or dust. Lead is persistent in the environment, and is not degraded. Due to their low water solubility and sequestration in bone, most lead compounds are not bio-concentrated in food chains.

In the past, organic lead compounds such as tetramethyl lead (TML) and tetraethyl lead (TEL) were widely used as antiknock agents in gasoline to control combustion in engine ignition chambers. This resulted in general population exposures, and occupational exposures during maintenance work in gasoline storage tanks. In most countries these have been substituted with substances such as methyl-tert-butyl-ether (MTBE) (Meyer *et al.*, 2008), and general population exposures have declined.

Toxicokinetics

Lead is a heavy metal with a relatively low melting point, and most inorganic lead compounds are insoluble in water. By comparison, organic TML and TEL are lipid soluble and slightly volatile. The way lead and other renal toxicants are absorbed, distributed, stored and excreted from the body (i.e. the toxickinetics) determines their toxicity.

All lead compounds are widely distributed in the body. Ninety percent of lead is stored in bone (Pb^{2+} probably substitutes for Ca^{2+}), with a half-life of 10–20 years. Smaller quantities are stored in soft tissue, including the kidneys, with a half-life of 20–40 days. Most lead is excreted in the urine. After cessation of lead exposure there are three phases of excretion with respective half-lives of 1 month, 1 year and 20 years. Organic lead compounds such as TML and TEL are also absorbed efficiently through the skin (Agency for Toxic Substances and Disease Registry, 2020).

Mechanisms of toxicity

Lead does not have any physiological function. It bonds covalently with the enzyme δ-aminolevulinic acid dehydratase (δALAD), which contributes to haem synthesis. By inhibiting this and other enzymes, it

Table 9. Effects of Lead on Haem Synthesis

Enzyme Inhibited	Biological Effect
δ-aminolevulinic acid dehydratase	↑ urinary δALAD
Coproporphyrinogen Oxidase	↑ urine coproporphyrin
Ferrochelatase	↑ erythrocyte protoporphyrin

produces anaemia and changes in body levels of several intermediates (Table 9) (Agency for Toxic Substances and Disease Registry, 2020).

Lead exposure increases erythrocyte protoporphyrin levels, zinc occupies the site normally occupied by iron, and the complex is commonly referred to as zinc protoporphyrin (ZPP).

Clinical features

Inorganic lead sometimes produces acute renal toxicity. The acute effects seem to be caused by the deposition of lead-protein complex in proximal tubular cells. There is a Fanconi type syndrome with proximal tubular nephropathy, glycosuria, aminoaciduria and phosphate loss (Agency for Toxic Substances and Disease Registry, 2020).

Chronic lead toxicity is characterised by progressive tubular atrophy, interstitial fibrosis, glomerulosclerosis, hypertension, hyperuricaemia, "saturnine" gout, and CKD. Increased levels of low molecular weight proteins and enzymes indicative of proximal tubular damage have been noted, but proteinuria is typically minimal.

In chronic poisoning subjects complain of fatigue, anorexia, vomiting, abdominal pain and altered bowel habit. A Burtonian blue line of lead sulphide on the gum margins may be seen, but is less common nowadays .

Health effects from lead exposure and co-conditions like diabetes, hypertension and cardio-vascular disease are synergistic (Agency for Toxic Substances and Disease Registry, 2020). Release of lead from bone and elevated blood levels can occur in acidosis, hypocalcaemia, hypothyroidism and old age (Rosin, 2009). Vitamin D receptor genotype may affect susceptibility to hypertension in people exposed to lead (Gidlow, 2015).

Investigations and health surveillance

Blood lead is the standard method of biological monitoring for exposure and toxicity. The level at a particular point in time will depend on several inter-related factors.

1. High environmental exposure in the preceding weeks and months.
2. At lower levels of contemporary exposure it will reflect the equilibrium between release of lead from bone and excretion from the body. The latter is largely from the kidneys, and will be impaired in CKD.
3. High bone lead levels will reflect exposure over decades (Hu *et al.*, 2007).

The various OELs for lead in the USA have been harmonised (Table 10), but for other substances may differ. Similarly, OELs in other countries often differ from these. These OELs usually prevent toxicity, but hypertension may occur at blood lead levels as low as 5–10 μg/100 mL (Gidlow, 2015).

While blood lead is a good parameter of recent exposure over weeks or months (Hu *et al.*, 2007), it a poor indicator of long-term

Table 10. Occupational Exposure Limits (OELs) for Inorganic Lead in the USA

OELs for Inorganic Pb	Organisation	Status
Permissible exposure limit (PEL) 0.05 mg/m^3 in air	Occupational Safety and Health Administration (OSHA, 2020)	Legally enforcible
Recommended exposure limit (REL) 0.05 mg/m^3 in air	NIOSH, 2020	Advisory, not legally enforcible
Threshold limit value (TLV) 0.05 mg/m^3 in air	American Conference of Governmental Industrial Hygienists (ACGIH, 2020)	Advisory, not legally enforcible
Biological exposure index (BEI) 200 μg/L (20 μg/dL) in blood	ACGIH, 2020	Advisory, not legally enforcible

body burden that is the main contributor to end-organ disease (Gidlow, 2015). This might be overcome by using serial estimations to calculate Cumulative Blood Lead index (Hu *et al.*, 2007).

Urinary δ-ALAD and blood zinc protoporphyrin are also used for biological effect monitoring, but are usually normal when blood lead is less than 60 μg/100 mL (SCOEL, 2002).

Body burden can be estimated using an EDTA lead mobilisation test (Sokas *et al.*, 1988; Hoet *et al.*, 2006). In epidemiological studies of general populations, K line X-ray fluorescence has been used since the 1990s as an adjunct to blood lead to estimate body burden (Hu *et al.*, 2007). Hu describes measurements in cortical bone of the tibia or patella taking 30 min with radiation exposures of less than 0.1 μSv. Total body burden is calculated and expressed as μgPb/g of bone mineral normalised to calcium counts. Measurements are reasonably precise but prone to error if the subject moves, or has excessive overlying adipose tissue. The method has also been used to monitor occupational exposure (Lee, 1999). Occupational Exposure Limits for μgPb/g of bone do not appear to have been developed, so single measurements are of limited use. However, monitoring body burden over a period of years in a large, stable occupational work-force would identify increasing body burden and hot-spots of exposure.

Mitigating exposure and treatment

The principal method of reducing lead toxicity is to prevent exposure using the hierarchy of control. Symptomatic lead toxicity can be treated with calcium disodium edetate or dimercapto succinic acid (DMSA) (Bradberry and Vale, 2009; Sakthithasan *et al.*, 2018).

Case Study 2: Lead Toxicity

A 55 year old British man was identified working on the demolition of a local power-station by a Health and Safety Executive Factory Inspector, and persuaded to consult a general practitioner for a blood lead estimation.

He had worked for decades as a demolition worker, and was exposed to lead fume when torch-cutting old steel structures coated with lead paint.

His work was sporadic, moving from site to site across the country, and his given address was a lodging house in a local port-area. He frequently changed address, and denied having a permanent residence. He was self-employed as a sub-contractor for different companies, and compliance with the UK Control of Lead at Work Regulations was lax. It was suspected that much of his work was "cash in hand," avoiding income tax payments to Her Majesty's Revenues & Customs.

He gave a history of gout, admitted to drinking 30 pints of beer a week, had mild hypertension (160/98), and was obese (Body Mass Index 34). He had a moderately low eGFR of 50 ml/min/1.73m^2, but no albuminuria. His blood lead was 55 μg/dl. The latter is just over the UK Health and Safety Executive Action Level of 50 μg/dl requiring investigation of control procedures, but below the Suspension Level of 60 μg/dl requiring removal from the workplace (Health and Safety Executive (HSE), 2002). His blood zinc protoporphyrin was normal.

He was reluctant to engage with medical services or Factory Inspectors. He had no academic qualifications or other skills, and feared both being suspended from work with loss of earnings, and prosecution for tax evasion.

He seemed to have mild lead toxicity with Saturnine gout, but it was not clear what proportion of his hypertension was related to lead, obesity or alcohol consumption. Because his lead exposure was chronic but episodic, his blood lead may have under-estimated his lead body burden, so a lead mobilisation test was planned.

Despite the free, integrated medical services in the UK, he was lost to medical and regulatory follow-up before the lead mobilisation test could be completed.

Mercury and Mercury Compounds

Exposures and prevalence of disease

Mercury occurs naturally in the earth's crust and is continually released into the environment (e.g. in volcanic eruptions). However, around two thirds of total atmospheric mercury is estimated to be derived from human activities. Mercury is not degraded to less harmful products in the environment and all forms are toxic. There

Table 11. Industrial Uses of Mercury Compounds (Agency for Toxic Substances and Disease Registry, 1999)

Mercury Compound	Physical Form	Use
Elemental mercury	Liquid–vapor	Electrolytic electrodes Temperature and pressure instruments electric lights Dental amalgams Batteries Laboratories Recycled materials
Mercuric chloride (i.e. mercury dichloride $HgCl_2$)	Solid–vapor	Chemical industry intermediates
Mercuric oxide HgO	Solid	Batteries (very small usage)
Mercury fulminate Hg $(CHNO)_2$	Solid	Detonators

is continuous cycling between organic and inorganic forms in the air, soil and water, where it enters the food chain (Ufelle and Barchowsy, 2019).

Elemental and inorganic compounds of mercury are used industrially, and these have different toxic effects (Table 11).

In the developed world, primary mercury production and industrial uses such as mercury cells in the chloralkali industry (to produce chlorine and sodium hydroxide from salt water) have been declining for several decades and occupational toxicity is rare (Agency for Toxic Substances and Disease Registry, 1999).

However, between 2010 and 2015 global anthropogenic emissions increased by 20%, and in Asia increased by 49%. Artisanal and small-scale occupational use of mercury is estimated to contribute 38% of emissions world-wide, largely in sub-Saharan Africa and South America (UNEP, 2019a; UNEP, 2019b). Artisan gold miners obtain ore by digging or panning, extract the gold using mercury to form an amalgam, and heat the amalgam to evaporate the mercury (Seccatore *et al.*, 2014; Tomicic *et al.*, 2011).

Little information is available on the global prevalence of occupational mercury toxicity. Recent studies of small populations exposed to industrial mercury demonstrated that rising urine (Zhang *et al.*,

2020) and blood (Afrifa *et al.*, 2017) mercury levels were associated with falling eGFR. However most eGFR remained within normal levels, and measurement of blood mercury would not have quantified long-term exposure.

Case Study 3: Mercury Exposure in Artisanal Gold Miners in Burkino Faso

In 2011, Tomicic et al studied 93 small-scale gold miners in Burkino Faso (Tomicic et al., 2011). They found that 69% of urine samples exceeded the then ACGIH Biological Exposure Index (BEI) of 35 µg mercury per gram creatinine, and many miners reported symptoms of mercury toxicity. Since then, the ACGIH has reduced the BEI has to 20 µg/g creatinine (ACGIH, 2020)

Non-occupational mercury poisoning can be an important problem in developing countries. Aquatic micro-organisms convert inorganic mercury to highly toxic short-chain organic compounds, which then ascend the food-chain and are consumed by people. For example, between 1953 and 1966, industrial mercury effluents released in Minimata Bay in Japan accumulated in seafood and caused widespread poisoning. In 1971–1972, grain treated with alkyl mercury compounds also caused mass poisoning in Iraq (Bakir et al., 1973). However, the relationship between body burden and CKD world-wide is not clear.

In developed countries environmental mercury levels are usually well controlled. Mercury in dental amalgam gives individuals with fillings continuous mercury exposure. This is usually below toxic levels (Bates, 2006; Ufelle and Barchowsy, 2019) but occasional significant exposures spanning recommended biological exposure levels are seen. Bruxism or gum-chewing are thought to be contributory (Barregard *et al.*, 1995).

Toxicokinetics

Mercury exists in three oxidation states: elemental mercury Hg^0, monovalent mercurous mercury Hg_2^{2+}, and divalent mercuric mercury Hg^{2+}. Elemental mercury is a metallic liquid at room temperature. Its vapor pressure of 0.0012 mm Hg at first sight appears low, but in poorly ventilated areas, evaporation can lead to toxicity. Mercury

Table 12. Toxicokinetics of Mercury Compounds (Ufelle and Barchowsy, 2019)

	Elemental Mercury	Mercuric Chloride	Organic Mercury
Absorption	Lung	Gut	Lung, gut and skin
Accumulation	Kidneys and CNS	Kidneys and CNS	Central nervous system, kidneys
Excretion	Urine	Urine	Faeces

also forms toxic inorganic and organic compounds. Most mercury compounds are readily decomposed by heat, light and weak reducing agents, releasing elemental mercury (Agency for Toxic Substances and Disease Registry, 1999).

Table 12 summarises the toxicokinetics of mercury and its compounds. Following absorption, elemental and divalent inorganic mercury are subject to oxidation-reduction interconversion in the body. Concentrations of methyl mercury in the renal cortex are especially high. In tissues, particularly the kidney, mercury cations bind to metallothionein, a low molecular weight protein. Mercuric mercury induces metallothionein synthesis in kidney tissue, and metallothionein sequestration probably acts as a form of detoxification.

Most elemental and inorganic mercury is shed via the urine, but following low level exposures only small amounts are excreted, with the remainder being retained.

Short chain organic compounds like methyl mercury are very resistant to biotransformation, with most excreted in the faeces after enterohepatic circulation. However, aryl and alkoxyalkyl organic compounds are more labile, are slowly broken down to inorganic forms, and excreted in the urine (Agency for Toxic Substances and Disease Registry, 2013).

Mechanisms of toxicity and clinical features

Elemental mercury toxicity

Chronic exposure to elemental mercury gives a classic triad of nephropathy, tremor and gingivitis. Kidney effects comprise glomerular and tubular damage. Animal experiments suggest a two-phase immunological insult. Firstly an anti-basement membrane glomerulonephritis, and secondly an immune complex glomerulonephritis (Klaunig and Kamendulis, 2008). In human poisoning various glomerular lesions can occur, including membranous glomerulonephritis and minimal change disease which can present as nephrotic syndrome (Miller *et al.*, 2013).

Multiple and severe central nervous system (CNS) effects may develop ("mercurialism") and can be permanent. There is increased flushing and sweating with neuropsychiatric changes ("erethism") and sometimes allergic skin reactions.

Mercury compounds: Toxicity

Mercuric chloride and other salts are very irritant, with corrosive effects following ingestion or skin contact. Occupational exposures rarely cause acute systemic toxicity. Deliberate ingestion of mercuric chloride leads to renal tubular damage, and high exposures result in acute renal papillary necrosis, oliguria and kidney failure (Ufelle and Barchowsy, 2019). In these circumstances, blood mercury levels are a useful marker of exposure (Baxter and Igisu, 2010).

Chronic exposure to divalent inorganic mercury compounds causes kidney and CNS similar to elemental mercury. They also cause allergic skin reactions. Chronic exposure to organic mercury, particularly alkyl mercury, gives severe and irreversible CNS effects.

Investigations and health surveillance

Biological monitoring of elemental and inorganic mercury exposure

Lauwerys and Hoet (Lauwerys and Hoet, 2001) and Mason (Mason *et al.*, 2001) detail biological monitoring using total inorganic mercury levels in urine. These reflect average exposure to both elemental and inorganic mercury over the previous 2–4 months.

The ACGIH recommends a Biological Exposure Index (BEI) of 20 ug/g creatinine, in urine collected before starting work-shifts (ACGIH, 2020). Urine mercury values are customarily corrected by laboratories for creatinine to minimise errors caused by variable water excretion and urine concentration. The rationale for early morning urine collection is that it minimises intra-individual variation in body burden, and contamination from work-place clothing etc.

Urine excretion is biphasic, with a peak level 10 days following high exposure and up to 6 months following low exposure. Thus results are easier to interpret following a prolonged period of routine occupational exposure.

Whole blood mercury reflects elemental and inorganic mercury exposure over recent days, and can therefore only be used to assess acute exposure.

Biological monitoring of organic mercury exposure

Exposure to short-chain alkyl mercury compounds such as methyl mercury is best monitored by measuring whole blood mercury. Single specimens can be collected at any time of the day. Dietary sources, e.g. fish can affect biological monitoring results for mercury.

Aryl and alkoxyalkyl organic mercury derivatives are more easily metabolised to inorganic mercury in the body, when compared with short-chain compounds, and measurement of both blood and urine mercury may be appropriate.

While the heavy metal content of hair is useful for estimating dietary exposures in general populations, its use is problematic in health surveillance of occupational exposures, because of incidental surface contamination of the scalp.

Biological effect monitoring of mercury exposure

Excretion of high molecular weight proteins like albumin (albuminuria) suggests glomerular damage. If high mercury exposures are possible, e.g. in the chloralkali industry, regular urine dip stick tests for protein provide a sensitive but relatively non-specific marker of morbidity, flagging the need for measurement of urine mercury.

Damage to the proximal tubule also increases urine excretion of low molecular weight proteins (Agency for Toxic Substances and Disease Registry, 1999). These have been proposed as parameters for biological effect monitoring for mercury, but seem to be used principally as research tools (Barregard *et al.*, 2008).

Employees with significant exposure to any form of mercury will need regular health surveillance. Those with eczema have a higher risk of skin absorption following dermal contact with mercury compounds, and should take careful hygiene precautions.

Mitigating exposure and treatment

Working surfaces for elemental mercury should be smooth and intact, to prevent the retention of spilled material. The latter can present a long-term hazard, and should be carefully cleared up. Small spillages may be removed using a vacuum device, but this must incorporate a mercury vapor filter, to avoid spreading air-borne contamination. Larger spills can be absorbed by sprinkling sulphur and leaving overnight to form an amalgam, or by using a commercial mercury spill kit. Waste mercury should only be disposed of via licensed contractors.

Chelation therapy with sodium 2,3-dimercaptopropane sulphonate (DMPS) or dimercapto succinic acid (DMSA) should be considered if blood or urine mercury levels exceed current reference ranges. For example, 25 nmol/L (5 μg/L) in blood and 6 nmol/mmol creatinine (10 μg/g creatinine] in urine. Expert advice must be sought before starting treatment (National Poisons Information Service, 2012).

Cadmium

Exposures and prevalance of disease

Cadmium is produced primarily from smelting zinc and other non-ferrous metals, and most is used in the manufacture of nickel-cadmium batteries (Table 13). Estimated world-wide production and usage fell after a peak in 1997, but between 1997 and 2010 rose in Asia (primarily in Korea, The People's Republic of China and Japan) (UNEP, 2010a).

In occupational settings, inhalation of cadmium oxide fumes is the principal route of exposure. Non-occupational exposures typically

Table 13. Uses and Occupational Exposure to Cadmium (UNEP, 2010a)

Industrial Uses of Cadmium	Incidental Occupational Exposure to Cadmium
Nickel cadmium batteries	Metal smelting
Platings and coatings	Welding and cutting cadmium coated Steels
Pigments in plastics, ceramics, inks, textiles etc.	Fossil fuels
Stabilisers in PVC and polymers	Cement
Specialised alloys	Phosphate fertilisers
Photo-electric cells and semi-conductors	

follow ingestion of contaminated food-crops and water (Ufelle and Barchowsy, 2019). Tobacco plants bio-concentrate cadmium, and smoking is an important source of exposure to cadmium oxide.

Gibb estimated that in 2015 food-borne cadmium caused more than 12,000 cases of CKD and more than 2,000 deaths world-wide (albeit with very wide uncertainty intervals (Gibb *et al.*, 2019). Little information is available on the global burden of disease caused by occupational exposures.

Toxicokinetics

Cadmium has a relatively low melting point, and fume or vapor produced in industrial processes rapidly reacts with air to produce cadmium oxide (Friberg and Elinder, 1992).

Absorption by inhalation is much more efficient than following ingestion, but increased gut absorption has been observed with low serum ferritin levels, so workers with iron deficiency (often women) may be more susceptible to toxicity. Cadmium accumulates in the renal cortex and the liver. It stimulates hepatic metallothionein synthesis, and formation of cadmium–metallothionein complex reduces its toxicity. Most cadmium is secreted in the urine bound to metallothionein (Ufelle and Barchowsy, 2019). Cadmium has a biphasic excretion with biological half-lives of approximately 4 months, and 10–30 years in the kidney (Hoet, 2010). Urine excretion of cadmium declines after the age of 50 or 60 years, and older individuals are also more susceptible to toxicity (SCOEL, 2017).

Mechanisms of toxicity and clinical features

The kidney is the principal toxicological target of cadmium, and exposed workers exhibit lower GFR (SCOEL, 2017). Proximal tubular damage results in a Fanconi-like syndrome with proteinuria, calcuria, aminoaciduria, glycosuria and phosphaturia. An increased incidence of kidney stones has been reported. In animal studies necrosis of the proximal tubules and interstitial fibrosis are seen.

Animal studies show that cadmium causes osteomalacia and osteoporosis, and epidemiological studies demonstrate increased rates of fracture in older women.

Case Study 4: Itai-itai Disease

The best known episode of cadmium poisoning was identified in the 1940s by local physicians in Japan. Sludge from a zinc mine polluted the Jinzu river basin and cadmium found its way into rice crops. Older Japanese women in the region developed pain and multiple bone fractures. They had renal tubular dysfunction (β2 microglobulinuria was a particular feature), pseudo-fractures typical of osteomalacia and severe osteoporosis This was associated with vitamin D and other deficiencies. It is not clear whether the effects were primarily caused by cadmium, or secondary to renal damage, and such changes are seldom seen in occupational settings (Kazantzis, 2004; SCOEL, 2017).

Inhalation of cadmium causes acute respiratory effects that can be severe (Ufelle and Barchowsy, 2019). The International Agency for Research on Cancer (IARC) classes cadmium as a human carcinogen for lung cancer, and possibly for the kidney and prostate as well (IARC, 2012).

Investigations and health surveillance

Urinary cadmium levels reflect exposure over 20 years, while blood cadmium levels reflect exposures over periods of both 20 years and 3 months (International Cadmium Association, 2018). With renal toxicity, tubular loss of metallothionein-cadmium complex is accelerated, and cadmium excretion increases (SCOEL, 2017).

Following proximal tubular damage, excretion of low molecular weight (LMW) proteins increases. Glomerular damage and excretion of high molecular weight proteins such as albumin and transferrin is less common. Urinary cadmium excretion is correlated with declines in GFR, and excretion of low molecular weight (LMW) proteins (Hoet, 2010; SCOEL, 2017; Bernard, 2004). Hoet maintained that low levels of microproteinuria (e.g. <1,500 μg β2-microglobulin per gram creatinine) may be reversible on cessation of exposure, but higher levels are not (Hoet, 2010). However, as noted above, there is a lack of robust longitudinal studies demonstrating that this progresses to CKD (De Broe *et al.*, 2010; Byber *et al.*, 2016; SCOEL, 2017).

Despite this uncertainty, the European Association of Metals/International Cadmium Association (2018) advocates using LMW proteins such as retinol binding protein and alpha-1 microglobulin for biological exposure monitoring (Table 14). Retinol binding protein is preferred because it is more stable for laboratory analysis, and more specific to renal tubular damage. β2-microglobulin is chemically unstable and is now regarded as unsuitable for surveillance purposes (Byber *et al.*, 2016). If the reference value is exceeded, or there is a consistent pattern of increase approaching the reference value, increased medical vigilance is recommended.

The ACGIH Biological Exposure Indices for cadmium and its inorganic compounds are 5 μg/g creatinine in urine, and 5 μg/L in blood (ACGIH, 2020). In distinction, because of evidence of renal effects at lower levels, the European Scientific Committee on

Table 14. Biological Effect Monitoring of Cadmium Using Urinary Retinol Binding Protein

Urine LMW Protein (μg/g Creatinine) (Bernard, 2004)	Health Effect
<300	None
300–1,000	No change in GFR, but incipient cadmium tubulopathy
1000–10,000	Irreversible tubular proteinuria that may lead to accelerated fall in GFR with age
>10,000	Nephropathy, usually with low GFR

Occupational Exposure Levels recommends a Biological Limit Value (BLV) of 2 μg/g creatinine in urine (SCOEL, 2017).

Treatment

Metal chelation with sodium calcium EDTA or DMSA may be effective in the first 24 h following acute cadmium toxicity, but this is difficult to demonstrate in prospective studies. Chelation does not appear to be effective in chronic toxicity (Smith, 2013; National Poisons Information Service, 2017).

Cystalline Silica (Quartz)

Exposures and prevalence of disease

Table 15 lists traditional occupational exposures to silica. A newer use is in the computing industry. For many decades, this has employed more cultured quartz than natural quartz. Cultured (electronic grade) quartz originates from lascas quartz mined mostly in Brazil and Madagascar, but then processed in China, Japan and Russia (Dolly, 2020). Its not clear whether the pathological effects of cultured quartz differ from those of natural quartz.

A meta analyis of more than 13,000 silica exposed workers published in 2017 identified 193 cases of glomerulonephritis with a modest Standardised Mortality Ratio of 1.28 (Möhner *et al.*, 2017). At the other end of the scale, Mourad and Ashour's study of 29 Egyptian pottery workers exposed to silica found that all had sub-clinical kidney disease with marked increases in urinary protein, enzyme and

Table 15. Occupational Exposure to Silica (IARC, 2018a)

Abrasives (multiple uses ranging from sand-blasting in ship-building to dentistry)
Mining/quarrying/tunneling
Working with stone in construction or processing
Manufacturing pottery and glass
Mould making and fettling in metal founding
Agricultural soil and chemicals
Manufacturing electronic components

Kidney Injury Molecule 1 excretion when compared with 35 controls (Mourad and Ashour, 2020).

Toxicokinetics

Silicon dioxide (silica) exists in non-toxic amorphous forms, and toxic crystalline forms such as quartz, cristobalite and tridymite. When bound to other minerals it is described as combined, but termed free, when it is not.

In occupational exposures most silica is absorbed by the respiratory route. Following exposure, high concentrations can be found in kidney tissue.

Mechanisms of toxicity and clinical features

Apart from its well-known pulmonary effects, case reports and large epidemiological studies show that occupational and environmental silica exposure is associated with nephritis/nephrosis, glomerulonephritis and stage 5 CKD, even in the absence of pulmonary silicosis. Silica in the kidney is believed to have a direct toxic effect, but there are also indirect effects related to autoimmune disease (Agency for Toxic Substances and Disease Registry, 2019a).

The IARC classifies quartz and cristobalite silica as a grade 1 carcinogen. There is sufficient evidence from both animal and human studies that it causes lung cancer. There is weaker evidence for renal cancer in epidemiological studies (IARC, 2018a).

Treatment

Treatment of silica induced kidney disease does not differ from standard treatments of CKD and kidney failure (Ghahramani, 2010; Vupputuri *et al.*, 2012).

Chromium

Exposures and prevalence of disease

Trivalent chromium (CrIII) is said to be an essential nutrient, but most chromium in the environment is derived from industrial processes.

Table 16. Industrial Uses of Hexavalent Chrome Compounds (IARC, 2018b)

Pigments in textiles, inks, paints and plastics
Corrosion inhibitors
Wood preservatives
Chrome plating
Casting, welding cutting and finishing metals containing chromium
Leather tanning
Impurity in Portland cement

Production is increasing, with exposures to workers, and populations near production plants (UNEP, 2013) (Table 16). There are several case reports of acute occupational kidney toxicity, but few reports of chronic kidney effects (Bonde and Vittinghus, 1996).

Toxicokinetics

Chromium exists in several valencies. Most natural occurring compounds are trivalent (CrIII), and for industrial use, hexavalent forms (CrVI) are manufactured by oxidation. The bulk of compounds used commercially contain hexavalent or trivalent chromium (Agency for Toxic Substances and Disease Registry, 2012).

Different hexavalent compounds have differing water solubilities and absorption characteristics. Hexavalent chromium compounds, such as chromium VI oxide (chromic acid) are well absorbed following inhalation. Rates of gut and skin absorption are lower, but can be enhanced by corrosive damage. Highest concentrations occur in the kidney, liver and bone. Hexavalent chromium is oxidised to trivalent forms in the body, and most is excreted in the urine (Agency for Toxic Substances and Disease Registry, 2012). Studies suggest triphasic excretion with half-lives of 7 h, 15–30 days, and 3 years or longer (Lauwerys and Hoet, 2001).

Mechanisms of toxicity and clinical features

Hexavalent chromium is far more toxic than the divalent and trivalent forms. Animal experiments administering hexavalent chromium have shown proximal tubular necrosis with disruption of the renal brush border membrane, glycosuria, mild albuminuria, and β-2 microglobulinuria (Murunga and Zawada, 2007; Wang *et al.*, 2011).

Accidental or deliberate ingestion of, and gross dermal exposure with hexavalent chromium compounds results in acute localised corrosive damage, circulatory collapse, hepatic dysfunction and intravascular haemolysis. Necrosis of the renal tubules and AKI commonly occurs 12–24 h following ingestion (National Poisons Information Service, 2019). Inhalation typically causes acute pulmonary edema that may be delayed for up to 72 h.

Most occupational exposures are of a lower order, and usually via the respiratory or dermal route. Peterson (Petersen *et al.*, 1994) reported a case of chronic interstitial nephropathy after high exposures to chromium, but systematic studies of workers chronically exposed to hexavalent chromium have produced equivocal results. Some show no renal effects, while others have demonstrated increased levels of SCr and urine levels of LMW proteins (Agency for Toxic Substances and Disease Registry, 2012). However, the significance of these observations for CKD is not clear.

The IARC classes' hexavalent chromium compounds as a group 1 carcinogen, with sufficient evidence for lung cancer in both animal experiments and human studies. There is also some evidence of upper-airway cancer (Agency for Toxic Substances and Disease Registry, 2012).

Investigations and health surveillance

The ACGIH have adopted a BEI for chromium VI (water soluble fume) of 25 μg/L total chromium in urine for end of shift at end of work week, and 10 μg/L increase during shift (ACGIH, 2020).

Treatment

Treatment of acute hexavalent chromium toxicity is by administration of supportive measures. No specific antidotes are available.

Organic Chemicals

Exposures and prevalence of disease

Kidney diseases follow both acute and chronic occupational exposure to organic chemicals such as petroleum products, solvents, halogen-

Table 17. Workers Routinely Exposed to Solvents (Brautbar *et al.*, 2006)

Mechanics
Painters
Metal workers
Pharmacists
Research technicians

ated hydrocarbons, alcohols and glycols (Table 17) (Murunga and Zawada, 2007). Epidemiological studies often generically class these exposures as "hydrocarbons" or "solvents." This is because occupational groups such as oil refinery workers are usually exposed to multiple chemicals over a period of years, and metal workers might employ a series of different de-greasing agents. In reality the different organic chemicals have a range of health effects, related to their intrinsic toxicity, dose and duration of exposure. In consequence, different renal effects have been described. These include direct toxic effects and immune-mediated diseases such as IgA nephropathy, anti-glomerular basement membrane disease, membranous glomerulonephritis and proliferative glomerulonephritis (Brautbar *et al.*, 2006; Murunga and Zawada, 2007). The following paragraphs will detail the effects of trichlorethylene as an example.

Trichlorethylene is widely used in industry; 73% as an intermediate in chemical manufacture, and 24% for metal degreasing in the automotive industry and metal component manufacture (in both liquid and vapor form). It is also used in textile processing and as a spot-on agent in dry cleaning. Use is declining in line with environmental regulation (Agency for Toxic Substances and Disease Registry, 2019b; IARC, 2014).

Case Study 5: Acute Interstitial Nephritis and Tubular Necrosis after Working With Trichlorethylene

David et al. (1989) reported a case of acute kidney injury in a 35 year old South African man using trichlorethylene to remove ink from computer ribbons for re-use. He wore gloves, but there was no extract ventilation in the factory.

He undertook this task for an unusually long period of eight hours. The next day he became irritable, and later vomited. In the following week he developed dependent oedema, loin tenderness and urinary frequency. Three weeks later he presented to hospital with hypertension and polyuria. Creatinine was 1148 μmol/L (reference value less than 130 μmol/L), with elevated serum gamma glutamyl transpeptidase and alanine amino transferase. Urinalysis revealed proteinuria, and copious red and white blood cells. Abdominal ultrasound scan showed some ascites. Renal biopsy demonstrated an interstitial eosinophilic infiltrate and tubular necrosis.

He was treated with furosemide and methyldopa. He made a good recovery — eight months later he had mild hypertension, but no renal abnormalities.

Toxicokinetics

Trichlorethylene C_2HCl_3 is a liquid at normal ambient temperatures, with a low boiling point (86.9°C), very high vapor pressure (100 Pa at 39°C, 69 mm Hg at 25°C), and a moderately high lipid solubility (Agency for Toxic Substances and Disease Registry, 2019b).

Because of these characteristics, it is rapidly absorbed via inhalation, the skin, and ingestion, so occupational exposures are often difficult to control. Most trichlorethylene metabolites are excreted in the urine, around a quarter as trichloracetic acid with a urine half-life of between 36 and 73 h.

Mechanisms of toxicity and clinical features

Some animal studies demonstrate a "toxic nephrosis" with abnormal tubular cells (tubulomegaly) and degeneration that might represent precursors of renal carcinoma. Perivascular interstitial inflammation and glomerulonephritis have also been documented (Agency for Toxic Substances and Disease Registry, 2019b).

It causes CNS depression, cardiac arrythmias and liver injury. Studies of occupationally exposed groups have identified increased excretion of tubular enzymes, and both low and high molecular weight proteins (albumin), reflecting tubular and glomerular damage respectively. A case-referent study of trichlorethylene and other hydrocarbon exposures in air-craft workers demonstrated a strong association with kidney failure (Radican *et al.*, 2006).

There is epidemiological evidence that trichlorethylene causes kidney cancer (renal cell carcinoma), and to a lesser extent liver cancer and non-Hodgkin's lymphoma. The IARC classifies trichlorethylene as a group 1 carcinogen .

Investigations and health surveillance

The ACGIH recommends a BEI (at end of shift, and end of work-week) of trichloracetic acid in urine of 15 mg/L, and trichloroethanol in blood of 0.5 mg/L (ACGIH, 2020).

Treatment

Treatment of acute toxicity is supportive.

Kidney and Renal Pelvis Cancers

Exposures and Prevalence of Disease

Renal cell carcinoma is estimated to cause 134,000 deaths each year. Most are clear cell carcinomas, but there are number of other histological types. The precise cause is usually unknown (Hsieh *et al.*, 2017). Only a limited number of occupational exposures have been shown to cause renal cancer. Far more cause bladder cancer (Markowitz, 2007), but these will not be dealt with here.

Case Study 6: Renal Cell Carcinoma Following Exposure To Trichlorethylene

In 2015, Lee et al. (2015) reported the case of a 52 year old Korean man. Since 1988, he had worked in an automobile plant. He spent ten years polishing crankshaft forging surfaces, and then 17 years painting. Trichlorethylene was used as a solvent in these processes. He smoked, but there were no other risk factors for renal cell carcinoma.

In 2003, a renal "cystoma" was found on routine ultrasound scan. This increased in size, and in 2011, a CT scan and renal biopsy revealed a renal cell carcinoma. He had a nephrectomy, and later returned to work, but was able to claim Industrial Accident Compensation.

Historically renal cell carcinoma was usually diagnosed after presentation with flank pain, gross haematuria and a palpable abdominal mass; but today, the majority are found incidentally following abdominal scans. They can also present with para-neoplastic syndromes giving hypercalcaemia, fever or erthrocytosis. The risk of metastatic disease following nephrectomy is around 30% (Hsieh *et al.*, 2017).

The IARC produces detailed monographs on carcinogenic risk that are intended to be definitive. However, much of the data comes from animal experiments, while case reports and epidemiological studies of human exposures are prone to confounding by many factors. In consequence, other organisations such as the National Institute for Occupational Safety and Health produce their own classifications (NIOSH, 2017, 2012) that might not agree with the IARC. For simplicity, only the IARC classifications are presented here (Table 18) (Table 19).

Occupational trichlorethylene exposure is described in detail above (IARC, 2014). Radiation exposure occurs in uranium miners and processors, nuclear power generation, recycling, medical services, industrial radiographers and military uses (IARC, 2000; Golden *et al.*, 2019; Rage *et al.*, 2018).

Non-occupational exposure to aristolochic acid causes Balkan endemic nephropathy after eating crops contaminated with the plant *Aristolochia clematitis* and in people using *Aristolochia fanghi* as a Chinese herbal medicine (Jelaković *et al.*, 2019). However it can also cause renal cancer in herbalists handling the plant (Yang *et al.*, 2013).

Table 18. IARC Classification of Carcinogens

Group 1 — Carcinogenic to humans
Group 2A — Probably carcinogenic to humans
Group 2B — Possibly carcinogenic to humans
Group 3 — Not classifiable (because of lack of information)
Group 4 — Not carcinogenic to humans

Table 19. Occupational Exposures Causing Kidney Cancer (IARC, 2020)

Substance/Process	Target Organ	IARC Group
Trichlorethylene	Kidney	1
X-radiation	Kidney	1
Gamma radiation	Kidney	1
Arsenic & inorganic arsenic compounds	Kidney	2
Cadmium & cadmium compounds	Kidney	2
Perfluorooctanoic acid	Kidney	2
Printing processes	Kidney	2
Welding fumes	Kidney	2
Aristolochic acid	Renal pelvis	2

Recent publications have linked kidney cancer to occupational exposure to asbestos (Peters *et al.*, 2018), gasoline or diesel exhaust (Peters *et al.*, 2018), plastics processing (Gerosa *et al.*, 2017), perchlorethylene (Purdue *et al.*, 2017) and in firefighting (Glass *et al.*, 2016).

Investigations and Health Surveillance

Many companies manufacturing or using these substances employ biological effect monitoring of exposed workers. For example, monitoring urine cell cytology, dip-stick tests for haematuria and other biomarkers. The Federal Drug Administration licenses several of these Point of Contact Tests, but because of their high sensitivity and low specificity, their use in health surveillance has been questioned (Markowitz, 2007).

Heat Exhaustion, Heat Stroke and Acute Kidney Injury

Exposures and Prevalence of Disease

Workers in hot environments are at risk of hyperthermia. Relevant occupations include agricultural workers, construction crew, military personnel, miners, metal smelters and firefighters (Xiang *et al.*,

2014). The WHO estimates that between 1998 and 2017 heat waves caused more than 166,000 deaths globally (WHO, 2020b). A large proportion of these were probably related to occupation. For example a meta-analysis by Flouris *et al.* found that heat stress was a major cause of productivity loss, and estimated that 15% of workers in hot environments suffered AKI or kidney disease (Flouris *et al.*, 2018). However, apart from developed countries like the USA, data on heat illness is not systematically compiled (Kjellstrom, 2016).

Acclimatisation

In hot conditions, normal thermoregulation gives cutaneous vasodilation with increased blood flow to the skin, sweating, and loss of salt and water. There is also tachycardia, increased cardiac output and respiratory effects. Workers in hot climates normally acclimatise in four to 14 days. Physical exertion and exposure to heat accelerates acclimatisation. There is improved cardio-vascular performance, increased rates of sweating, and aldosterone-mediated salt conservation by sweat glands and the kidneys. De-acclimatisation can occur within a few days of withdrawing from hot environments (Oakley, 2010; Warrell *et al.*, 2010; Brearley *et al.*, 2016).

Heat Exhaustion

Clinical features

Impaired thermoregulation or salt/water balance predisposes to heat exhaustion. This is common in people who are physically unfit, unacclimatised, dehydrated, obese, or have pyrexial illnesses; also in kidney disease, heart disease or diabetes (with autonomic dysfunction). Its also associated with diuretics, beta-blockers, calcium-channel blockers, alcohol, cocaine, amphetamines, hallucinogens, and drug withdrawal.

Symptoms include intense thirst, weakness, malaise, anxiety, dizziness, paranesthesia and headache. There may be a moderate pyrexia, dehydration, hot/dry skin because of reduced sweating, and reduced cardiac/urine output. Heart rate correlates well with heat stress (Oakley, 2010; Danzl, 2018).

Investigations and health surveillance

Core temperature is very difficult to measure accurately, and ingested telemetric devices are the most accurate (Department of Health and Human Services, 2016). Serum sodium tends to be normal, but can sometimes fall following high rates of water replacement without electrolytes ("miner's cramp").

In occupational settings Wet Bulb Globe Temperatures and psychometric charts are commonly used as an index of heat stress, although other indices have been suggested. For further information on assessment and control for heat exposure, see Youle (2005), and NIOSH (Department of Health and Human Services, 2016).

Mitigation of exposure and treatment

The use of personal protective equipment typically adds to heat stress. A compromise is often needed between heat shielding, reflectant properties and vapor permeability.

Adequate water and dietary salt is needed, with perhaps a ceiling of 10–12 L of fluid during an extended working day. Workers need appropriate education, and urine color charts can be used to self-assess the degree of hydration. In desert environments like the Middle East, extra precautions during the hot summer months are necessary.

Most national authorities do not set maximum limits for workplace temperatures and recommendations tend to focus on comfort levels rather than safety (HSE, 2015).

Victims should be placed in a recumbent position in a cool environment to normalise blood pressure. Oral fluids and electrolytes are often adequate, but intravenous fluids are sometimes needed. Between five and 10 liters of oral or intravenous fluids in the first 24 h may be required. (Warrell *et al.*, 2010; Leon and Bouchama, 2015).

Case Study 7: Meso-American Nephropathy (MeN)

In the 1990s, physicians in El Salvador noticed an increasing incidence of renal failure in young men working on sugar cane plantations. Since the 2000s, the term meso-american nephropathy has been used for chronic kidney disease of unknown origin (CKDu) in central America and south East Mexico. The prevalence of CKDu in countries like El Salvador and Nicaragua is extremely high. Access to dialysis and transplant is limited, and mortality is also very high. It typically occurs in men aged 20–60 years working on cane plantations on the Pacific Coast, where they are the predominant industry (Correa-Rotter et al., 2014, Correa-Rotter and García-Trabanino, 2019). An alternative term is heat stress nephropathy (Glaser et al., 2016). CKDu also has a high incidence in other crop-workers in Sri Lanka and India, and a rival label is chronic kidney disease of unknown cause in agricultural communities (CINAC) (Johnson et al., 2019; Jayasumana, 2019). Its not clear which of these labels will stand the test of time.

Sugar-cane is used as a human and animal feed-stuff, and a bio-fuel. Between 2001 and 2018 global production increased by 39% (Leite et al., 2018; International Sugar Organization, 2020). Cane workers can undertake heavy manual work for 4–12 hours a day in temperatures of 34°C to 42°C, and lose 2.6 kg of weight by dehydration. Pure drinking water may be difficult to obtain, and instead may be substituted with high-energy high-osmolar sugar drinks (Correa-Rotter et al., 2014; Nerbass et al., 2017).

This plausible circumstantial evidence and numerous small case-series (Leite et al., 2018) link meso-American nephropathy to continual occupational heat stress and dehydration. Sub-clinical kidney injury could follow hyperosmolarity with increased vasopressin excretion, sub-clinical rhabdomyolysis, or crystalluria (Johnson et al., 2019).

MeN can present with acute interstitial nephritis, or chronic interstitial disease, tubular nephropathy, inflammation and interstitial fibrosis. Proteinuria is absent or mild, and hyperuricaemia is common (Johnson et al., 2019).

However, large longitudinal case series monitoring kidney function and histology, or case-referent studies to confirm the aetiology of MeN have not been completed. Similarly public health surveillance in these regions is poorly developed. In consequence the theory has been contested (Herath et al., 2018). Other factors may be implicated such as use of non-steroidal anti-inflammatory drugs (NSAIDs), genetic predisposition, infectious disease, heavy metals, minerals and pesticides. Sugar cane is commonly burned before or after harvesting (Leite et al., 2018; Bodin et al., 2016; Wesseling et al., 2016), and inhalation of fine particulate hydrocarbon and crystalline silica (Le Blond et al., 2017) could be contributory. The condition may be multi-factorial.

Despite uncertain causation, it is wise to mitigate occupational dehydration by education programmes, and limiting working hours, and the frequent use of NSAIDs should be discouraged (Correa-Rotter et al., 2014; Johnson et al., 2019; Correa-Rotter and García-Trabanino, 2019). Reducing working hours is often impractical in poor countries where workers are paid according to the amount of sugar produced (Nerbass et al., 2017). Increasing mechanisation should result in a lower incidence of dehydration, but in 2016, 60% of the global cane crop was still harvested by hand (International Sugar Journal, 2016).

Heat Stroke and Acute Kidney Injury

Pathological mechanisms and clinical features

Heat exhaustion and heat stroke represent a continuum of illness, without a clear boundary. The latter is a very severe condition characterised by rapid onset and thermo-regulatory failure. Diagnosis is largely clinical, based on the triad of a core temperature of more than 40°C, neurological abnormalities and a history of heat exposure. Differentiation from other life-threatening conditions like septicaemia may be very difficult (Danzl, 2018).

Case Study 8: Heat Stroke in an Aluminium Smelter Worker

In 2019, Wesdock and Donoghue (Wesdock and Donoghue, 2019) reported the case of a 34 year old man exposed to high temperatures working in an American pot-room. He complained of muscle cramps, and at the end of a 12-hour shift developed generalised convulsions, followed by agitation and combativeness. Initial oral temperature was 36.5°C, but his core temperature was not measured. Microscopic urinalysis showed a "large amount of blood."

He had severe rhabdomyolysis, kidney and liver injury, and Enterococcus faecalis septicaemia. He required five days intensive care treatment. His anion gap was 31 mmol/L (reference range 7–14). Creatinine phosphokinase peaked on the second day at more than 22,000 units/L (36–174), and aspartate aminotransferase on the fourth day at 1,478 units/L (10–40). He spent a further eight days in hospital, and on discharge had polyneuropathy of his lower limbs.

He had returned to work after a seven-day rest, without any schedule of acclimatisation. He was relatively inexperienced, having worked at the plant for less than five months. Other pre-disposing factors included mild attention-deficit-hyperactivity disorder, hypertension, and obesity.

Table 20 summarises the usual presentations of the two principal forms of heat stroke, classical and exertional. The latter is commonest in occupational settings, and is typically behavioural in origin.

There is an exaggerated inflammatory response and multi-organ failure is common. With diversion of blood from the gut to the periphery, and gut injury, the absorption of gut endotoxins may also contribute to the inflammatory response (Leon and Bouchama, 2015).

The incidence of AKI is 5% in classic heat stroke, and 25% in exertional heat stroke. There is often rhabdomyolysis and tubular necrosis. The urine contains red and white cells, hyaline and granular casts (Leon and Bouchama, 2015).

Treatment

Treatment consists of rapid cooling to 38°C–39°C. The evidence for the relative effectiveness of different cooling methods is incomplete, but immediate immersion in iced water is increasingly recommended (Gaudio and Grissom, 2016). Pharmaceutical treatment to reduce temperature is not useful (Gaudio and Grissom, 2016). Aggressive supportive treatment including intubation is usually needed (Epstein and Yanovich, 2019).

Following resuscitation, a quiet interval of 12–24 h may be followed by further deterioration, despite aggressive treatment in the

Table 20. Features of Classic & Exertional Heat Stroke (Epstein and Yanovich, 2019)

Feature	Classic Heat Stroke	Exertional Heat Stroke
Age group	Very young and elderly	Young and active
Occurrence	Heat waves	Sporadic
Activity	Sedentary	Strenous
Health status	Usually poor	Usually good
Mechanism	High environmental heat	Excessive heat production
Sweating	May be absent	Usually present
Central nervous system dysfunction	Common	Common
Acid-base disturbance	Respiratory alkalosis	Metabolic acidosis
Rhabdomyolysis	Unusual	Frequent
Liver dysfunction	Mild	Marked/Severe
Kidney failure	Uncommon	Common
Acute respiratory distress syndrome	Common	Common
Multi-organ failure	Common	More severe
Creatine kinase	Mild elevation	Marked elevation
Calcium	Normal	Low
Potassium	Normal	Usually high

following days or weeks (Bouchama and Knochel, 2002; Leon and Bouchama, 2015).

The hospital mortality rate for exertional heat stroke ranges from 3% to 5%, and for classic heat stroke from 10% to 60%. Survivors may sustain permanent neurological and other organ damage (Leon and Bouchama, 2015).

Conclusion

The renal tract can be affected by occupational exposures. The better recognised examples of these exposures are described above. Preventive measures to reduce hazardous exposures can minimise the likelihood of health effects including kidney damage. Where health surveillance is indicated for such exposures, several markers of kidney function have been described, with guidance for interpretation.

References

ACGIH. (2020) *TLVs and BEIs.* [Online] Available from: https://www.acgih.org/science/tlv-bei-guidelines/. [Accessed on 10 May 2021].

Afrifa J, Essien-Baidoo S, Ephraim RKD, Nkrumah D, Dankyira DO. (2017) Reduced eGFR, elevated urine protein and low level of personal protective equipment compliance among artisanal small scale gold miners at Bibiani-Ghana: a cross-sectional study. *BMC Public Health* **17**: 601.

Agency for Toxic Substances and Disease Registry. (2020) *Toxicological profile for lead.* [Online] Available from: https://www.atsdr.cdc.gov/toxprofiles/tp13.pdf. [Accessed on 10 May 2021].

Agency for Toxic Substances and Disease Registry. (2019a) *Toxicological profile for silica.* [Online] Available from: https://www.atsdr.cdc.gov/toxprofiles/tp211.pdf. [Accessed on 10 May 2021].

Agency for Toxic Substances and Disease Registry. (2019b) *Toxicological profile for trichlorethylene.* [Online] Available from: https://www.atsdr.cdc.gov/toxprofiles/tp19.pdf. [Accessed on 10 May 2021].

Agency for Toxic Substances and Disease Registry. (2013) *Addendum to the toxicological profile for mercury (alkyl and dialkyl compounds).* [Online] Available from: https://www.atsdr.cdc.gov/toxprofiles/mercury_organic_addendum.pdf. [Accessed on 10 May 2021].

Agency for Toxic Substances and Disease Registry. (2012) *Toxicological profile for chromium.* [Online] Available from: https://www.atsdr.cdc.gov/toxprofiles/tp7.pdf. [Accessed on 10 May 2021].

Agency for Toxic Substances and Disease Registry. (2007) *Toxicological profile for arsenic.* [Online] Available from: https://www.atsdr.cdc.gov/toxprofiles/tp2.pdf. [Accessed on 10 May 2021].

Agency for Toxic Substances and Disease Registry. (1999) *Toxicological profile for mercury.* [Online] Available from: https://wwwn.cdc.gov/TSP/ToxProfiles/ToxProfiles.aspx?id=115&tid=24. [Accessed on 10 May 2021].

Bakir F, Damluji SF, Amin-Zaki L, Murtadha M, Khalidi A, Al-Rawi nY, Tikriti S, Dahahir HI, Clarkson TW, Smith JC, Doherty RA. (1973) Methylmercury poisoning in Iraq. *Science* **181**: 230–241.

Barregard L, Trachtenberg F, Mckinlay S. (2008) Renal effects of dental amalgam in children: The New England children's amalgam trial. *Environ Health Perspect* **116**: 394–399.

Barregard L, Sallsten G, Jarvholm B. (1995) People with high mercury uptake from their own dental amalgam fillings. *Occup Environ Med* **52**: 124–128.

Bates MN. (2006) Mercury amalgam dental fillings: An epidemiologic assessment. *Int J Hyg Environ Health* **209**: 309–316.

Baxter PJ, Igisu H. (2010) Mercury. In: Harrington, M., Baxter, P.J., Tar-Ching, A.W., Cockcroft, A., Durrington, P., Malcolm, J (eds.), *Hunter's diseases of occupations* (10th Ed). London, CRC Press.

Bernard A. (2004) Renal dysfunction induced by cadmium: Biomarkers of critical effects. *Biometals* **17**: 519–523.

Bodin T, García-Trabanino R, Weiss I, Jarquín E, Glaser J, Jakobsson K, Lucas RA, Wesseling C, Hogstedt C, Wegman DH, WE Program Working Group. (2016) Intervention to reduce heat stress and improve efficiency among sugarcane workers in El Salvador: Phase 1. *Occup Environ Med* **73**(6): 409–416. Available from: https://doi.org/10.1136/oemed-2016-103555.

Bonde JP, Vittinghus E. (1996) Urinary excretion of proteins among metal welders. *Hum Exp Toxicol* **15**: 1–4.

Bouchama A, Knochel JP. (2002) Heat stroke. *N Engl J Med* **346**: 1978–1988.

Bradberry S, Vale A. (2009) A comparison of sodium calcium edetate (edetate calcium disodium) and succimer (DMSA) in the treatment of inorganic lead poisoning. *Clin Toxicol (Phila)* **47**: 841–858.

Brautbar N, Wu MP, Gabel E, Regev L. (2006) Occupational kidney cancer: Exposure to industrial solvents. *Ann N Y Acad Sci* **1076**: 753–764.

Brearley MB, Norton I, Rush D, Hutton M, Smith S, Ward L, Fuentes H. (2016) Influence of chronic heat acclimatization on occupational thermal strain in tropical field conditions. *J Occup Environ Med* **58**: 1250–1256.

Byber K, Lison D, Verougstraete V, Dressel H, Hotz P. (2016) Cadmium or cadmium compounds and chronic kidney disease in workers and the general population: A systematic review. *Crit Rev Toxicol* **46**: 191–240.

Centers For Disease Control & Prevention. (2020) *National report on human exposure to environmental chemicals.* [Online] Available from: https://www.cdc.gov/exposurereport/index.html. [Accessed on 10 May 2021].

Correa-Rotter R, García-Trabanino R. (2019) Mesoamerican nephropathy. *Semin Nephrol* **39**: 263–271.

Correa-Rotter R, Wesseling C, Johnson RJ. (2014) CKD of unknown origin in Central America: The case for a Mesoamerican nephropathy. *Am J Kidney Dis* **63**: 506–520.

Danzl DF. (2018) Heat-Related Illnesses. In: Jameson, J.L., Fauci, A.S., Kasper, D.L., Hauser, S.L., Longo, D.L, Loscalzo, J. (eds.), *Harrison's Principles of Internal Medicine* (19th Ed). New York, McGraw-Hill Education.

David NJ, Wolman R, Milne FJ, Van Niekerk I. (1989) Acute renal failure due to trichloroethylene poisoning. *Br J Ind Med* **46**: 347–349.

De Broe ME, D'haese PC, Elseviers MM. (2010) Chronic tubulointerstitial nephritis. In: Warrell, D.A., Cox, T.M, Firth, J.D. (eds.), *Oxford textbook of medicine* (5th Ed). Oxford, Oxford University Press.

Department Of Health And Human Services. (2016) Criteria for a recommended standard: occupational exposure to heat and cold environments: Draft revised criteria 2016. [Online] Available from: https://www.cdc.gov/niosh/docs/2016-106/pdfs/2016-106.pdf. [Accessed on 10 May 2021].

Dolly TP. (2020) *2017 Minerals yearbook (advance release)*, Reston, Virginia, United States Geological Survey.

Duff S, Murray PT. (2020) Defining early recovery of acute kidney injury. *Clin J Am Soc Nephrol* **15**(9): 1358–1360.

Ekong EB, Jaar BG, Weaver VM. (2006) Lead-related nephrotoxicity: A review of the epidemiologic evidence. *Kidney Int* **70**: 2074–2084.

Epstein Y, Yanovich R. (2019) Heatstroke. *N Engl J Med* **380**: 2449–2459.

Flouris AD, Dinas PC, Ioannou LG, Nybo L, Havenith G, Kenny GP, Kjellstrom T. (2018) Workers' health and productivity under occupational heat strain: A systematic review and meta-analysis. *Lancet Planet Health* **2**: e521–e531.

Friberg L, Elinder CG. (1992) *Environmental health criteria 134, cadmium.* [Online] Available from: http://www.inchem.org/documents/ehc/ehc/ehc134.htm. [Accessed on 10 May 2021].

Gaudio FG, Grissom CK. (2016) Cooling methods in heat stroke. *J Emerg Med* **50**: 607–16.

GBD Chronic Kidney Disease Collaboration. (2020) Global, regional, and national burden of chronic kidney disease, 1990–2017: A systematic analysis for the Global Burden of Disease Study 2017. *Lancet (Lond)* **395**(10225): 709–733. Available from: https://doi.org/10.1016/S0140-6736(20)30045-3.

Gerosa A, Scarnato C, Marchesini B, Ietri E, Pavone VLM. (2017) Mortality study in a cohort of workers employed in the hot working processing of plastics and rubber. *Epidemiol Prev* **41**: 125–133.

Ghahramani N. (2010) Silica nephropathy. *Int J Occup Environ Med* **1**: 108–115.

Gibb HJ, Barchowsky A, Bellinger D, Bolger PM, Carrington C, Havelaar AH, Oberoi S, Zang Y, O'Leary K, Devleesschauwer B. (2019) Estimates of the 2015 global and regional disease burden from four foodborne metals—arsenic, cadmium, lead and methylmercury. *Environ Res* **174**: 188–194. Available from: https://doi.org/10.1016/j.envres.2018.12.062.

Gidlow DA. (2015) Lead toxicity. *Occup Med (Lond)* **65**: 348–356.

Glaser J, Lemery J, Rajagopalan B, Diaz HF, García-Trabanino R, Taduri G, Madero M, Amarasinghe M, Abraham G, Anutrakulchai S, Jha V, Stenvinkel P, Roncal-Jimenez C, Lanaspa MA, Correa-Rotter R, Sheikh-Hamad D, Burdmann EA, Andres-Hernando A, Milagres T, Weiss I, Johnson RJ. (2016) Climate change and the emergent epidemic of CKD from heat stress in rural communities: The case for heat stress nephropathy. *Clin J Am Socf Nephrol* **11**(8): 1472–1483. Available from: https://doi.org/10.2215/CJN.13841215.

Glass DC, Del Monaco A, Pircher S, Vander Hoorn S, Sim MR. (2016) Mortality and cancer incidence at a fire training college. *Occup Med (Lond)* **66**: 536–542.

Golden AP, Ellis ED, Cohen SS, Mumma MT, Leggett RW, Wallace PW, Girardi D, Watkins JP, Shore RE, Boice JD. (2019) Updated mortality analysis of the Mallinckrodt uranium processing workers, 1942–2012. *Int J Radiat Biol* 1–21. Advance online publication. Available from: https://doi.org/10.1080/09553002.2019.1569773.

Gwini S, Macfarlane E, Del Monaco A, Mclean D, Pisaniello D, Benke GP, Sim MR. (2012) Cancer incidence, mortality, and blood lead levels among workers exposed to inorganic lead. *Ann Epidemiol* **22**: 270–276.

Office For Disability Issues. (2015) *Equality Act 2010 Guidance*. [Online] Available from: https://www.gov.uk/guidance/equality-act-2010-guidance. [Accessed on 10 May 2021].

Hall YN, Himmelfarb J. (2017) The CKD Classification system in the precision medicine era. *Clin J Am Soc Nephrol* **12**(2): 346–348.

Herath C, Jayasumana C, De Silva PCMS, De Silva PHC, Siribaddana S, De Broe ME. (2018) Kidney diseases in agricultural communities: A case against heat-stress nephropathy. *Kidney Int Rep* **3**: 271–280.

Hoet P. (2010) Cadmium. In: Harrington, M., Baxter, P.J., Tar-Ching, A.W., Cockcroft, A., Durrington, P., Malcolm, J. (eds.), *Hunter's Diseases of Occupations* (10th Ed). London, CRC Press.

Hoet P, Buchet JP, Decerf L, Lavalleye B, Haufroid V, Lison D. (2006) Clinical evaluation of a lead mobilization test using the chelating agent dimercaptosuccinic acid. *Clin Chem* **52**: 88–96.

HSE. (2002) *Control of Lead at Work, Control of Lead at Work Regulations 2002: Approved Code of Practice and Guidance*. [Online] London, HSE Books. Available from: https://www.hse.gov.uk/pUbns/priced/l132.pdf.

HSE. (2015) *Temperature.* [Online] Available from: http://www.hse.gov.uk/temperature/. [Accessed on 10 May 2021].

Hsieh JJ, Purdue MP, Signoretti S, Swanton C, Albiges L, Schmidinger M, Heng DY, Larkin J, Ficarra V. (2017) Renal cell carcinoma. *Nature reviews. Disease primers* **3**: 17009. Available from: https://doi.org/10.1038/nrdp.2017.9.

Hu H, Shih R, Rothenberg S, Schwartz BS. (2007) The epidemiology of lead toxicity in adults: Measuring dose and consideration of other methodologic issues. *Environ Health Perspect* **115**: 455–462.

IARC. (2000) *Ionizing Radiation, Part 1: X- and Gamma (Υ)-radiation, and Neutrons IARC Monographs on the Evaluation of Carcinogenic Risks to Humans-Volume 75.* [Online] Available from: https://publications.iarc.fr/Book-And-Report-Series/Iarc-Monographs-On-The-Identification-Of-Carcinogenic-Hazards-To-Humans/Ionizing-Radiation-Part-1-X--And-Gamma-%CE%B3--Radiation-And-Neutrons-2000. [Accessed on 10 May 2021].

IARC. (2012) Arsenic, metals, fibres and dusts. *IARC Monographs on the Evaulation of Carcinogenic Risks to Humans, v. 100C.* Lyon, IARC.

IARC. (2014) *IARC Monograph 106 on the Evaluation of Carcinogenic Risk to Humans. Trichlorethylene, Tetrachlorethylene and Some Other Chlorinated Solvents.*, Lyon, IARC

IARC. (2018a) *Silica Dust, Crystalline, in the Form of Quartz or Cristobalite.* [Online] Available from: https://monographs.iarc.who.int/wp-content/uploads/2018/06/mono100C-14.pdf. [Accessed on 10 May 2021].

IARC. (2018b) *Chromium (VI) Compounds.* [Online] Available from: https://monographs.iarc.who.int/wp-content/uploads/2018/06/mono100C-9.pdf. [Accessed on 10 May 2021].

IARC. (2020) *List of Classifications by Cancer Site with Sufficient or Limited Evidence in Humans, IARC Monographs Volumes 1-127.* [Online] Available: https://monographs.iarc.fr/wp-content/uploads/2019/07/Classifications_by_cancer_site.pdf. [Accessed on 10 May 2021].

Ikizler TA, Parikh CR, Himmelfarb J, Chinchilli VM, Liu KD, Coca SG, Garg AX, Hsu CY, Siew ED, Wurfel MM, Ware LB, Faulkner GB, Tan TC, Kaufman JS, Kimmel PL, Go AS, ASSESS-AKI Study Investigators.

(2021) A prospective cohort study of acute kidney injury and kidney outcomes, cardiovascular events, and death. *Kidney Int* **99**(2): 456–465. Available from: https://doi.org/10.1016/j.kint.2020.06.032.

International Cadmium Association. (2018) *Management of Risks Related to Chronic Occupational Exposure to Cadmium and its Compounds (2018.2 Revision).* [Online] Available from: https://www.cadmium.org/doc/news_18/2018-2-icda-guidance-document.pdf. [Accessed on 10 May 2021].

International Lead Association. (2020) *Lead Production and Statistics.* [Online] Available from: https://ila-lead.org/resources/lead-production-statistics/. [Accessed on 10 May 2021].

International Sugar Organization. (2020). *About Sugar.* [Online] Available from: https://www.isosugar.org/sugarsector/sugar. [Accessed on 10 May 2021].

International Sugar Journal. (2016) *Only 40% of Cane Crop Mechanized Globally.* [Online] Available from: https://internationalsugarjournal.com/only-40-of-cane-crop-mechanized-globally/. [Accessed on 10 May 2021].

Jameson JL, Fauci AS, Kasper DL, Hauser SL, Longo DL, Loscalzo J. (2018) *Harrison's Principles of Internal Medicine*, London, McGraw Hill Medical.

Jayasumana C. (2019) Chronic Interstitial Nephritis in Agricultural Communities (CINAC) in Sri Lanka. *Semin Nephrol* **39**: 278–283.

Jelaković B, Dika Ž, Arlt VM, Stiborova M, Pavlović NM, Nikolić J, Colet JM, Vanherweghem JL, Nortier JL. (2019) Balkan endemic nephropathy and the causative role of aristolochic acid. *Sem Nephrol* **39**(3): 284–296. Available from: https://doi.org/10.1016/j.semnephrol.2019.02.007.

Johnson RJ, Wesseling C, Newman LS. (2019) Chronic kidney disease of unknown cause in agricultural communities. *N Engl J Med* **380**: 1843–1852.

Kaneko M, Kazatani T, Shikata H. (2020) Occupational lead poisoning in a patient with acute abdomen and normocytic anemia. *Intern Med (Tokyo, Japan)* **59**: 1565–1570.

Kazantzis G. (2004) Cadmium, osteoporosis and calcium metabolism. *Biometals* **17**: 493–8.

Khwaja A. (2012) KDIGO clinical practice guidelines for acute kidney injury. *Nephron Clin Pract* **120**(4): c179–184.

Kjellstrom T. (2016) Impact of climate conditions on occupational health and related economic losses: A new feature of global and urban health in the context of climate change. *Asia Pac J Public Health* **28**: 28s–37s.

Klaunig JE, Kamendulis LM. (2008) Chemical carcinogens. In: Klaassen, C.D. (ed.), *Casarett & Doull's toxicology* (7th Ed). London, McGraw-Hill.

Lauwerys RR, Hoet P. (2001) *Industrial Chemical Exposure: Guidelines for Biological Monitoring*. Boca Raton, Florida, Lewis Publishers.

Le Blond JS, Woskie S, Horwell CJ, Williamson BJ. (2017) Particulate matter produced during commercial sugarcane harvesting and processing: A respiratory health hazard? *Atmos Environ* **149**: 34–46.

Lee BK. (1999) The role of biological monitoring in the health management of lead-exposed workers. *Toxicol Lett* **108**: 149–60.

Lee JH, Kim I, Seok H, Park I, Hwang J, Park JO, Won JU, Roh J. (2015) Case report of renal cell carcinoma in automobile manufacturing factory worker due to trichloroethylene exposure in Korea. *Ann Occup Environ Med* **27**: 19. Available from: https://doi.org/10.1186/s40557-015-0068-x.

Leite MR, Zanetta DMT, Trevisan IB, Burdmann EA, Santos UP. (2018) Sugarcane cutting work, risks, and health effects: A literature review. *Rev Saude Publica* **52**: 80.

Leon LR, Bouchama A. (2015) Heat stroke. *Compr Physiol* **5**: 611–47.

Levey AS, Coresh J, Tighiouart H, Greene T, Inker LA. (2020a) Measured and estimated glomerular filtration rate: Current status and future directions. *Nature reviews. Nephrology* **16**(1): 51–64. Available from: https://doi.org/10.1038/s41581-019-0191-y.

Levey AS, de Jong PE, Coresh J, El Nahas M, Astor BC, Matsushita K, Gansevoort RT, Kasiske BL, Eckardt KU. (2011) The definition, classification, and prognosis of chronic kidney disease: A KDIGO Controversies Conference report. *Kidney Int* **80**(1): 17–28. Available from: https://doi.org/10.1038/ki.2010.483.

Levey AS, Eckardt KU, Dorman NM, Christiansen SL, Hoorn EJ, Ingelfinger JR, Inker LA, Levin A, Mehrotra R, Palevsky PM, Perazella MA, Tong A, Allison SJ, Bockenhauer D, Briggs JP, Bromberg JS, Davenport A, Feldman HI, Fouque D, Gansevoort RT, Winkelmayer WC. (2020b) Nomenclature for kidney function and disease: Report of a Kidney Disease: Improving Global Outcomes (KDIGO) Consensus Conference. *Kidney Int* **97**(6): 1117–1129. Available from: https://doi.org/10.1016/j.kint.2020.02.010.

Levey AS, Levin A. (2017) A Rebuttal to "The CKD Classification System in the Precision Medicine Era." *Clin J Am Soc Nephrol* **12**(10): 1711–1713.

Markowitz SB. (2007). Occupational bladder cancer. In: Rom, W.M., Markowitz, S.B. (eds.), *Environmental and ocupational medicine* (4th Ed). London, Wolters Kluwer.

Mason HJ, Hindell P, Williams NR. (2001) Biological monitoring and exposure to mercury. *Occup Med (Lond)* **51**: 2–11.

Mcelvenny DM, Miller BG, Maccalman LA, Sleeuwenhoek A, Tongeren MV, Shepherd K, Darnton AJ, Cherrie JW. (2015) Mortality of a cohort of workers in Great Britain with blood lead measurements. *Occup Environ Med* **71** Suppl 1(9): A47.

Meyer PA, Brown MJ, Falk H. (2008) Global approach to reducing lead exposure and poisoning. *Mutat Res* **659**: 166–75.

Miller S, Pallan S, Gangji AS, Lukic D, Clase CM. (2013) Mercury-associated nephrotic syndrome: A case report and systematic review of the literature. *Am J Kidney Dis* **62**: 135–8.

Mourad BH, Ashour YA. (2020) Demonstration of subclinical early nephrotoxicity induced by occupational exposure to silica among workers in pottery industry. *Int J Occup Environ Med* **11**: 85–94.

Murunga E, Zawada ET. (2007) Environmental and occupational causes of toxic injury to the kidneys and urinary tract. In: Rom, W.M., Markowitz, S.B. (eds.), *Environmental and occupational medicine* (4th Ed). London, Wolters Kluwer.

Möhner M, Pohrt A, Gellissen J. (2017) Occupational exposure to respirable crystalline silica and chronic non-malignant renal disease: Systematic review and meta-analysis. *Int Arch Occup Environ Health* **90**: 555–574.

National Poisons Information Service. (2012) *Mercury Chelation Therapy — Antidotes.* [Online] Available from https://www.toxbase.org. [Accessed on 20 November 2020].

National Poisons Information Service. (2017) *Cadmium Compounds.* [Online] Available from https://www.toxbase.org. [Accessed on 20 November 2020].

National Poisons Information Service. (2019) *Chromic Acid (Chromium VI Oxide).* [Online] Available from https://www.toxbase.org. [Accessed on 20 November 2020].

Nerbass FB, Pecoits-Filho R, Clark WF, Sontrop JM, Mcintyre CW, Moist L. (2017) Occupational Heat Stress and Kidney Health: From Farms to Factories. *Kidney Int Rep* **2**: 998–1008.

NIOSH. (2012) *Occupational Cancer, Carcinogen List.* [Online] Available from: https://www.cdc.gov/niosh/topics/cancer/npotocca.html. [Accessed on 10 May 2021].

NIOSH. (2015) *Hierarchy of Controls.* [Online] Available from: https://www.cdc.gov/niosh/topics/hierarchy/default.html. [Accessed on 10 May 2021].

NIOSH. (2017) *Niosh Chemical Carcinogen Policy.* [Online] Available from: https://www.cdc.gov/niosh/docs/2017-100/default.html. [Accessed on 10 May 2021].

NIOSH. (2020) *NIOSH pocket guide to chemical hazards.* [Online] Available from: https://www.cdc.gov/niosh/npg/default.html. [Accessed on 10 May 2021].

Oakley EHN. (2010) Heat and cold. In: Harrington, M., Baxter, P.J., Tar-Ching, A.W., Cockcroft, A., Durrington, P., Malcolm, J. (eds.), *Hunter's Diseases of Occupations* (10th Ed). London, CRC Press.

OSHA. (2020) *Permissible Exposure Limits — Annotated Tables.* [Online] Available from: https://www.osha.gov/annotated-pels. [Accessed on 10 May 2021].

Peters, C. E., Parent, M. E., Harris, S. A., Kachuri, L., Latifovic, L., Bogaert, L, Villeneuve, P. J. (2018) Workplace exposure to asbestos and the risk of kidney cancer in Canadian men. *Can J Public Health* **109**: 464–472.

Petersen R, Mikkelsen S, Thomsen OF. (1994) Chronic interstitial nephropathy after plasma cutting in stainless steel. *Occup Environ Med* **51**: 259–261.

Purdue MP, Stewart PA, Friesen MC, Colt JS, Locke SJ, Hein MJ, Waters MA, Graubard BI, Davis F, Ruterbusch J, Schwartz K, Chow WH, Rothman N, Hofmann JN. (2017) Occupational exposure to chlorinated solvents and kidney cancer: A case-control study. *Occup Environ Med* **74**(4): 268–274. Available from: https://doi.org/10.1136/oemed-2016-103849.

Radican L, Wartenberg D, Rhoads GG, Schneider D, Wedeen R, Stewart P, Blair A. (2006) A retrospective occupational cohort study of end-stage renal disease in aircraft workers exposed to trichloroethylene and other hydrocarbons. *J Occup Environ Med* **48**: 1–12.

Rage E, Caër-Lorho S, Laurier D. (2018) Low radon exposure and mortality among Jouac uranium miners: An update of the French cohort (1946–2007). *J Radiol Prot* **38**: 92–108.

Rosin A. (2009) The long-term consequences of exposure to lead. *Isr Med Assoc J* **11**: 689–694.

Sakthithasan K, lévy P, Poupon J, Garnier R. (2018) A comparative study of edetate calcium disodium and dimercaptosuccinic acid in the treatment of lead poisoning in adults. *Clin Toxicol (Phila)* **56**: 1143–1149.

Schnellmann RG. (2019) Toxic responses of the kidney. In: Klaassen, C.D. (ed.), *Casarett & Doull's Toxicology, The Basic Science of Poisons.* London, McGraw Hill Medical.

SCOEL. (2002) *Recommendations from the Scientific Committee on Occupational Exposure Limits for Lead and its Inorganic Compounds.* [Online] Available from: https://op.europa.eu/en/publication-detail/-/publication/ea927655-f429-41cf-ad7a-c070a8751cab. [Accessed on 10 May 2021].

SCOEL. (2017) *Cadmium and its Inorganic Compounds.* [Online] Available from: https://op.europa.eu/en/publication-detail/-/publication/3325374b-0a14-11e7-8a35-01aa75ed71a1. [Accessed on 10 May 2021].

Seccatore J, Veiga M, Origliasso C, Marin T, De Tomi G. (2014) An estimation of the artisanal small-scale production of gold in the world. *Sci Total Environ* **496**: 662–667.

Sharp VJ, Barnes KT, Erickson BA. (2013) Assessment of asymptomatic microscopic hematuria in adults. *Am Fam Physician* **88**(11): 747–754.

Smith SW. (2013) The role of chelation in the treatment of other metal poisonings. *J Med Toxicol* **9**: 355–369.

Sokas RK, Atleson J, Keogh JP. (1988) Shortened forms of provocative lead chelation. *J Occup Med* **30**: 420–424.

Tomicic C, Vernez D, Belem T, Berode M. (2011) Human mercury exposure associated with small-scale gold mining in Burkina Faso. *Int Arch Occup Environ Health* **84**: 539–546.

Ufelle AC, Barchowsy A. (2019) Toxic effects of metals. In: Klaassen, C.D. (ed.), *Cassarett & Doull's Toxicology: The Basic Science of Poisons.* London, McGraw Hill Education.

UNEP. (2010a) *Final Review of Scientific Information on Cadmium.* [Online] Available from: https://wedocs.unep.org/xmlui/handle/20.500.11822/27636. [Accessed on 10 May 2021].

UNEP. (2010b) *Final Review of Scientific Information on Lead.* [Online] Available from: https://wedocs.unep.org/handle/20.500.11822/27635. [Accessed on 10 May 2021].

UNEP. (2013) *Environmental Risks and Challenges of Anthropogenic Metals Flows and Cycles.* [Online] Available from: https://wedocs.unep.org/handle/20.500.11822/8451. [Accessed on 10 May 2021].

UNEP. (2019a) *Global Mercury Assessment 2018.* [Online] Available from: https://www.unep.org/resources/publication/global-mercury-assessment-2018. [Accessed on 10 May 2021].

UNEP. (2019b) *Technical Background Report to the Global Mecury Assessment 2018.* [Online] Available from: https://web.unep.org/globalmercurypartnership/technical-background-report-global-mercury-assessment-2018. [Accessed on 10 May 2020].

Vupputuri S, Parks CG, Nylander-French LA, Owen-Smith A, Hogan SL, Sandler DP. (2012) Occupational silica exposure and chronic kidney disease. *Ren Fail* **34**: 40–46.

Wang T, Jia G, Zhang J, Ma Y, Feng W, Liu L, Zhang N, Yan L, Wang X, Zhang X, Liu Z, Du X, Zhen S. (2011) Renal impairment caused by chronic occupational chromate exposure. *Int Arch Occup Environ Health* **84**: 393–401.

Warrell, DA, Cox TM, Firth, JD. (2010) *Oxford Textbook of Medicine* (Fifth Edition), Oxford, Oxford University Press.

Wesdock JC, Donoghue AM. (2019) Life-threatening heat-related illness with severe hyponatremia in an aluminum smelter worker. *Am J Ind Med* **62**: 1068–1075.

Wesseling C, Aragón A, González M, Weiss I, Glaser J, Rivard CJ, Roncal-Jiménez C, Correa-Rotter R, Johnson RJ. (2016) Heat stress, hydration and uric acid: A cross-sectional study in workers of three occupations in a hotspot of Mesoamerican nephropathy in Nicaragua. *BMJ Open* **6**(12): e011034. Available from: https://doi.org/10.1136/bmjopen-2016-011034.

WHO. (2020a) *Lead Poisoning and Health.* [Online] Available from: https://www.who.int/news-room/fact-sheets/detail/lead-poisoning-and-health. [Accessed on 10 May 2021].

WHO. (2020b) *Heatwaves.* [Online] Available from: https://www.who.int/health-topics/heatwaves#tab=tab_1. [Accessed on 10 May 2021].

Xiang J, Bi P, Pisaniello D, Hansen A. (2014) Health impacts of workplace heat exposure: An epidemiological review. *Ind Health* **52**: 91–101.

Yang HY, Wang JD, Lo TC, Chen PC. (2013) Occupational exposure to herbs containing aristolochic acids increases the risk of urothelial carcinoma in Chinese herbalists. *J Urol* **189**: 48–52.

Ye X, Wong O. (2006) Lead exposure, lead poisoning, and lead regulatory standards in China, 1990–2005. *Regul Toxicol Pharmacol* **46**: 157–162.

Youle A. (2005) The thermal environment. In: Gardiner, K., Harrington, J.M. (eds.), *Occupational Hygiene* (3rd Ed). Oxford, Blackwell Publishing.

Zhang C, Gan C, Ding L, Xiong M, Zhang A, Li P. (2020) Maternal inorganic mercury exposure and renal effects in the Wanshan mercury mining area, southwest China. *Ecotoxicol Environ Saf* **189**: 109987.

Zhang F, Bai Y, Zhu B, Zhu W, Ye M. (2016) Group and insidious tetraethyl lead poisoning occurred in industry of plastic weaving: A case report. *J Thorac Dis* **8**(5): E325–E329.

Zhang X, Wang Z, Li T. (2010) The current status of occupational health in China. *Environ Health Prev Med* **15**: 263–270.

Chapter 12

Cardiovascular Disorders

Eduard Shantsila, Alena Shantsila,† Mikhail S. Dzeshka‡ and Gregory Y.H. Lip§,¶*

Introduction

Despite significant reduction in cardiovascular and cerebrovascular mortality over the past decades, cardiac deaths in people of working age are still common in both developing and developed countries. Advances in cardiovascular health are largely attributed to major improvements in risk factor control, such as smoking cessation, blood pressure and cholesterol lowering and better diabetes control. Expanding evidence-based pharmacological and invasive treatments as well as up-to-date risk stratification tools for everyday clinical practice also play an important role.

*Faculty of Health and Life Sciences and Liverpool Centre for Cardiovascular Science, University of Liverpool, UK.
†Liverpool Centre for Cardiovascular Science, University of Liverpool, Liverpool, UK.
‡Grodno State Medical University, Grodno, Belarus.
§Liverpool Centre for Cardiovascular Science, University of Liverpool and Liverpool Heart & Chest Hospital, Liverpool, UK.
¶Aalborg Thrombosis Research Unit, Department of Clinical Medicine, Faculty of Health, Aalborg University, Aalborg, Denmark.

Prevalence of Cardiovascular Disease and Associated Risk Factors in the Population

While cardiovascular mortality is decreasing, the prevalence of the cardiac pathology is actually increasing due to improved survival. Cardiovascular risk factors are common and need attention (Mozaffarian *et al.*, 2015). For example, despite reduction in the prevalence of smoking in Americans from 24.1% to 17.9%, the habit is still common. Only approximately half of adults have appropriate aerobic physical activity and the prevalence of obesity is increasing. In addition, over 40% of the population have total cholesterol levels exceeding 200 mg/dL (5.2 mmol/L) of whom a substantial proportion is not aware of hypercholesterolaemia, related cardiovascular risk and hypolipidaemic therapy. High blood pressure was reported in 32.6% of the population and of those with hypertension only 54.1% had their blood pressure well controlled, leading to 18.9 deaths per 100,000 (Mozaffarian *et al.*, 2015).

As a result, in the year 2011 the death rate from cardiovascular causes was up to 230 per 100,000 of population. This corresponds to approximately one cardiovascular death of every three deaths in the United States (US), notwithstanding a 30.8% reduction during the last decade. About 20% of deaths due to cardiovascular causes were under 65 years old, much below the average life expectancy of 78.7 years for the US (Mozaffarian *et al.*, 2015). The total prevalence of coronary heart disease was 6.2% (projected to increase to 18% by 2030) of which 2.8% developed myocardial infarction.

A total of 2.6% of the US population suffered from stroke. The relative rate of stroke-related death decreased by 35.1 in 2001 through 2011, but remained high accounting approximately for one of every 20 deaths in 2011 (37.9 per 100,000). Heart failure developed in 2.2% of the population, and the prevalence of heart failure is expected to increase by 46% by 2030 (Mozaffarian *et al.*, 2015).

Arrhythmic events also require attention since only about 10% patients survive from arrhythmia cardiac arrest. Atrial fibrillation (AF) is associated with a five-fold elevated risk of strokes, which are more frequently fatal and debilitating compared to those without AF (Mozaffarian *et al.*, 2015).

Assessment of Cardiovascular Risk

Given that cardiovascular diseases are a major contributor to mortality and disability, continuous efforts are made to further improve primary and secondary prevention of cardiovascular diseases and their complications. Assessment of cardiovascular risk is an essential part of prevention of cardiovascular diseases in general population. Smoking cessation, physical activity, blood pressure control, reduction of body weight, and management of dyslipidaemia (specifically of increased non-high density lipoproteins (non-HDL) cholesterol) are the most powerful interventions to prevent atherosclerotic cardiovascular events. Lowering non-HDL cholesterol generally requires administration of statins as 80% of body cholesterol is produced and only 20% are consumed from diet. The paradigm for their use for primary prevention of cardiovascular has shifted to embrace much bigger populations of people who are now eligible for initiation of the treatment (Stone *et al.*, 2015). National cardiovascular societies in different countries adopted such risk prediction tools. These tools are derived from large registries involving national cohorts and therefore perform best and reflect current risks and their relative importance in specified countries.

Four community-based cohorts from the major epidemiological cardiovascular studies broadly representative of the US population have been analysed. These are the Framingham Heart Study, the Atherosclerosis Risk in Communities (ARIC) study, the Cardiovascular Health Study (CHS), and the Coronary Artery Risk Development in Young Adults (CARDIA) study, to derive pooled cohort equations for estimation of 10-year risk of atherosclerotic cardiovascular disease (Goff *et al.*, 2014). These equations replaced previously widely adopted Framingham 10-year risk score that was based on one study only. The Framingham Heart Study provided valuable information with respect to factors associated with the development of atherosclerotic cardiovascular disease, but it has several acknowledged limitations. For example, underrepresentation of ethnic groups (it involved exclusively white participants) as well as weaknesses of the end-points used. The end-points were initially developed for prediction of coronary heart disease including stable and unstable angina, myocardial infarction, and coronary death. Later the end-points were updated to additionally predict stroke, stroke-related death and heart failure. The end-points thus include some unreliable endpoints, which resulted in possible misclassification of risk strata (Shah, 2010).

Currently used pooled cohort equations supply physicians with a tool to predict race- and sex-specific risk of developing nonfatal myocardial infarction, coronary death, fatal or nonfatal stroke based on age, total cholesterol, HDL cholesterol, and systolic blood pressure (Goff *et al.*, 2014). Nonetheless, the Framingham Risk Score, only modified for a family history of premature coronary disease, is still used for cardiovascular disease risk assessment, e.g. in Canada (Anderson *et al.*, 2013).

Population QRISK2 and QRISK3 assessment tools have been developed for the United Kingdom (UK) to evaluate the 10-year risk of stroke/transient ischaemic attack, myocardial infarction/heart attacks, and angina. It includes consideration of smoking status, history of diabetes, family history of early angina or heart attack, chronic kidney disease, AF, hypertension, rheumatoid arthritis, cholesterol/HDL ratio, systolic blood pressure, and body mass index. The important advantage of the QRISK tools is availability of regular updates and calibrations for better prediction of cardiovascular event rate in the UK (Collins and Altman, 2012). Also, SCORE charts have been developed separately for low-risk and high-risk countries in Europe to determine the risk of fatal cardiovascular disease based on age, gender, smoking status, systolic blood pressure and total cholesterol level (Perk *et al.*, 2012).

The utilisation of multiple risk stratification reflects a lack of a single 'one size fits all' tool so far. This is due to significant diversity of risk factor profile, genetic and cultural factors in different regions, which also have dynamic rather than fixed patterns thus requiring regular updates. Moreover, all of them provide physicians with estimated risk rather than the actual probability of cardiovascular disease development.

Therefore, risk classification tools are subject to further improvement by adding new risk factors identified, including epidemiological characteristics, imaging or circulatory biomarkers, which were found to offer independent predictive value. For example, the American College of Cardiology/American Heart Association Guideline on the Assessment of Cardiovascular Risk offers an opportunity to consider family history of premature cardiovascular disease in first-degree relatives (i.e. occurring at less than 55 years old in men and less than 65 year old for women), high-sensitive C-reactive protein (≥2 mg/dL), coronary artery calcium score (≥300 Agatston units or ≥75th percentile for age, sex, and ethnicity), and ankle-brachial index (<0.9). These additional factors aim to provide a better quantitative individual risk assessment for decision making regarding statins prescription for primary prevention. Many other risk factors have been tested, such as elevated apolipoprotein B, chronic kidney disease, microalbuminuria, and cardio-respiratory fitness, but the benefits of their addition to the score systems need further evidence and evaluation (Goff *et al.*, 2014). There are pros and cons for both simplified but easily accessible in routine clinical practice, and complex but more personalised risk assessment tools. These should be chosen based on clinical circumstances and resource availability.

Work and Cardiovascular Disease

Whilst cardiovascular risk assessment has been extensively studied for multiple lifestyle risk factors and biomarkers the extent of cardiovascular risk posed by occupational exposures remains less addressed. Also, as cardiac disorders are common, especially in the older members of workforce, it would be important to establish how the occupational risks influence the heart disease state and progression to minimise risks involved. Again, more remains to be done in the field.

There are various physical, chemical, biological, ergonomic, and psychosocial hazards, which are linked to development and/or exacerbation of arterial hypertension, coronary heart disease and arrhythmia. Tremendous variability of occupational risk factors and their combinations makes development and validation of specific scoring tools problematic. Few of the putative occupational cardiovascular risk factors have been adequately assessed to establish their independent impact for risk of cardiovascular disease. This is in part due to a shortage of epidemiological studies to evaluate occupational risk factors.

Baseline risk of cardiovascular disease is important when evaluating fitness for particular jobs, especially those which may trigger accelerated progression of atherosclerosis, unmask subclinical changes, and cause development of cardiovascular disease. In patients with pre-existing cardiovascular disease, occupational risk factors can result in further exacerbation in the clinical course of cardiovascular disease. However, data on particular characteristics of the work environment of patients are often not inquired by physicians despite many patients feeling that their illness may be related to work conditions or aggravated by factors at their workplace. An occupational history or even a job title is often missing from medical records.

Chemical Hazards

Polycyclic Aromatic Hydrocarbons

There is a range of chemical hazards, which are known to be associated with cardiovascular disease. Polycyclic aromatic hydrocarbons are present in vehicle exhausts, asphalt, bitumen, coal tar, wild fires, agricultural burning, soil, charbroiled meat and tobacco smoke, i.e. they appear as by-products of organic compound combustion. Other sources include oil spills, forest fires, use of technologies which do not utilise fuel efficiently, cook ovens, and foundries, and other natural and anthropogenic sources causing environmental pollution (Ball and Truskewycz, 2013).

In the US National Health and Nutrition Examination Surveys (NHANES) carried out in 2011–2012, urinary polycyclic aromatic hydrocarbons used as biomarkers of exposure to extrinsic polycyclic aromatic hydrocarbon were shown to be associated with cardiovascular diseases. For instance, 4-hydroxyphenanthrene was associated with a higher risk of hypertension (odds ratio [OR] 1.33, 95% confidence interval [CI] 1.00–1.76) and 1-hydroxypyrene was associated with an increased risk of myocardial infaction (OR 1.47, 95% CI 1.05–2.06) (Shiue, 2015). Also higher levels of 1-hydroxypyrene were observed in patients with acute myocardial infarction compared to controls, and elevated 1-hydroxypyrene concentrations correlated with markers of oxidative stress (e.g. malondialdehyde, catalase, beta-carotene) and inflammation (e.g. C-reactive protein) (Freitas *et al.*, 2014). These detrimental effects can be contributed to by the metabolism of polycyclic aromatic hydrocarbons via binding to aryl hydrocarbon receptors during which reactive oxygen species and other radicals are generated (Ball and Truskewycz, 2013; Pan *et al.*, 2008).

Combustion-derived air pollutants may also be an occupational risk. Diesel exhaust in diesel-powered trains exposes to black carbon and ultrafine particles affected heart rate variability and increased levels of DNA strand breaks in blood cells after a 3-day exposure (Anderson *et al.*, 2019). Apparently, time and intensity of exposure to these factors are critical for occurrence of cardiovascular changes. For example, there was a significant association between long-term (but not medium-term) exposure to polycyclic aromatic hydrocarbons at the place of residence and the prevalence of hypertension among individuals from the Mano a Mano cohort (OR 1.40, 95% CI 1.01–1.94) (Bangia *et al.*, 2015). In an animal model of short-term exposure to benzopyrene, circadian dynamics of blood pressure was affected, in particular insufficient blood pressure decrease (dipping) at night time (Gentner and Weber, 2011). However, the question whether these associations were causal or mechanistic was not addressed. A probability of overlap with pathogenic effects of other pollutants was acknowledged through all the studies.

Both experimental models and a clinical study showed increased risk of congenital heart defects associated occupational exposure to polycyclic aromatic hydrocarbons during pregnancy. In the National Birth Defects Prevention Study (NBDPS) (1997–2011) an adjusted analysis, that compared mother from highest quartile of exposure to polycyclic aromatic hydrocarbons during early pregnancy had more children with the conotruncal heart defects group (OR 1.41; 95% CI 1.00–2.00), and with tetralogy of Fallot (OR 1.83; 95% CI 1.21–2.78) compared to mothers with no such exposure (Patel *et al.*, 2020). This is a significant call for considerations for provision of adequate protection or safer roles for women of childbearing potential in industries working with polycyclic aromatic hydrocarbons.

Polyhalogenated Hydrocarbons

Polyhalogenated hydrocarbons are one of the major representatives of persistent organic pollutants, known for their ability to persist in the environment. They are generally of low water and high lipid solubility, and undergo bio magnification in the food chain (Magliano *et al.*, 2014). There is a wide range of polyhalogenated hydrocarbons (e.g. polychlorinated biphenyls, polybrominated biphenyls, 2, 3, 7, 8-tetrachlorodibenzo-p-dioxin, polychlorinated dibenzo-p-dioxin D and hexachlorobenzene) used in the chemical industry. Substances with more chlorine atoms are generally considered to be more toxic. Serum concentrations of octachlorodibenzo-p-dioxin and polychlorinated biphenyls were found to be associated with a reduction of left ventricular ejection fraction in residents of Uppsala, Sweden (Sjoberg *et al.*, 2013) that was likely mediated by activation of oxidative stress and inflammation (Kopf *et al.*, 2008; Vogel *et al.*, 2007). An association was shown between dietary intake of polychlorinated biphenyls and a higher risk of developing hypertension (hazard ratio [HR] for the 5th quintile versus 1st quintile 1.43, 95% CI 1.09–1.88) (Donat-Vargas *et al.*, 2015). Incidentally, the data from many studies are also suggestive of a link between exposure to polyhalogenated hydrocarbons and diabetes mellitus (Magliano *et al.*, 2014). In an analysis of two pooled Asian cohorts exposed to polychlorinated biphenyls and dibenzofurans, a 30% higher mortality risk was detected compared to unexposed controls (Li *et al.*, 2015).

Inorganic Arsenic

Arsenic is a natural element of the earth's crust. Knowledge about sequelae of exposure to inorganic arsenic was derived mostly from data on environmental exposure (mostly via drinking water from wells where the groundwater is in contact with this metalloid, or consuming food grown in contaminated soil or water) rather than occupational sources (e.g. in some mines, the wood industry, tin and copper workers, coal-fired power plants, ore smelting, battery assembly, and in electronics). In non-occupational settings exposures may vary depending on location (Moon *et al.*, 2012).

Arsenic is metabolised within hours and excreted via the kidneys as monomethylarsonic acid, dimethyarsinic acid, and inorganic arsenic. Urinary arsenic is considered as a reliable marker of arsenic exposure, however various metabolites of arsenic are of different toxicity, with monomethylarsonate being the most toxic (Stea *et al.*, 2014). Arsenic levels can also be determined in nails and hair, but are used mainly for forensic purposes rather than for assessing occupational exposure.

The consequences of exposure to arsenic depend on dose, duration, and frequency of exposure, and smoking status. Arsenic effects include neurologic symptoms, respiratory effects, and malignancies (Stea *et al.*, 2014). Multiple mechanisms of cardiovascular damage caused by arsenic exposure have been suggested, e.g. oxidative stress, genetic mutations and inhibition of nucleic acids repair, interference with sulfhydryl groups of proteins and enzymes, decrease in synthesis of macroergic phosphates, disturbance of intercellular communications, induction of tumor necrosis factor-α and endothelial dysfunction (Stea *et al.*, 2014; Mo *et al.*, 2011; Wade *et al.*, 2015). Arsenic exposure was found to be associated with gene expression in heart encoding ion channels (increased expression of KCNA5, decreased expression of CACNA1, KCNH2, KCNQ1 and KCNE1) and therefore can change QT-interval duration, induce ventricular arrhythmias and cause sudden cardiac death (Mo *et al.*, 2011; Chen *et al.*, 2013).

Water concentrations of arsenic below 100 μg/L are not associated with overt adverse effects (Tsuji *et al.*, 2014). However emerging data indicate elevated cardiovascular risk even within this "safe" range. In a study from China, every 10 μg/L increase in arsenic concentrations in water was associated with a 19% increase in risk of cardiovascular diseases (angina, myocardial infarction or cardiomyopathy) (Wade *et al.*, 2015). In another study there was a 2.2-fold higher risk of cardiovascular disease for a life-time arsenic in water exposure of 20–30 μg/L and a 9.1-fold higher risk when arsenic concentrations in drinking water were over 45 μg/L (James *et al.*, 2015). In fact, a recent meta-analysis showed a significant risk of cardiovascular disease across low to high levels of arsenic exposure (Moon *et al.*, 2017).

In a systematic review of 31 studies arsenic exposure in drinking water (>50 μg/L) was associated with increased risks for cardiovascular disease (RR 1.32, 95% CI 1.05–1.67), coronary heart disease

(RR 1.89, 95% CI 1.33–2.69), peripheral arterial disease (RR 2.17, 95% CI 1.47–3.20), and stroke (RR 1.08, 95% CI 0.98–1.19) (20). A dose-response analysis of twelve published studies ($n = 408\,945$) showed that water arsenic concentration of 20 μg/L compared to 10 μg/L resulted in modest but significant increase in cardiovascular mortality, incidence of coronary artery disease and stroke (Moon *et al.*, 2017).

Extrapolating results of environmental research to occupational exposure to arsenic indicate that even under relatively low concentrations, the toxic effects accumulate over time predisposing to cardiac autonomic dysregulation and cardiovascular disease (Karakulak *et al.*, 2017). Of interest, work related exposure to low arsenic levels did not affect levels of total cholesterol, LDL, HDL, or triglycerides, but did affect Lp(a), Apo-A1, and Apo-B fraction, thus leading to dyslipidaemia not reflected by routine clinical tests (Ledda *et al.*, 2018).

Lead

Exposure to lead has decreased due to implementation of industrial hygiene controls, improvement of technology, and discontinuation of leaded petrol. However, lead is still widely used in battery manufacture, badge and jewellery enamelling and other vitreous enamelling operations, glass making, manufacture of pigments and colours, manufacture of lead compounds (salts), shipbuilding, ship repairing and breaking, painting, food-can soldering, and soldering joints of drinking water pipe systems (McElvenny *et al.*, 2015). Consuming lead-contaminated food or water, breathing lead-polluted air, or even skin contact with organic lead can result in accumulation of lead in the body.

Blood lead levels reflect a balance between circulating lead and body stores of the metal. Prolonged chronic exposure to lead can be evaluated with bigger accuracy by bone X-ray fluorescence (Solenkova *et al.*, 2014). The effect of lead exposure on the cardiovascular system also depends on co-exposure with other metals, which may exhibit antagonism or synergism of action in terms of blood pressure regulation, cardiac contractility or electrical activity (Wildemann *et al.*, 2015).

A study of over nine thousand workers from Great Britain, showed a positive relationship between blood lead levels and cardiovascular mortality (HR 1.30, 95% CI 1.17–1.44) and an increased risk of ischaemic heart disease (HR 1.30, 95% CI 1.17–1.43) (McElvenny *et al.*, 2015). In a study of patients with blood lead levels below 10 µg/dL, assessed in the Third National Health and Nutrition Examination Survey, there was a significant increase in cardiovascular mortality in adults with blood lead levels over 3.6 µg/dL compared to those with blood lead levels below 1.9 µg/dL (Menke *et al.*, 2006).

Data from the Korea Occupational Safety and Health Agency, which included lead-exposed male workers showed a clear increase in ischaemic heart disease (admission HR 1.78, 95% CI 1.17–2.72), angina pectoris (admission HR 1.93, 95% CI 1.13–3.29) and cerebral infarction (admission HR 2.24, 95% CI 1.14–4.39) among workers with a blood lead levels ≥20 µg/dL than those with a blood lead levels ≤10 µg/dL (Min and Ahn, 2017). A cumulative analysis of three cohorts of lead-exposed workers (US, Finland, UK) including over 88,000 workers confirmed that median blood lead levels of 26 µg/dL or higher were associated with increased rates of stroke and heart disease (Steenland *et al.*, 2017). A study of 58,368 male US workers followed for a median of 19 years further confirmed increased mortality from ischaemic heart disease in those with occupational lead exposure (Barry and Steenland, 2019).

Multiple studies have established a link between lead exposure and hypertension. Acute lead exposure was demonstrated to increase blood pressure via activation of the renin-angiotensin system, but in case of chronic exposure only a weak association was shown. Two meta-analyses addressed this topic. In one meta-analysis, for each 10 µg/g increase in tibia lead concentration, the systolic blood pressure increased by 0.26 mmHg (95% CI 0.02–0.50) and the diastolic blood pressure increased by 0.02 mmHg (95% CI –0.15–0.19) (Navas-Acien *et al.*, 2008). A broadly similar association was obtained for blood lead level. Doubling of the blood lead concentrations led to a 1.0 mmHg (95% CI 0.5–1.4) increase in systolic blood pressure and 0.6 mmHg (95% CI 0.4–0.8) rise in the diastolic blood pressure (Nawrot *et al.*, 2002). Again, studies of effects of lead on blood pressure have not been entirely consistent and one study found no correlation between lead exposure and hypertension at all (Taheri *et al.*, 2014).

The Trial to Assess Chelation Therapy assessed therapeutic potential of EDTA chelation in people with lead exposure and history of myocardial infarction and showed improvement in rates cardiovascular events, particularly in patients with diabetes. However, lead levels were not measured in this study and further studies are needed in the field (Glicklich *et al.*, 2020).

Carbon Disulfide

Carbon disulfide (CS_2) is used as a reagent for viscose rayon production. Rayon workers are exposed to CS_2 via respiration and skin absorption. The occupational exposure limits for CS_2 are between one and 10 ppm (parts per million). Cardiovascular effects are secondary to long-term exposure to CS_2, and similarly to many other hazardous chemical substances. This is mediated by an increase in oxidative stress and an accelerated progression of atherosclerosis (Wronska-Nofer *et al.*, 2007). Exposure to CS_2 was found to be associated with dyslipidaemia (Di Lorenzo *et al.*, 2003), carotid intima-media thickness (Schramm *et al.*, 2016), diastolic and systolic blood pressure, electrocardiogram abnormalities and kidney dysfunction (Chen *et al.*, 2009).

Case Study 1: Effects of Carbon Disulfide Exposure during Rayon Manufacturing

A 45 year-old man developed dyslipidaemia, and cardiac abnormalities and features of diabetic nephropathy and nephrotic syndrome despite no history of diabetes (Klemmer and Harris, 2000). He had been exposed to toxic levels of CS_2 during work in a rayon manufacturing plant. His condition progressed to end-stage renal failure with background hypertension and evidence of focal sclerosing glomerulonephritis, which were deemed related to CS_2 exposure.

A recent analysis of chemical occupational risks conducted on request of the Swedish government concluded that exposure to carbon disulphide increases risk of stroke and cardiac disease and thus exposed workers need appropriate health protection (Swedish Council on Health Technology Assessment, 2017).

Carbon Monoxide

Carbon monoxide (CO) is a colourless, odourless, tasteless, and non-irritating toxic gas produced by incomplete combustion of organic compounds. CO is one of the most frequent causes of occupational fatality due to acute gaseous inhalation. The toxicity of CO is a sequel of a higher affinity of CO for haemoglobin than oxygen. This leads to displacement of oxygen from haemoglobin, formation of carboxy-haemoglobin (COHb) and development of tissue hypoxia. As a result, workers exposed to CO have a higher prevalence of ischaemic heart disease (Koskela *et al.*, 2000). Exposure to CO at workplaces results in 2–8% of COHb in blood, whilst in smokers it is higher (5–15%) (Price, 2004). The higher the blood COHb concentration the lower the coronary ischaemic threshold. Motor vehicles have been the most frequent source of fatal CO exposure, followed by heating systems (especially those using coal as fuel in homes) and generators (Henn *et al.*, 2013). Carboxyhaemoglobin in blood can be used for evaluation of exposure to CO, as well as automatic sensors for CO in air which can be installed in working areas (Mikov *et al.*, 2000; Erdogan *et al.*, 2004).

A recent large review concluded that occupational CO exposure increases risks of heart disease but could not provide such evidence in relation to risk of stroke or hypertension (Swedish Council on Health Technology Assessment, 2017).

Cobalt

Exposure to cobalt in occupational settings occurs in the hard metal industries (for example, tool production and grinding), coal mining, metal mining, smelting and refining, cobalt dye painters, and cobalt chemical production. More recently, cobalt plays an important role in manufacturing of batteries for electric vehicles, with particular concerns expressed about the working conditions at the stage of its mining. In non-occupational settings, people with cobalt-chromium joint implants, those living near plants using cobalt or in areas where cobalt-containing fertilisers are used, or using cobalt-containing supplements or large amounts of vitamin B12 may develop symptoms and signs of cobalt toxicity (Perez and Tang, 2015).

Experimental exposure to cobalt resulted in reduction of superoxide dismutase activity, decrease in mitochondrial ATP production rate and reduction in the respiratory chain capacity (Clyne *et al.*, 2001). The effect of exposure to cobalt can be assessed by measuring blood or urinary concentration of cobalt. Blood levels of 300 µg/L or lower are considered safe with no known relationship to disease.

Earlier reports indicated that cobalt toxicity was associated with a risk of development of heart dysfunction or even phenotypical presentation of dilated cardiomyopathy (at cobalt blood levels of 700–800 µg/L or higher) (Perez and Tang, 2015; Finley *et al.*, 2012). There is a suspicion of cobalt causing cardiomyopathy, but definitive epidemiological evidence is lacking (Lantin *et al.*, 2013). Several very suspicious fatal cases have been reported.

Case Study 2: Cardiac Shock and Cobalt Cardiomyopathy

A 48 year-old man developed a fatal cardiac shock under anaesthesia during an abdominal surgery. On autopsy he was found cardiac compatible with cobalt cardiomyopathy and very high myocardial cobalt levels. His job involved operation of the powdered metal with exposure to cobalt (Kennedy et al., *1981).*

However, a recent prospective echocardiographic study of 93 exposed and 49 non-exposed workers re-examined over a six year period found no evidence of cardiac damage beyond expected for age and traditional cardiovascular risk factors (Linna *et al.*, 2020).

Consequently, at present there is no reliable evidence of heart related hazards for people with occupational exposure to cobalt (Linna *et al.*, 2020). This is good news for the industry involving use of cobalt.

Warfarin and Other Vitamin K Antagonists

Warfarin is an anticoagulant that interferes with the synthesis of vitamin K-dependent clotting factors (II, VII, IX, X), and therefore it is widely used for prevention of thrombotic complications in patients with AF, prosthetic heart valves, pulmonary embolism, and deep vein thrombosis (Dzeshka and Lip, 2014).

Occupational exposure to warfarin in pharmaceutical manufacturing companies may occur via air, skin contact, and ingestion. The major signs of overexposure to warfarin include haemorrhage, e.g. epistaxis, gingival bleeding, widespread bruising, ecchymosis, haematomas under the skin or around joints, haematuria, menorrhagia, gastrointestinal bleeding, rectal bleeding and bleeding into any internal organ. Life-threatening bleeding can occur as a result of acute poisoning (Xu *et al.*, 2013). The international normalised ratio (INR) is used for assessment of anticoagulant effect of warfarin as a result of warfarin exposure, and vitamin K can be used as an antidote for over-exposure (Dzeshka and Lip, 2014).

Warfarin was also used commercially as a rodenticide. However, with the emergence of warfarin-resistant strains of rats, other anticoagulant rodenticides have been developed, e.g. brodifacoum, bromadiolone, difenacoum, flocoumafen, chlorophacinone and diphacinone. These newer rodenticides have been termed "superwarfarins" due to their higher potency and duration of action resulting from a greater affinity for vitamin K-epoxide reductase, an ability to disrupt the vitamin K-epoxide cycle at several stages, hepatic accumulation, high lipid solubility and enterohepatic circulation (Watt *et al.*, 2005). Anecdotal cases of occupational exposure to warfarin have been reported (Svendsen *et al.*, 2002; Moery and Pontious, 2009). Exposure to anticoagulants should be considered in the absence of an obvious cause for bleeding.

Nitrates

Nitroglycerine and ethylene glycol dinitrate (nitroglycol) were used for explosives production. Overexposure can also occur among construction workers using dynamite. Exposure is particularly high during mixing and filling cartridges of explosives, since nitrates are volatile and capable of fast absorption via skin and airways.

Prolonged exposure can cause vasodilation and compensatory activation of vasoconstrictive systems, which counteract nitrates, e.g.

renin-angiotensin system. In cases when vasoconstriction was not balanced by the vasodilation it resulted in coronary spasm, angina, myocardial infarction and even sudden death (also described as "Monday morning sudden death") (Price, 2004; Warren, 1988).

Occupational exposure to nitrates with severe health effects is rare. However, there is a significant association between prenatal exposure to nitrates in drinking water and the risk of congenital cardiac anomalies which may indicate that exposure to nitrates may be best minimised in women of childbearing age (Biaisdell *et al.*, 2019).

Physical Hazards

Noise

Noise is a well-recognised occupational hazard at workplaces in most countries. Effects of noise can be divided into auditory (hearing loss) and non-auditory (variety of pathologic effects resulting from general non-specific stress triggered by noise exposure). The latter include psychological consequences (agitation, annoyance or even depression), disturbed fragmented night sleep, endocrine impairment, and also cardiovascular effects (hypertension, heart rate increase) (Hammer *et al.*, 2014). Noise may act either directly via synaptic interactions, or indirectly through the emotional and cognitive (subjective) perception of sound (Munzel *et al.*, 2014). Occupational exposure limits to control noise exposure at workplaces have been set at around 85 dB(A) in most countries.

Studies that addressed cardiovascular effects of noise exposure in different settings have produced inconsistent findings. Some studies showed a transient increase of blood pressure after exposure to noise. For example, there was a transient 6 mmHg and 3 mmHg elevation of systolic and diastolic blood pressure, respectively, in normotensive workers at a metallurgical factory exposed to noise levels of >85 dB(A) compared to those exposed to <80 dB(A) (Fogari *et al.*, 2001). However, no persistent blood pressure elevation was established. Recently, analysis of 4,548 participants from the National Health and Nutrition Examination Survey concluded that evidence was not consistent to support the link between occupational noise exposure and blood pressure (Gan and Mannino, 2018).

In other studies, there was no association between blood pressure and noise exposure (Krista-Boneh *et al.*, 1995). Impact of noise exposure on blood pressure also showed age dependence with more apparent effect in younger workers (Green *et al.*, 1991). Importantly, as exposure to noise is known to interfere with the quality of night sleep (Gitanjali and Ananth, 2003), it was also associated with the night-time elevation of blood pressure (Chang *et al.*, 2003). When workers at a metal manufacturing factory were classified according to extent of noise exposure, those exposed to noise of 85 dB(A) or higher persistently (workers at worksite) as well as exposed intermittently (inspectors, technical support) were found to have higher systolic blood pressure (approximately 4 and 2 mmHg, respectively) than office workers exposed to noise below 85 dB(A) (Lee *et al.*, 2009).

A meta-analysis of historical data from the 1970s–1990s showed a significant association between occupational noise and hypertension (RR 1.14, 95% CI 1.01–1.29 per 5 dB(A) increase) (van Kempen *et al.*, 2002). Recently more attention has been paid to environmental exposure to noise, which is usually continuous and chronic. Results from various studies consistently demonstrate a negative and independent role of noise in cardiovascular disorders. Increase in noise exposure per 5 dB(A) was shown to be associated with a 3.9% (95% CI 0.0–8.0%) increase of thoracic aorta calcification, a measure of subclinical atherosclerosis (Kalsch *et al.*, 2014). The adverse impact of noise exposure on the cardiovascular system can be further augmented by other concomitant risk factors, e.g. shift work, organic solvents (Attarchi *et al.*, 2013; Attarchi *et al.*, 2012).

Accumulating data point towards association between occupational noise exposure and prevalent coronary heart disease. A large Chinese study suggested dose-response effect between hearing loss and coronary heart disease prevalence (Fang *et al.*, 2018). A prospective cohort Swedish study of occupational noise exposure showed increased risk for coronary heart disease but not a stroke in relation to noise levels 75 dB or higher (Eriksson *et al.*, 2018). A different large Swedish study of 85,169 seafarers showed no increased mortality on passenger ferries but younger male seafarers on different types of vessels had increased mortality from cardiovascular disease, which was attributable to noise exposure (Eriksson *et al.*, 2020). These findings are consistent with a study of 194,501 Swedish construction workers in whom moderate and high noise exposure was associated with increased risk of myocardial infarction mortality (but also with increased stroke mortality (Pettersson *et al.*, 2020). In a recent systematic review, despite methodological limitations, occupational noise was a risk factor for ischaemic heart disease (Dzhambov and Dimitrova, 2016a) Although mechanisms of such associations are not yet clear, they could be contributed by an evidence of linear association between noise exposure and increase in heart rate (Burns *et al.*, 2016).

Vibration

Exposure to noise coincides with exposure to vibration frequently in a variety of professions (metal and mining workers, crane and truck drivers, forestry workers and carpenters). There are two major ways of vibration transmission in occupational settings: whole body vibration and hand-arm vibration. The latter is associated with impairment of peripheral circulation due to endothelial dysfunction, increased vascular resistance, and vasoconstriction.

A higher prevalence of ischaemic heart disease was found in individuals exposed to vibration than in non-exposed people (Tamaian and Cocarla, 1998). Occupational vibration was a risk factor for prevalent heart disease in Bulgaria (Dzhambov and Dimitrova, 2016b). Operators of vibrating machines were prone to myocardial infarction in the cohort of the Vasternorrland heart epidemiology programme (OR 1.6, 95% CI 1.1–2.4). Overall outcomes of vibration exposure depend on lifetime duration of the exposure. It is likely to be dependent on frequency of vibration and co-exposure to other occupational hazards (e.g. noise, dust) (Bjor *et al.*, 2006, 2010 Maikala *et al.*, 2006).

Temperature Extremes

Exposure both to heat and cold can be detrimental to the cardiovascular system. Arguably global warming could potentially have an impact on the traditional patterns of environmental exposure for jobs done in open environments, such as minting and agriculture. Heat exposure frequently occurs in workers of metallurgical industry, sailors operating in tropical waters, outdoor workers in countries with very high seasonal heat.

Cardiac responses to the heat include tachycardia since circulated blood acts as a cooling fluid transporting heat from the central body to peripheral tissues and skin where the heat is disseminated to the air. To facilitate this process, cardiac output increases by an increase of stroke volume and tachycardia. Physical activity during exposure to heat further increases the heart rate. Also reduction of volume of circulated blood (hypohydration) due to sweating creates an additional load on the cardiovascular system and increases cardiac strain (Sett and Sahu, 2014; Sahu *et al.*, 2013; Rodahl, 2003). Workers in countries with hot desert environments, e.g. in the Middle East, can be exposed to environmental temperatures as high as 50 degrees Centigrade. The risks of cardiovascular and other health effects can be high, and have been mitigated by campaigns on awareness and advice on reducing the likelihood of heat stress in such locations.

The risk of cardiovascular disease is also elevated in case of exposure to cold. Relevant environments are the frozen food industry, cold storage units, mining, offshore oil and gas facilities in the Arctic and Antarctic environments (Nayha, 2002). Chronic exposure to cold is associated with hypertension, increased cholesterol levels, haematological changes (e.g. raised platelet count) (Lin *et al.*, 2013).

Psychosocial Stress

High job demands, excessive workload, limited resources, poor supervision, lack of support, mismatch between expectations and actual work requirements, lack of reciprocity between efforts at work and rewards received (i.e. effort-reward imbalance), and job insecurity are all risk factors for the development of work-related stress. People with low coping potential, type A behaviour personality (defined as rigidly organised, ambitious, highly status-conscious, taking on more than they can handle, wanting other people to 'get to the point,' and concern with time management) are also at higher risk of work-related stress. Work-related stress is also experienced by individuals where workplace downsizing, restructuring of companies, and increased use of flexible forms of employment, collectively result in everyday fear of job loss.

There is a range of professions associated with a high prevalence of work-related stress (e.g. teaching and in healthcare). Work-related stress results in low level job satisfaction, emotional exhaustion, depersonalisation, and burnout. Cardiovascular effects from stress and related factors such as long working hours, include elevation of blood pressure, heart rate, and coronary heart disease (Xu *et al.*, 2015).

Severe stress has been also related to risk of cardiac arrest and sudden cardiac death (Glozier *et al.*, 2013). In Japan the term "Karoshi" has been used to refer to "death from over-work" in recognition of this observed association (Li, 2016). The association could be difficult to prove but cases of successful claims have been reported.

Case Study 3: Sudden Death After High Intensity Work

An apparently healthy 55-year-old Chinese man died suddenly after 11 days of high intensity work with cement bags (Liu et al., 2015). The cement factory was sued and compensation was awarded despite some difficulty of providing evidence of the causative links between the work related stress and death.

However even less extensive stress seen in Western style work patterns can also pose cardiovascular risk. Data from 64,394 individuals primarily obtained from Finland, Sweden and UK showed that job strain was related to shorter healthy life expectancy with overall difference of 1.7 years between high and low strain jobs, which was higher in men (2.0 years) than in women (1.5 years) (Magnusson Hanson *et al.*, 2018).

Changes in work organisation, bullying and exposure to workplace violence appear to be particularly detrimental for cardiovascular health. In a Sweden and Denmark of 79,201 responders 9% reported workplace bullying and 13% reported exposure to workplace violence with both stressors being associated with high risk of cardiovascular disease (HR of 1.59, 95% CI 1.28–1.98 for bullying HR of 1.25, 95% CI 1.12–1.40 of workplace violence exposure (Xu *et al.*, 2019). A multivariable analysis done in 14,788 employees showed doubling in risk of cardiovascular disease in the year following change in the work unit compared to no change and there was a clear excess in cardiovascular disease risk following exposure to any organisational change (HR 1.48, 95% CI 0.91–2.43) (Jensen *et al.*, 2020).

Of interest, including perceived stress as mediator in the analysis model did not really change the estimates, leaving the body adaptation to the new arrangement as the likely culprit. In fact, this accords to the Canadian Community Health Survey (CCHS) — of 13,291 respondents where job control and psychological demands have not been associated with incident myocardial infarction and congestive heart failure over a 15-year observation period (Smith *et al.*, 2020).

Individual attributes of employees may play a role. The Taiwan Bus Driver Cohort Study that involved 1,650 professional drivers found that high over commitment scores were attributed to over 70% increase in cardiovascular risk (Wu *et al.*, 2019). However, the field would benefit from further research on factors linking occupational stress of cardiovascular risk.

Cardiovascular Assessment

Fitness for Work in Remote Locations

Residing outside major urban centres is often linked to lower utilisation of specialised health care services and higher mortality than the general population (Magliano *et al.*, 2015; Vanasse *et al.*, 2010). Mortality from myocardial infarction is particularly affected by the area where patients reside since primary percutaneous coronary intervention (PCI) is a treatment of choice for a majority of patients with acute coronary syndrome. However, facilities for PCI are not available in all hospitals, and transfer between hospitals is required.

Given that employment in remote locations results in poorer access to specialised medical care, such individuals are at higher risk of adverse cardiovascular events compared to those who have access to specialised medical care within an appropriate time frame recommended by contemporary guidelines. Thus, pre-placement medical assessments can be performed with an evaluation of individual cardiovascular risk and risks related to working in remote locations. This will allow informed decision making with respect to employment, both for employees and employers.

Firefighters

Firefighters are exposed to multiple hazards including toxic fumes, smoke, products of combustion, flames, high temperatures, loud noise, limited visibility, risk of collapse of affected buildings, and stressful, dynamically changing, chaotic and unpredictable work environments (Smith, 2011). Working at scenes of fire also poses high demands to the cardiovascular system due to strenuous physical activity. The latter results in severe tachycardia and increase in blood pressure, which may continue for extended periods of time. Insulated protective equipment combined with heat exposure also leads to sweating, dehydration, reduced volume of circulated blood (up 15%) and haemoconcentration (Smith, 2011).

As a result, the leading cause of duty-related mortality among firefighters is cardiovascular disease with a high percentage (up to 45%) of sudden cardiac deaths. In turn, a majority of sudden cardiac deaths are attributable to coronary heart disease, and this is more common in older firefighters, predominately during firefighting itself and less often during other activities such as minor rescue work, extrications, natural disasters, and dealing with spills of hazardous substances (Smith *et al.*, 2013, Soteriades *et al.*, 2011). Outside the firefighting activity, these employees often remain physically inactive and are subject to common cardiovascular risk factors such as smoking, obesity, dyslipidaemia and blood pressure elevation (Yang *et al.*, 2013, Baur *et al.*, 2011).

To minimise the risks, risk factor screening and healthy lifestyle programmes should be implemented with a focus on optimal body mass index, prohibition or cessation of smoking, restriction from participating in strenuous emergency duties for firefighters with established coronary heart disease or other structural heart disease, and mandatory retirement from active duties (Kales and Smith, 2014; Yang *et al.*, 2013; Wynn and Hawdon, 2012; Kales and Smith, 2014), with clearly defined criteria. Better cardiorespiratory fitness measured by maximal exercise tolerance is inversely associated with all-cause mortality and cardiovascular mortality (Baur *et al.*, 2011).

Prior to employment firefighters undergo a series of functional tests aimed at evaluating muscular strength and cardiorespiratory fitness to meet the physical and safety requirements. For example, a maximum oxygen consumption (VO_2 max) of 42 ml/kg/min (or 12 metabolic equivalents (METs)) is used as a minimum cardiorespiratory fitness standard for fire fighters in the UK (Wynn and Hawdon, 2012).

Fitness to Drive

Driving is an essential skill in the modern mobile world. Issuing a driving permission (license) is based on the "safety first" principle. The principle assumes that the prospective driver is capable of driving safely by taking responsibility for himself, passengers and other road users sufficient to prevent road traffic accidents. Driving can be particularly challenging if a driver is unfamiliar with new routes, where there is limited visibility, and in busy road traffic. These factors may cause substantial stress and lead to sympathetic activation with tachycardia and dysrhythmia, elevation of blood pressure, and other stress-related physiological changes. Whilst these changes are usually within physiological range, they can exceed the safe threshold in predisposed people, such as in those with background cardiovascular pathology.

Furthermore, given that a variety of cardiovascular diseases can result in different degree of functional impairment, including reduction in cognitive function, loss of consciousness, severe pain, temporary or permanent ceasing of driving may be required (Alosco *et al.*, 2015; Banning and Ng, 2013; Sorajja *et al.*, 2009). Stricter criteria are used for professional drivers, such as truck and bus drivers, because of greater size and weight of their vehicle, often greater length of time spent driving, and more dramatic consequences in the event of an accident (Driver and Vehicle Licensing Agency, 2021).

Cardiovascular conditions are accountable for approximately 8% of all road traffic accidents (Banning and Ng, 2013). Medical standards of fitness to drive were issued by national authorities to aid decision making in evaluation of safety of driving after diagnosis of a cardiovascular disease and related pharmacological, interventional or surgical treatment.

For example, in the UK, the Driver and Vehicle Licensing Agency (DVLA) indicates the following criteria for fitness to drive motor cars. Driving is allowed when symptoms of angina are well controlled, hypertension if antihypertensive drugs do not cause any symptoms, in patients with carotid atherosclerosis, peripheral vascular disease, chronic aortic dissection, valvular and congenital heart disease, hypertrophic and dilated cardiomyopathy, heart failure and even after heart transplantation given no other disqualifying conditions were revealed (Driver and Vehicle Licensing Agency, 2021).

Permission to drive should be withheld for the following duration for car and motorcycle license:

(a) 1 week after elective PCI or successful coronary intervention in patients with acute coronary syndrome if left ventricular ejection fraction is over 40% and no other intervention is planned (in case of unsuccessful coronary angioplasty, the 4-week timeframe is typically applied);
(b) 4 weeks after coronary artery bypass grafting and heart valve surgery;
(c) 1 week after implantation of a pacemaker or cardiac resynchronisation therapy device with pacing only function (CRT-P);
(d) 2 days after successful catheter ablation of arrhythmia, but a longer 4-week period is specified for ventricular tachycardia when there is impaired ventricular function and congenital heart disease even after corrective surgery.

Driving is not allowed for patients with symptomatic aortic stenosis, angina episodes at rest and stress-provoked angina, for people an aortic aneurysm of more than 6.5 cm diameter, and those after insertion of left ventricular assist device (Driver and Vehicle Licensing Agency, 2021).

Much stricter rules are usually applied for holders of bus, coach or lorry licences.

The rules are a subject of change and the latest national recommendations should always be consulted and advice from appropriate specialist or the agency be sought if in doubt. "Safety first" rule should be applied in these situations.

Perhaps the most complicated issues in clinical judgment on fitness to drive occur in patients with arrhythmias. Supraventricular and ventricular tachycardias are most common causes of loss of or impaired consciousness after vasovagal syncopes (the latter are considered to be generally benign and do not require any driving restrictions) (Banning and Ng, 2013; Sorajja and Shen, 2010). Indeed, life-threatening arrhythmias, such as ventricular tachycardia/ventricular fibrillation pose the patients at highest risk of driving incapacity with high probability of consequent road traffic accident.

Implantation of cardioverter-defibrillator (ICD) or cardiac resynchronisation therapy device with defibrillation function (CRT-D) also may cause syncope particularly within the first 6 months. Therefore driving should cease for at least 1 month after ICD implantation indicated for primary prevention in patients with a high risk of ventricular tachycardia/ventricular fibrillation or after ICD implantation for secondary prevention if tachycardia does not lead to haemodynamic instability, left ventricular ejection fraction is over 35%, no fast tachycardia episodes are induced during an electrophysiological study, and tachycardia is effectively terminated by ICD shocks twice after implantation (Driver and Vehicle Licensing Agency, 2021). If ventricular tachycardia leads to haemodynamic instability during 6 months after implantation and 6 months after ICD shock delivery or symptomatic anti-tachycardia pacing, the patient is not allowed to drive (Driver and Vehicle Licensing Agency, 2021).

Fitness for Scuba Diving

Diving, either recreational or professional is being considered a non-strenuous physical activity since the buoyancy force of the water results in a lower perceived body weight. Despite this, diving can be detrimental to the cardiovascular system. Increased ambient pressure (one bar or 750 mmHg for each 10 m depth) leads to several haemodynamic changes, such as reduction of pulmonary air volume, increased venous blood return to the heart, higher solubility and saturation of blood with gases (particularly, nitrogen), increased secretion of atrial natriuretic peptide and decreased synthesis of antidiuretic hormone leading to forced diuresis and reduction of volume of circulated blood (Eichhorn and Leyk, 2015; Marabotti *et al.*, 2013).

Professional divers are usually required to have a detailed assessment of their past medical history with comprehensive examination which often includes a 24-h electrocardiogram, blood pressure monitoring, and echocardiography. Exercise testing, and even heart catheterisation may be indicated depending on symptoms and results of the non-invasive tests, and the nature of the diving environment. As such assessments requiring specialist qualifications as a decision of fitness for professional scuba diving might not always be done in primary care setting and specialist (for example, cardiology) referral may be needed. Patients with hypertension but optimally controlled blood pressure, those after myocardial infarction but with preserved left ventricular function and no symptoms, controlled supraventricular arrhythmias, appropriately programmed pacemakers able to withstand high ambient pressure may be fit for scuba diving (Eichhorn and Leyk, 2015). Patients with implanted ICD and CRT devices, haemodynamic instability, poorly controlled blood pressure, left ventricular systolic dysfunction must not scuba dive. Divers aged 40 years or older require more frequent check-ups because of an increased risk of cardiac death during diving (Eichhorn and Leyk, 2015).

Decompression illness is one of the most common complications affecting the cardiovascular system in divers. It develops during inappropriate fast ascent to the surface which is accompanied by a reduction of the ambient pressure and formation of gas bubbles (particularly, nitrogen). This may take place in tissues causing decompression sickness, or intravascularly resulting in arterial gas embolism, and potentially loss of consciousness and death (Liou *et al.*, 2015). During slow ascents with stops of appropriate duration at different depths, minor quantities of gas bubbles can be formed but they are eliminated by the lungs. Patients with patent foramen ovale are prone to developing more severe decompression illness and require a longer duration of hyperbaric oxygen therapy (Liou *et al.*, 2015). Patients with unexpected decompression illness, migraine with aura, a family history of patent foramen ovale or atrial septal defect and those with other forms of congenital heart disease are considered to be at higher risk during scuba diving, and can be screened for patent foramen ovale with bubble contrast transthoracic echocardiography (Liou *et al.*, 2015; Smart *et al.*, 2015).

Fitness to Work as a Security Guard or Law Enforcement Officer

Security guards are typically employed to guard property against theft and vandalism and to control access to premises. Police officers maintain order and enforce the law during public events. Such workers can be subjected to multiple occupational hazards depending on the jobs and work tasks. There is a likelihood of traumatic injury, electric injury, psychophysical exhaustion, and exposure to unfavourable climatic conditions, high pressure, noise, vibration, ionising and non-ionising radiation and fumes from firearms and transport vehicles. The risk of emotional, psychosomatic and behavioural stress-related disorders such as burnout syndrome, post-traumatic stress disorder are recognised sequalae. Given the extended list of multiple hazards, a careful assessment of individual risks is mandatory and this should be the basis for the selection of appropriately fit employees. It is also essential to conduct regular risk assessment, provide adequate protection devices, and refer individuals for prompt diagnosis and treatment when required (Candura *et al.*, 2006). Physical workload and emotional stress can be particularly relevant to this job with a specific hazard of potential of occasional rather than routine exposure of both hazards. In view of this it is important that the assessments during the selection and periodic reviews are designed to detect risks posed by such extreme exposures.

Return to Work

An opportunity to return to work after the onset or following exacerbation of cardiovascular disease is an important consideration for individuals of working age. Involvement in a productive, rewarding job is crucial for self-fulfilment and self-assertion and is directly related to their mental health and quality of life (Coggon and Palmer, 2010; Nordgren and Soderlund, 2015). However, decisions regarding return to work depend on a variety of factors. Depending on job specifications, symptoms of angina, ventricular arrhythmias, impaired systolic and diastolic function, and the presence of clinical, imaging and laboratory prognostic markers and co-morbidities may all affect a decision on fitness (Price, 2004).

Patient attitudes and expectations should not be ignored. Willingness to return to work vary widely (Fiabane *et al.*, 2015). Cardiac events at the workplace with a fear of further exacerbation of the disease, longer periods of sickness absence, demanding jobs, poor work conditions, and availability of redeployment and/or retraining, depressive symptoms, job insecurity, a necessity for cardiac rehabilitation, and benefits of staying on sick leave or taking early retirement, along with other factors do affect patient decision whether to return to work or not (Biering *et al.*, 2015; Worcester *et al.*, 2014; Coggon and Palmer, 2010; Price, 2004). Detailed information and clear advice should be provided to all patients to encourage and facilitate their safe return to a suitable work role with workplace adjustments provided if required.

Conclusion

Occupational hazards are important risk factors for the development or exacerbation of cardiovascular diseases, which are largely preventable by following the hierarchy of control of workplace hazards. Identifying patients whose illness is caused or aggravated by work is of paramount importance for their effective clinical management. Importantly, occupational hazards can potentiate the effects of common cardiovascular risk factors. Therefore, promoting a healthy life style, modification of dietary habits, smoking cessation, control of blood pressure and lipids, and manageable workload are essential for primary and secondary prevention of cardiovascular diseases among workers.

References

Alosco ML, Penn MS, Spitznagel MB, Cleveland MJ, Ott BR, Gunstad J. (2015) Reduced Physical Fitness in Patients With Heart Failure as a Possible Risk Factor for Impaired Driving Performance. *Am J Occup Ther* **69**(2): 6902260010p1-8. Available from: doi: 10.5014/ajot.2015.013573. [Accessed on 25 April 2021].

Andersen MHG, Frederiksen M, Saber AT, Wils RS, Fonseca AS, Koponen IK, Johannesson S, Roursgaard M, Loft S, Møller P, Vogel U. (2019) Health effects of exposure to diesel exhaust in diesel-powered trains. *Part Fibre Toxicol* **16**(1): 21. Available from: doi: 10.1186/s12989-019-0306-4. [Accessed on 25 April 2021].

Anderson TJ, Gregoire J, Hegele RA, Couture P, Mancini GB, McPherson R. (2013) Update of the Canadian Cardiovascular Society guidelines for the diagnosis and treatment of dyslipidemia for the prevention of cardiovascular disease in the adult. *Can J Cardiol* **29**(2): 151–167. Available from: doi: 10.1016/j.cjca.2012.11.032. [Accessed on 25 April 2021].

Attarchi M, Dehghan F, Safakhah F, Nojomi M, Mohammadi S. (2012) Effect of exposure to occupational noise and shift working on blood pressure in rubber manufacturing company workers. *Ind Health* **50**(3): 205–213. [Accessed on 25 April 2021].

Attarchi M, Golabadi M, Labbafinejad Y, Mohammadi S. (2013) Combined effects of exposure to occupational noise and mixed organic solvents on blood pressure in car manufacturing company workers. *Am J Ind Med* **56**(2): 243–251. Available from: doi: 10.1002/ajim.22086. [Accessed 25 April 2021].

Ball A, Truskewycz A. (2013) Polyaromatic hydrocarbon exposure: An ecological impact ambiguity. *Environ Sci Pollut Res Int* **20**(7): 4311–4326. Available from: doi: 10.1007/s11356-013-1620-2. [Accessed on 25 April 2021].

Bangia KS, Symanski E, Strom SS, Bondy M. (2015) A cross-sectional analysis of polycyclic aromatic hydrocarbons and diesel particulate matter exposures and hypertension among individuals of Mexican origin. *Environ Health* **14**: 51. Available from: doi: 10.1186/s12940-015-0039-2. [Accessed on 25 April 2021].

Banning AS, Ng GA. (2013) Driving and arrhythmia: A review of scientific basis for international guidelines. *Eur Heart J* **34**(3): 236–244. Available from: doi: 10.1093/eurheartj/ehs356. [Accessed 25 April 2021].

Barry V, Steenland K. (2019) Lead exposure and mortality among U.S. workers in a surveillance program: Results from 10 additional years of follow-up. *Environ Res* **177**: 108625. Available from: doi: 10.1016/j.envres.2019.108625. [Accessed on 25 April 2021].

Baur DM, Christophi CA, Tsismenakis AJ, Cook EF, Kales SN. (2011) Cardiorespiratory fitness predicts cardiovascular risk profiles in career firefighters. *J Occup Environ Med* **53**(10): 1155–1160. Available from: doi: 10.1097/JOM.0b013e31822c9e47. [Accessed on 25 April 2021].

Biering K, Lund T, Andersen JH, Hjollund NH. (2015) Effect of psychosocial work environment on sickness absence among patients treated for ischemic heart disease. *J Occup Rehabil* **25**(4): 776–782. Available from: doi: 10.1007/s10926-015-9587-0. [Accessed on 25 April 2021].

Bjor B, Burstrom L, Eriksson K, Jonsson H, Nathanaelsson L, Nilsson T. (2010) Mortality from myocardial infarction in relation to exposure to vibration and dust among a cohort of iron-ore miners in Sweden. *Occup Environ Med* **67**(3): 154–158. [Accessed on 25 April 2021].

Bjor B, Burstrom L, Nilsson T, Reuterwall C. (2006) Vibration exposure and myocardial infarction incidence: The VHEEP case-control study. *Occup Med* **56**(5): 338–344. Available from: doi: 10.1093/occmed/kql024. [Accessed 25 April 2021].

Blaisdell J, Turyk ME, Almberg KS, Jones RM, Stayner LT. (2019) Prenatal exposure to nitrate in drinking water and the risk of congenital anomalies. *Environ Res* **176**: 108553. Available from: doi: 10.1016/j.envres.2019.108553. [Accessed 25 April 2021].

Burns KN, Sun K, Fobil JN, Neitzel RL. (2016) Heart Rate, Stress, and Occupational Noise Exposure among Electronic Waste Recycling Workers. *Int J Environ Res Public Health* **13**(1): 140. Available from: doi: 10.3390/ijerph13010140 [Accessed 25 April 2021].

Candura SM, Verni P, Minelli CM, Rosso GL, Cappelli MI, Strambi S. (2006) Occupational risks among public safety and security forces. *G Ital Med Lav Ergon* **28**(1): 53–62. [Accessed on 25 April 2021].

Chang TY, Jain RM, Wang CS, Chan CC. (2003) Effects of occupational noise exposure on blood pressure. *J Occup Environ Med* **45**(12): 1289–1296. Available from: doi: 10.1097/01.jom.0000100003.59731.3d. [Accessed on 25 April 2021].

Chen, J., Li, Y. J., Yang, W. P. (2009) Effects of carbon disulfide on blood pressure and electrocardiogram for workers exposed to levels below the national maximum allowable concentration. *Chinese J Ind Hygiene Occup Dis* **27**(11): 644–648. [Accessed on 25 April 2021].

Chen Y, Wu F, Parvez F, Ahmed A, Eunus M, McClintock TR. (2013) Arsenic exposure from drinking water and QT-interval prolongation: Results from the Health Effects of Arsenic Longitudinal Study. *Environ Health Perspect* **121**(4): 427–432. Available from: doi: 10.1289/ehp.1205197. [Accessed 25 April 2021].

Clyne N, Hofman-Bang C, Haga Y, Hatori N, Marklund SL, Pehrsson SK. (2001) Chronic cobalt exposure affects antioxidants and ATP production in rat myocardium. *Scand J Clin Lab Invest* **61**(8): 609–614. [Accessed on 25 April 2021].

Coggon D, Palmer KT. (2010) Assessing fitness for work and writing a "fit note." *BMJ* **341**, c6305. Available from: doi: 10.1136/bmj.c6305. [Accessed on 25 April 2021].

Collins GS, Altman DG. (2012) Predicting the 10 year risk of cardiovascular disease in the United Kingdom: Independent and external validation of an updated version of QRISK2. *BMJ* **344**: e4181. Available from: doi: 10.1136/bmj.e4181. [Accessed on 25 April 2021].

Di Lorenzo L, Basso A, Pesola G, Balice M, Tempesta M, Lasorsa G. (2003) Exposure to low doses of CS2 and cardiovascular risk factors. *G Ital Med Lav Ergon* Suppl(3): 112–113. [Accessed on 25 April 2021].

Donat-Vargas C, Gea A, Sayon-Orea C, de la Fuente-Arrillaga C, Martinez-Gonzalez MA, Bes-Rastrollo M. (2015) Association between dietary intake of polychlorinated biphenyls and the incidence of hypertension in a Spanish cohort: the Seguimiento Universidad de Navarra project. *Hypertension* **65**(4): 714–721. Available from: doi: 10.1161/HYPERTENSIONAHA.114.04435. [Accessed on 25 April 2021].

Driver And Vehicle Licensing Agency. (2021) *Assessing fitness to drive: A guide for medical professionals.* [Online] Available from: https://www.gov.uk/government/publications/assessing-fitness-to-drive-a-guide-for-medical-professionals [Accessed on 25 April 2021].

Dzeshka MS, Lip GY. (2014) Antithrombotic and anticoagulant therapy for atrial fibrillation. *Cardiol Clin* **32**(4): 585–599. Available from: doi: 10.1016/j.ccl.2014.07.009. [Accessed on 25 April 2021].

Dzhambov AM, Dimitrova DD. (2016a) Occupational noise and ischemic heart disease: A systematic review. *Noise Health* **18**(83): 167–177. Available from: doi: 10.4103/1463-1741.189241. [Accessed on 25 April 2021].

Dzhambov AM, Dimitrova DD. (2016b) Heart disease attributed to occupational noise, vibration and other co-exposure: Self-reported population-based survey among Bulgarian workers. *Med Pr* **67**(4): 435–445. Available from: doi: 10.13075/mp.5893.00437. [Accessed on 25 April 2021].

Eichhorn L, Leyk D. (2015) Diving medicine in clinical practice. *Dtsch Arztebl Int* **112**(9): 147–157. Available from: doi: 10.3238/arztebl.2015.0147. [Accessed on 25 April 2021].

Erdogan MS, Islam SS, Chaudhari A, Ducatman AM. (2004) Occupational carbon monoxide poisoning among West Virginia workers' compensation claims: diagnosis, treatment duration, and utilization. *J Occup Environ Med* **46**(6): 577–583. [Accessed on 25 April 2021].

Eriksson HP, Forsell K, Andersson E. (2020) Mortality from cardiovascular disease in a cohort of Swedish seafarers. *Int Arch Occup Environ Health* **93**(3): 345–353. Available from: doi: 10.1007/s00420-019-01486-5. [Accessed 25 April 2021].

Eriksson HP, Andersson E, Schiöler L, Söderberg M, Sjöström M, Rosengren A, Torén K. (2018) Longitudinal study of occupational noise exposure and joint effects with job strain and risk for coronary heart disease and stroke in Swedish men. *BMJ Open* **8**(4): e019160. Available from: doi: 10.1136/bmjopen-2017-019160. [Accessed 25 April 2021].

Fang Q, Wang Z, Zhan Y, Li D, Zhang K, Zhou T, Yang H, Zhang C, Li X, Min X, Chen W, Guo H, He MA, Kong W, Wu T, Zhang X. (2018) Hearing loss is associated with increased CHD risk and unfavorable CHD-related biomarkers in the Dongfeng-Tongji cohort. *Atherosclerosis* **271**: 70–76. Available from: doi: 10.1016/j.atherosclerosis.2018.01.048. [Accessed on 25 April 2021].

Fiabane E, Giorgi I, Candura SM, Argentero P. (2015) Return to work after coronary revascularization procedures and a patient's job satisfaction: A prospective study. *Int J Occup Med Environ Health* **28**(1): 52–61. Available from: doi: 10.2478/s13382-014-0313-5. [Accessed 25 April 2021].

Finley BL, Monnot AD, Gaffney SH, Paustenbach DJ. (2012) Dose-response relationships for blood cobalt concentrations and health effects: A review of the literature and application of a biokinetic model. *J Toxicol Environ Health B Crit Rev* **15**(8): 493–523. Available from: doi: 10.1080/10937404.2012.744287. [Accessed on 25 April 2021].

Fogari R, Zoppi A, Corradi L, Marasi G, Vanasia A, Zanchetti A. (2001) Transient but not sustained blood pressure increments by occupational noise. An ambulatory blood pressure measurement study. *J Hypertens* **19**(6): 1021–1027. [Accessed on 25 April 2021].

Freitas F, Brucker N, Durgante J, Bubols G, Bulcao R, Moro A. (2014) Urinary 1-hydroxypyrene is associated with oxidative stress and inflammatory biomarkers in acute Myocardial Infarction. *Int J Environ Res Public Health* **11**(9): 9024–9037. Available from: doi: 10.3390/ijerph110909024. [Accessed on 25 April 2021].

Gan WQ, Mannino DM. (2018) Occupational noise exposure, bilateral high-frequency hearing loss, and blood pressure. *J Occup Environ Med* **60**(5): 462–468. Available from: doi: 10.1097/JOM.0000000000001232. [Accessed on 25 April 2021].

Gentner NJ, Weber LP. (2011) Intranasal benzo[a]pyrene alters circadian blood pressure patterns and causes lung inflammation in rats. *Arch Toxicol* **85**(4): 337–346. Available from: doi: 10.1007/s00204-010-0589-6. [Accessed on 25 April 2021].

Glicklich D, Shin CT, Frishman WH. (2020) Heavy metal toxicity in chronic renal failure and cardiovascular disease: Possible role for chelation therapy. *Cardiol Rev* **28**(6): 312–318. Available from: doi: 10.1097/CRD.0000000000000304. [Accessed on 25 April 2021].

Gitanjali B, Ananth R. (2003) Effect of acute exposure to loud occupational noise during daytime on the nocturnal sleep architecture, heart rate, and cortisol secretion in healthy volunteers. *J Occup Health* **45**(3): 146–152. [Accessed on 25 April 2021].

Glozier N, Tofler GH, Colquhoun DM, Bunker SJ, Clarke DM, Hare DL. (2013) Psychosocial risk factors for coronary heart disease. *Med J Aus* **199**(3): 179–180. [Accessed on 25 April 2021].

Goff DC, Jr, Lloyd-Jones DM, Bennett G, Coady S, D'Agostino RB, Sr Gibbons R. (2014) ACC/AHA guideline on the assessment of cardiovascular risk: A report of the American College of Cardiology/American Heart Association Task Force on Practice Guidelines. *J Am Coll Cardiol* **63**(25 Pt B): 2935–2959. Available from: doi: 10.1016/j.jacc.2013.11.005. [Accessed on 25 April 2021].

Green MS, Schwartz K, Harari G, Najenson T. (1991) Industrial noise exposure and ambulatory blood pressure and heart rate. *J Occup Med* **33**(8): 879–883. [Accessed on 25 April 2021].

Hammer MS, Swinburn TK, Neitzel RL. (2014) Environmental noise pollution in the United States: Developing an effective public health response. *Environ Health Perspect* **122**(2): 115–119. Available from: doi: 10.1289/ehp.1307272. [Accessed on 25 April 2021].

Henn SA, Bell JL, Sussell AL, Konda S. (2013) Occupational carbon monoxide fatalities in the US from unintentional non-fire related exposures, 1992–2008. *Am J Ind Med* **56**(11): 1280–1289. Available from: doi: 10.1002/ajim.22226. [Accessed on 25 April 2021].

James KA, Byers T, Hokanson JE, Meliker JR, Zerbe GO, Marshall JA. (2015) Association between lifetime exposure to inorganic arsenic in drinking water and coronary heart disease in Colorado residents. *Environ Health Perspect* **123**(2): 128–134. Available from: doi: 10.1289/ehp.1307839. [Accessed on 25 April 2021].

Jensen JH, Flachs EM, Skakon J, Rod NH, Bonde JP, Kawachi I. (2020) Work-unit organizational changes and risk of cardiovascular disease:

A prospective study of public healthcare employees in Denmark. *Int Arch Occup Environ Health* **93**(4): 409–419. Available from: doi: 10.1007/s00420-019-01493-6. [Accessed on 25 April 2021].

Kales SN, Smith DL. (2014) Sudden cardiac death in the fire service. *Occup Med* **64**(4): 228–230. Available from: doi: 10.1093/occmed/kqu057. [Accessed on 25 April 2021].

Kalsch H, Hennig F, Moebus S, Mohlenkamp S, Dragano N, Jakobs H. (2014) Are air pollution and traffic noise independently associated with atherosclerosis: The Heinz Nixdorf Recall Study. *Eur Heart J* **35**(13): 853–860. Available from: doi: 10.1093/eurheartj/eht426. [Accessed on 25 April 2021].

Karakulak UN, Gunduzoz M, Ayturk M, Tek Ozturk M, Tutkun E, Yilmaz OH. (2017) Assessment of heart rate response to exercise and recovery during treadmill testing in arsenic-exposed workers. *Ann Noninvasive Electrocardiol* **22**(5): e12437. Available from: doi: 10.1111/anec.12437 [Accessed on 25 April 2021].

Kennedy A, Dornan JD, King R. (1981) Fatal myocardial disease associated with industrial exposure to cobalt. *Lancet* **1**(8217): 412–414. [Accessed on 25 April 2021].

Klemmer PJ, Harris AA. (2000) Carbon disulfide nephropathy. *Am J Kidney Dis* **36**(3): 626–69. [Accessed on 25 April 2021].

Kopf PG, Huwe JK, Walker MK. (2008) Hypertension, cardiac hypertrophy, and impaired vascular relaxation induced by 2,3,7,8-tetrachlorodibenzo-p-dioxin are associated with increased superoxide. *Cardiovasc Toxicol* **8**(4): 181–193. Available from: doi: 10.1007/s12012-008-9027-x. [Accessed on 25 April 2021].

Koskela RS, Mutanen P, Sorsa JA, Klockars M. (2000) Factors predictive of ischemic heart disease mortality in foundry workers exposed to carbon monoxide. *Am J Epidemiol* **152**(7): 628–632. [Accessed on 25 April 2021].

Kristal-Boneh E, Melamed S, Harari G, Green MS. (1995) Acute and chronic effects of noise exposure on blood pressure and heart rate among industrial employees: The Cordis Study. *Arch Environ Health* **50**(4): 298–304. Available from: doi: 10.1080/00039896.1995.9935958. [Accessed on 25 April 2021].

Lantin AC, Vermeulen J, Mallants A, Vanoverschelde JL, Speybroeck N, Swennen B. (2013) Occupational exposure to cobalt is not associated with incipient signs of dilated cardiomyopathy in a Belgian refinery. *Occup Environ Med* **70**(6): 386–392. Available from: doi: 10.1136/oemed-2012-100930. [Accessed on 25 April 2021].

Ledda C, Lavicoli I, Bracci M, Avola R, Senia P, Santarelli L, Pomara C, Rapisarda V. (2018) Serum lipid, lipoprotein and apolipoprotein profiles in workers exposed to low arsenic levels: Lipid profiles and occupational arsenic exposure. *Toxicol Lett* **282**: 49–56. Available from: doi: 10.1016/j.toxlet.2017.10.014. [Accessed on 25 April 2021].

Lee JH, Kang W, Yaang SR, Choy N, Lee CR. (2009) Cohort study for the effect of chronic noise exposure on blood pressure among male workers in Busan, Korea. *Am J Ind Med* **52**(6): 509–517. Available from: doi: 10.1002/ajim.20692. [Accessed on 25 April 2021].

Li J. (2016) Karoshi: An international work-related hazard? *Int J Cardiol* **206**: 139–140. Available from: doi: 10.1016/j.ijcard.2016.01.092. [Accessed on 25 April 2021].

Li MC, Chen PC, Tsai PC, Furue M, Onozuka D, Hagihara A. (2015). Mortality after exposure to polychlorinated biphenyls and polychlorinated dibenzofurans: A meta-analysis of two highly exposed cohorts. *Int J Cancer J Int Du Cancer* **137**(6): 1427–1432. Available from: doi: 10.1002/ijc.29504. [Accessed on 25 April 2021].

Lin YK, Chang CK, Wang YC, Ho TJ. (2013) Acute and prolonged adverse effects of temperature on mortality from cardiovascular diseases. *PLOS One* **8**(12): e82678. Available from: doi: 10.1371/journal.pone.0082678. [Accessed 25 April 2021].

Linna A, Uitti J, Oksa P, Toivio P, Virtanen V, Lindholm H, Halkosaari M, Sauni R. (2020) Effects of occupational cobalt exposure on the heart in the production of cobalt and cobalt compounds: A 6-year follow-up. *Int Arch Occup Environ Health* **93**(3): 365–374. Available from: doi: 10.1007/s00420-019-01488-3. [Accessed on 25 April 2021].

Liou K, Wolfers D, Turner R, Bennett M, Allan R, Jepson N. (2015) Patent foramen ovale influences the presentation of decompression illness in SCUBA divers. *Heart Lung Circ* **24**(1): 26–31. Available from: doi: 10.1016/j.hlc.2014.07.057. [Accessed on 25 April 2021].

Liu NG, Wang T, Huang P, Qing ZQ, Zhang JH, Chen YJ. (2015) Karoshi Related to Labor Intensity and Risk of Cardiovascular Events: A Case Report. *Fa Yi Xue Za Zhi* **31**(5): 343–346. [Accessed on 25 April 2021].

Magliano DJ, Cohen K, Harding JL, Shaw JE. (2015) Residential distance from major urban areas, diabetes and cardiovascular mortality in Australia. *Diabetes Res Clin Pract* **109**(2): 271–278. Available from: doi: 10.1016/j.diabres.2015.05.029. [Accessed on 25 April 2021].

Magliano DJ, Loh VH, Harding JL, Botton J, Shaw JE. (2014) Persistent organic pollutants and diabetes: a review of the epidemiological evidence. *Diabetes Metab* **40**(1): 1–14. Available from: doi: 10.1016/j.diabet.2013.09.006. [Accessed on 25 April 2021].

Magnusson Hanson LL, Westerlund H, Chungkham HS, Vahtera J, Rod NH, Alexanderson K, Goldberg M, Kivimäki M, Stenholm S, Platts LG, Zins M, Head J. (2018) Job strain and loss of healthy life years between ages 50 and 75 by sex and occupational position: Analyses of 64,934 individuals from four prospective cohort studies. *Occup Environ Med* **75**(7): 486–493. Available from: doi: 10.1136/oemed-2017-104644 [Accessed on 25 April 2021].

Maikala RV, King S, Bhambhani YN. (2006) Acute physiological responses in healthy men during whole-body vibration. *Int Arch Occup Environ Health* **79**(2): 103–114. Available from: doi: 10.1007/s00420-005-0029-8. [Accessed on 25 April 2021].

Marabotti C, Scalzini A, Menicucci D, Passera M, Bedini R, L'Abbate A. (2013) Cardiovascular changes during SCUBA diving: An underwater Doppler echocardiographic study. *Acta Physiologica* **209**(1): 62–68. Available from: doi: 10.1111/apha.12112. [Accessed on 25 April 2021].

McElvenny DM, Miller BG, MacCalman LA, Sleeuwenhoek A, van Tongeren M, Shepherd K. (2015) Mortality of a cohort of workers in Great Britain with blood lead measurements. *Occup Environ Med* **72**(9): 625–632. Available from: doi: 10.1136/oemed-2014-102637. [Accessed on 25 April 2021].

Menke A, Muntner P, Batuman V, Silbergeld EK, Guallar E. (2006) Blood lead below 0.48 micromol/L (10 microg/dL) and mortality among US adults. *Circulation* **114**(13): 1388–1394. Available from: doi: 10.1161/CIRCULATIONAHA.106.628321. [Accessed on 25 April 2021].

Mikov I, Draskovic D, Savic M, Arsic M, Todorovski Z, Glavaski M. (2000) Occupational intoxication with carbon monoxide. *Arch Environ Health* **55**(6): 455–456. Available from: doi: 10.1080/00039890009604046. [Accessed on 25 April 2021].

Min YS, Ahn YS. (2017) The association between blood lead levels and cardiovascular diseases among lead-exposed male workers. *Scand J Work Environ Health* **43**(4): 385–390. Available from: doi: 10.5271/sjweh.3631. [Accessed on 25 April 2021].

Mo J, Xia Y, Wade TJ, DeMarini DM, Davidson M, Mumford J. (2011) Altered gene expression by low-dose arsenic exposure in humans and cultured cardiomyocytes: assessment by real-time PCR arrays. *Int J Environ Res Public Health* **8**(6): 2090–2108. Available from: doi: 10.3390/ijerph8062090. [Accessed on 25 April 2021].

Moery S, Pontious JM (2009) Coagulopathy associated with superwarfarin exposure. *J Okla State Med Assoc* **102**(10): 323–325 [Accessed on 25 April 2021].

Moon K, Guallar E, Navas-Acien A. (2012) Arsenic exposure and cardiovascular disease: An updated systematic review. *Curr Atheroscler Rep* **14**(6): 542–555. Available from: doi: 10.1007/s11883-012-0280-x. [Accessed on 25 April 2021].

Moon KA, Oberoi S, Barchowsky A, Chen Y, Guallar E, Nachman KE, Rahman M, Sohel N, D'Ippoliti D, Wade TJ, James KA, Farzan SF, Karagas MR, Ahsan H, Navas-Acien A. (2017) A dose-response meta-analysis of chronic arsenic exposure and incident cardiovascular disease. *Int J Epidemiol* **46**(6): 1924–1939. Available from: doi: 10.1093/ije/dyx202. [Accessed on 25 April 2021].

Mozaffarian D, Benjamin EJ, Go AS, Arnett DK, Blaha MJ, Cushman M. (2015) Heart disease and stroke statistics--2015 update: A report from the American Heart Association. *Circulation* **131**(4): e29–322. Available from: doi: 10.1161/CIR.0000000000000152. [Accessed on 25 April 2021].

Munzel T, Gori T, Babisch W, Basner M. (2014) Cardiovascular effects of environmental noise exposure. *Eur Heart J* **35**(13): 829–836. Available from: doi: 10.1093/eurheartj/ehu030. [Accessed on 25 April 2021].

Navas-Acien A, Schwartz BS, Rothenberg SJ, Hu H, Silbergeld EK, Guallar E. (2008) Bone lead levels and blood pressure endpoints: A meta-analysis. *Epidemiology* **19**(3): 496–504. Available from: doi: 10.1097/EDE.0b013e31816a2400. [Accessed on 25 April 2021].

Nawrot TS, Thijs L, Den Hond EM, Roels HA, Staessen JA. (2002) An epidemiological re-appraisal of the association between blood pressure and blood lead: A meta-analysis. *J Hum Hypertens* **16**(2): 123–131. Available from: doi: 10.1038/sj.jhh.1001300. [Accessed on 25 April 2021].

Nayha S. (2002) Cold and the risk of cardiovascular diseases. A review. *Int J Circumpolar Health* **61**(4): 373–380. [Accessed on 25 April 2021].

Nordgren L, Soderlund A. (2015) Being on sick leave due to heart failure: Self-rated health, encounters with healthcare professionals and social insurance officers and self-estimated ability to return to work. *Psychol Health Med* **20**(5): 582–593. Available from: doi: 10.1080/13548506.2015.1007148. [Accessed on 25 April 2021].

Pan CH, Chan CC, Huang YL, Wu KY. (2008) Urinary 1-hydroxypyrene and malondialdehyde in male workers in Chinese restaurants.

Occup Environ Med 65(11): 732–735. Available from: doi: 10.1136/oem.2007.036970. [Accessed on 25 April 2021].

Patel J, Nembhard WN, Politis MD, Rocheleau CM, Langlois PH, Shaw GM, Romitti PA, Gilboa SM, Desrosiers TA, Insaf T, Lupo PJ. (2020) National Birth Defects Prevention Study. Maternal occupational exposure to polycyclic aromatic hydrocarbons and the risk of isolated congenital heart defects among offspring. *Environ Res* **186**: 109550. Available from: doi: 10.1016/j.envres.2020.109550. [Accessed on 25 April 2021].

Perez AL, Tang WH. (2015) Contribution of environmental toxins in the pathogenesis of idiopathic cardiomyopathies. *Curr Treat Options Cardiovas Med* **17**(5): 381. Available from: doi: 10.1007/s11936-015-0381-2. [Accessed on 25 April 2021].

Perk J, De Backer G, Gohlke H, Graham I, Reiner Z, Verschuren M. (2012) European Guidelines on cardiovascular disease prevention in clinical practice (version 2012). The Fifth Joint Task Force of the European Society of Cardiology and Other Societies on Cardiovascular Disease Prevention in Clinical Practice (constituted by representatives of nine societies and by invited experts). *Eur Heart J* **33**(13): 1635–1701. Available from: doi: 10.1093/eurheartj/ehs092. [Accessed on 25 April 2021].

Pettersson H, Olsson D, Järvholm B. (2020) Occupational exposure to noise and cold environment and the risk of death due to myocardial infarction and stroke. *Int Arch Occup Environ Health* **93**(5): 571–575. Available from: doi: 10.1007/s00420-019-01513-5. [Accessed on 25 April 2021].

Price AE. (2004) Heart disease and work. *Heart* **90**(9): 1077–1084. Available from: doi: 10.1136/hrt.2003.029298. [Accessed on 25 April 2021].

Rodahl K. (2003) Occupational health conditions in extreme environments. *Ann Occup Hygiene* **47**(3): 241–252. [Accessed on 25 April 2021].

Sahu S, Sett M, Kjellstrom T. (2013) Heat exposure, cardiovascular stress and work productivity in rice harvesters in India: Implications for a climate change future. *Ind Health* **51**(4): 424–431. [Accessed 25 April 2021].

Schramm A, Uter W, Brandt M, Goen T, Kohrmann M, Baumeister T. (2016) Increased intima-media thickness in rayon workers after long-term exposure to carbon disulfide. *Int Arch Occup Environ Health* **89**(3): 513–519. Available from: doi: 10.1007/s00420-015-1091-5. [Accessed on 25 April 2021].

Sett M, Sahu S. (2014) Effects of occupational heat exposure on female brick workers in West Bengal, India. *Global Health Action* 7: 21923. Available from: doi: 10.3402/gha.v7.21923. [Accessed on 25 April 2021].

Shah PK. (2010) Screening asymptomatic subjects for subclinical atherosclerosis: Can we, does it matter, and should we? *J Am Coll Cardiol* **56**(2): 98–105. Available from: doi: 10.1016/j.jacc.2009.09.081. [Accessed on 25 April 2021].

Shiue I. (2015) Are urinary polyaromatic hydrocarbons associated with adult hypertension, heart attack, and cancer? USA NHANES, 2011–2012. *Environ Sci Pollution Res Int* **22**(21). Available from: doi: 10.1007/s11356-015-4922-8. [Accessed on 25 April 2021].

Simoes MR, Ribeiro Junior RF, Vescovi MV, de Jesus HC, Padilha AS, Stefanon I. (2011) Acute lead exposure increases arterial pressure: Role of the renin-angiotensin system. *PLOS One* **6**(4): e18730. Available from: doi: 10.1371/journal.pone.0018730. [Accessed on 25 April 2021].

Sjoberg Lind Y, Lind PM, Salihovic S, van Bavel B, Lind L. (2013) Circulating levels of persistent organic pollutants (POPs) are associated with left ventricular systolic and diastolic dysfunction in the elderly. *Environ Res* **123**: 39–45. Available from: doi: 10.1016/j.envres.2013.02.007. [Accessed on 25 April 2021].

Smart D, Mitchell S, Wilmshurst P, Turner M, Banham N. (2015) Joint position statement on persistent foramen ovale (PFO) and diving. South Paci fi c Underwater Medicine Society (SPUMS) and the United Kingdom Sports Diving Medical Committee (UKSDMC). *Diving Hyperb Med* **45**(2): 129–131. [Accessed on 25 April 2021].

Smith, DL. (2011) Firefighter fitness: Improving performance and preventing injuries and fatalities. *Curr Sports Med Rep* **10**(3): 167–172. Available from: doi: 10.1249/JSR.0b013e31821a9fec. [Accessed on 25 April 2021].

Smith DL, Barr DA, Kales SN. (2013) Extreme sacrifice: Sudden cardiac death in the US Fire Service. *Extreme Physiol Med* **2**(1): 6. Available from: doi: 10.1186/2046-7648-2-6. [Accessed on 25 April 2021].

Smith P, Gilbert-Ouimet M, Brisson C, Glazier RH, Mustard CA. (2020) Examining the relationship between the demand-control model and incident myocardial infarction and congestive heart failure in a representative sample of the employed women and men in Ontario, Canada, over a 15-year period. *Can J Public Health* **112**(2): 280–288. Available from: doi: 10.17269/s41997-020-00378-3. [Accessed on 25 April 2021].

Solenkova NV, Newman JD, Berger JS, Thurston G, Hochman JS, Lamas GA. (2014) Metal pollutants and cardiovascular disease: Mechanisms and consequences of exposure. *Am Heart J* **168**(6): 812–822. Available from doi: 10.1016/j.ahj.2014.07.007. [Accessed on 25 April 2021].

Sorajja D, Nesbitt GC, Hodge DO, Low PA, Hammill SC, Gersh BJ. (2009) Syncope while driving: Clinical characteristics, causes, and prognosis. *Circulation* **120**(11): 928–934. Available from: doi: 10.1161/CIRCULATIONAHA.108.827626. [Accessed on 25 April 2021].

Sorajja D, Shen WK. (2010) Driving guidelines and restrictions in patients with a history of cardiac arrhythmias, syncope,or implantable devices. *Curr Treat Options Cardiovasc Med* **12**(5): 443–456. Available from: doi: 10.1007/s11936-010-0088-3. [Accessed on 25 April 2021].

Soteriades ES, Smith DL, Tsismenakis AJ, Baur DM, Kales SN. (2011) Cardiovascular disease in US firefighters: A systematic review. *Cardiol Rev* **19**(4): 202–215. Available from: doi: 10.1097/CRD.0b013e318215c105. [Accessed on 25 April 2021].

Stea F, Bianchi F, Cori L, Sicari R. (2014) Cardiovascular effects of arsenic: Clinical and epidemiological findings. *Environ Sci Pollut Res Int* **21**(1): 244–251. Available from: doi: 10.1007/s11356-013-2113-z. [Accessed on 25 April 2021].

Steenland K, Barry V, Anttila A, Sallmén M, McElvenny D, Todd AC, Straif K. (2017) A cohort mortality study of lead-exposed workers in the USA, Finland and the UK. *Occup Environ Med* **74**(11): 785–791. Available from: doi: 10.1136/oemed-2017-104311. [Accessed on 25 April 2021].

Stone NJ, Robinson JG, Lichtenstein AH, Bairey Merz CN, Blum CB, Eckel RH. (2013) ACC/AHA guideline on the treatment of blood cholesterol to reduce atherosclerotic cardiovascular risk in adults: A report of the American College of Cardiology/American Heart Association Task Force on Practice Guidelines. *J Am Coll Cardiol* **63**(25 Pt B): 2889–2934. Available from doi: 10.1016/j.jacc.2013.11.002. [Accessed on 25 April 2021].

Svendsen SW, Kolstad HA, Steesby E. (2002) Bleeding problems associated with occupational exposure to anticoagulant rodenticides. *Int Arch Occup Environ Health* **75**(7): 515–517. Available from: doi: 10.1007/s00420-002-0339-z. [Accessed on 25 April 2021].

Swedish Council on Health Technology Assessment. (2017) *Occupational Health and Safety — Chemical Exposure: A Systematic Review and Assessment of the Social, Medical and Ethical Aspects.* [Online] Available from: https://www.sbu.se/261e. [Accessed on 25 April 2021].

Taheri L, Sadeghi M, Sanei H, Rabiei K, Arabzadeh S, Golshahi J. (2014) The relation between occupational exposure to lead and blood pressure among employed normotensive men. *J Res Med Sci* **19**(6): 490–194.

Tamaian LD, Cocarla A. (1998) Occupational Exposure to Vibration and Ischemic Heart Disease. *J Occup Health* **40**(1):173–176. Available from: doi: 10.1539/joh.40.73. [Accessed on 25 April 2021].

Tsuji JS, Perez V, Garry MR, Alexander DD. (2014) Association of low-level arsenic exposure in drinking water with cardiovascular disease: A systematic review and risk assessment. *Toxicology* **323**: 78–94. Available from: doi: 10.1016/j.tox.2014.06.008. [Accessed on 25 April 2021].

van Kempen EE, Kruize H, Boshuizen HC, Ameling CB, Staatsen BA, de Hollander AE. (2002) The association between noise exposure and blood pressure and ischemic heart disease: A meta-analysis. *Environ Health Perspect* **110**(3): 307–317. [Accessed on 25 April 2021].

Vanasse A, Courteau J, Cohen AA, Orzanco MG, Drouin C. (2010) Rural-urban disparities in the management and health issues of chronic diseases in Quebec (Canada) in the early 2000s. *Rural And Remote Health* **10**(4): 1548. [Accessed 25 April 2021].

Vogel CF, Nishimura N, Sciullo E, Wong P, Li W, Matsumura F. (2007) Modulation of the chemokines KC and MCP-1 by 2,3,7,8-tetrachlorodibenzo-p-dioxin (TCDD) in mice. *Arch Biochem Biophys* **461**(2): 169–175. Available from: doi: 10.1016/j.abb.2007.01.015. [Accessed on 25 April 2021].

Wade TJ, Xia Y, Mumford J, Wu K, Le XC, Sams E. (2015) Cardiovascular disease and arsenic exposure in Inner Mongolia, China: A case control study. *Environ Health* **14**(1): 35. Available from: doi: 10.1186/s12940-015-0022-y. [Accessed on 25 April 2021].

Warren JV. (1988) Monday morning sudden death. *Trans Am Clin Climatol Assoc* **99**: 10–16. [Accessed on 25 April 2021].

Watt BE, Proudfoot AT, Bradberry SM, Vale JA. (2005) Anticoagulant rodenticides. *Toxicol Rev* **24**(4): 259–269. [Accessed on 25 April 2021].

Wildemann TM, Weber LP, Siciliano SD. (2015) Combined exposure to lead, inorganic mercury and methylmercury shows deviation from additivity for cardiovascular toxicity in rats. *J App Toxicol* **35**(8): 918–926. Available from: DOI:10.1002/jat.3092. [Accessed on 25 April 2021].

Worcester MU, Elliott PC, Turner A, Pereira JJ, Murphy BM, Le Grande MR. (2014) Resumption of work after acute coronary syndrome or coronary artery bypass graft surgery. *Heart Lung Circ* **23**(5): 444–453.

Available from: doi: 10.1016/j.hlc.2013.10.093. [Accessed on 25 April 2021].

Wronska-Nofer T, Nofer JR, Stetkiewicz J, Wierzbicka M, Bolinska H, Fobker M. (2007). Evidence for oxidative stress at elevated plasma thiol levels in chronic exposure to carbon disulfide (CS2) and coronary heart disease. *Nutr Metab Cardiovasc Dis* **17**(7): 546–553. Available from: doi: 10.1016/j.numecd.2006.03.002. [Accessed on 25 April 2021].

Wu WT, Tsai SS, Wang CC, Lin YJ, Wu TN, Shih TS, Liou SH. (2019) Professional Driver's Job Stress and 8-year Risk of Cardiovascular Disease: The Taiwan Bus Driver Cohort Study. *Epidemiology* Suppl **1**: S39–S47. Available from: doi: 10.1097/EDE.0000000000001003. [Accessed on 25 April 2021].

Wynn P, Hawdon P. (2012) Cardiorespiratory fitness selection standard and occupational outcomes in trainee firefighters. *Occup Med* **62**(2): 123–128. Available from: doi: 10.1093/occmed/kqr206. [Accessed on 25 April 2021].

Xu JN, Fu ZH, Yu WL, Wang QK, Tan F. (2013) Establishment of occupational exposure limit for warfarin in China. *Biomed Environ Sci* **26**(6): 513–516. Available from: 10.3967/0895-3988.2013.06.015. [Accessed on 25 April 2021].

Xu S, Huang Y, Xiao J, Zhu W, Wang L, Tang H. (2015) The association between job strain and coronary heart disease: A meta-analysis of prospective cohort studies. *Ann Med* **47**(6): 512–518. Available from: doi: 10.3109/07853890.2015.1075658. [Accessed on 25 April 2021].

Xu T, Magnusson Hanson LL, Lange T, Starkopf L, Westerlund H, Madsen IEH, Rugulies R, Pentti J, Stenholm S, Vahtera J, Hansen ÅM, Virtanen M, Kivimäki M, Rod NH. (2019) Workplace bullying and workplace violence as risk factors for cardiovascular disease: A multi-cohort study. *Eur Heart J* **40**(14): 1124–1134. Available from: doi: 10.1093/eurheartj/ehy683. [Accessed on 25 April 2021].

Yang J, Teehan D, Farioli A, Baur DM, Smith D, Kales SN. (2013) Sudden cardiac death among firefighters </=45 years of age in the United States. *Am J Cardiol* **112**(12): 1962–1967. Available from: doi: 10.1016/j.amjcard.2013.08.029. [Accessed on 25 April 2021].

Chapter 13

Hepatobiliary and Gastrointestinal Disorders

Retneswari Masilamani, Jayakumar Gurusamy*[†] *and Rosmawati Mohamed*[‡]

Introduction

Occupational exposures can affect the hepatobiliary system and the gastrointestinal (GI) tract, although few disorders of the GI system, except infections, are caused or exacerbated by the work environment. Disorders of both these systems though can have a significant effect on work. Ingestion of corrosive chemicals will have a direct effect on the upper GI tract and the GI tract also functions as a means for absorption of ingested toxic substances. However, there are in-built defence mechanisms of the GI tract that can reduce the likelihood of systemic absorption. Some compounds are poorly absorbed through the GI tract, and others may be removed by diarrhoea and/or vomiting. Systemic absorption of chemicals leads to its distribution to other sites, and can result in effects on other target organs. The liver is an important organ for the detoxification of systemically absorbed chemicals, and is therefore also a prime site for toxic damage.

*Faculty of Medicine and Health Sciences, Universiti Tunku Abdul Rahman, Selangor, Malaysia.

[†] Faculty of Medicine, Manipal University College Malaysia.

[‡] University of Malaya, Kuala Lumpur, Malaysia.

The efficacy of detoxification by the liver varies depending on the substances involved. It is possible that attempts at detoxification can result in metabolites that may have other toxic or carcinogenic properties, e.g. conversion of a pro-carcinogen into a direct carcinogen. Interaction between occupational and non-occupational chemical agents can also result in additive or synergistic effects on the liver. Alcohol (ethanol) ingestion and exposure to chlorinated organic solvents is one example. In the evaluation of liver and GI damage from exposure to chemicals, information on non-occupational risk factors such as alcohol consumption and medications is essential.

Pathophysiology

The Hepatic Response to Toxic Exposures

Two basic precepts should be remembered when considering the response of a target organ to external assault. First, humans evolved in an environment of clean air but contaminated food and water. Thus, the GI system has a better protective mechanism than the respiratory system. Secondly, the more specialised the target organ, the more limited is its range of responses to external damage.

In the case of the liver, its metabolic role means that it can double as a detoxification factory to some extent. Furthermore, the relatively unspecialised nature of its cellular function means that its power of regeneration following damage is formidable. However, this ability to regenerate at a cellular level is not matched by a similar ability to repair lost architecture, and so continued damage can lead to cirrhosis. To continue the analogy: the liver can replace the bricks but not necessarily use them to recreate the same-shaped building.

The liver is the largest visceral organ and has a major role in body metabolism. It produces bile, which assists in digestion of fats, and the liver itself processes amino acids, glucose, fatty acids and glycerol. It also manufactures some essential proteins concerned with blood coagulation and body water regulation. The liver also has a further function of detoxification, though it does not have a toxicological lexicon to distinguish poison from food. It performs its digestive functions on the majority of toxic chemicals through its widely varied enzymic activity in two main ways: degradation and conjugation.

In general, the main object is to produce water-soluble by-products which are then capable of being used as nutrient material, or in the case of foreign (non-nutrient) agents, rendering them capable of urinary excretion. Whilst some foreign materials particularly the metallic poisons such as lead, cadmium and mercury are directly toxic, others only achieve their toxic potential after metabolic transformation. For example, carbon tetrachloride (CCl_4) becomes toxic only when it has been acted upon by a hydroxylation enzyme system to produce the highly reactive, CCl_3 radical.

The degradation enzyme systems are chemical reactions involving oxidation, reduction or hydration, and as in the case of CCl_4, can result in unstable intermediates capable of damaging the hepatocytes. Conjugation is a more complex reaction usually involving glucuronic acid but again the objective is to produce the polar and less fat-soluble compounds. The metabolism of trichloroethylene is a good example. Following absorption, trichloroethylene is converted to chloral hydrate, which is further metabolised by one of two routes. One involves rapid reduction to trichloroethanol and the other is a slower oxidation to trichloroacetic acid (TCA). Trichloroethanol is not water-soluble and further metabolic transformation by conjugation with glucuronic acid is required to produce a water-soluble conjugate capable of being excreted through the urinary tract.

The liver also possesses two other characteristics of relevance to its role in detoxification. The first is the phenomenon of enzyme induction. Inducing agents are factors that increase the levels of the relevant metabolic enzymes and thus improve, or speed the detoxification process, (or enhance the production of secondary toxins). In small doses, many toxic chemicals can cause enzyme induction. Ethanol, phenobarbitone and the pesticide DDT are prime examples. Heavy drinkers may be more susceptible than others to the toxic effects of chlorinated hydrocarbon exposure because of damage to liver cells from ethanol resulting in a reduced liver capacity to metabolise other hepatotoxic chemicals.

The other characteristic of note concerns the liver architecture itself. Not only is it less well regenerated than the individual hepatocytes but the structure of the hepatic lobule means that the liver cells closest to the hepatic venules receive blood with a lower oxygen content than those closest to the portal tracts. The centrilobular hepatocytes are therefore more vulnerable to toxic (and anoxic) conditions than the periportal cells. Centrilobular necrosis is thus an early sign of hepatic damage.

Finally, pre-existing liver disease might render the liver less capable of dealing with some new xenobiotic assault and this is of particular importance when undertaking health assessments of workers who during their job, may be potentially exposed to hepatotoxins (Moorman *et al.*, 2020). Ethanol, non-alcoholic fatty liver disease and chronic viral hepatitis (B and C) are the most important causes of chronic liver disease (Table 1).

There is limited data to date to support the view that pre-existing liver disease will impact or enhance liver injury caused by occupational toxins.

Mechanisms for Liver Disease

Liver diseases arising from occupational and environmental exposures have been associated with the entire spectrum of acute liver injury and chronic liver injury encompassing a clinical presentation ranging from asymptomatic liver enzyme elevation, to acute liver failure, cirrhosis and cancer. The presenting features of liver disease seen by an occupational physician do not differ remarkably in its presenting features from those seen by a gastroenterologist or hepatologist in daily practice.

The features depend on the underlying pathology, e.g. whether there is acute or chronic liver damage, and whether there is hepatocyte (high liver transaminases) or bile duct injury (high alkaline phosphatase), liver failure or malignancy. In the early stage of liver disease, symptoms may be vague, e.g. poor appetite, mild upper abdominal discomfort and tiredness. Jaundice is often not apparent until the late stage of chronic liver injury or in acute severe liver injury where sufficient liver function has been compromised. When this happens, other clinical effects may also manifest because of liver structure and function being compromised. Clinical features of cirrhosis include oedema and ascites from portal hypertension, gynecomastia from inability of the liver to metabolise oestrogens, and haematemesis from oesophageal varices. Although the reduced production of coagulation factors leads to elevated prothrombin time, cirrhosis is associated with a procoagulant state and spontaneous bleeding in acute liver failure is rare.

Rapid discovery, commercialisation and globalisation resulted in innumerable new chemicals introduced into the market daily and the potential impact of all these chemicals are not known. It has been reported that 30% of the total workplace chemicals in the National Institute of Occupational Safety and Health Pocket Guideline can be hepatoxic.

Hepatotoxicity is characterised by organic and functional damage of the liver. The main pathogenic mechanisms are inflammation, dysfunction of cytochrome P450, mitochondrial dysfunction and oxidative stress. The principal mechanisms of hepatotoxicity are: (1) Disruption of the hepatocyte with a decrease in ATP levels; (2) Disruption of the transport proteins interrupting bile flow; (3) Cytolytic T-cell activation, the P450 enzyme stimulating a multifaceted immune response; (4) Apoptosis of hepatocytes causing cell death and bile duct injury from metabolites excreted into the bile ducts. Most of the hepatotoxicity is caused by exposure to solvents at the workplace (Fig. 1) (Malaguarnera *et al.*, 2012; Luster *et al.*, 2000; Luster *et al.*, 2001).

Inflammation plays an important role in classical chemical-induced hepatoxicity and repair. Hepatic non-parenchymal cells, the Kupffer, sinusoidal endothelial, and fat-storing or Ito (stellate) cells, and recruited leukocytes, contribute to the pathogenesis of hepatic toxicity. In response to a direct action of the chemical, the Kupffer cells are activated resulting in the production of proinflammatory cytokines such as interleukin (IL)-1, IL-6 and tumour necrosis factor (TNF) α, and chemokine receptor chemokines.

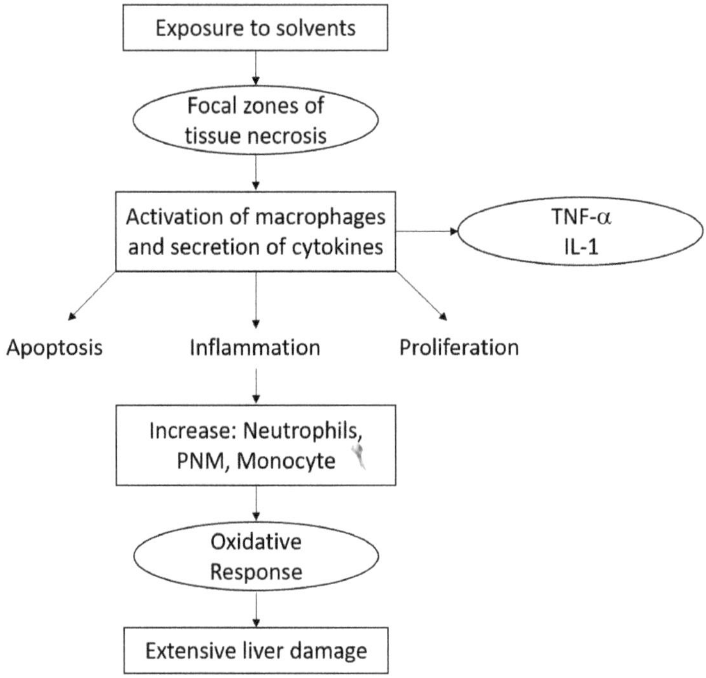

Fig. 1. Inflammation process in chemical-induced hepatotoxicity. TNF: Tumour necrosis factor; IL: Interleukin; PMN: Prime neutrophils.

The most common enzyme system for oxidation of xenobiotics is cytochrome P450, also known as CYP450 monooxygenase, hydroxylase or oxidase which plays an important role in the biotransformation of a wide variety of exogenous and endogenous substrates through P450 isoform CYP2E1. CYP2E1 dependent ethanol metabolism produces oxidative stress through generation of reactive oxygen species (ROS), a possible mechanism by which solvents are hepatotoxic. It has been shown that all conditions resulting in reduced activity of cytochrome P450, reduce the ability to detoxify solvents and, alternatively, increase the percentage of fat in the liver (e.g. malnutrition). In the study of toxic hepatitis there is a need to evaluate the potential inhibition and inductions of some of the substances

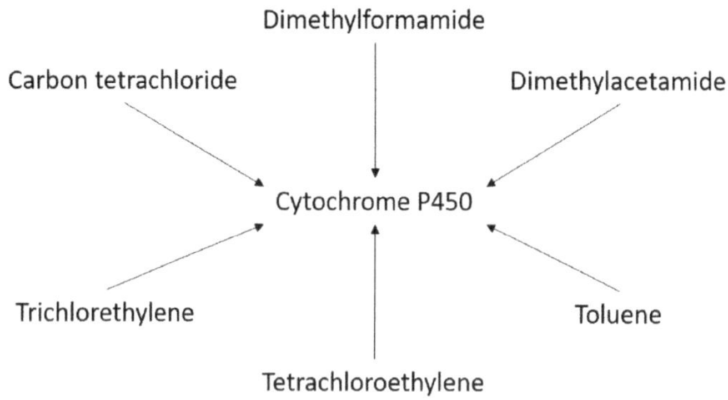

Fig. 2. Effects of solvents on cytochrome P450 (Malaguarnera *et al.*, 2012).

involved and assess the potential interaction with the myriad of drugs that are substrates of CYP (Fig. 2).

Various endogenous and exogenous substances impair mitochondrial β-oxidation to cause micro-vesicular steatosis through oxidative stress and damage to mitochondrial proteins, lipids, and DNA. In humans, these oxidative lesions cause mitochondrial DNA (mtDNA) deletions.

The oxidative damage caused by free radicals is thought to be a basic mechanism underlying many pathological conditions, including hepatotoxicity by solvents (Malaguarnera *et al.*, 2012).

Agents Causing Liver Injury

The main occupational exposures that have been associated with liver disease are chemicals and infectious agents. Acute liver injury may be easily recognised while the chronic conditions may be obscured due to insidious onset, being asymptomatic with normal values of conventional markers and confounded by other concurrent conditions. Thus, diagnosis of such chronic injuries can be challenging, one of exclusion and require an interdisciplinary approach. The awareness of clinicians on the aetiology of liver injury is limited while under-diagnosis and poor notification hinders the incidence and prevalence of occupational liver disease (OLD) being quantified. A variety of chemicals have been linked to OLDs, including several solvents, and mixtures, pesticides, and metals.

Table 1 shows liver diseases classified into acute liver injury and chronic liver injury as in the Clinical Practice Guidelines (CPGs) for OLDs, prepared by the European Association for the Study of the Liver (EASL) in 2019 (Colombo *et al.*, 2019).

Acute Liver Injury

Acute liver injury in occupational workers has been further classified based on the CPG by EASL, into hepatocellular, cholestatic and mixed, according to liver biochemistry during the first laboratory assessment at recognition.

Hepatocellular necrosis

Most forms of acute occupational hepatic injury in humans involve the hepatic parenchyma and manifest hepatocellular jaundice. The hepatocyte cytotoxicity and resulting necrosis characterise acute liver injury with or without lobular inflammation.

Commonly used chemicals at work or industries which cause hepatocellular necrosis include CCl_4, chloroform, toluene, trinitrotoluene, PCBs, chloronaphthalene, DMF, hydrazine, 2-nitropropane, phosphorus, dimethylacetamide, halothane, trichloroethanol, tetrachloroethane, 1,4-dichlorobenzene.

Halogenated hydrocarbons

This is the most important group of hepatotoxic chemicals causing acute liver injury. Many have been in widespread use in industry mostly as chlorinated derivatives of aliphatic or aromatic bases. As a rough rule of thumb, for the chlorinated benzene derivatives, increasing the extent of chlorination tends to lower the overall toxicity

Table 1. Pathological Patterns and Morphological Features of Liver Disease Associated with Workplace-Related Toxicants (Colombo *et al.*, 2019)

Pathological Patterns	Morphological Features	Toxicants
Acute Liver Injury		
Hepatocellular	Hepatocellular necrosis ± lobular inflammation	CCl_4, chloroform, toluene, Trinitro toluene, polychlorinated biphenyls (PCB), chloronaphthalene, dimethylformamide (DMF), hydrazine, 2-nitropropane, phosphorus, Dimethyacetamide, halothane, trichloroethylene, tetrachloroethane, 1,4-dichlorobenzene
Cholestatic/mixed	Microvesicular steatosis	DMF
	Cholestasis, cholangitis Combined features	Methylenedianiline Nitrobenzene, paraquat, methylenedianiline
Toxicant-associated fatty liver disease (TAFLD)	Steatosis (macro/ microvesicular) Steato-hepatitis (steatosis + lobular inflammation + hepatocellular ballooning)	Chloroalkenes (PCE, trichloroethylene), vinyl chloride monomer (VCM), chloroform, CCl_4, volatile organic compounds (benzene, toluene, styrene, xylene), dioxins, chlordecone, DMF, hydrazine, arsenic, mercury, persistent organic pollutants (POP), pesticides, and some nitro-organic compounds
Vascular	Sinusoidal obstruction syndrome Peliosis	VCM, dioxin, pyrrolizidine alkaloids, arsenic, copper sulfate VCM
Chronic Liver injury		
Fibrosis	Periportal fibrosis Extensive fibrosis/ cirrhosis	VCM, PCBs, chloronaphthalene, Tetrachloroethane VCM
Vascular	Porto-sinusoidal vascular disease (previously hepatoportal sclerosis)	VCM, sprays containing copper sulphate and lime
Tumors		
Epithelial		
Hepatocellular carcinoma Cholangiocarcinoma		Arsenic, dimethylnitrosamine 1,2-Dichloropropane, dichloromethane
Vascular		
Angiosarcoma		VCM, Arsenic
Epithelioid hemangioendothelioma		VCM

whereas for saturated aliphatic and some aromatic hydrocarbons, the reverse is true.

Chloroform is an example of an aliphatic agent belonging to this group of hepatotoxic agents. The use of chloroform as an anaesthetic in the past, has been abandoned due to its toxicity, which can cause hepatocellular necrosis and steatosis in acute exposures and liver cirrhosis following chronic exposure. Chloroform is mainly used as a raw material in the production of hydrochlorofluorocarbon-22 (HCFC-22), in the pharmaceutical industry (in the extraction of penicillin and other antibiotics), and as a solvent, degreasing agent, or chemical intermediary in industries like adhesives, pesticides, fats and oils (Table 2).

Table 2. Workplace-Related Hepatic Toxicants and Sources of Exposure (Colombo *et al.*, 2019)

Toxicant	Uses and Source of Exposure
Arsenic	Pesticide; impurity in smelting processes
CCl_4	Chemical manufacturing; cleaning fluid; dry cleaning; degreasing agent; refrigerant; pesticide
Chlordecone	Pesticide
Chlorinated hydrocarbons	Degreasers and cleaning solvent; refrigeration
Chloroform	Pharmaceutical industry; dyes and pesticides; reagent
1,4-Dichlorobenzene	Insecticide
Dimethylacetamide	Industrial solvent; production of acrylic fibres
Dimethylformamide	Industrial solvent, chemical manufacturing (acrylic fibres and plastic); paints
Dimethylnitrosamine	Waste product of rocket fuel manufacturing
Dioxin	Pesticide
Halothane	Anaesthesiology
Hexachlorobenzene	Fungicide
Hydrazine	Rocket fuel; preparation of gas precursors in airbags; oxygen scavenger
Methylene dianiline	Production workers; intermediate for polyurethane foam insulation

Table 2. (*Continued*)

Toxicant	Uses and Source of Exposure
2-Nitropropane	Paint; adhesive; coatings
Paraquat	Insecticide
Phosphorus	Munition
Polychlorinated biphenyls	Production; electrical utility (coolants, insulating fluids)
1,1,2,2-Tetrachloroethane	Aircraft manufacturing; formerly in paints and pesticides; dry cleaning; leather treatment
Toluene	Paints; coatings; adhesives; inks; cleaning agents; dyes
Trichloroethylene	Glue and cleaning solvent; grease remover; decaffeination of coffee
Trinitrotoluene	Munition
Vinyl chloride	Plastic (Polyvinylchloride and rubber manufacturing
Xylene	Resins; gums; paints; adhesives; inks; gasoline

Though chloroform use has been significantly reduced and even banned in certain western countries, its use in Asian countries is still prevalent, as illustrated in Case Study 1.

Case Study 1: Chloroform Exposure and Hepatotoxicity

Two women aged 34 and 41 years, who worked in a medical endoscopic device factory for approximately 40–45 days, were admitted to hospital for complaints of nausea, vomiting, abdominal discomfort, dark urine and were found to be jaundiced. Workplace chloroform exposure preceded the patients' recognition of symptoms. Their liver enzyme levels increased to more than 3 times the upper limit of the normal range. Other causes of hepatitis were ruled out.

Occupational history and workplace inspection revealed both worked in the cleanroom, assembling medical endoscopic devices, and used 99% chloroform as an adhesive and 98% ethanol as a cleanser. They poured chloroform from large bottles into 50-mL vessels and subsequently immersed the device in the chloroform adhesive or applied chloroform to the devices. Both gave no history of consuming drugs or smoking and rarely consumed alcohol. Both wore cleanroom garments without wearing personal protective equipment. The cleanroom maintained particulate-free air through use of high-efficiency particulate air (HEPA) filters, devoid of any air circulation system. The concentration of ethanol was within the recommended occupational exposure limit. Particulate levels in cleanrooms were maintained for quality of products manufactured.

The final investigation revealed that the presence of only a HEPA filter with inadequate ventilation system caused excessive chloroform accumulation in the cleanroom, resulting in severe hepatotoxicity. Both workers recovered and liver enzymes decreased to normal levels. They were discharged but did not return to work (Kang et al., 2014).

Emphasis on an appropriate ventilation system in cleanroom worksites require more attention as even small amounts of volatile compounds can accumulate in high concentrations in cleanrooms and cause severe hepatotoxicity. Chemical health risk assessment and regular medical surveillance of workers should be strictly advocated.

For the aromatic derivatives, chlorinated naphthalene and the chlorodiphenyls are particularly potent causes of acute liver injury. The toxicity of polychlorinated biphenyls (PCBs) and polychlorinated dibenzofurans (PCDFs) is dependent on the number and also on the location of chlorine atoms in the molecule.

Aliphatic halogenated hydrocarbons are capable of producing severe acute liver injury. CCl_4 is the classic example, and this may be a direct result of trichloromethyl free radical generation, (CCl_3). It is used in chemical manufacturing, dry cleaning, as a cleaning fluid, degreasing agent, refrigerant and pesticide (Table 2). The damage is first noted in the endoplasmic reticulum with vacuolation and ribosome detachment. Whilst the mitochondria remain intact, lipid droplets appear intracellularly and gross fatty changes occur in the lobular mid-zone. The toxicity of CCl_4 is enhanced by earlier treatment with enzyme-inducing drugs but diminished by a previous low protein diet. Death from exposure to CCl_4 is usually caused by renal failure rather than hepatic failure. The hepatotoxic effects of other chemicals in this group are usually less marked, but their fat solubility ensures widespread dissemination in the bone marrow and central nervous system where the clinical effects of toxicity may be more obvious or the long-term sequelae more serious.

Trichloroethylene and tetrachloroethane exposure have also been known to cause acute liver failure. On prolonged exposure it can lead to chronic liver injury and fibrosis. On an equivalent amount basis, 1,1,1-trichloroethane is probably one of the least toxic of the halogenated hydrocarbon solvents in common industrial use. Trichloroethylene is used as a glue, cleaning solvent and grease remover.

Dimethylformamide

DMF is a colourless organic solvent, extensively used in the manufacturing of synthetic leathers, films, fibres and surface coatings, in the pharmaceutical industry for pesticide formulation and polyurethane materials. The expansion of chemical, pharmaceutical and electronic industries has shown a remarkably increased global utilisation of this chemical in the 80s, and several cases of severe hepatotoxicity have been reported till the new millennium. The most prevalent disorders found in workers exposed to DMF were toxic hepatitis, fibrosis, cirrhosis, and cancer (Kim and Kim, 2011). The extent of damage from DMF exposure paralleled with increases of the amount of DMF utilisation in industries. Though these occurrences set regulations and guidelines in place, still cases occur due to poor education and management negligence.

DMF has shown to cause hepatocellular necrosis, cholestatic or mixed effects, and toxicant associated fatty liver disease which have previously been reported extensively in the literature even till 2011. Other than these toxic hepatitis cases, two very rare liver conditions have been reported following DMF exposures at work. One is a case of autoimmune hepatitis (Jang *et al.*, 2020) and the other is acute liver failure (Lei *et al.*, 2017).

Case Study 2: Autoimmune Hepatitis (AIH) and Dimethylformamide (DMF)

A 31-year-old man, who started working in a glove factory since July 2015, was admitted in late August 2015 for nausea, fatigue, and hand cramping and found to be jaundiced. He had intermittently put his bare hands in a diluted solution of DMF for the first 15 days at work though he received occupational safety education. He reported to have been healthy prior to his current job and was a regular blood donor, who did not consume any drugs or excessive alcohol.

The laboratory findings revealed elevated aspartate aminotransferase (ALT), alanine aminotransferase (ALT), positive antinuclear antibodies (ANA) and smooth muscle antibodies (SMA), immunoglobulin G (IgG) and, a liver biopsy showed portoperiportal lymphoplasmacytic infiltration and interface activity with confluent centrilobular necrosis, which was compatible with severe AIH. Wilson's disease was excluded. He was treated with a combination therapy of prednisolone and azathioprine, until March 2019 followed by a tapering of immunosuppressive therapy. He had no symptoms during this phase and liver biochemistry was within normal limits till April 2020.

The absence of previously reported cases and experimental data on the pathogenic mechanism of DMF causing AIH, made it difficult to establish that this was DMF-induced AIH. The points in favour of the diagnosis were a previously healthy man with normal liver test results, an occupational history of DMF exposure (dipping his hands in the chemical without using gloves), the time sequence of exposure before developing AIH and exclusion of other causes of hepatitis, which strongly supported the diagnosis of AIH (Jang et al., 2020).

Compared to other forms of autoimmune liver disease (AILD), AIH is characterised by a hepatocellular pattern of elevated levels of liver enzymes, positive tests for non-disease-specific antinuclear antibodies (ANA) and/or smooth muscle antibodies (SMA), which are the histological hallmark of AIH interface hepatitis on liver biopsy, and an optimal response to steroids in most patients.

Toxic hepatitis due to exposure to hepatotoxins at work is generally detected by standard liver biochemistry, revealing inflammation and necrosis of the liver. The toxicity is related to the cytochrome P450 enzyme system. The aetiology of AIH is unknown and the pathogenesis proposed is secondary failure of immune tolerance in a genetically susceptible individual leading to a T-cell mediated inflammation caused by environmental exposures namely; toxins, infections and medication. AIH is rare, characterised by the presence of autoantibodies, an elevated blood immunoglobulin G (IgG) level and typical pathological features including interface hepatitis with portal lymphoplasmacytic infiltrates with optimal response to steroids in most patients.

The limitations in this case were: no measurement of DMF exposure at his workplace, no detection of urine metabolite for DMF at the early phase of diagnosis, and his HLA typing was not performed due to cost. This case points to the importance of a high index of suspicion by hepatologists and occupational physicians for early diagnosis as timely treatment with immunosuppressive therapy can lead to complete remission. It also averts progression of disease to acute liver failure, cirrhosis with complications such as end-stage liver disease or hepatocellular carcinoma (Wang *et al.*, 2020). Workplace safety education, chemical health risk assessment, and periodic medical examinations among workers who handle DMF should be strictly instituted.

Case Study 3: Dimethylformamide (DMF) and Acute Liver Failure

A 38-year-old healthy female with no history of alcohol consumption, started her job at a synthetic leather factory that manufactured belts using DMF as a solvent in late 2014. One week into working, a routine physical check-up, laboratory tests and an abdominal ultrasound, showed results of all within normal levels.

After 2.5 months of working, she sought treatment for fatigue, poor appetite, abdominal distention, nausea and jaundice. With no improvement, she went to another hospital where she was found conscious with stable vital signs. She was jaundiced with abdominal shifting dullness and had oedema of both lower limbs. Laboratory investigations revealed high serum bile acid level of 435 μmol/l (normal range, 0–12 μmol/l) and hyaluronidase >2,000 ng/ml (normal range, 0–100 ng/ml). Viral infections Hepatitis A — C and drug related diseases were excluded.

Treatment strategies for DMF-induced hepatic dysfunction included hepatoprotection, plasma, blood platelet and albumin transfusions. An artificial liver support system (ALSS) was instituted as patient's condition deteriorated. Patient recovered after 2.5 months.

Workplace inspection revealed patient worked in a wet process for 10 hours a day using large quantities of DMF in a poorly ventilated room with no personal protective devices. Several co-workers had similar symptoms and received supportive treatment and returned to work. In this case, a diagnosis of DMF-induced acute hepatic failure was based on clinical history (no history of medication use or alcohol intake), symptoms and signs, abnormal liver function, negative hepatitis viral series and high DMF concentrations in the work environment. Several co-workers also suffered from liver dysfunction (Lei et al., 2017).

The mortality of DMF-induced acute severe hepatitis is high with no specific treatment for DMF-induced acute hepatic failure, though ALSS has shown to be effective in clinical treatment. This calls for vigilance among occupational physicians and hepatologists to suspect acute renal failure in patients who report working in a factory handling DMF. Health education, usage of appropriate personal protective equipment, good ventilation and regular workplace monitoring, chemical health risk assessment, and medical surveillance should be instituted. DMF has also been reported to cause microvesicular steatosis; foamy changes in the hepatocyte cytoplasm as tiny fat droplets with a preserved nucleus in the centre.

Other chemicals known to cause hepatocellular necrosis with cholestatic lesions due to workplace exposures are methylenedianiline causing cholestasis and cholangitis. Paraquat, a toxic herbicide, commonly used in under-developed and developing countries, and nitrobenzene have reported combined features.

Alcohols

Alcohols are metabolised by the liver and the effect of ethanol on the liver is the best known and understood. Exposure is primarily dependent upon lifestyle, with limits being suggested for sensible alcohol consumption. The current United Kingdom (UK) revised guidelines for alcohol intake advise ingestion of less than 14 units a week for women and men (a unit is equivalent to half a pint of beer (250 mL); a measure of spirits (25 mL); a measure of fortified wine (50 mL) or a glass of ordinary wine (80 mL)) (Rosenberg *et al.*, 2018). This is equivalent to drinking no more than six pints of average-strength beer (4% ABV) or seven medium-sized glasses of wine (175 mL, 12% ABV) a week. It is best to spread the 14 units over a period of 3 days or more. The Australian revised guidelines for alcohol intake for healthy men and women, is to drink no more than 10 standard drinks per week and no more than four standard drinks on any one day. A standard drink contains 10 g of alcohol (Australian Department of Health, 2020). The advice for pregnant women and those trying to conceive is that alcohol intake should be avoided. Advice is also provided on not mixing alcohol with medications or recreational drugs, nor drinking and driving or when operating machinery, and to be discouraged for those with mental health problems such as depression.

Fatty liver is common in those who have a prolonged history of excessive alcohol intake and this can progress to a liver fibrosis and eventually liver cirrhosis. Steatohepatitis with inflammation called alcoholic hepatitis can also occur on the background of liver fibrosis from alcohol, clinically presenting with jaundice. Genetic susceptibility has been suggested as an explanation for the different amounts of alcohol required to cause liver effects between individuals (Stickel *et al.*, 2017). Ethyl alcohol is metabolised to acetaldehyde and then to acetate. Highly reactive free radicals are also produced, and the liver damage from alcohol consumption is thought to be due to acetaldehyde and the free radicals. A high proportion of individuals of Chinese ethnic origin have a genetically determined lack of alcohol dehydrogenase and aldehyde dehydrogenase (Matsumura *et al.*, 2019). An increase in blood levels of unmetabolised acetaldehyde causes "facial flushing," tachycardia, and headaches (Lee *et al.*, 2014). These symptoms may discourage further alcohol intake, and thus can act as a protective factor against acute alcohol effects.

Non-alcoholic fatty liver disease (NAFLD) has emerged as the leading cause of chronic liver disease worldwide (Younossi *et al.*, 2018). It is estimated that one in four people globally has fatty liver disease and the prevalence of NAFLD parallels the prevalence of metabolic syndrome (MetS) and its components. The effects of xenobiotic in non-alcoholic fatty liver diseases have been described in Fig. 3 (Klaunig *et al.*, 2018). A panel of international experts

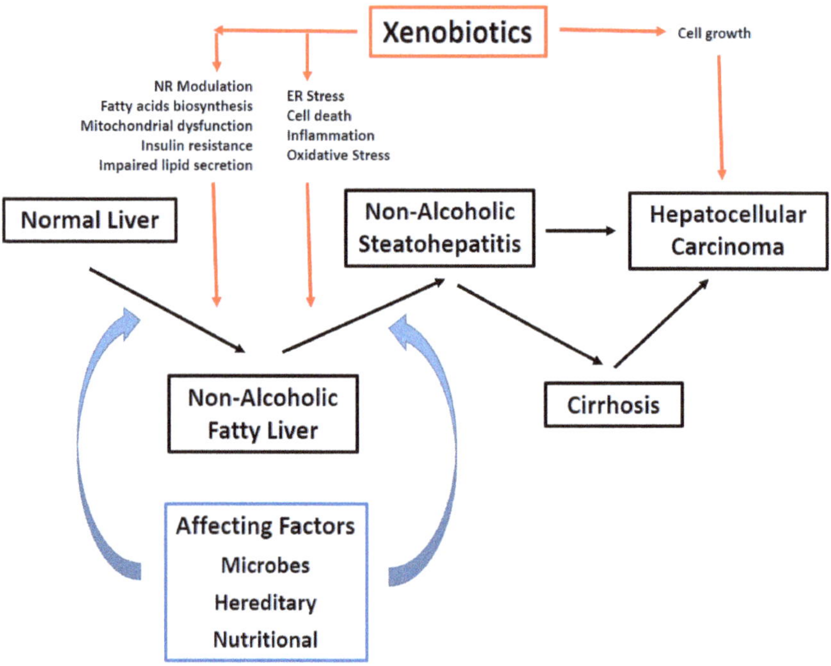

Fig. 3. The effects of xenobiotic in non-alcoholic fatty liver diseases. ER — endoplasmic reticulum; NR — nuclear receptor.

recently proposed the nomenclature of NAFLD should be updated to metabolic (dysfunction) associated fatty liver disease (MAFLD). In addition to evidence of hepatic steatosis, the definition for the diagnosis of MAFLD requires one of the following three criteria, namely, overweight or obesity, presence of type 2 diabetes mellitus, or evidence of metabolic dysregulation (Eslam *et al.*, 2020). MAFLD is a heterogeneous entity and can coexist with other liver diseases.

Fatty liver disease caused by occupational and environmental chemical exposure is termed "toxicant-associated steatohepatitis" (TASH) (Wahlang *et al.*, 2019), which is characterised by hepatic steatosis, and inflammation. Fatty liver has been related to the occupational exposure to organic solvents. TASH has been described in highly exposed VCM workers. Environmental agents which have been shown to be associated with TASH include persistent organic pollutants (POPs), volatile organic chemicals (VOCs), metals (arsenic, lead, mercury, cadmium) and pesticides (Lang and Beier, 2018).

In severe cases of TASH, fatty liver is characterised by steatosis, inflammatory infiltrates, ballooning hepatocytes and in some cases fibrosis and cirrhosis It is pathologically indistinguishable from NASH, even occurring in lean individuals (Lundqvist *et al.*, 1999; Malaguarnera *et al.*, 2012).

Nitro-compounds

Nitrated compounds, particularly the aromatic ones, can cause hepatocellular damage. Trinitrotoluene is used in the ammunition industry as explosives. It has caused fatalities either from acute liver injury, centrilobular necrosis or aplastic anaemia. Nitrobenzene also causes jaundice, from hepatocellular damage and from excessive haemolysis. 1,1-Dimethylhyrazine is used as a rocket fuel and can cause necrosis while 1,2-dimethylhydrazine has no commercial applications and is classified as a Group 2A carcinogen (probably carcinogenic to humans) by the International Agency for Research on Cancer (IARC).

Metals and metalloids

Metals and metalloids reported to cause hepatic damage in humans include arsenic, selenium, thallium and phosphorus. Yellow phosphorus used in the manufacture of "strike-anywhere" matches is largely of historical interest. It was used because of its ability to ignite readily; hence it was also included in napalm (used in the Vietnam War). Occupational health notoriety was achieved when workers in the East End of London (Bow) developed "phossy jaw" from their work exposure to the element. It also caused acute yellow atrophy of the liver. Phosphorus compounds are used today for the production of pesticides (organophosphates), fireworks, and detergents, and its toxicity has been exploited in rodent control. Control of occupational exposure to the ingredients for these products in modern factories today have diminished the likelihood of "phossy jaw" and acute yellow atrophy.

Biochemical Definition for Acute Liver Injury

Standard liver biochemistry is used to reflect necro-inflammatory processes in hepatic injury caused by occupational exposure to potential

Table 3. Threshold of Liver Enzymes Used to Define Acute Liver Injury and Pattern of Damage According to Ratio (R)

Criteria to Define Liver Injury (any one of the following)	Pattern of Liver Injury, According to R Value (ALT/ULN)/(ALP/ULN); AST can Replace ALT When ALT is Unavailable
ALT level ≥5x ULN	Hepatocellular pattern: $R \geq 5$
ALP level ≥2x ULN (particularly if concomitantly elevated gamma-glutamyl transpeptidase (GGT) in the absence of bone disease)	Cholestatic pattern: $R \leq 2$
ALT level ≥3x ULN and simultaneous TB level >2x ULN	Mixed pattern: R value is >2 and <5

ALP: alkaline phosphatase; ALT: alanine aminotransferase; AST: aspartate aminotransferase; TB: total bilirubin; ULN: upper limit of normal.

hepatotoxins. These biomarkers are not specific for any form of toxic liver disease, lack mechanistic insight and may not reveal prognostic significance. Due to similarities observed in clinical and histopathological features of hepatic injury between occupational exposure to hepatoxins and occupational exposure to chemicals and drugs, thresholds of liver enzymes were introduced by the EASL CPGs for drug-induced liver injury and the Clinical Practice Guidelines for occupational diseases (Andrade *et al.*, 2019; Colombo *et al.*, 2019) to define acute liver injury following occupational exposure to hepatotoxins (Table 3).

- In patients with abnormal baseline liver blood tests, upper limit of normality (ULN) is replaced by the mean baseline values obtained prior to the exposure to the suspect chemical, and the increases in Alanine Aminotransferase (ALT), Alkaline Phosphatase (ALP) and Total Bilirubin (TB) should be proportionate to this modified baseline.

Chronic Liver Injury

Fibrosis and vascular

Fibrosis of the liver is the outcome of insults by different toxicants leading to chronic hepatitis, subacute necrosis or steatohepatitis.

Periportal fibrosis and cirrhosis have been reported following occupational exposure to VCM.

Other sub-categories of chronic liver injury are vascular disorders, sinusoidal obstruction syndrome, peliosis and porto-sinusoidal vascular disease (previously known as hepatoportal sclerosis). Porto-sinusoidal vascular disease has been documented to be caused by VCM.

Tumours

Although VCM is well known to cause angiosarcoma, its prevalence has drastically reduced due to good control measures at the workplace in developed countries. However, the occurrence of angiosarcoma due to VCM can still be anticipated in the future due to the lack of enforcement in under-developed and developing countries.

Drug induced liver injury (DILI)

DILI is traditionally classified as intrinsic (or direct) versus idiosyncratic. Drug Induced Liver Injury (DILI) is not directly related to occupational exposures. It is deliberated here to emphasis the challenges posed, namely low incidence, absence of specific biomarkers, the hepatotoxic potential of multidrug regimens used in clinical practice and presentation with a variety of clinical and pathological phenotypes which can result in illness, hospitalisation and even life-threatening liver failure, death or need for liver transplantation (Andrade *et al.*, 2019).

Idiosyncratic liver injury occasionally occurs following drug absorption. Examples of drugs involved are co-amoxiclav, isoniazid, halothane, methyldopa and propylthiouracil (Andrade *et al.*, 2019). Some of the drugs in combination apparently act synergistically to cause liver damage, e.g. alcohol and acetaminophen, and rifampicin and isoniazid. Genetic factors, immunological responses and variable reactions to toxic metabolites have all been invoked to explain the effects. A good example of a drug hypersensitivity reaction affecting the liver is that of halothane administration to patients for anaesthesia resulting in acute liver injury in a small proportion of patients.

The key feature of idiosyncratic DILI with most drugs is the critical role of the adaptive immune system. Key in the development of an adaptive immune response is the role of restricted human leukocyte antigen (HLA) associations (Andrade *et al.*, 2019). The release of hepatic proteins causes further liver damage (Dara *et al.*, 2016). Occupational exposure to anaesthetic agents in nurses and other intensive care staff have not been associated with liver injury. Acetaminophen, is a potent hepatotoxin as it is metabolised by two pathways, both increasing its solubility in water. One pathway generates a highly reactive quinone which requires rapid glutathione conjugation and the liver has limited supplies of glutathione. Once exhausted the reactive electrophilic quinone damages hepatocytes and causes cell necrosis and potentially toxic liver failure (Ramachandran and Jaeschke, 2018).

Infectious Agents

Table 4 lists the main infectious agents which can cause liver damage and the occupational groups at risk. Laboratory workers who have to process organisms for research or diagnostic purposes, or work on potentially infected biological samples, may be exposed to a variety of infectious agents in the course of work activity. Research staff in genetic engineering laboratories and laboratory and post-mortem technicians in the healthcare industry are also at risk.

The hepatitis viruses (Hepatitis A, B, C, D and E) cause acute hepatitis and in some cases of hepatitis B (+/− D) and C, this may progress to chronic liver disease (Teo, 1992). Although acute hepatitis C is rare, it contributes towards more than 70 million cases of chronic liver diseases globally (Pawlotsky *et al.*, 2020).

Hepatitis A is an enterovirus transmitted by the oro-faecal route (Shin and Jeong, 2018). It appears to be an occupational health hazard for sewage workers. Outbreaks have also occurred in institutions for the mentally handicapped. A formalin-inactivated vaccine is available to protect against this infection. Primary immunisation involves a single dose given intramuscularly with a booster administered any time between 6 to 12 months later (Zhang L, 2020).

Table 4. Infectious Agents Affecting the Liver

Infectious Agents/Diseases	Occupations at Risk
Dengue Hemorrhagic Fever	Forestry workers
Hepatitis A	Sewer workers
Hepatitis B	Pathologists, laboratory staff, other healthcare personnel
Hepatitis C	Healthcare and laboratory staff
Leptospirosis (*L. icterohaemorrhagiae, L. hardjo*)	Sewer workers, veterinary surgeons and cattle workers
Malaria (*Plasmodium falciparum, vivax, malariae*)	Workers who have to travel and work in endemic areas
Melioidosis (*Burkholderia pseudomallei*)	Farmers
Yellow Fever	Workers who have to travel and work in endemic areas
Q Fever (*Coxiella burneti*)	Farm workers
Schistosomiasis (*S. mansoni, S. japonicum*)	Agricultural workers, civil construction (e.g. dams, irrigation projects)
Coronavirus disease 2019 (COVID 19)	Healthcare workers

Hepatitis B causes infection that can result in full recovery or can lead to chronic infection in 10% of adults. Chronic infection carries a risk of primary liver cancer which is higher in the presence of cirrhosis and high viral loads. There is a residual risk of transmission of the infection to others through contact with blood or body fluids or from sexual activity.

Hepatitis C is now thought to be responsible for more than 75% of what was previously termed post transfusion non-A, non-B hepatitis. Treatment with 6–12 months of Interferon therapy, (which was associated with significant side-effects including depression affecting ability to work), is being replaced by shorter courses of well tolerated oral direct acting antiviral agents with high cure rates of >90%.

Hepatitis D and E seem less likely to be occupationally acquired. Hepatitis D can only exist/replicate in the presence of hepatitis B infection.

In the COVID-19 pandemic, hepatic dysfunction has been seen in 14–53% of patients with COVID-19, particularly in those with severe disease. Cases of acute liver injury have been reported and are associated with higher mortality. Hepatic involvement in COVID-19 could be related to the direct cytopathic effect of the virus, an uncontrolled immune reaction, sepsis or drug-induced liver injury (Jothimani *et al.*, 2020).

Case Study 4: A Healthcare Worker with Markers of Hepatitis B Infection

A 24-year-old female nurse working in a surgical ward was found to be HBsAg positive two weeks after a needle-stick injury. She completed three doses of Hepatitis B vaccine as part of the neonatal immunisation schedule for hepatitis B. When she joined the nursing school, her HBsAg was negative but due to her low anti-HBs level, she received a booster dose of Hepatitis B vaccine with good anti-HBs response of 241 mIU.

Her HBsAg remained positive six weeks after the needle-stick injury with persistently low anti-HBs of 3.66 mIU but HBc Ab and HBV DNA were persistently not detected. She was allowed to continue working in the surgical ward but was asked to be excluded from assisting or performing exposure-prone procedures. Repeat HBsAg at six months after the needle-stick injury was negative and remained negative a year later.

A HBsAg positive surgical ward nurse may not be involved in exposure-prone procedures (EPPs). Phlebotomy, and procedures where the operator's hands are always clearly visible are not considered EPPs. In this case the nurse is unlikely to pose a significant risk from regular work in a surgical ward, and can be allowed to continue in her vocation. However, in some countries, there are national laws whereby a work visa will only be granted to, a foreign healthcare worker if they can demonstrate an absence of Hepatitis B, Hepatitis C and HIV. If the nurse was undertaking EPPs and was found to have significant viraemia, an important consideration is whether treatment of hepatitis B infection would allow the nurse or health care personnel to continue to do EPPs. Treatment with either entecavir or tenofovir, to reduce viral load to low or undetectable levels will allow them to perform EPP with regular viral load testing.

Hepatic Carcinogens

Occupational groups such as workers in the restaurant and beverage trade, journalists and seafarers have an increased risk of primary liver cancer (hepatocellular carcinoma). This is likely to be due to consumption of alcoholic drinks — ethyl alcohol, (ethanol), being a recognised liver carcinogen and has been designated a Group 1 human carcinogen by the IARC. A dose–response association has been established for cancer types caused by alcohol consumption. Agents causing primary hepatocellular tumours can be arbitrarily separated from hepatotoxic agents (Table 5). The latter group can, in some cases, cause sufficient damage over a long enough time to lead to cirrhosis. Liver cirrhosis is a well-known risk factor for primary liver cancer (Torre *et al.*, 2015). Liver cirrhosis, the end-stage of every chronic liver disease, is not only the major risk factor for the development of hepatocellular carcinoma but also a limiting factor for anticancer therapy of liver and non-hepatic malignancies (Pinter *et al.*, 2016).

Angiosarcoma of the liver is a rare malignancy consisting of malignant endothelial cells supported by a reticular framework. The classic occupational example of angiosarcoma of the liver is due to VCM. In 1987, the IARC concluded that VCM exposure causes

Table 5. Summary of IARC Evaluation Reports on the Carcinogenicity of Vinyl Chloride, Arsenic, Trichloroethylene, Perchloroethylene, Polychlorinated Biphenyls, and 1,1,1-Trichloro-2,2-Bis(p-chlorophenyl) Ethane (DDT) (Uccello *et al.*, 2012)

	Year of Publication	Group Assigned by IARC	Summary of IARC Evaluation on Overall and Liver Carcinogenicity
Vinyl chloride	2008	Group 1 (carcinogenic to humans)	There is sufficient evidence for the carcinogenicity of vinyl chloride because it has been found to induce angiosarcomas of the liver and hepatocellular carcinomas in both humans and experimental animals.

(*Continued*)

Table 5. (*Continued*)

	Year of Publication	Group Assigned by IARC	Summary of IARC Evaluation on Overall and Liver Carcinogenicity
Arsenic	2004	Group 1 (carcinogenic to humans)	There is sufficient evidence in humans that arsenic in drinking water causes cancers of the urinary bladder, lung, and skin; however, the interpretation of the findings on liver cancer mortality has several methodological limitations. Moreover, the studies on inorganic arsenic provide limited evidence for carcinogenicity in experimental animals.
Trichloroethylene	1995	Group 2A (probably carcinogenic to humans)	Evidence from several epidemiological studies suggests that trichloroethylene may enhance the risks for non-Hodgkin's lymphoma and cancers of the liver and biliary tract. Trichloroethylene can also induce liver tumours in rodents through peroxisome proliferation and other mechanisms.
Perchloroethylene	1995	Group 2A (probably carcinogenic to humans)	There is consistent evidence for positive associations between exposure to tetrachloroethylene and the risks for non-Hodgkin's lymphoma and oesophageal and cervical cancer. Although tetrachloroethylene is known to induce hepatocellular carcinomas in experimental animals, evidence of liver tumour induction in humans is inconsistent.

Table 5. (*Continued*)

	Year of Publication	Group Assigned by IARC	Summary of IARC Evaluation on Overall and Liver Carcinogenicity
Polychlorinated Biphenyls	1987	Group 2A (probably carcinogenic to humans)	Evidence for carcinogenicity in humans is limited. An increased risk from hepatobiliary cancer has been found in different studies, which were biased. On the other hand, evidence for carcinogenicity in animals is sufficient. Administration of certain polychlorinated biphenyls produced benign and malignant liver neoplasms in mice and rats.
Dichloro-diphenyl-trichloroethane (DDT)	1991	Group 2B (possibly carcinogenic to humans)	There is inadequate evidence for the carcinogenicity of DDT in humans. Evidence for the carcinogenicity of DDT in experimental animals is sufficient, particularly for liver tumours

hepatocellular carcinoma (HCC), a statement that was confirmed in 2012 following the re-analysis of VCM-exposed European and United States (US) workers (Colombo, 2020; IARC, 2012). Thorium therapy has also resulted in cholangiocarcinomata (this bile duct tumour has been linked with parasitic infestations such as *Clonorchis sinensis* and *Opistorchis viverrini*). Chronic exposure to inorganic arsenical compounds is also thought to cause angiosarcoma of the liver (Neugut *et al.*, 1986).

Vinyl Chloride Monomer (VCM) and Angiosarcoma of the Liver

VCM was first synthesised in 1835 and has been in commercial production for the past sixty years. Nearly all the monomer is used in the production of vinyl chloride homo-polymer and co-polymer resins. In the early days of production, control of the gaseous VCM was not particularly stringent. This may have been in part due to the mistaken belief that VCM was relatively safe, as it had been trialled at one time for possible use as an anaesthetic agent. Concentrations in the vicinity of the polymerisation reactor vessels frequently reached 3,000 ppm and during the process of cleaning the chambers, the workforce might have been exposed to levels of 4,000 ppm. By the mid-1960's, certain curious effects of exposure had been noted in the workers who cleaned the reactor vessels. A number of them had developed acro-osteolysis, some had Raynaud's phenomenon and a few periportal liver fibrosis.

Introduction of measures to control the workplace concentration of VCM was swift. In 1975, Occupational Safety and Health Administration (OSHA) implemented a time-weighted VC exposure limit of 1 ppm and mandated medical surveillance of VC workers. By the late 1980's, the number of new cases of angiosarcoma reported had peaked and was beginning to decline. In total, perhaps less than 100 cases have occurred world-wide but the effect of the VCM story on the chemical industry invoked a salutary lesson. No chemical agent can be considered "safe" until proven to be so, and no new chemical since this episode has been assumed to be without potentially serious hazard.

Case Study 5: Vinyl Chloride Monomer (VCM) and Angiosarcoma of the Liver

A 73-year-old man with a history of hypertension and congestive cardiac failure was admitted at a hospital for progressive jaundice of unknown aetiology. During prior hospitalisations, multiple hepatic nodular lesions of uncertain nature had been reported at various imaging exams. Two ultrasound-guided liver biopsies had already been performed, leading to a diagnosis of nodular regenerative hyperplasia of uncertain interpretation (Marletta et al., 2020). After admission to the hospital, laboratory tests revealed increased direct bilirubin levels (9.59 mg/dl), while liver enzymes were within the recognised normal ranges. Moreover, search for autoantibodies and serologic tests for hepatotropic viruses were negative and no anomaly was noted for blood iron parameters. Abdominal contrast-enhanced ultra sound revealed multiple hyperechoic, anaechoic, and isoechoic hepatic nodules.

Abdominal contrast-enhancement computerised tomography (CT) and magnetic resonance imaging (MRI) revealed increased liver volume, with left lobe hypertrophy and heterogeneous appearance of the parenchyma: multiple confluent lesions with numerous blanks were detected. These atypical radiological findings were utterly unspecific for any particular disease; not only for their diffuse and bilobar massive spreading throughout the liver but also for the involvement of both central and peripheral areas of the hepatic parenchyma. Liver biopsy histological findings were suspicious for a vascular lesion. The patient eventually succumbed to the illness. A chronic occupational vinyl chloride exposure was retrospectively discovered. Based on the clinical data with atypical presentations and the morphologic features, the diagnosis of multifocal hepatic angiosarcoma was established.

Hepatic angiosarcoma is a rare entity, accounting for less than the 2% of all the primary malignant hepatic neoplasms, with about 200 cases worldwide diagnosed every year. VCM, Thorotrast (thorium dioxide), and arsenic are known risk factors for HAS (Chaudhary et al., 2015). Hepatic angiosarcoma due to environmental exposure has a prolonged latency period of 10–40 years (Kumar et al., 2020). The long latent period makes it challenging for recognition of the aetiological cause. The cornerstone for recognition of the aetiologic cause is a detailed occupational history and environmental monitoring.

Diagnosis of Occupational Liver Disease

The diagnosis of OLD remains tricky to establish. OLDs rarely display pathognomonic signs, have long latent period and are often multi causal in aetiology. Diagnosis is made more challenging with non-retrievable records of patients' workplace exposure levels. A schematic approach to the assessment and diagnosis of OLD is shown in Fig. 4 (Colombo *et al.*, 2019).

As in the case of the diagnosis of angiosarcoma due to occupational exposure to VCM, a good occupational history is essential to

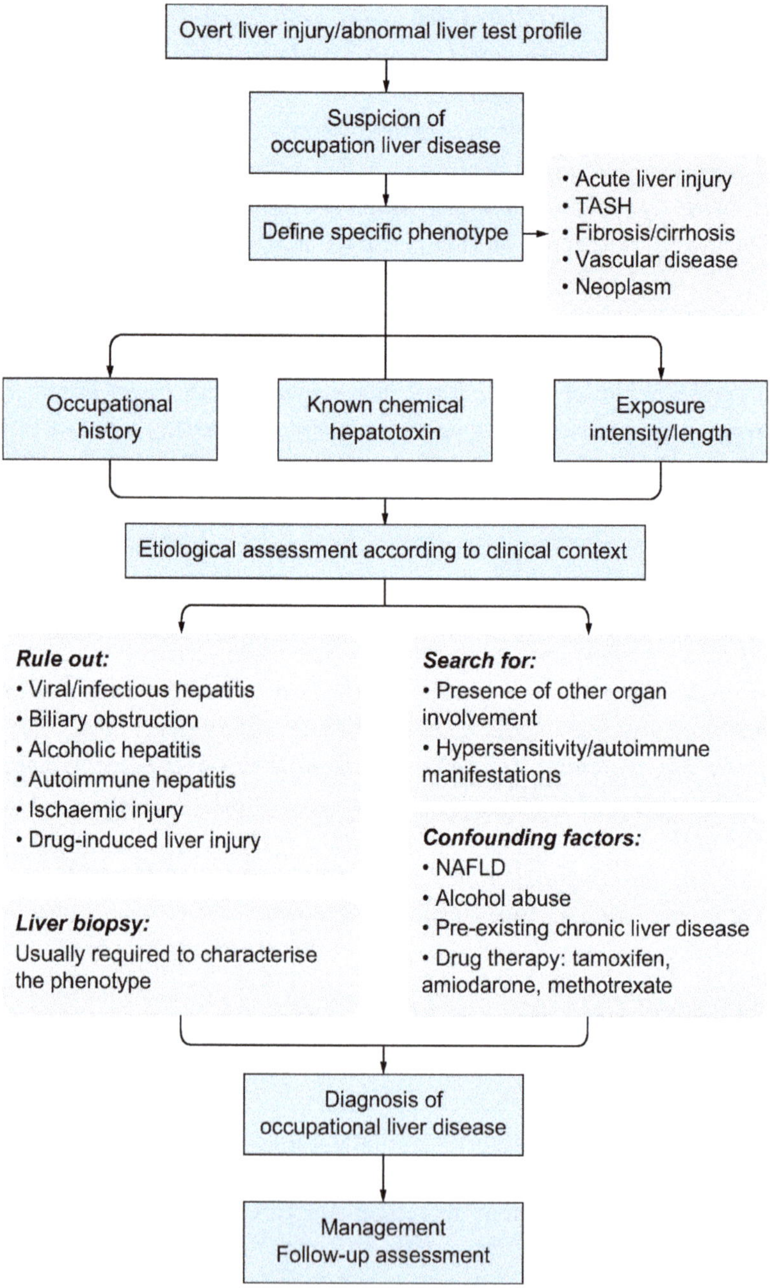

Fig. 4. Schematic approach to the assessment and diagnosis of OLD.

Box 1. Critical Information to be Obtained from the Patient with a Suspicion of OLD.

1. A chronological summary of all work activities and their duration.
2. A detailed description of the workplace, job and of a typical working day.
3. An inventory of all chemicals that are present and how they are used. Sometimes this information can be obtained from the management.
4. Details of any measures to limit chemical exposure such as: workplace ventilation and the nature of protective measures that are taken (requirement to wear special clothing and gloves, the use of masks, goggles and other devices).
5. Enquiring if programmes of industrial hygiene, biological monitoring and medical surveillance are or have been in place and retrieve the result, if necessary, keeping in mind however that compliance with occupational exposure limits do not necessarily protect all workers from adverse effects.
6. Enquire as to whether co-workers have similar symptoms and signs to those of a patient with suspected OLD. This may involve questioning and even examining co-workers. If several cases come to light, it may be possible to demonstrate an exposure-response relationship.
7. Enquire if compensation procedures have been undertaken and results are available.
8. Exposures to chemicals other than those present at workplaces, associated for instance with environmental air pollution, hobbies, recreational habits and others should be ruled out.

raise an index of suspicion regarding the work relatedness of the illness (Box 1). As practiced in United States, Europe and in some other countries, a recognised occupational physician is critical in assisting to diagnose occupational diseases. The occupational physicians will work with other stakeholders like the pathologists, occupational hygienists, hepatologists and others. Medical surveillance, biological and environmental monitoring, promotive as well as preventive measures are the backbone to minimise or prevent occupational diseases. Additionally, occupational physician's role in walk through surveys is an important aspect to understand and recognise the hazards and risks at the workplace.

Exposure Assessment

Liver injury markers such as ALT, AST and GGT or miRNAs, merely represent liver damage and, although they may be used for classification of the type of liver damage, they do not offer any insight into the aetiology underlying this damage (McGill *et al.*, 2017).

Urine and blood are the most commonly used biological matrices for biomonitoring. However, for both matrices, the window of detection of the toxicants themselves or their metabolites are quite limited (typically maximally in the range of days). For a more extended historical window, segmental hair analysis could be used or, alternatively, adducts in blood could be monitored (Delahaye *et al.*, 2017; Sabbioni and Turesky, 2017).

Adducts with haemoglobin are detectable up to >100 days following exposure, as their disappearance is linked to the lifespan of red blood cells, which is about four months. Although the markers that can be assessed this way are highly selective, there are still confounding factors like smoking (Thier *et al.*, 2001; De Smedt *et al.*, 2014).

Confirming Occupational Exposure

A key element in the investigation of possible OLD is the confirmation of exposure to a hepatotoxic agent. This may be suspected from the history provided by the patient. An occupational history of poor systems of work leading to frequent skin contact with organic solvents or working in poorly-ventilated areas with solvent vapor is important as a clue to the aetiology of the disease. Work involving unventilated exposure to gases is also relevant. This was the case in the workers who had to clean out the polymerisation chambers where VCM was being polymerised to polyvinyl chloride (PVC). High levels of residual VCM gas were present. Lack of provision and/or use of personal protective equipment are also a relevant factor in the occupational history.

Environmental hygiene records may be available which could confirm high levels of exposure to the suspected hepatotoxic chemicals. Evaluation of hygiene records will require comparison of the readings against some occupational exposure standard. In the UK, the Health Safety Executive produces an annual update on such standards (document EH40/00). In the US, such standards are available from the American Conference of Governmental Industrial Hygienists (ACGIH) in the form of a booklet on threshold limit values and biological exposure indices (ACGIH, 2021). The US OSHA also produces permissible exposure levels (PELs) for exposure to chemicals in the workplace. In Germany, equivalent standards are produced by the Deutsche Forschungsgemeinschaft. These documents will help in interpretation of hygiene measurements regarding the extent of exposure. However, the basis of the standards set is not necessarily on data pertaining to the likelihood of liver damage. Some of the standards are based on toxic effects on other target organs, and others are produced by extrapolation from animal studies with introduction of different safety factors, or from case reports which unfortunately often lack good exposure data.

Occasionally, biological monitoring results may be available to indicate absorption of hepatotoxins from several different sources of exposure. Chlorinated hydrocarbons such as trichloroethylene, perchloroethylene, and 1,1,1-trichloroethane can be detected from analysis of blood and breath samples. Trichloroethylene is metabolised to TCA and trichloroethanol, both of which are detectable in urine as an indicator of exposure. In contrast, only a small fraction of perchloroethylene is metabolised to TCA. Hence detection of TCA in urine is of limited value for perchloroethylene exposure, except possibly for end-of-shift samples taken at the end of a working week when urinary levels may be expected to be at the highest level. Other examples of biological monitoring data for hepatotoxic chemicals are venous blood levels of aromatic compounds such as toluene and styrene, or urinary levels of metabolites such as hippuric acid in those exposed to toluene, methyl hippuric acid for xylene exposure, and mandelic acid in workers exposed to styrene. Documentation of excessive exposure with an appropriate time interval between exposure and effect are essential in deciding on an occupational cause for liver damage.

Differential Diagnoses

Although there appears to be a bewildering array of workplace hepatotoxins, the clinicians faced with a patient with liver disease is, in most cases, dealing with a non-occupational aetiology. Cases of acute hepatitis or acute liver failure are usually due to viruses, drugs or autoimmune liver disease. The acute nature of the disease means that the only occupational aetiology that usually could be countenanced is a history of accidental acute overexposure to a known hepatotoxin. The absence of such a history would, in the vast majority of cases, preclude an occupational aetiology.

The jaundiced patient likewise is more likely to have an acute viral hepatitis, biliary obstruction or have been taking drugs capable of causing drug induced liver injury, than to have liver disease of occupational aetiology. Nevertheless, there is no substitute for a good occupational history and if a suspicion exists, laboratory investigations may provide evidence of toxic exposure.

The patient presenting with cirrhosis is a similar example. The aetiology depends quite heavily on geographic location. In the Western world, alcohol, chronic hepatitis B or C or non-alcoholic fatty liver disease account for most of the cases. Other rarer causes include autoimmune liver disease, haemochromatosis and chronic intrahepatic biliary diseases including primary sclerosing cholangitis and primary biliary cirrhosis (recently renamed primary biliary cholangitis). In the Far East, hepatitis B and C would be a much more likely cause, although public health steps have been taken to offer widespread immunisation against hepatitis B. It would be the exclusion of alcohol, risk factors for non-alcoholic fatty liver disease and a negative hepatitis B and C screening that should spur the clinician to delve further into possible occupational exposures but the chances of finding a relevant workplace exposure are, thankfully, small these days. A sizeable minority of cirrhosis though remains cryptogenic.

Clinical Investigations

Detection of abnormal liver structure

Investigation of structural abnormalities of the liver by biopsy, special radiological ultrasound, have been used mainly in the clinical evaluation of patients with liver damage. Non-invasive assessments of liver fibrosis are also now used clinically such as serum biomarkers and transient elastography. These investigations are not warranted for regular health surveillance of occupational groups.

Liver function tests

Standard liver function tests include determination of serum levels of a range of liver enzymes that may be released from the liver and may be physiological during increased liver activity, from damaged hepatocytes or inflamed, damaged or obstructed bile ducts. This includes GGT, ALT and AST, (from hepatocytes) ALP, (from bile ducts) and lactate dehydrogenase (LDH), (many liver sources, mainly intracellular). In addition, serum bilirubin, albumin, and prothrombin time are also measured. Of all these parameters, the one most used for exposure to chemical agents is GGT, and this is usually in the context of detecting excessive alcohol consumption. This may be in an occupational or non-occupational setting. GGT has been attempted as a biological effect measure for exposure to organic solvents and other hepatotoxic chemicals. The main limitation in its use is its high sensitivity and low specificity as an indicator of liver injury. GGT levels are often raised in chronic liver injury of a non-alcohol cause. Of the other enzymes mentioned, raised LDH levels are not specific to liver cell injury. Raised serum levels may also occur from sources such as the heart, liver, muscle, kidney, lung and blood.

In a study of VCM-exposed workers, 13 of 271 workers had persistent liver function abnormalities (Ho *et al.*, 1991). These abnormalities include raised GGT alone, or with either raised AST or ALT, or had in addition raised ALP. Some workers showed an improvement in liver function within six months of removal from further VCM exposure. Follow-up of the patients showed no consistent pattern of liver function abnormalities. Another investigation into workers exposed to relatively low levels of VCM and ethylene dichloride showed raised ALT and AST levels, but not GGT (Cheng *et al.*, 1999). Hsieh and co-workers in Taiwan reported a possible synergistic effect between those with hepatitis B and C infection and occupational exposure to VCM and 1, 2-ethylene dichloride (Hsieh *et al.*, 2003). A possible synergistic effect for liver function abnormalities between hepatitis B infection and exposure to dimethylformamide was also reported (Luo *et al.*, 2001). The laboratory findings from the different studies point to the difficulty of using liver function tests for biological effect monitoring of individuals exposed to VCM.

D-glucaric acid excretion

The excretion of urinary D-glucaric acid has been proposed as an indicator for biological effect monitoring in operating theatre workers exposed to anaesthetic agents (Franco and Fonte, 1994). Absorption of anaesthetic gases can lead to induction of liver microsomal enzymes such as the mixed function oxidases. Halothane, nitrous oxide, and isoflurane are anaesthetic agents that can increase urinary D-glucaric acid.

Compensation for Liver Disease

Most countries have lists of agents that can cause occupational disease and for which State compensation is payable. In the United Kingdom, Hepatitis B is by far the most important infectious agent resulting in tens of cases per year. For the chemical hepatotoxins, there are only a handful of claims in any year.

Viral hepatitis is a prescribed occupational disease in the UK and benefits may be paid under the Industrial Injuries Compensation Scheme, where viral hepatitis occurs following occupational contact with human blood or blood products or a source of viral hepatitis in a prescribed occupation. The latter contacts could include patients suffering from Hepatitis B, or carriers of the disease.

Angiosarcoma of the liver, as well as acro-osteolysis of the terminal phalanges of the fingers and non-cirrhotic portal fibrosis are conditions which are listed in the UK prescribed diseases list (Department for Work and Pensions, 2009; Industrial Injuries Advisory Council, 1993). The relevant occupational activity for consideration of benefits under this scheme is work involving or work near the polymerisation of VCM.

Liver damage from exposure to CCl_4 or chloroform fumes or vapor is also listed as a prescribed disease in the U.K., compensable within a prescribed occupation.

Fitness for Return to Work

Employees with liver disease should be protected where possible from workplace exposure to hepatotoxins to a greater extent than other employees unless there is good clinical and laboratory evidence that their previous liver disease has resolved.

A specialist should optimise the care of patients with cirrhosis and decompensated liver disease before work is resumed. In patients with oesophageal varices, there is no restriction on occupation once the varices have been treated. Patients with ascites may experience difficulties with lifting, bending, or stooping. The complications arising from alcoholism, especially ascites, hepatic impairment, and depression, will require individual assessment, to determine whether the patient is disabled. Patients with chronic or intermittent encephalopathy should not be employed in intellectually demanding work or jobs requiring a high degree of vigilance, including safety, critical work or operating machinery. Individuals suffering from hepatic cirrhosis with chronic encephalopathy or those who are cognitively impaired must not drive (Madan and Hellier, 2019).

For specific hepatic infections such as Hepatitis B an elevated viral load of $>10^3$ IU/ml represent a risk of person-to-person transmission. This is relevant for health care workers involved in exposure prone procedures.

Managing Workers with Intestinal Stomas

Patients with ileostomies and colostomies may be seen by occupational physicians for advice on fitness for work. The advice given is often varied, and concerns may revolve around suitability for jobs requiring food handling, problems with manual handling, working in hot environments and perceived increased sickness absence.

According to the American Society of Colon and Rectal Surgeons, once a person has recovered from surgery, the ostomy should not limit the return to work. Return to work depends on the individual's recovery, ease of pouch management and how physical the job is due to the increased risk of hernia. When returning to work after stoma surgery, workers are likely to be apprehensive about possible leaks and how the routine of work may affect them. Before starting back to work they may wish to consider a trial run as the preparation for work and leaving the house may take them longer than they expected. They may need to think about work clothing or work uniform and if it allows them to empty their stoma bag easily. They will need to consider the changing facilities and location of the toilet facilities at work and they may need to purchase a small portable changing bag that they can take discreetly to the toilets (Madan and Hellier, 2019).

With good personal hygiene and proper systems of work, there is no increased risk of spread of infection from or to a stoma patient from work activity. Lifting heavy objects or excessive bending may damage the stoma and some patients working in hot environments may experience some difficulty. In hot climates, as in the tropics and in the desert climate of the Middle East, adequate occupational advice should include instructions on rehydration (Wyke *et al.*, 1989). The key to living an active life is embracing a "new normal," and that daily norm means return to work.

A patient is ready to return to work when he/she is:

1. Able to empty the pouch without assistance.
2. Able to change the pouch without too much difficulty.
3. Able to commute to work comfortably.
4. Able to handle leaks or replacement of pouch.
5. Physically and mentally able to work.

Exposures Affecting Other Parts of the Gastrointestinal Tract

Oesophagitis, Peptic Ulcer and Gastritis

Ingestion of corrosive chemicals causes severe oesophageal and gastric damage. The extent of damage depends in part on the specific chemical involved, the pH of the solutions ingested, the amount ingested, and the presence of food in the upper GI tract. Severe gastric damage from chemicals is more likely to result from intentional ingestion as in suicide attempts, rather than inadvertent occupational exposures.

Ingestion of small quantities of workplace chemicals can follow poor hygiene practices at work, such as eating or drinking at worksites where chemicals are handled, or consuming food and drinks without adequate cleaning of the hands after contact with chemicals.

Hexavalent chromium Cr(VI), is widely used in numerous industrial processes; including chrome pigment production, chrome plating, stainless steel manufacturing, and leather tanning (Langard and Costa, 2014). The carcinogenic potential of oral exposure to Cr(VI) in human is supported by a number of new studies. However, due to extracellular reduction of Cr(VI) to Cr(III) in the GI system, oral exposure results in a lower amount of Cr(VI) that gets into target cells compared to inhalation exposure (Sun *et al.*, 2015). According to the US EPA, mutagenic carcinogens have no threshold.

Carbon disulphide used in the viscose rayon industry has been described as causing GI and metabolic disturbances in addition to the neurotoxic and cardio toxic effects. A mortality cohort study was carried out on 2,291 workers with chronic occupational CS_2 poisoning diagnosed during the years 1970–1990. The general population of Poland was the reference population. With respect to neoplastic diseases, the analysis in male subjects showed a statistically significant excess of deaths from colon cancer (standard mortality ratio = 233; nine cases). All these cases were noted in workers of the two oldest rayon plants. A detailed future analysis is required to derive further conclusions (Peplonska *et al.*, 1996).

A nationwide population-based cohort study was conducted among healthcare workers (HCW) in Taiwan to evaluate the risk for peptic ulcer disease (PUD) in physicians, nurses, pharmacists, and other HCWs. The study found nurses and other HCWs had a significantly higher risk than the general population. Physicians and nurses had a higher PUD risk than other HCWs. Physicians specialised in internal medicine, surgery, Ob/Gyn, and family medicine had higher risks than did those in other specialties; however, emergency physicians had a lower risk. The possible explanations for the increased risk for PUD may be working hours, job stress, shift work, and coping skills. Additional study is needed to clarify the mechanism (Lin *et al.*, 2015).

Policemen and firefighters experience high work-related stress and burnout. A number of studies reported the correlation between job characteristics and the risk of PUD across various industries (Huerta-Franco *et al.*, 2013; Pietroiusti *et al.*, 2006).

The interaction effects of burnout and job support on PUD among firefighters and policemen indicated in another study in Taiwan the overall prevalence rates of PUD by self-report and diagnosis by physicians were 8.3% and 6.5% for policemen and 7.1% and 5.5% for firefighters, respectively. The interaction effect between burnout and job support was correlated with the prevalence of PUD (Lin *et al.*, 2019).

Shift workers have an increased incidence of digestive disorders and peptic ulcers. However, the specific contributions of diet, smoking, alcohol intake, stress and irregular mealtimes to the condition in these workers have not been determined (Waterhouse *et al.*, 1992). In a study conducted by Saberi *et al.*, the prevalence of GI symptoms in shift working nurses was 81.9% and in day working nurses was 52.2% (Saberi and Moravveji, 2010). In Yoo *et al.*'s study in Korea, the prevalence of GI symptoms was 40.1% among female shift-working textile workers (Yoo, 1994).

Pancreatitis and Pancreatic Cancer

Pancreatitis is known to be associated with gallstones, heavy alcohol consumption, and some medications (Forsmark *et al.*, 2016). Effects on the pancreas from occupational exposures are rare. Organophosphates are commonly used as insecticides in agriculture and are potent toxicants. Patients with organophosphorus poisoning may present with subclinical features of acute pancreatitis (Goud *et al.*, 2012).

Pancreatic cancer has a high case-fatality rate. Based on a comprehensive meta-analysis of studies published between 1969 and May 1998 and more recent studies published between 1998 and 2010, a review in 2012 concluded that the strongest and most consistent findings linking occupational exposures with pancreatic cancer risk to date are for chlorinated hydrocarbons and PAHs. Some of the specific chlorinated hydrocarbon compounds linked to pancreatic cancer are trichloroethylene, PCB, methylene chloride, vinyl chloride, and tetrachloroethylene; and the most commonly reported industries associated with chlorinated hydrocarbons are dry cleaning and metal-related work (Andreotti and Silverman, 2012). Another study conducted in Spain on specific occupational exposures and risk of exocrine pancreatic cancer (EPC) was conducted. A higher risk of EPC was associated with having worked as "miners, shot firers, stone cutters and carvers," "machinery mechanics and fitters," "building trades workers" and "motor vehicle drivers" in men, "office clerks" in women, and "waiters" in both sexes. The study revealed that occupational exposure to chlorinated hydrocarbon solvents were associated with exocrine pancreatic cancer (Santibañez *et al.*, 2010).

Peritoneal Mesothelioma and Cancer of the Colon

Mesothelioma affects mostly older individuals who have been occupationally exposed to asbestos. The global mesothelioma incidence and mortality rates are unknown, because data are not available from developing countries that continue to use large amounts of asbestos. The incidence rate of mesothelioma has decreased in Australia, the United States, and Western Europe, where the use of asbestos was banned or strictly regulated in the 1970s and 1980s, demonstrating the value of these preventive measures. However, in these same countries, the overall number of deaths from mesothelioma has not decreased as the size of the population and the percentage of old people have increased (Carbone *et al.*, 2019). The accumulating evidence implicate that all forms of asbestos exposure appear to minimally increase the risk of stomach cancer as well as possibly other GI cancers involving the larynx, oesophagus, intestines and colorectal regions. As compared to the pulmonary effects, however, these effects appear much less robust and not all studies demonstrate a positive association suggesting that the risk is small (Kim *et al.*, 2013).

Case Study 6: Asbestos Exposure and Malignant Peritoneal Mesothelioma

A case of malignant peritoneal mesothelioma was reported in a 53-year-old former construction worker with prior asbestos exposure. The clinical presentation was a 3-month history of dyspeptic complaints. As initial workup, abdominal ultrasound and upper gastrointestinal endoscopy were performed. Chronic gastritis due to Helicobacter pylori was detected, which was promptly treated but without symptom relief. Abdominal ultrasound showed small volume ascites with hyperechogenic foci, which was later confirmed on computed tomography scan showing the presence of peritoneal nodules in the greater omentum and mesentery. A thorough investigation was conducted based on the suspicion of peritoneal carcinomatosis. A non-peritoneal primary tumour was not found. Ascitic cytology and immunocytochemical studies were suggestive of mesothelioma (de Sousa et al., 2020).

A 2016 World Health Organisation report described an average 40-year latency period for asbestosis, lung cancer and mesothelioma in Polish workers (Świątkowska *et al.*, 2016). The dose-response for peritoneal mesothelioma from asbestos has not been established, and thus to be precautionary, all exposures to asbestos at any dose must be considered potentially causative. It is of interest that investigators detected asbestos-associated cases of mesothelioma in women from nonoccupational sources — that is, bystander, incidental, or take-home exposures (Lemen, 2016). Control of exposure to asbestos, in particular at the workplace, remains the main approach for the prevention of peritoneal mesothelioma.

Other Gastrointestinal Effects

Gastroenteritis is common in laboratory technicians working in research and hospital laboratories, particularly those handling and processing microorganisms regularly. Sewer workers have a higher prevalence of GI disorders.

Case Study 7: Typhoid Fever in a Food Handler

For the first time in 16 years, a food-borne outbreak of typhoid fever due to Salmonella enterica serotype Typhi was reported in Japan. Seven people without travel history to an endemic region were diagnosed with typhoid fever between September and October 2014. Each patient diagnosed with typhoid and/or paratyphoid fever reported to a local health centre for government surveillance, where each patient was interviewed for history of travel and meal. All seven patients had consumed food in an Indian buffet, including curry with rice, tandoori chicken, and fresh vegetables, at a restaurant in the centre of Tokyo. None of the seven patients had a travel history to an endemic country, except patient 1, who had travelled to Nepal six months earlier but demonstrated no symptoms of typhoid fever on return. The index patient moved from Nepal to Japan in January 2013 and had frequent travel history to Nepal, the last time of which was in February 2014 (Kobayashi et al., 2016).

Typhoid fever which is also known as enteric fever is an acute febrile illness that is caused by the bacteria Salmonella enterica serovar typhi. Salmonella typhi is a Gram-negative bacterium that infects the intestinal tract of man and can enter blood circulation too (Gbodo and Anumudu, 2019). Annually about 200 cases of typhoid fever are seen in the UK mostly in people after visiting relatives or friends in developing countries with the peak incidence being in the autumn months. Watery diarrhoea occurs 12–72 hours after infection, accompanied by abdominal pain, vomiting, and fever. The illness lasts a few days and is usually self-limiting (Madan and Hellier, 2019).

Return to work for patients who recovered from typhoid should be after three consecutive negative stool cultures (and urine in patients with schistosomiasis) at least 24 h apart and at least 48 h after completion of antimicrobials. Household members of people with a Typhoid Fever diagnosis must also have three consecutive negative stool cultures, as above, before a food handler is allowed to return to food handling duties. Hand hygiene education must occur before return to work. Good hand hygiene must be practiced at all times (Iowa Department of Public Health, 2015). The recognition of the critical and synergistic role of water and sanitation improvements in concert with vaccine introduction emphasise the importance of improving our understanding of the sources, patterns, and modes of transmission of Salmonella Typhi in diverse settings (Crump, 2019). Some local authorities require a food handler declaration of health to be completed by all food handlers on return to work following absence due to ill health or overseas travel. Typhoid vaccination is made mandatory for all food handlers in some developing countries. A public health order may be taken out against a case who refuses to comply where public health laws are in place. Silent or healthy carriers of Typhoid fever is another challenging task for physicians. Historical data of Mary Mallon, a cook and a healthy carrier of Salmonella typhi with her nickname of "Typhoid Mary" had become synonymous with the spread of the disease. By the time she died, New York health officials had identified more than 400 other healthy carriers of Salmonella typhi. Mary Mallon is always a reference when mentioning the compliance of the laws concerning public health issues (Marineli *et al.*, 2013).

Working with Hepatobiliary and Gastrointestinal Disorders

As has been described above, few disorders of the GI system are caused or exacerbated by the work environment and the liver is only involved when undertaking its usual function of detoxification and does not distinguish between occupational or environmental agents. Similarly, with infective agents, which may be work acquired and perhaps more importantly blood borne where the health care environment could well be the source of contamination. Perhaps more commonly, hepatobiliary and liver disorders may limit the capacity of an individual to undertake the duties of their job and the symptoms and treatment of some disorders such as inflammatory bowel disease may lead to the employee requiring long periods of absence from work, especially when recovering from surgery.

Conditions likely to cause employment problems or risks to individuals and the public include the following (Madan and Hellier, 2019):

- Inflammatory bowel disease;
- Ulcerative colitis;
- Crohn's disease;
- Ileostomy and ileo-anal pouch;
- Irritable bowel disease;
- Gastroenteritis and GI infections;
- Viral hepatitis A;
- Cirrhosis of the liver;
- Obesity.

Detailed discussion of the adjustments and modifications required for each of these conditions is outside the scope of this chapter but the reader is referred to the above reference in the 6th edition of "Fitness for Work — the medical aspects" published by Oxford University Press. A final case history though may emphasise the important role of the occupational physician.

Conclusion

There are a wide variety of aetiological agents encountered in the course of work activities that can cause damage to the liver and GI tract. A detailed occupational history in chronological order from the first job of the patient to the current work with documentation of exposure, an understanding of the nature and properties of chemical and physical agents, and consideration of the differential diagnoses will aid the clinician in reaching the correct diagnosis. The appropriate treatment can then be provided and relevant preventive measures taken. Often, the identification and removal of the offending workplace exposure is important to inhibit progression of occupational diseases. Hepatobiliary and liver disorders are not uncommonly encountered at the workplace where the cause cannot be assigned to the nature of the job or the exposures encountered at the workplace. Some may well be self-limiting, but others may have a long latent period. The skills of an occupational physician are essential for diagnosis of work-related liver diseases, to ensure job modifications and adjustments for the comfort of the employee and sustain job continuity.

References

ACGIH. (2016) *TVI/BEI Guidelines.* [Online] Available from: https://www.acgih.org/science/tlv-bei-guidelines. [Accessed on 18 April 2021].

Andrade RJ, Aithal GP, Björnsson ES, Kaplowitz N, Kullak-Ublick GA, Larrey D, Karlsen TH. (2019) European Association for the Study of the Liver. EASL clinical practice guidelines: Drug-induced liver injury. *J Hepatol* **70**: 1222–61.

Andreotti G, Silverman DT. (2012) Occupational risk factors and pancreatic cancer: A review of recent findings. *Mol Carcinog* **51**: 98–108. Available from: doi:10.1002/mc.20779.

Australian Department of Health. (2020) *How much alcohol is safe to drink?* [Online] Available from: https:// www.health.gov.au/using-our-web-sites/about-our-website. [Accessed on 18 April 2020].

Carbone M, Adusumilli PS, Alexander Jr, HR, Baas P, Bardelli F, Bononi A, Bueno R, Felley-Bosco E, Galateau-Salle F, Jablons D, Mansfield AS. (2019) Mesothelioma: Scientific clues for prevention, diagnosis, and therapy. *CA-Cancer J Clin* **69**: 402–29.

Chaudhary P, Bhadana U, Singh RAK, Ahuja A. (2015) Primary hepatic angiosarcoma. *Eur J Surg Oncol* **41**: 1137–43. Available from: https://doi.org/10.1016/j.ejso.2015.04.022.

Cheng TJ, Huang ML, You NC, Du CL, Chau TT. (1999) Abnormal liver function in workers exposed to low levels of ethylene dichloride and vinyl chloride monomer. *J Occup Environ Med* **41**(12): 1128–1133.

Colombo M. (2020) EASL clinical practice guidelines for the management of occupational liver diseases. *Liver Int* **40**: 136–41.

Colombo M, La Vecchia C, Lotti M, Lucena MI, Stove C, Paradis V. (2019) European Association for the Study of the Liver. EASL Clinical Practice Guideline: Occupational liver diseases. *J Hepatol* **71**: 1022–1037.

Crump JA. (2019) Progress in typhoid fever epidemiology. *Clin Infect Dis* **68**: S4–9.

Dara L, Liu ZX, Kaplowitz N. (2016) Mechanisms of adaptation and progression in idiosyncratic drug induced liver injury, clinical implications. *Liver Int* **36**: 158–165.

Delahaye L, Janssens B, Stove C. (2017) Alternative sampling strategies for the assessment of biomarkers of exposure. *Curr Opin Toxicol* **4**: 43–51.

Department for Work and Pensions. (2009) *DB1 — A guide to Industrial injuries disablement benefits.* [Online] Available from: https://www.gov.uk/government/publications/industrial-injuries-disablement-benefits-technical-guidance/industrial-injuries-disablement-benefits-technical-guidance.

De Smedt T, De Cremer K, Vleminckx C, Fierens S, Mertens B, Van Overmeire I, Bader M, De Paepe P, Göen T, Nemery B, Schettgen T. (2014) Acrylonitrile exposure in the general population following a major train accident in Belgium: A human biomonitoring study. *Toxicol Lett* **231**: 344–351.

De Sousa SM, Pereira F, Duarte M, Marques M, Vázquez D, Marques C. (2020) Malignant peritoneal mesothelioma as a rare cause of dyspeptic complaints and ascites: A diagnostic challenge. *GE — Portuguese J Gastroenterol* **27**: 197–202.

Eslam M, Newsome PN, Anstee QM, Targher G, Gomez MR, Zelber-Sagi S, Wong VW, Dufour JF, Schattenberg J, Arrese M, Valenti L. (2020) A new definition for metabolic associated fatty liver disease: An international expert consensus statement. *J Hepatol* **73**: 202–209.

Franco G, Fonte R. (1994) Advances in evaluating liver response to operating theatre work: Urinary D-glucaric acid as an index of effect. *Occup Med* **44**: 12–16.

Forsmark CE, Vege SS, Wilcox CM. (201) Acute Pancreatitis. *N Engl J Med* **375**: 1972–1981.

Gbodo EE, Anumudu CK. (2019) Prevalence of *Salmonella typhi* infection among food handlers in ImoState University Owerri Nigeria and its Environs. *Int J Trop Dis* 7: 315. Available from: doi: 10.4172/2329-891X.1000315.

Goud M, Nayal B, Deepa K, Devi OS, Devaki RN, Anitha M. (2012) A case of acute pancreatitis with occupational exposure to organophosphorus compound. *Int J Toxicol* **19**: 223.

Ho SF, Phoon WH, Gan SL, Chan YK. (1991) Persistent liver dysfunction among workers at a vinyl chloride monomer polymerization plant. *J Soc Occup Med* **41**: 10–16.

Hsieh HI, Wang JD, Chen PC, Cheng TJ. (2003) Synergistic effect of hepatitis virus infection and occupational exposures to vinyl chloride monomer and ethylene dichloride on serum amino transaminase activity. *Occup Environ Med* **60**: 774–778.

Huerta-Franco MR, Vargas-Luna M, Tienda P, Delgadillo-Holtfort I, Balleza-Ordaz M, Flores-Hernandez C. (2013) Effects of occupational stress on the gastrointestinal tract. *World J Gastrointest Pathophysiol* **4**:108–118. Available from: doi: 10.4291/wjgp.v4.i4.108.

Iowa Department of Public Health. (2015) *Typhoid Fever. Guide to Surveillance, Investigation, and Reporting.* [Online] Available from: https://wiki.idph.iowa.gov/Portals/3/userfiles/5/Files/Typhoid%20Fever%20Chapter.pdf. [Accessed on 18 April 2021].

IARC Working Group on the Evaluation of Carcinogenic Risks to Humans. (2012) *Chemical Agents and Related Occupations. IARC Monographs on the Evaluation of Carcinogenic Risks to Humans.* Lyon, France, International Agency for Research on Cancer.

Industrial Injuries Advisory Council. (1993) *Periodic Report 1993. A Review of Recent Activity of the Industrial Injuries Advisory Council Concerning Work Related Ill Health*. London, The Stationery Office Books.

Jang BO, Choi GH, Jang HY, Ahn S, Choi JK, Kim S, Lee K, Jang ES, Kim JW, Jeong SH. (2020) A case of autoimmune hepatitis after occupational exposure to n, n-dimethylformamide. *J Korean Med Sci* **35**: e288. Available from: https://doi.org/10.3346/jkms.2020.35.e228.

Jothimani D, Venugopal R, Abedin MF, Kaliamoorthy I, Rela M. (2020) COVID-19 and Liver. *J Hepatol* **73**: 1231–1240.

Kang YJ, Ahn J, Hwang YI. (2014) Acute liver injury in two workers exposed to chloroform in cleanrooms: A case report. *Ann Occup Environ Med* **26**: 49. Available from: doi.org/10.1186/s40557-014-0049-5.

Kim TH, Kim SG. (2011) Clinical outcomes of occupational exposure to n, n-dimethylformamide: Perspectives from experimental toxicology. *Saf Health Work* **2**: 97–104.

Kim SJ, Williams D, Cheresh P, Kamp DW. (2013) Asbestos-induced gastrointestinal cancer: An update. *J Gastrointest Dig Syst* **3**: 135. Available from: doi: 10.4172/2161-069X.1000135.

Klaunig JE, Li X, Wang Z. (2018) Role of xenobiotics in the induction and progression of fatty liver disease. *Toxicol Res* **7**: 664–680.

Kobayashi T, Kutsuna S, Hayakawa K, Kato Y, Ohmagari N, Uryu H, Yamada R, Kashiwa N, Nei T, Ehara A, Takei R. (2016) An outbreak of food-borne typhoid fever due to *Salmonella enterica* serotype *typhi* in japan reported for the first time in 16 years. *Am J Trop Med Hygiene* **94**: 289–291.

Kumar A, Sharma B, Samant H. (2020) Liver Angiosarcoma. In: *StatPearls*. Treasure Island, Florida, StatPearls Publishing.

Lang AL, Beier JI. (2018) Interaction of volatile organic compounds and underlying liver disease: A new paradigm for risk. *Biol Chem* **399**: 1237–48. Available from: doi: 10.1515/hsz-2017-0324.

Langard S, Costa M. (2014) Chromium. In: Nordberg, G.F., Fowler, B.A, Nordberg, M. (eds.), *Handbook on the Toxicology of Metals*. Cambridge, Massachusetts, United States, Academic Press.

Lee H, Kim SS, You KS, Park W, Yang JH, Kim M, Hayman LL. (2014) Asian flushing: Genetic and sociocultural factors of alcoholism among east asians. *Gastroenterol Nurs* **37**: 327–336.

Lei Y, Xiao S, Chen S, Zhang H, Li H, Lu Y. (2017) N, N-dimethylformamide-induced acute hepatic failure: A case report and literature review. *Exp Ther Med* **14**: 5659–5663.

Lemen RA. (2016) Mesothelioma from asbestos exposures: Epidemiologic patterns and impact in the United States. *J Toxicol Environ Health* **19**: 250–265.

Lin PY, Wang JY, Shih DP, Kuo HW, Liang WM. (2019) The interaction effects of burnout and job support on peptic ulcer disease (PUD) among Firefighters and Policemen. *Int J Environ Res Public Health* **16**: 2369.

Lin HY, Weng SF, Lin HJ, Hsu CC, Wang JJ, Su SB, Guo HR, Huang CC. (2015) Peptic ulcer disease in healthcare workers: A nationwide population-based cohort study. *PLOS One* **10**: e0135456.

Lundqvist G, Flodin U, Axelson O. (1999) A case-control study of fatty liver disease and organic solvent exposure. *Am J Ind Med* **35**: 132–136.

Luo JC, Kuo HW, Cheng TJ, Chang MJ. (2001) Abnormal liver function associated with occupational exposure to dimethylformamide and hepatitis B virus. *J Occup Environ Med* **43**: 474–482.

Luster MI, Simeonova PP, Gallucci RM, Matheson JM, Yucesoy B. (2000) Immunotoxicology: Role of inflammation in chemical-induced hepatotoxicity. *Int J Immunopharmacol* **22**(12): 1143–1147.

Luster MI, Simeonova PP, Gallucci RM, Bruccoleri A, Blazka ME, Yucesoy B. (2001) Role of inflammation in chemical-induced hepatotoxicity. *Toxicol Lett* **120**(1–3): 317–321.

Madan I, Hellier S. (2019) Gastrointestinal and liver disorders. In: Hobson, J, Smedley, J. (eds.), *Fitness for Work: The Medical Aspects (*6th Ed). Oxford University Press, USA.

Malaguarnera G, Cataudella E, Giordano M, Nunnari G, Chisari G, Malaguarnera M. (2012) Toxic hepatitis in occupational exposure to solvents. *World J Gastroenterol* **18**: 2756–2766.

Marletta S, Cavallo E, Ammendola S, Stefanizzi L, Mastrosimini MG, D'Onofrio M, Brunelli M, Caliò A, Pecori S, Dalbeni A, Ruzzenente A. (2020) Multifocal hepatic angiosarcoma with atypical presentation: Case report and literature review. *J Gastrointest Cancer* 7: 1–5. Available from: https://doi.org/10.1007/s12029-020-00504-x.

Marineli F, Tsoucalas G, Karamanou M, Androutsos G. (2013) Mary Mallon (1869–1938) and the history of typhoid fever. *Ann Gastroenterol* **26**(2): 132–134.

Matsumura Y, Stiles KM, Reid J, Frenk EZ, Cronin S, Pagovich OE, Crystal RG. (2019) Gene therapy correction of aldehyde dehydrogenase 2 deficiency. *Mol Ther Methods Clin Dev* **15**: 72–82.

McGill MR, Woolbright BL, Weemhoff JL, Jaeschke H. (2017) Mechanistic biomarkers in liver diseases. In: Patel, V.B, Preedy, V.R. (eds.), *Biomarkers in Liver Disease*. Dordrecht, Netherlands, Springer.

Moorman AC, de Perio MA, Goldschmidt R, Chu C, Kuhar D, Henderson DK, Naggie S, Kamili S, Spradling PR, Gordon SC, Russi MB, Teshale EH. (2020) Testing and clinical management of health care personnel potentially exposed to Hepatitis C virus — CDC Guidance, United States, 2020. *MMWR Recomm Rep* **69**(No. RR-6): 1–8. Available from: doi: http://dx.doi.org/10.15585/mmwr.rr6906a1.

Neugut AI, Wylie P, Brandt-Rauf PW. (1986) Occupational cancers of the gastrointestinal tract, Part II: Pancreas, liver, and biliary tract. In: *Occupational Cancer and Carcinogenesis — State of the Art Reviews,* 2, pp. 137–154.

Pawlotsky JM, Negro F, Aghemo A, Berenguer M, Dalgard O, Dusheiko G, Marra F, Puoti M, Wedemeyer H, European Association for the study of the liver. (2020) EASL recommendations on treatment of hepatitis C: Final update of the series. *J Hepatol* **73**: 1170–1218.

Pepłońska BE, Szeszenia-Dąbrowska NE, Sobala WO, Wilczyńska UR. (1996) A mortality study of workers with reported chronic occupational carbon disulfide poisoning. *Int J Occup Environ Health* **4**: 291–299.

Pietroiusti A, Forlini A, Magrini A, Galante A, Coppeta L, Gemma G, Romeo E, Bergamaschi A. (2006) Shift work increases the frequency of duodenal ulcer in H pylori infected workers. *Occup Environ Med* **63**: 773–775.

Pinter M, Trauner M, Peck-Radosavljevic M, Sieghart W. (2016) Cancer and liver cirrhosis: Implications on prognosis and management. *ESMO Open* **1**: e000042. Available from: doi:10.1136/esmoopen-2016-000042.

Ramachandran A, Jaeschke H. (2018) Acetaminophen toxicity: Novel insights into mechanisms and future perspectives. *Gene Expression. J Liver Res* **18**: 19–30. Available from: https://doi.org/10.3727/105221617X15084371374138.

Rosenberg G, Bauld L, Hooper L, Buykx P, Holmes J, Vohra J. (2018) New national alcohol guidelines in the UK: Public awareness, understanding and behavioural intentions. *J Public Health* **40**: 549–56. Available from: https://doi.org/10.1093/pubmed/fdx126.

Sabbioni G, Turesky RJ. (2017) Biomonitoring human albumin adducts: The past, the present, and the future. *Chem Res Toxicol* **30**: 332–366.

Saberi HR, Moravveji AR. (2010) Gastrointestinal complaints in shift-working and day-working nurses in Iran. *J Circadian Rhythms* **8**: 9.

Santibañez M, Vioque J, Alguacil J, De La Hera MG, Moreno-Osset E, Carrato A, Porta M, Kauppinen T. (2010) Occupational exposures and risk of pancreatic cancer. *Eur J Epidemiol* **25**: 721–730.

Shin EC, Jeong SH. (2018) Natural history, clinical manifestations, and pathogenesis of hepatitis A. *Cold Spring Harb Perspect Med* **8**: a031708. Available from: doi: 10.1101/cshperspect.a031708.

Stickel F, Moreno C, Hampe J, Morgan MY. (2017) The genetics of alcohol dependence and alcohol-related liver disease. *J Hepatol* **66**: 195–211.

Sun H, Brocato J, Costa M. (2015) Oral chromium exposure and toxicity. *Curr Environ Health Rep* **2**: 295–303. Available from: https://link.springer.com/article/10.1007/s40572-015-0054-z.

Świątkowska B, Szeszenia-Dąbrowska N, Wilczyńska U. (2016) Medical monitoring of asbestos-exposed workers: Experience from Poland. *Bull World Health Organ* **94**: 599.

Thier R, Lewalter J, Selinski S, Bolt HM. (2001) Re-evaluation of the effect of smoking on the methylation of N-terminal valine in haemoglobin. *Arch Toxicol* **75**: 270–273.

Torre LA, Bray F, Siegel RL, Ferlay J, Lortet□Tieulent J, Jemal A. (2015) Global cancer statistics, 2012. *CA Cancer J Clin* **65**: 87–108.

Uccello M, Malaguarnera G, Corriere T, Biondi A, Basile F, Malaguarnera M. (2012) Risk of hepatocellular carcinoma in workers exposed to chemicals. *Hepat Mon* **12**: e5943. Available from: doi: 10.5812/hepatmon.5943.

Wahlang B, Jin J, Beier JI, Hardesty JE, Daly EF, Schnegelberger RD, Falkner KC, Prough RA, Kirpich IA, Cave MC. (2019) Mechanisms of environmental contributions to fatty liver disease. *Curr Environ Health Rep* **6**: 80–94.

Wang S, Toy M, Hang Pham TT, So S. (2020) Causes and trends in liver disease and hepatocellular carcinoma among men and women who received liver transplants in the US, 2010–2019. *PloS one* **18**: e0239393.

Waterhouse JM, Folkard S, Minors DS. (1992) *Shift Work, Health, and Safety. An Overview of the Scientific Literature 1987–90. HSE Research Report 31/1992.* HMSO.

Wyke RJ, Aw TC, Allan RN, Harrington JM. (1989) Employment prospects for patients with intestinal stomas: The attitude of occupational physicians. *J Soc Occ Med* **39**: 19–24.

Yoo KH. (1994) Sleeping patterns and gastrointestinal disorders according to the shift works in female textile workers. *J Prevent Med Public Health* **27**: 74–83.

Younossi Z, Anstee QM, Marietti M, Hardy T, Henry L, Eslam M, George J, Bugianesi E. (2018) Global burden of NAFLD and NASH: Trends, predictions, risk factors and prevention. *Nat Rev Gastroenterol Hepatol* **15**: 11.

Zhang L. (2020) Hepatitis A Vaccination. *Hum Vaccin Immunother* **16**: 1565–1573. Available from: doi: 10.1080/21645515.2020.1769389.

Chapter 14

Eye Injuries and Other Disorders

Livia Teo[*,†], *Tien Yin Wong*[*,†] *and Laurence Shen Lim*[*,†]

Case Study 1: Intraocular Foreign Body

A 21 year old construction worker was struck in the right eye by a large piece of metal while he was hammering. He felt a sudden drop in his vision and quickly presented to the accident and emergency department. On examination, his visual acuity was 6/60 in his right eye, and 6/6 in his left. There was gross hyphema in the anterior chamber of his left eye. The intraocular pressure was raised to 25 mmHg. X-ray of the right orbit showed no orbital fracture or intraocular foreign body. He was admitted for observation and management. When the hyphema had partially cleared, examination of his retina showed multiple areas of retinal haemorrhage and edema (commotio retinae) (Fig. 9). His visual acuity improved to 6/18 at discharge. On questioning, he admitted being non-compliant with use of eye protective device at the worksite.

Case Study 2: Penetrating Eye Injury

A 33 year old electrician was connecting wires in the ceiling when the end of a wire poked his left eye. Although he felt no pain or visual loss,

*Duke-NUS Medical School, Singapore.
†Singapore National Eye Centre, Singapore.
Corresponding author: Laurence Lim Shen (laurence.lim.s@snec.com.sg).

he consulted a family doctor after work, and was referred to the accident and emergency department. On examination, his visual acuity was 6/6 in both eyes. There was a vertical 2 mm U-shaped partial thickness corneal laceration in his left eye (Figs. 1 and 2). The rest of the eye examination was unremarkable and X-ray of the left orbit revealed no intraocular foreign body. He was started on prophylactic topical antibiotic eye drops and followed up at the outpatient clinic. At three-month follow-up, his visual acuity remained 6/6 and a corneal scar was seen at the site of the laceration.

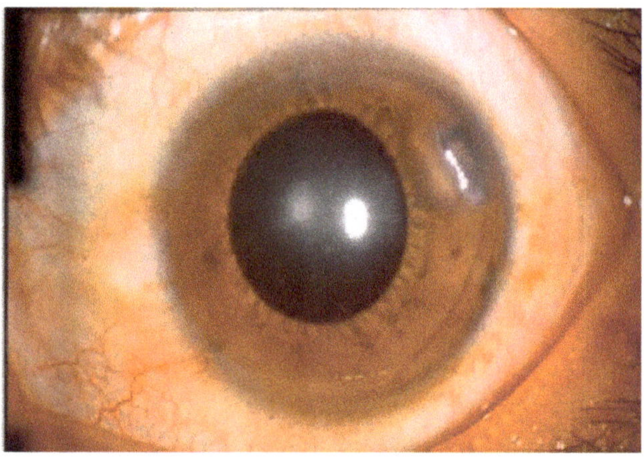

Fig. 1. Partial thickness U-shaped corneal laceration.

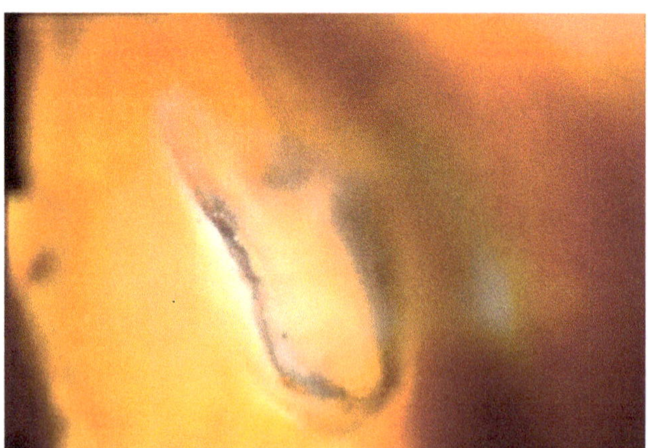

Fig. 2. Partial thickness U-shaped corneal laceration.

Introduction

Occupational eye injuries and other disorders are important for three reasons. First, they cause disproportionately more morbidity than similar injuries elsewhere. A small foreign body lodged in the cornea can inflict significant discomfort and potentially lead to sight-threatening complications (e.g. corneal infection). Second, they occur in the adult working population and therefore carry significant socioeconomic implications, including time off work, loss of income and long-term disability in cases of blindness. Third, work practice legislation and environmental modification offer potential for primary prevention, which is no possible in other settings (e.g. injuries at home).

In this chapter, we will first discuss occupational eye injuries, the most common and important work-related eye problem seen in clinical practice and then briefly deal with less common non-traumatic work-related ocular disorders.

Occupational Eye Injury

Epidemiology

Work-related eye injuries are significant causes of ocular morbidity. In the United States, these injuries are major components of the approximately 2.5 million ocular injuries that are estimated to occur each year (National Society to Prevent Blindness, 1980). Various case series and eye registry data in the US have indicated that between 14% and –48% of all ocular trauma are work-related (Dannenberg *et al.*, 1992; White *et al.*, 1989; Schein *et al.*, 1988; Morris *et al.*, 1987; Baker *et al.*, 1996). In Australia, a study estimated that 42% of ocular injuries were work-related (Fong and Taouk, 1995) while in the United Kingdom, another study puts the proportion of occupationally related eye injury at 70% (MacEwen, 1989). A prospective case series from a hospital in New South Wales, Australia, estimated that the incidence of eye trauma was 334.4 per 100,000 thousand person-years, of which 45.8% was work related (Northey *et al.*, 2014). The wide variations in estimates result partly from a lack of well-defined populations at risk in all these studies and inability therefore to calculate incidence rates, which is a better indication of risk of injury.

Data on the incidence rates of eye injury in the workplace are limited (Wong and Tielsch, 2009; Tielsch, 1995). The 2002 National Health Interview Survey (NHIS) revealed that the overall lifetime prevalence rate of work-related eye injuries was 4.4% amongst 28,913 working adults aged 18 years of older (Forrest and Cali, 2009). One source of data are from hospitalisation records, which typically captures severe injuries requiring hospital admissions. A retrospective chart review of 812 consecutive patients with open globe injuries treated at the Massachusetts Eye and Ear Infirmary between 1999 and 2008 found that 18% were attributable to workplace injuries (Kanoff *et al.*, 2010). A study based on hospital discharge data estimated an annual incidence of 1.7 and 3.0 ocular injuries per 100,000 employed persons when ocular trauma was the principal reason and secondary reason for hospital admission, respectively (Baker *et al.*, 1996). Less severe injuries not requiring hospitalisation are not captured in that study. However, from a public health perspective, perhaps less severe injuries are even more important, as they are more prevalent, can potentially lead to blinding complications (e.g. trauma-related corneal ulcers) and incur both cost of medical care (direct costs) and time lost from work (indirect costs). Of equal significance is the fact that minor eye injuries are often preventable by the use of simple protective eyewear or by modifying worksite environments. The National Institute for Occupational Safety and Health estimated that more than 80% of work-related eye injuries could be classified as minor (Centers for Disease Control, 1984). Studies that include severe injuries exclusively are therefore only partially representative of the size and impact of the problem.

Incidence rates regarding less severe work-related injuries are less readily available. One study based on persons treated at the emergency departments in Dane County, Wisconsin estimated an incidence of 55 work-related eye injuries per 100,000 persons, 20–30 times higher than the severe injuries requiring hospital admission reported in Baker's study (Karlson and Klein, 1986). Population-based studies yield an even higher rate; one study in New England observed that the annual incidence of work-related eye injuries to be approximately 600 per 100,000 persons (Glynn *et al.*, 1988).

The epidemiology of work-related ocular trauma has also been reported in other countries. In Italy, a national insurance database which registers all casualties that cause work disabilities exceeding 3 days estimated an annual incidence of 370 injuries per 100,000 (Cruciani *et al.*, 1997). In Scotland, the incidence of hospitalised ocular trauma was estimated to be 8.14 per 100,000 persons, of which about 70% were work-related injuries (Desai *et al.*, 1996).

Data on work-related ocular trauma from Asian populations, which has previously been lacking compared to Western populations (Négrel and Thylefors, 1998), has begun to emerge from a number of large population based studies. A prospective survey at the emergency department of a large hospital in Singapore indicated that half of all ophthalmic cases presenting to the department were due to trauma, of which 70% were work-related (Voon *et al.*, 1998). Grinding, cutting metal and drilling were the specific activities in more than 90% of these injuries. More alarming was the fact that less than 20% use some form of eye protective devices, with another 30% provided protective equipment, but did not use them at the time of injury (Voon *et al.*, 1998). In India, the Aravind Comprehensive Eye Survey of 5,150 adult subjects (Nirmalan *et al.*, 2004), elicited a history of ocular trauma in either eye from 4.5% of the population, with agricultural labor the commonest setting (46.9%). Similarly, the Andhra Pradesh Eye Disease Study reported the age- and gender adjusted prevalence of a history of ocular trauma as 7.5% in the rural setting, of which 55.9% was work related, and 3.9% in the urban setting (Dandona *et al.*, 2000; Krishnaiah *et al.*, 2006). Extrapolation of these estimates to the Indian population gives an indication of the magnitude of the problem, with approximately six million people with a history of work related ocular trauma and more than 600,000 blinded as a result.

Data from the Singapore Malay Eye Study are consistent with the estimates in an urban setting, with a history of ocular trauma given in 5%. Interestingly, more than 90% of those with a history of ocular trauma worked indoors (Loon *et al.*, 2009). The only estimate to data of the incidence of ocular trauma in Asia is from rural Nepal. In this study, the crude incidence of ocular trauma was 0.51 per 1,000 population at risk per year (Khatry *et al.*, 2004). Of these, 68% were classified as 'severe' at initial presentation and 75% of these were lacerating injuries.

Demographic Distribution

Like other work-related diseases, ocular injuries occur most often in the young, working adult population (Baker *et al.*, 1992). In particular, they tend to occur in the 20–30 years age group. This has been observed consistently in both descriptive (Dannenberg *et al.*, 1992; Schein *et al.*, 1988; Morris *et al.*, 1987; MacEwen, 1989) and controlled epidemiological studies (Tielsch *et al.*, 1989; Wong and Tielsch, 1999; Brian *et al.*, 2011; Jafari *et al.*, 2010). Three quarters of work-related open globe injury reported in one study were among persons under 40 years of age (Dannenberg *et al.*, 1992). This high incidence may reflect the placement of younger workers in more hazardous jobs, their increased susceptibility from lack of regard for safety practices or, simply, inexperience. The 2002 NHIS however reported that the age-specific prevalence rates were 2%, 3.8%, 4.9%, 6.0%, 5.4%, 4.0%, and 3.1% for ages 18–24, 25–34, 35–44, 45–54, 55–64, 65–74, and 75+ years respectively, with the highest prevalence reported for the 45–54 age group (Forrest and Cali, 2009).

The higher risk in males has been found in every population-based study of ocular injuries, with incidence or prevalence rate ratios of male to female between two and over five (Serinken *et al.*, 2013; Goel *et al.*, 2013; Klopfer *et al.*, 1992). Again, the higher risk in males reflects either the placement of male workers in more hazardous jobs or higher risks in males due to a lack of regard for safety practices compared to females. One study in the military found that males had consistently higher risks of injuries compared to females with the same specific occupation and job tasks (Smith *et al.*, 2005). It is also interesting to note that differences between the genders disappear in older workers, perhaps related to changing risk behaviours in older males.

There are ethnic variations reported as well. However, the key variable is probably the socio-economic status rather than ethnicity *per se*. In Baker's study in California, the highest risk of hospitalised work-related ocular injury occurred in young men of Hispanic origin

(Baker *et al.*, 1996). In the 2002 NHIS, workers with less than high-school education and who were of non-Hispanic white ethnicity were more likely to sustain injuries (Forrest and Cali, 2009). In Singapore, half of the work-related injuries seen at the emergency setting were in non-resident foreign workers from Bangladesh, China and India (Voon *et al.*, 1998). Direct evidence of a role for socio-economic status has also been identified in some population based studies. In the urban population of the Andhra Pradesh Eye Disease Study (Dandona *et al.*, 2000), lower socio-economic status was a risk factor for ocular injury, while alcohol consumption was identified as a risk factor in the Singapore Malay Eye Study. Tobacco use was a risk factor identified amongst among welders in coastal south India (Kumar and Dharanipriya, 2014).

Industry-specific rates

There is a wealth of data on industry-specific rates of ocular injury. In one study, Schein and associates at the Massachusetts Eye and Ear Infirmary observed that 63% of occupationally related injuries occurred among workers in the construction industry and 18% among auto repair workers (Schein *et al.*, 1988).

A survey on 1,552 firemen in the United Kingdom fire service indicated an annual incidence of 3,500 ocular injuries per 100,000 firefighters (Owen *et al.*, 1995). In Finland, industry-specific data showed that iron and steel, fabricated metal manufacturing and excavating and foundation industries have the highest annual incidence of ocular injuries at 680 per 100,000 workers (Saari and Parvi, 1984). In a study of the chemical industry, an incidence of 2,300 per 100,000 worker-years was observed, which reflects the high risks in this occupational group (Jones and Grifffith, 1992). In Australia, automotive industry workers had the highest relative incidence of open-globe injuries compared to other occupations but these workers were also the least likely to wear safety eye-wear (Fong and Taouk, 1995). Another study in a large US automotive corporation estimated an annual incidence rate of 1,500 eye injuries per 100,000 employees (Wong *et al.*, 1998).

Other high-risk occupations highlighted in recent years include professional sports such as basketball, baseball and boxing (Vinger and Vinger, 1994). However, almost any professional sport can benefit from primary prevention with simple eye protective devices. A classic and often cited example is the 90% decline in incidence of ice-hockey related ocular injury in Canada following the introduction of mandatory usage of appropriate helmets and eye protection (Pashby, 1985; Pashby *et al.*, 1975). Similarly, the military is a special occupational group at high risk of ocular injury both during wartime (Wong and Seet, 1997; Zhang *et al.*, 2009) as well as in peacetime (Wong and Tielsch, 1999), but these injuries are likewise eminently preventable with proper eye protection. In the Israeli Defense Force, not a single eye injury occurred amongst soldiers wearing proper goggles (Belkin *et al.*, 1982).

In the rural developing world context, agricultural labor is one of the commonest cause of work-related ocular trauma. 25.9% of injuries in Nepal occurred in farmers, and 27.4% percent of injuries took place in the fields and farms (Khatry *et al.*, 2004). Vegetable matter was also the commonest instrument of injury in Andhra Pradesh (45.3%) (Krishnaiah *et al.*, 2006) and 66.8% of those reporting ocular trauma in the Aravind Comprehensive Eye Survey were agricultural laborers (Nirmalan *et al.*, 2004). In Nigeria, 37.2% of ocular injuries in geriatric subjects occurred on the farm, with 41.1% due to sticks or twigs (Onakpoya *et al.*, 2010). In Thailand, agricultural workers are more likely to sustain work-related open-globe injuries (Chaikitmongkol *et al.*, 2015). In Western Uttar Pradesh, India, 221 out of 718 agricultural workers surveyed had sustained corneal injuries, of whom four had had multiple injuries. A survey of migrant farm workers in North Carolina showed that the incidence rate of lost work-time injuries of 23.8/10,000 worker years, far exceeding the national average of 6.9/10,000 worker years (Quandt *et al.*, 2012).

Types and Causes of Injuries

The types and causes of injuries vary depending on the severity of injury. For severe work-related trauma requiring hospitalisation, one study found that the most common types were open globe injury (46%), adnexal wounds (20%), orbital fractures (11%), and traumatic hyphema (11%) (Baker *et al.*, 1999). The most common causes of these injuries were foreign-body or projectile objects (19%), transport vehicles (18%), cutting or piercing objects (17%), and assaults (9%).

The spectrum is slightly different for less severe trauma not requiring hospital admission. For example, at the emergency department setting, the most common types in one study were superficial foreign bodies (58.2%), corneal abrasion (25.1%) and blunt trauma (12.5%). The most common causes were grinding (31%), foreign objects from cutting metal or drilling (21%) or construction-related activities (12%) (Voon *et al.*, 1998).

Economic Impact

Beyond acute medical care, work-related ocular injuries may cause both short term and long-term morbidity. Schein *et al.* observed that patients with open globe injuries had an average of 70 days of medical leave from work (Schein *et al.*, 1988). In another study in the automotive industry, almost one third of the injuries resulted in an inability of the worker to resume his normal duties at the company (Wong and Tielsch, 1999). In terms of disability, nearly 10% of hospitalised injuries require long-term nursing or rehabilitation services (Baker *et al.*, 1999).

The overall economic impact of eye injuries in terms of cost has been difficult to estimate (Munoz, 1984). Less severe injuries are usually not reported, although they can account for enormous indirect costs (time off work). Based on US claims data, the average cost per claim for ocular injuries varied from $171 to $331 per claim (McCall and Horwitz, 2006). For severe injuries, Baker's study on hospitalised work-related injury estimated annual hospital charges (excluding professional fees) of $14.6 million in the US when work-related ocular trauma was the principal admitting diagnosis and $40 million when ocular trauma was either a principal or secondary diagnosis (Baker *et al.*, 1999). In addition, up to 40% of those with the open globe injuries sustained at work could be pursuing costly legal action against their employers (Schein *et al.*, 1988). Work-related trauma in underdeveloped countries, where agricultural labor is the main occupation, may lead to lower absolute costs, but the individual economic burden is arguably greater as the visual outcome is frequently poorer and alternative sheltered employment is usually not readily available.

Clinical Presentation

From a clinical management perspective, no two eyes are traumatised in an identical manner. There may be extreme variability and unpredictability. However, there are several specific features that distinguish work-related eye injuries from non-work related injuries. First, work-related injuries tend to be more severe. For example, blunt trauma may be associated with blow-out fractures (fractures involving the orbital walls without involvement of the rim), traumatic hyphema (haemorrhage in the anterior chamber), angle damage (leading subsequently to glaucoma, sometimes decades later) lens dislocation (Fig. 3) and vitreous haemorrhage. Second, metallic intraocular foreign bodies (IOFBs) are common and have to be excluded in any work-related open-globe injuries. Third, thermal, chemical and radiation injuries, rarely seen in non-occupational settings, are fairly important aetiological agents in work-related injuries. Lastly, injuries from contaminated

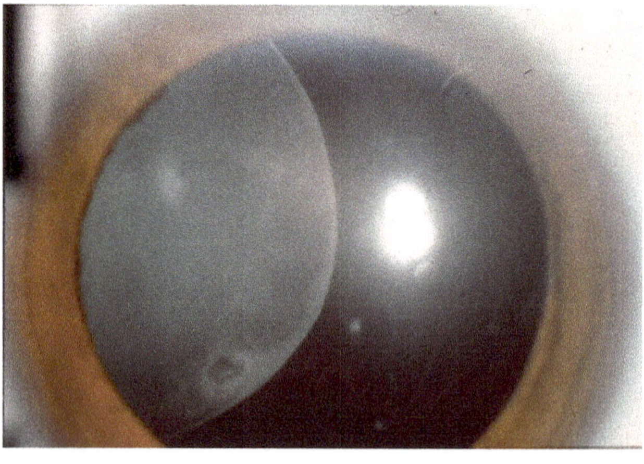

Fig. 3. Dislocated lens from blunt trauma.

work-related instruments, and vegetative matter in particular, are frequently complicated by severe infections by bacteria (e.g. *Bacillus cereus*) and fungi that may be more blinding than the initial injury.

Clinically, work-related ocular trauma can be classified according to type of injury (e.g. blunt versus open-globe), location of injury (e.g. anterior versus posterior segment of the eye) and aetiology of injury (e.g. mechanical versus chemical or thermal). The Birmingham Eye Trauma Terminology (BETT) has been introduced to standardise ocular trauma reporting and has gained general acceptance (Kuhn *et al.*, 2002). Ocular injuries are classified as closed or open globe injuries. Closed globe injuries in turn are sub classified as contusions and lamellar (partial thickness) lacerations. Open globe injuries may be ruptures, in which a full thickness breach occurs secondary to blunt trauma, or lacerations due to a sharp object. Lacerations may take one of three forms — penetrating injuries without an exit wound, perforations with entry and exit wounds, or retained IOFBs.

Most open-globe or penetrating injuries occur directly at the site of impact when secondary to a sharp instrument and opposite the site of impact when secondary to blunt trauma. The clinical features and complications vary. The more severe open globe injuries are usually easy to visualise and are accompanied by reduced visual acuity, a shallow anterior chamber, hyphaema, a change in the shape of the pupil and an open wound in either the cornea or sclera.

In blunt injuries, compression and deformation of the eye are unusual occurrences because of the protection afforded the eye by the surrounding bones of the orbit, particularly the orbital rim. However, even though no actual tissue loss occurs, the force of the blow may cause extensive injury to many of the delicate structures of the eye. These same structures usually have only a limited ability to recover and repair the damage.

Surgical management is targeted towards primary repair for even the most severe injuries, with enucleation (removal of the globe) indicated only if the globe is totally disorganised with loss of retinal tissue and if pre-operative written consent has been obtained from an alert, sober, patient. Frequently, secondary surgical procedures are required on an elective basis after the initial acute management.

History

A detailed history is extremely important in all work-related ocular injuries in the assessment of the extent of damage, potential for foreign bodies and complications (e.g. infection) and in the determination of appropriate investigative studies. The circumstances surrounding the injury are often important in future medico-legal actions. When, where, and how the injury occurred should be reported in the patient's own words. A note should be made concerning whether the patient was wearing any type of ocular protection and the names of any witnesses should be recorded. A detailed description of the mechanism of injury (blunt or sharp), details about the size, composition and velocity of the object (e.g. nail) and activities (e.g. hammering) producing the injury is important, because radiologic studies are indicated if there is any possibility of an IOFB. An account of the events that occurred in the time interval between the injury and examination may suggest that additional damage or complication (e.g. infection) may have occurred.

The patient's pre-injury ocular status should be documented. Pertinent information includes a history of previous eye injury, surgery, or amblyopia. This is especially important in work-related eye injuries when disability compensation may become an issue later on.

Clinical Examination

The visual acuity should be measured in both eyes before any therapy is initiated. Pupil reactions to light (which may indicate optic nerve damage) should be elicited. The extent of injury (with drawings and photographs if possible) should be documented. If possible, maximal dilation of the pupil and ophthalmoscopy is indicated at the time of the initial examination because cataractous opacification of the lens or progressive vitreous haemorrhage may obscure fundus details within hours of the injury, precluding further examination. Ocular ultrasound is another alternative to evaluate eyes with opaque media. However, in patients with penetrating globe injuries, clinical maneuvers during physical examination may lead to further extrusion of intraocular contents. In these circumstances, physical examination should be confined to measuring acuity only. If the vitreous cavity and retina cannot be visualised, radiologic studies are indicated to rule out an IOFB. Plain orbital X-rays with look-up and look-down views may reveal the presence of a radio-opaque orbital or IOFB. If IOFB is suspected but the radiological or ultrasound investigations are negative, a CT scan of the orbit may be indicated.

In subjects where no injury is immediately apparent, certain signs mandate a high index of suspicion. These include an unusually deep or shallow anterior chamber, bullous subconjunctival haemorrhage in which the posterior extent is not visualised, gross hyphema, an afferent pupillary defect, irregular pupil, and poor ocular motility.

Pre-Operative Management

The injured globe should immediately be protected with a hard shield that is supported by the bony parts of the face. An improvised shield can be fashioned from a variety of everyday objects including plastic or cardboard cups. Analgesia may reduce the patient's anxiety, thereby relieving lid blepharospasm and further pressure on the globe. The instillation of prophylactic antibiotic drops should probably be deferred until wound closure has been achieved to reduce manipulation of the globe as well as potential preservative toxicity. Cultures of the wound also involve additional manipulation and are probably best performed in the operating room. Broad-spectrum prophylactic systemic antibiotic coverage is recommended in wounds caused by contaminated material or if the possibility of an IOFB exists. The timing of surgery will be related to the patient's history of last known food or fluid intake because general anesthesia is preferred. The anesthetist should be informed of the nature of the injury and a request to avoid depolarising neuromuscular blocking agents like succinylcholine made as there is a theoretical risk of extrusion of globe contents. Although no documented cases of systemic tetanus following injuries to the globe are present in the literature, this possibility must always be considered and prophylactic tetanus treatment is preferred.

Informed Consent

Since even the simplest open globe injuries may be associated with severe intraocular damage, a serious discussion with the patient and employers with regard to prognosis is extremely important pre-operatively and a full informed consent taken. This is again of particular importance in work-related injuries when medico-legal compensation may be a future issue. The ocular trauma score (OTS) is a clinical instrument that may use in prognostication and counselling (Kuhn *et al.*, 2002). The OTS is calculated from the following variables: initial vision, and the presence of globe rupture, perforating injury, endophthalmitis, retinal detachment, and an afferent pupillary defect. Based on the raw score, the patient may then be assigned to a prognostic category that gives estimates of the likelihood of achieving a certain level of final visual acuity. For example, a patient in category 1, the most severe category, has a 74% chance of no light perception acuity and only a 1% chance of achieving a final acuity of ≥6/12. In contrast a patient in the best prognostic category has a 0% chance of no light perception vision and a 94% chance of ≥6/12 vision. In a recent publication from Mexico, the OTS has been shown to be ascertainable in 98.9% of ocular injuries (Lima-Gomez *et al.*, 2010). Recent studies from both Caucasian and Asian populations have confirmed the utility of the OTS. A study on 31 open-globe injuries seen over three years in Hungary found the final visual outcome to be correlated with the initial OTS with a high degree of statistical significance ($p = 0.000095$) (Maneschg *et al.*, 2011), and similar outcomes have been noted in Korea (Han and Yu, 2010).

Appropriate translation to the native languages of the worker is necessary. Both the patient and employer must understand that (1) the goal of surgery is adequate wound closure with restoration of the integrity of the globe, (2) vision will be affected, complications such as bleeding and infection may occur and removal of the eye may be needed, (3) the healing period may be long and that additional operations to maximise visual potential may be indicated, and (4) long term follow-up, for years after the injury is required because of the risk of late glaucoma and retinal detachment. It is worth emphasising to the employer that the injured worker may be unable to return quickly to his or her present job.

Management

Injuries to the Cornea and Sclera

The primary goal in repairing cornea and scleral lacerations is to achieve a watertight globe with structural integrity. Secondary goals include removing any disrupted lens fragments and vitreous, repositioning any uveal tissue, relieving vitreous incarceration, removing any IOFB, and restoring normal anatomic relationships with a minimum of globe distortion. A methodical surgical strategy is essential for injury repair.

Partial thickness corneal injuries usually result in a shelved flap of edematous cornea that is in relatively good apposition with the surrounding tissue. Firm patching will often lead to re-epithelialisation and complications are rare. If the visual axis is involved, secondary scarring may reduce visual acuity, but surgery is only indicated if the tissue is irregular and poorly opposed. Occasionally, a soft contact lens (bandage contact lens) may be used to reduce irritation and promote re-epithelialisation of the area.

Full thickness corneal lacerations can be in the form of puncture wounds or linear, irregular, or avulsing lacerations. These injuries may be self-sealing or associated with a shallow or flat anterior chamber. Incarceration or prolapse of intraocular tissue further complicates management. Full thickness corneal lacerations are at risk of endophthalmitis and patients should be routinely admitted for management. For small, self-sealing full thickness corneal lacerations, a bandage contact lens may be sufficient to protect and support the wound as it heals. Corneal glue (cyanoacrylate surgical adhesive) can also be applied under topical anesthesia. If leakage persists for more than 24 h or there is progressive shallowing of the anterior chamber, more definitive surgical treatment should be undertaken. On the other hand, large, non-shelving lacerations associated with a flat anterior chamber or incarcerated tissue usually require surgery to close the wound, to

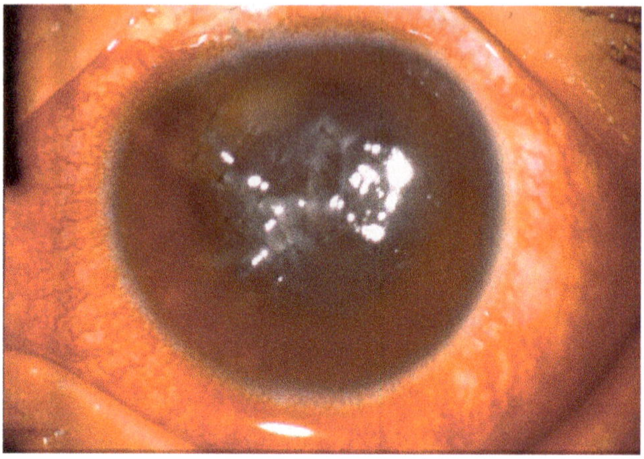

Fig. 4. Surgical repair of full thickness corneal laceration in a 25-year-old shipyard worker who was hit by a flying metal piece while drilling.

remove all incarcerated tissue and to re-form the anterior chamber (Fig. 4).

Injuries to the Lens

It is often difficult to diagnose lens damage or disruption in association with a corneal laceration, especially if the pupil is not maximally dilated and if blood and fibrin are present in the anterior chamber. In principle, removal of a damaged or cataractous lens rarely needs to be done in the emergency setting. However, in certain scenarios, mainly where a large breach in the anterior or posterior lens capsule has occurred, primary lens removal may be advantageous. If the anterior lens capsule is clearly damaged with flocculent lens material in the anterior chamber, or if the posterior capsule is disrupted and there is vitreous presenting in the anterior chamber, it may be preferable to complete all surgical interventions at one setting. On the other hand, a small lens opacity with an intact capsule and no liberated material may be removed at a later date. If any doubt regarding lens clarity exists, however, the lens should be left in place at the acute setting. Various surgical techniques are available for the removal of the lens. Intraocular lens implantation in the primary trauma setting is controversial because of the risk of endophthalmitis. The patient's age, the visual and refractive status of the fellow eye, and the ability to use an aphakic contact lens postoperatively are factors in the decision.

Hyphema

Blood in the anterior chamber (hyphema) may lead to a number of secondary complications (Fig. 5). Even a small amount of blood in the anterior chamber is significant because it indicates the possibility of serious intraocular damage.

Secondary (delayed) haemorrhage may occur at the time of clot retraction. If the haemorrhage is extensive, the blood may totally fill the anterior chamber and completely replace the aqueous (8-ball or blackball hyphema). The extravasated blood will turn from bright red to black as the aqueous circulation ceases and the haemoglobin becomes deoxygenated.

The main complications are glaucoma and corneal blood staining. Multiple mechanisms may lead to secondary glaucoma, which are usually difficult to manage. Blood breakdown products from hyphema

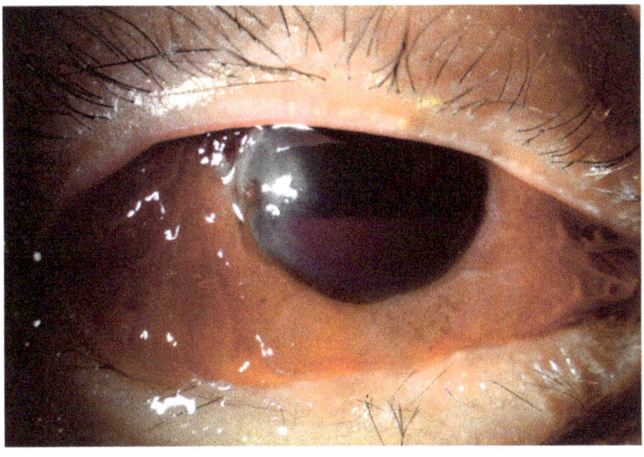

Fig. 5. Traumatic gross hyphema, sustained by a 21-year-old construction worker while hammering. A globe rupture must be excluded in all cases of severe blunt trauma, particularly when there is a bullous subconjunctival haemorrhage as in this case.

may diffuse into the cornea, causing corneal blood staining (reddish orange opacification of the stroma). Blood staining may eventually clear; however, permanent staining is not uncommon, and may be severe enough to require subsequent corneal transplantation. Medical management is directed at control of intraocular pressure while waiting for spontaneous resolution. Surgical intervention is sometimes needed when this does not occur and optic nerve damage from glaucoma is likely.

Intraocular Foreign Body

An IOFB should always be excluded in work-related eye injuries as they are particularly common after activities involving striking metal on metal. Typically, the foreign body is small and the eye may not show obvious signs of trauma. Entry wounds through the cornea may be small and self-sealing, and subconjunctival bleeding or edema may cover those through the sclera. The entry site and intraocular site of damage may help delineate the trajectory and resting place of an IOFB. The IOFB is usually in one of the following locations: anterior chamber, lens (creating a focal cataract) (Fig. 6), vitreous cavity (Fig. 7) or embedded in the retina (Fig. 8).

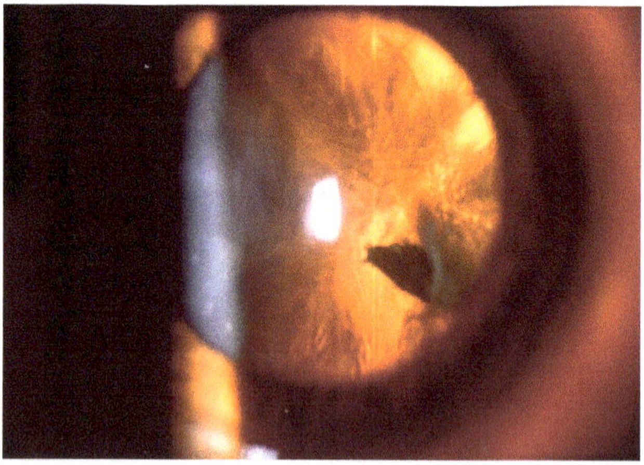

Fig. 6. IOFB located in the lens. The surrounding lens usually turns cataractous within hours. In this instance, both the foreign body and the lens should be removed.

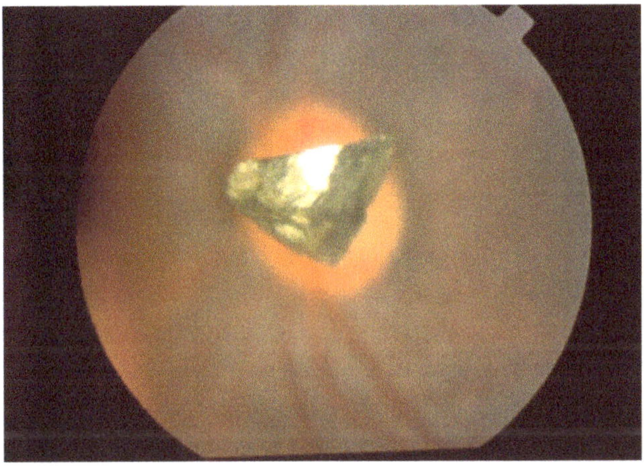

Fig. 7. IOFB located within the vitreous. Removal of the foreign body may involve a complex posterior segment surgery (vitrectomy).

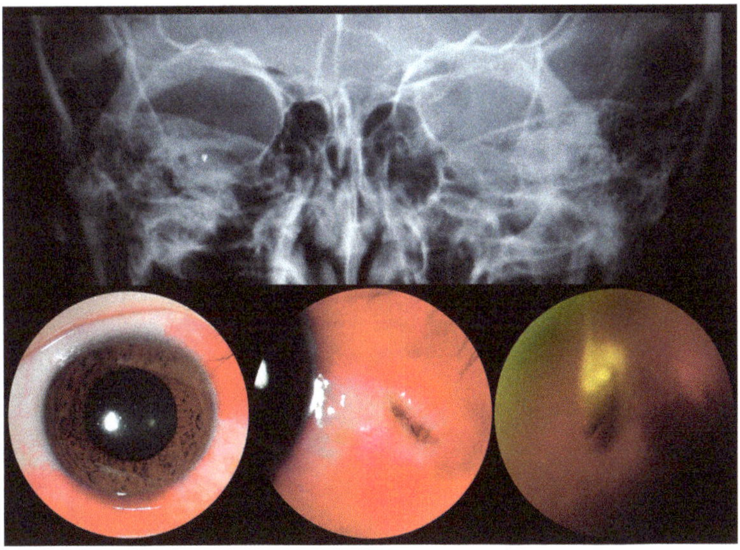

Fig. 8. Metallic foreign body impacted on the retina. Orbital X-ray shows radio-opaque foreign body in right orbit. The entry site through the sclera is visible in the middle panel of the second row.

The composition of the foreign body involved determines the urgency of its removal. Some materials (e.g. iron and copper) may be toxic and stimulate inflammation and/or siderois bulbi with long term loss of vision, while others (e.g. vegetable matter) may pose a risk for severe infection. Contamination with *Bacillus cereus* in particular is well known to cause a fulminant endophthalmitis that may cause blindness in a matter of hours. These items should be removed promptly. On the other hand, inert substances such as plastic and glass may be well tolerated and left in place in certain situations. Surgery to remove IOFBs generally involves intra-ocular surgery with vitrectomy techniques, in which various grasping and cutting instruments, and occasionally intraocular magnets, are used to extract the IOFB and clear debris and inflammatory material.

Injuries to the Retina

Severe work-related blunt trauma commonly produces posterior segment injuries including retinal edema (known as Berlin's edema or commotio retinae), retinal haemorrhage, vitreous haemorrhage, retinal tears, choroidal tears and retinal detachment (Fig. 9). Even for mild

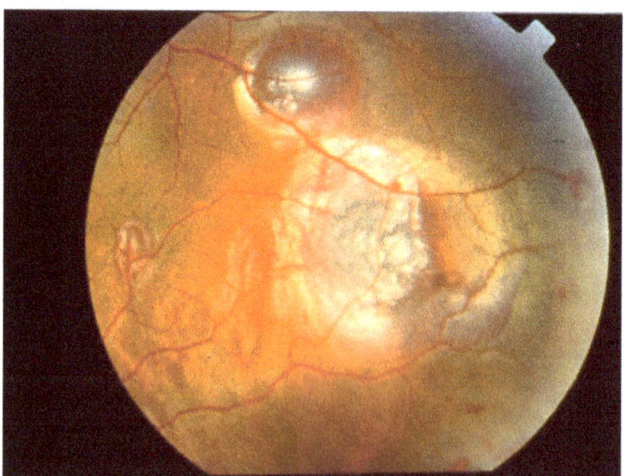

Fig. 9. Retinal photograph showing retinal haemorrhage and edema (Commotio retinae) in a 21-year-old construction worker who sustained severe blunt trauma while hammering.

blunt posterior segment trauma such as retinal edema, visual acuity is often affected and late pigmentary scarring may occur in the macular area, while peripheral areas of involvement may be the sites for future retinal tears. Choroidal tears may lead to the development of choroidal neovascular membranes that cause retinal scarring.

Penetrating injuries involving the posterior segment carry a less favorable prognosis than blunt trauma. The primary mechanical damage of vital structures by such injuries may be so great that useful vision is instantly destroyed. Major advances in the management of all posterior segment injuries are the development of microsurgery and vitrectomy. The latter, a closed intraocular procedure in which the surgeon can remove blood, debris or IOFB and repair retinal tears or detachment, has led to improvement in the prognosis of previously untreatable posterior segment injuries.

Injuries to the Ocular Adnexa

As the first line of protection for the globe, the eyelids are often involved in both blunt and penetrating trauma to the eye, avulsions as well as orbital trauma which are commonly associated with significant ocular trauma. In cases of occult ocular penetraion, a relatively inoccuous eyelid wound may be the only sign of a more sinister injury. Lacerations of the eyelid are classified according to where the lid margin is involved. Lacerations involving the lid margin may require surgical closure in layers to reconstitute the eyelid anatomy, and are usually best handled by a specialist. Lacerations which do not involve the lid margin may not require suturing. In the assessment of medial eyelid lacerations, particular attention should be paid to the lacrimal apparatus. Eyelid lacerations medial to the lacrimal punctum, may sever the lacrimal canaliculi (Fig. 10).

If the severed ends are not reanastamosed, it might lead to subsequent canalicular stenosis and epiphora. In the primary setting, identification of the severed ends of the canaliculus and suturing over a stent can help to reduce the incidence of subsequent stenosis.

Blunt trauma to the ocular region may also be associated with orbital fractures. The patient might complain of a periorbital haemorrhage and diplopia (double vision) due to misalignment of the globes.

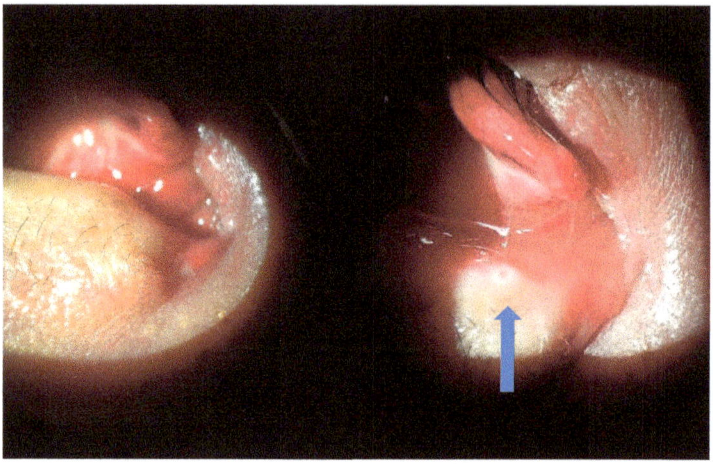

Fig. 10. Eyelid laceration on the medial end of the right lower lid. When the lower lid is pulled downwards, the blue arrow points to the right lower lid punctum. The eyelid laceration is medial the punctum and the canaliculus was lacerated in thie case.

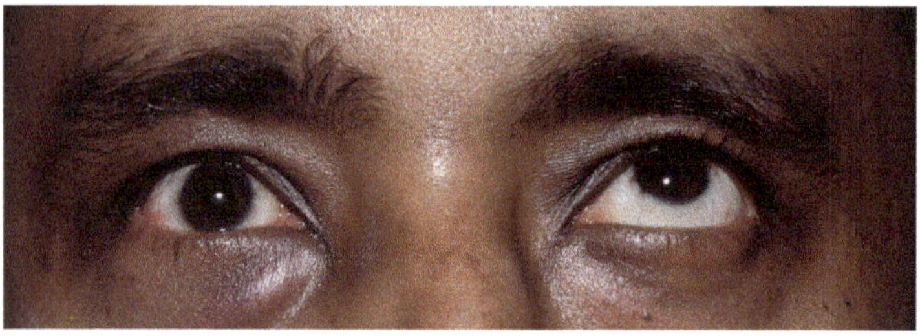

Fig. 11. This patient sustained a right orbital fracture with prolapse of the orbital tissue into the fracture. As a result, he is unable to look up with his right eye.

Ocular motility might be limited in the presence of an orbital fracture (Fig. 11).

If there is clinical suspicion of an orbital fracture, an orbital X-ray (Waters view) can be performed. There can be opacification of the maxillary sinus suggesting blood has collected there in the setting of trauma and orbital fracture (Fig. 12).

A CT of the orbital area can be performed to confirm the presence and assess the extent of the orbital fracture (Fig. 13).

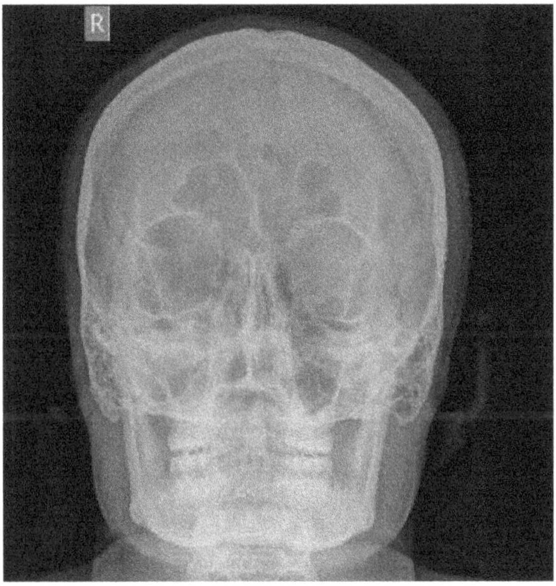

Fig. 12. There is opacification of the right maxillary sinus.

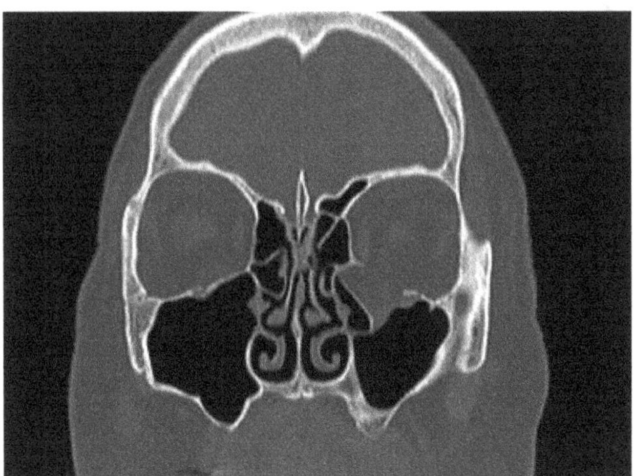

Fig. 13. A bone window CT scan showing a left orbital floor fracture.

Not all orbital fractures require surgical repair. If there is no diplopia, the fracture is small and/ or there is no enophthalmos (sinking in) of the involved eye, one can potentially opt for conservative management.

Enucleation

In all trauma cases, repair of the globe should be attempted. However, there are some severe work-related injuries (e.g. industrial accidents involving trauma from heavy machinery) which are beyond repair. Enucleation (removal of the globe) at the time of the original surgical procedure (primary enucleation) should be considered only in the event of total disruption of the globe; this includes those patients in whom large amounts of intraocular contents have been extruded or who have large scleral lacerations or ruptures associated with tissue loss that are completely irreparable. Initial primary repair permits evaluation of the total ocular status in the immediate postoperative period, with possible secondary enucleation at a later date. Thus, the patient is allowed a period of mental recovery to a more alert and oriented state. Also, both the patient and the employer recognise that the surgeon is making all possible efforts to salvage the injured globe. Should primary enucleation be considered, appropriate informed consent must be obtained. However, in cases where enucleation is delayed, the patient should be advised on the small but well recognised risk of sympathetic ophthalmia, a condition in which an autoimmune reaction triggered by the trauma causes severe and blinding inflammation in the fellow uninjured eye.

Post-Operative Management

The goals of postoperative management are directed at (1) controlling infection, (2) suppressing inflammation, and (3) visual rehabilitation.

To prevent infection, postoperatively, the eye should be protected by an eye-shield and a topical broad-spectrum antibiotic should be prescribed. Patients admitted to the hospital should receive 4–5 days of treatment with intravenous antibiotics, usually a cephalosporin or vancomycin and an aminoglycoside. Most cases of bacterial endophthalmitis present by the fifth postoperative day.

One must weigh the anti-inflammatory advantages against the risk of infection with corticosteroid use. Intensive corticosteroid use in early wound healing may also diminish the rate of stromal healing as well as the tensile strength of the wound. Topical corticosteroid should therefore be used cautiously to control inflammation only once infection is ruled out, usually 48 h after the operation and continued until the eye is white and quiet.

Visual rehabilitation depends on the severity of the trauma. In certain cases, secondary operations such as corneal grafts may be indicated to improve vision when the eye is quiet and free of infection.

Chemical, Thermal, Electrical and Radiation Injuries

Chemical Injuries

Chemical injuries are common in a wide array of occupational settings, involving workers not just in the chemical industry (Griffith and Jones, 1994; Bulbulia *et al.*, 1995) but in other industries as well (Hong *et al.*, 2010). The spectrum of ocular damage can be minor or severe, depending on the type of chemical, the quantity, concentration, duration of exposure, the directness of exposure, the lipid solubility, anionic affinity and, most importantly, the pH of the chemical.

For acid injuries, an instantaneous coagulative necrosis and precipitation of protein in the epithelium helps neutralise the acid and acts as a barrier to further penetration of the acid, limiting the intraocular damage. In addition, the tear film can act as a buffer against acids (unless the amount of acid is excessive or the pH is less than 3.0). Explosions of car batteries due to spark ignition of oxygen and hydrogen gas mixtures released by sulfuric acid have become one of the most common types of acid injuries in mechanics and other workers involved in the automotive industry, and add an element of thermal injury (charring). While usually only superficial injuries occur, severe cases may result in corneal scarring, cataract and glaucoma.

On the other hand, alkali injuries are extremely dangerous. Alkali denatures proteins and saponifies lipids, which produces an immediate swelling of the epithelium followed by desquamation (rather than precipitation of protein as in the acid burn). Thus, the alkali is allowed direct access to the corneal stroma, through which it can penetrate rapidly via the corneal endothelium into the eye. In addition, alkali coagulates conjunctival and scleral blood vessels, which causes ischaemic damage. When alkali gains access to the interior of the eye, it destroys lens and ciliary epithelial cells and causes extensive inflammation. Clinically, the conjunctiva has a porcelain-white appearance due to coagulation of the blood vessels. Later in the course of the injury, the inflammatory process further destroys corneal tissues, leading to extensive corneal ulceration and perforation. Alkali injury to the conjunctiva and lids also leads to scarring, dry eyes and other deformities.

Chemical injuries are one of few true ocular emergencies and should be treated immediately without delay to prevent blindness. Ideally, the employers should have a protocol for dealing with these types of injuries at the work-site. The single most important management is extensive and continuous eye irrigation at the time of injury. This could even be in the form of an eye wash with clean running tap water at the site of the accident prior to medical evacuation. Cement injuries are a special case of alkali injuries, as the particulate matter is difficult to remove by simple irrigation, and require meticulous forniceal sweeping and removal of all cement particles. Further management is directed at preventing complications (e.g. infection and glaucoma) and promoting re-epithelialisation.

Thermal and Electrical Burns

The blink reflex usually protects the eye from most burn injuries. The cornea and conjunctiva may suffer extensive effects of secondary exposure when the lids and face are burned severely. The management of thermal burns is similar in many respects to chemical injuries from acids, with the primary aim at promoting epithelial healing of the ocular surface.

Electrical injuries, especially if in the area of the head, can cause cataracts. Industrial accidents affect mainly the anterior superficial lens cortex whereas non-industrial electrical burns (e.g. lightning strikes) affect both the anterior and posterior parts of the lens. In extreme cases, there may be anterior uveitis or even anterior tissue necrosis.

Radiation Injuries

Radiation injuries are uncommon in non-occupational settings. The spectrum of ocular injuries depends on the type of radiation. Radiation may be either non-ionising or ionising. Ocular injuries from ionising radiation are less common and are only applicable to workers in the medical profession of radiology. On the other hand, many more workers are exposed to different types of non-ionising radiation, including long-wave radiation in the broadcast radio industry, microwave radiation in radar and communication industries, infrared radiation emitted from furnaces in glass and metal industries, visible radiation from sunlight in agricultural and construction industries and ultraviolet radiation from sunlight and welding in metal industries. Ultraviolet light sources in laboratories may also cause corneal burns. In addition, injuries from industrial lasers (either ultraviolet, visible or infrared radiation) are becoming increasingly important.

Microwave radiation causes thermal injuries to various ocular structures. Infrared waves can cause true exfoliation of the lens capsule (Glassblower cataracts) as well as other effects. Visible light of sufficient intensity can cause chorioretinal burns, and is potentially sight threatening if the burns involve the macula. Ocular effects of ionising radiation include conjunctival and corneal telangiectasis and keratinisation. Retinal microvasculopathy, vitreous haemorrhage and optic atrophy have also been reported in severe cases, and usually present many years after the exposure. Ultraviolet radiation exposure has been implicated in many ocular conditions, such as conjunctivitis, keratitis and even macular damage. Welder's arc eye is a common condition and refers to an acute, painful, but frequently transient keratoconjunctivitis from ultraviolet radiation exposure in welders without adequate eye protection (Chou and Cullen, 1996; Davies *et al.*, 2007).

Case Study 3: Arc Eye

A 30 year old welder presented to the emergency department late at night complaining of severe tearing and pain in one eye. He had been welding earlier in the day but was well when he stopped work and only felt the pain several hours later. On examination, the conjunctiva was diffusely injected and the cornea showed multiple punctate erosions that stained with fluorescein. He was prescribed topical lubricants and the eye was patched. On review the next day, his symptoms had resolved.

Recently, attention has focused on the risks associated with ionising radiation amongst interventional cardiology staff. A cohort study of 81 interventional cardiology staff showed that the incidence of lens opacity was 79% amongst staff with exposure, compared to 7.1% amongst those without (relative risk 11.06) (Bitarafan *et al.*, 2015). Another survey reported a relative risk of 2.2–2.6 for staff in the field (Ciraj-Bjelac *et al.*, 2012).

Other Occupational Eye Disorders

Non-trauma related occupational eye disorders usually result from long-term exposure to various chemicals, infectious agents or radiation. Almost all industrial chemicals (including halides, solvents, insecticides, fungicides, herbicides and fertilisers) have been implicated in allergic conjunctivitis, keratitis, photophobia and other non-specific ocular irritation (Ansari, 1997; Marshall and Meetz, 1995; Yokota *et al.*, 1999; Ireland *et al.*, 1994).

In addition to acute radiation eye injuries, long-term exposure to radiation can lead to chronic ocular conditions such as corneal diseases, cataracts and age-related macular degeneration (Vano *et al.*, 1998; Milacic, 2009). Microwave has been shown to produce cataracts in animals experimentally but has not been demonstrated convincingly in humans (Kurz and Einaugler, 1968; Appleton *et al.*, 1975). However, the evidence for ultraviolet radiation as a risk factor for ocular diseases is strong. Among the many different effects of this type of radiation, the two most important are cataract and pterygium (Dolin and Johnson, 1994; Moran and Hollows, 1984). Taylor and colleagues effectively demonstrated the association with cortical cataract and ptergyium among Chesapeake Bay watermen (Taylor, 1982; Taylor *et al.*, 1989). A high prevalence of pterygium have been reported in postmen (Tang *et al.*, 1999), welders (Karai and Horiguchi, 1984; Norn and Franck, 1991) and patients engaged in outdoor activities (Viso *et al.*, 2010). In the Tanjong Pagar study in Singapore, participants who were outdoor workers, or laborers and agricultural workers, were more likely to have pterygium and nuclear cataracts respectively (Wong *et al.*, 2001; Foster *et al.*, 2003). These studies suggest that cataract and pterygium can be considered as work-related disorders in persons with long-term direct exposure to ultraviolet light (e.g. welders) (Tenkate *et al.*, 2019; Modense and Gobba, 2018; Okuno *et al.*, 2010) or indirect exposure via sunlight (e.g. occupations requiring extensive outdoor work). There is also emerging evidence of a relationship between sunlight and ultraviolet radiation exposure and an increased risk of age-related macular degeneration (Plestina-Borjan and Klinger-Lasic, 2007; Peate, 2007).

Adult onset myopia has been linked to occupations associated with an increased frequency of "near-work activities" (Simensen and Thorud, 1994). For example, one study documented the onset and progression of adult myopia among clinical microscopists (McBrien and Adams, 1997). A population-based survey of refractive errors observed a higher prevalence of myopia among professionals and clerks relative to other occupations (Wensor *et al.*, 1999). Similarly, in the Tanjong Pagar Study in Singapore, greater education, near work related occupations, and higher income were associated with myopic refractive errors (Wong *et al.*, 2002).

Other occupations are associated with higher risks of specific ocular disorders. For example, a higher risk of fungal infection of the cornea has long been associated with agricultural occupations (Lin *et al.*, 1999).

"Computer Vision Syndrome" is a clinical entity that has gained significant public attention in recent years due to the rapid digitisation of many workplaces (Munshi *et al.*, 2017). Symptoms include dry eyes, asthenopia, headaches, as well as induced refractive errors, and it has been identified as a common cause of unexplained visual disturbances (Bogdănici *et al.*, 2017). The main risk factors for this condition include duration of usage of digital devices, the brightness of the display, as well as the ambient hudmidity and illumination (Al Tawil *et al.*, 2020). Computer vision syndrome is extremely prevalent, with estimates of up to 90% of adult workers who use screens for at least three hours a day experiencing symptoms (Randolph, 2017). The management of this condition revolved primarily around prevention through education. Common strategies include the 20-20-20 rule: workers are encouraged to take a 20-s break to view something 20 feet away every 20 min. Other preventive measures include proper placement of screens to avaoid ambient glare, ergonomic workstations, and apropriate viewing distances.

Eye Protection and Prevention

Modern injury prevention theory does not support the claim that injuries are "accidents" or "bad luck" (Baker *et al.*, 1992). Most work-related ocular injuries occur in well-defined predictable and consistent settings and are hence potentially preventable.

There are a number of preventive strategies available. First, the exposure itself may be altered. For example, toxic chemicals can be redesigned or substituted by less toxic alternatives. Radiation doses may be reduced to decrease the risk of radiation injuries. Second, the work environment may be modified to reduce ocular hazards. Static shielding equipment's like transparent plastic boards may prevent foreign body and other mechanical injuries. Similarly, radiation barrier shields will decrease the risk of radiation injuries. Efficient exhaust systems that draw toxic fumes from the work area will help prevent chemical injuries. Appropriate provisions for first aid such as irrigating solutions and eye shields should also be in place at the workplace to reduce the morbidity from ocular injuries.

Third, personal ocular protective equipment is available to prevent nearly all types of injuries. This may range from general head and face protectors to goggles designed to prevent specific types of injuries (e.g. laser protective goggles) (Davies *et al.*, 2007; Okuno *et al.*, 2010; Hoskin *et al.*, 2019). Multiple studies have shown that adequate eye protective equipment in the workplace can prevent many serious eye injuries and makes economic sense (Wong and Tielsch, 2009). The efficacy of workplace eduation programmes promoting the use of eye protection has been variable. A randomised trial of worker education programmes has been conducted in quarry workers in India. An enhanced education programmed with repeated sessions of instruction over 6 months was able to increase compliance by 25% at 6 months, with corresponding reductions in eye trauma by 12% (Adams *et al.*, 2013). This study demonstrates that periodic reinforcement is necessary to improve compliance. Another study demonstrated that a personal experience of injury was more likely to result in compliance. Workers who had experienced injuries reported an increase in the proportion of work-time they used eye protection from a median of 20% to 100%. (Blackburn *et al.*, 2012) Most of the workers (66%) were more likely to use eye protection after sustaining an injury, and workers not using eye protection at the time of injury were more likely to use eye protection in the future.

A major problem is compliance among workers. This is partly related to poorly designed and uncomfortable eyewear as well as a lack of organisational emphasis on ocular safety, as typified in the military (Scott, 2011; Morley *et al.*, 2010). Interestingly, a survey on the depiction of protective eyewear use in the mass media showed that adequate protective eyewear was shown in only 12% of exposure scenes (Glazier *et al.*, 2010). Likewise, other studies have shown that 44–45% of workers sustained injuries despite wearing some form of eye protection (Ramakrishnan *et al.*, 2012; Thompson and Mollan, 2009). More attention should be directed to the development of ergonomic protective eyewear for use in occupational settings. Specific criteria for protective eyewear must be developed. Polycarbonate plastic lenses and frames which are sturdy and impact resistant provide optimal protection while lens-less goggles, street wear and spectacle correction glasses do not provide adequate eye protection (Simmons *et al.*, 1984). Other important design features include appropriate venting (indirect), and side shields (Peate, 2007). There must be increasing active participation from all ophthalmologists and occupational physicians in the prevention of work-related eye injuries, including addressing particular industrial needs, identifying high-risk workers and continued education to the public of the need for protective eyewear.

Conclusion

Occupational eye injuries can have diverse presentations but remain an important cause of workplace morbidity. The provision of appropriate eye protection, as well as education on their use, are effective in reducing incidence rates and further regulatory intervention in this regard is warranted.

References

Adams JS, Raju R, Solomon V. (2013) Increasing compliance with protective eyewear to reduce ocular injuries in stone-quarry workers in Tamil Nadu, India: A pragmatic, cluster randomised trial of a single education session versus an enhanced education package delivered over six months. *Injury* **44**: 118–125.

Al Tawil L, Aldokhayel S, Zeitouni L, Qadoumi T, Hussein S, Ahamed SS. (2020) Prevalence of self-reported computer vision syndrome symptoms and its associated factors among university students. *Eur J Ophthalmol* **30**(1): 189–195. Available from: doi: 10.1177/1120672118815110. Ansari EA. (1997) Ocular injury with xylene — a report of two cases. *Hum Exp Toxicol* **16**: 273–275.

Appleton B, Hirsch S, Kinion RO, Soles M, McCrossan GC, Neidlinger RM. (1975) Microwave lens effects in humans. II. Results of five-year survey. *Arch Ophthalmol* **93**: 257–258.

Baker SP, O"neill B, Ginsburg MJ, Li, G. (1992) *Occupational Injury. The injury fact book.* New York, Oxford University Press.

Baker RS, Wilson MR, Flowers CW, Lee DA, Wheeler NC. (1996) Demographic factors in a population-based survey of hospitalized, work-related, ocular injury. *Am J Ophthalmol* **122**: 213–219.

Baker RS, Wilson RM, Flowers CW, Lee DA, Wheeler NC. (1999) A population-based survey of hospitalized work-related ocular injury: Diagnoses, cause of injury, resource utilization, and hospitalization outcome. *Ophthalmic Epidemiol* **6**: 159–169.

Belkin M, Treister G, Dotan S. (1984) Eye injuries and ocular protection in the Lebanon War, 1982. *Isr J Med Sci* **20**: 333–338.

Bitarafan RA, Noohi F, Hashemi H. (2015) Ionizing radiation-induced cataract in interventional cardiology staff. *Res Cardiovasc Med* **4**: e25148.

Blackburn JL, Levitan EB, MacLennan PA, Owsley C, McGwin Jr, G. (2012) Changes in eye protection behavior following an occupational eye injury. *Workplace Health Saf* **60**(9): 393–400. Available from: doi: 10.1177/216507991206000904.

Brian G, Toit R, Ramke J, Szetu J. (2011) Population-based study of self-reported ocular trauma in Fiji. *Clin Experiment Ophthalmol* **39**(5): 441–448.

Bulbulia A, Shaik R, Khan N, Vayej S, Kistnasamy B, Page T. (1995) Ocular health status of chemical industrial workers. *Optom Vis Sci* **72**: 233–240.

Bogdănici CM, Săndulache DE, Nechita CA. (2017) Eyesight quality and Computer Vision Syndrome. *Rom J Ophthalmol* **61**(2): 112–116. Available from: doi:10.22336/rjo.2017.21.

Centers for Disease Control. (1984) Leading work-related diseases and injuries — United States. *MMWR* **33**: 213–215.

Chaikitmongkol V, Leeungurasatien T, Sengupta S. (2015) Work-related eye injuries: Important occupational health problem in Northern Thailand. *Asia Pac J Ophthalmol (Phila)* **4**: 155–160.

Chou BR, Cullen AP. (1996) Ocular hazards of industrial spot welding. *Optom Vis Sci* **73**: 424–427.

Ciraj-Bjelac O, Rehani M, Minamoto A, Sim KH, Liew HB, Vano E. (2012) Radiation-induced eye lens changes and risk for cataract in interventional cardiology. *Cardiology* **123**: 168–171.

Cruciani F, Lucchetta F, Regine F, Salandri AG, Abdolrahimzadeh B, Balacco GC. (1997) Work-related accidents of ophthalmologic interest in Italy during 1986–1991. *Ophthalmologica* **211**: 251–255.

Dandona L, Dandona R, Srinivas M, John RK, McCarty CA, Rao, GN. (2000) Ocular trauma in an urban population in southern India: The Andhra Pradesh eye disease study. *Clin Experiment Ophthalmol* **28**: 350–356.

Dannenberg AL, Parver LM, Brechner RJ, Khoo L. (1992) Penetration eye injuries in the workplace. The National Eye Trauma System Registry. *Arch Ophthalmol* **110**: 843–848.

Davies KG, Asanga U, Nku CO, Osim EE. (2007) Effect of chronic exposure to welding light on Calabar welders. *Niger J Physiol Sci* **22**: 55–58.

Desai P, MacEwen CJ, Baines P, Minassian DC. (1996) Incidence of cases of ocular trauma admitted to hospital and incidence of blinding outcome. *Br J Ophthalmol* **80**: 592–596.

Dolin PJ, Johnson GJ. (1994) Solar ultraviolet radiation and ocular disease: A review of the epidemiological and experimental evidence. *Ophthalmic Epidemiol* **1**: 155–164.

Fong LP, Taouk Y. (1995) The role of eye protection in work-related eye injuries. *Aust N Z J Ophthalmol* **23**: 101–106.

Forrest KY, Cali JM. (2009) Epidemiology of lifetime work-related eye injuries in the U.S. population associated with one or more lost days of work. *Ophthalmic Epidemiol* **16**: 156–162.

Foster PJ, Wong TY, Machin D, Johnson GJ, Seah SK. (2003) Risk factors for nuclear, cortical and posterior subcapsular cataracts in the Chinese population of Singapore: The Tanjong Pagar survey. *Br J Ophthalmol* **87**: 1112–1120.

Glazier R, Slade M, Mayer H. (2010) The depiction of protective eyewear use in popular television programs. *J Trauma* **70**(4): 965–969.

Glynn RJ, Seddon JM, Berlin BM. (1988) The incidence of eye injuries in New England adults. *Arch Ophthalmol* **106**: 785–789.

Goel R, Malik KP, Goel A, Sharma N, Aggarwal A. (2013) Agriculture related corneal injuries. *Nepal J Ophthalmol* **5**: 45–49.

Griffith GA, Jones NP. (1994) Eye injury and eye protection: A survey of the chemical industry. *Occup Med (Lond)* **44**: 37–40.

Han SB, Yu HG. (2010) Visual outcome after open globe injury and its predictive factors in Korea. *J Trauma* **69**: E66–E72.

Hong J, Qiu T, Wei A, Sun X, Xu J. (2010) Clinical characteristics and visual outcome of severe ocular chemical injuries in Shanghai. *Ophthalmology* **117**: 2268–2272.

Hoskin AK, Mackey DA, Keay L, Agrawal R, Watson S. (2019) Eye Injuries across history and the evolution of eye protection. *Acta Ophthalmol* **97**(6): 637–643.Available from: doi: 10.1111/aos.14086.

Ireland B, Acquavella J, Farrell T, Anne M, Fuhreman T. (1994) Evaluation of ocular health among alachlor manufacturing workers. *J Occup Med* **36**: 738–742.

Jafari AK, Anvari F, Ameri A, Bozorgui S, Shahverdi N. (2010) Epidemiology and sociodemographic aspects of ocular traumatic injuries in Iran. *Int Ophthalmol* **30**: 691–696.

Jones NP, Griffith GA. (1992) Eye injuries at work: A prospective population-based survey within the chemical industry. *Eye* **6**: 381–385.

Kanoff JM, Turalba AV, Andreoli MT, Andreoli CM. (2010) Characteristics and outcomes of work-related open globe injuries. *Am J Ophthalmol* **150**: 265–269.

Karai I, Horiguchi S. (1984) Pterygium in welders. *Br J Ophthalmol* **68**: 347–349.

Karlson TA, Klein BE. (1986) The incidence of acute hospital-treated eye injuries. *Arch Ophthalmol* **104**: 1473–1476.

Khatry SK, Lewis AE, Schein OD, Thapa MD, Pradhan EK, Katz J. (2004) The epidemiology of ocular trauma in rural Nepal. *Br J Ophthalmol* **88**: 456–460.

Klopfer J, Tielsch JM, Vitale S, See LC, Canner JK. (1992) Ocular trauma in the United States. Eye injuries resulting in hospitalization, 1984 through 1987. *Arch Ophthalmol* **110**: 838–842.

Krishnaiah S, Nirmalan PK, Shamanna BR, Srinivas M, Rao GN, Thomas R. (2006) Ocular trauma in a rural population of southern India: The Andhra Pradesh Eye Disease Study. *Ophthalmology* **113**: 1159–1164.

Kuhn F, Morris R, Witherspoon CD. (2002) Birmingham Eye Trauma Terminology (BETT): Terminology and classification of mechanical eye injuries. *Ophthalmol Clin North Am* **15**: 139–143.

Kuhn F, Maisiak R, Mann L, Mester V, Morris R, Witherspoon CD. (2002) The Ocular Trauma Score (OTS). *Ophthalmol Clin North Am* **15**: 163–165.

Kumar SG, Dharanipriya A. (2014) Prevalence and pattern of occupational injuries at workplace among welders in coastal south India. *Indian J Occup Environ Med* **18**: 135–139.

Kurz GH, Einaugler RB. (1968) Cataract secondary to microwave radiation. *Am J Ophthalmol* **66**: 866–869.

Lima-Gomez V, Blanco-Hernandez DM, Rojas-Dosal JA. (2010) Ocular trauma score at the initial evaluation of ocular trauma. *Cir Cir* **78**: 209–213.

Lin SH, Lin CP, Wang HZ, Tsai RK, Ho CK. (1999) Fungal corneal ulcers of onion harvesters in southern Taiwan. *Occup Environ Med* **56**: 423–425.

Loon SC, Tay WT, Saw SM, Wang JJ, Wong TY. (2009) Prevalence and risk factors of ocular trauma in an urban south-east Asian population: The Singapore Malay Eye Study. *Clin Exp Ophthalmol* **37**(4): 362–367. Available from: doi: 10.1111/j.1442-9071.2009.02035.x. PMID: 19594562.

MacEwen CJ. (1989) Eye injuries: A prospective survey of 5671 cases. *Br J Ophthalmol* **73**: 888–894.

Maneschg OA, Resch M, Papp A, Nemeth J. (2011) Prognostic factors and visual outcome for open globe injuries with intraocular foreign bodies. *Klin Monbl Augenheilkd* **228**(9): 801–807.

Marshall EC, Meetz RE. (1995) Ocular health status of chemical industrial workers. *Optom Vis Sci* **72**: 686–687.

McBrien NA, Adams DW. (1997) A longitudinal investigation of adult-onset and adult-progression of myopia in an occupational group. Refractive and biometric findings. *Invest Ophthalmol Vis Sci* **38**: 321–333.

McCall BP, Horwitz IB. (2006) Assessment of occupational eye injury risk and severity: An analysis of Rhode Island workers' compensation data 1998–2002. *Am J Ind Med* **49**(1): 45–53. Available from: doi:10.1002/ajim.20234. PMID: 16362940.Milacic S. (2009) Risk of occupational radiation-induced cataract in medical workers. *Med Lav* **100**: 178–186.

Modenese A, Gobba F. (2018) Cataract frequency and subtypes involved in workers assessed for their solar radiation exposure: A systematic review. *Acta Ophthalmol* **96**(8): 779–788. Available from: doi: 10.1111/aos.13734.Moran DJ, Hollows FC. (1984) Pterygium and ultraviolet radiation: A positive correlation. *Br J Ophthalmol* **68**: 343–346.

Morley MG, Nguyen JK, Heier JS, Shingleton BJ, Pasternak JF, Bower KS. (2010) Blast eye injuries: A review for first responders. *Disaster Med Public Health Prep* **4**: 154–160.

Morris RE, Witherspoon CD, Helms HA, Feist RM, Byrne JB. (1987) Eye injury registry of Alabama (preliminary report): Demographics and prognosis of severe eye injury. *South Med J* **80**: 810–816.

Munoz E. (1984) Economic costs of trauma, United States, 1982. *J Trauma* **24**: 237–244.

Munshi S, Ashley Varghese A, Dhar-Munshi S. (2017) Computer vision syndrome — A common cause of unexplained visual symptoms in the modern era. *Int J Clin Pract* **71**(7). Available from: doi: 10.1111/ijcp.12962.

National Society to Prevent Blindness. (1980) *National Society to Prevent Blindness: Fact Sheet.* New York, National Society to Prevent Blindness.

Négrel AD, Thylefors B. (1998) The global impact of eye injuries. *Ophthalmic Epidemiol* **5**(3): 143–169. Available from: doi: 10.1076/opep.5.3.143.8364.

Nirmalan PK, Katz J, Tielsch JM. (2004) Ocular trauma in a rural south Indian population: The Aravind Comprehensive Eye Survey. *Ophthalmology* **111**: 1778–1781.

Norn M, Franck C. (1991) Long-term changes in the outer part of the eye in welders. Prevalence of spheroid degeneration, pinguecula, pterygium, and corneal cicatrices. *Acta Ophthalmol (Copenh)* **69**: 382–386.

Northey LC, Bhardwaj G, Curran S, McGirr J. (2014) Eye trauma epidemiology in regional Australia. *Ophthalmic Epidemiol* **21**: 237–246.

Okuno T, Ojima J, Saito H. (2010) Blue-light hazard from CO2 arc welding of mild steel. *Ann Occup Hyg* **54**: 293–298.

Onakpoya OH, Adeoye A, Adeoti CO, Ajite K. (2010) Epidemiology of ocular trauma among the elderly in a developing country. *Ophthalmic Epidemiol* **17**: 315–320.

Owen CG, Margrain TH, Woodward EG. (1995) Aetiology and prevalence of eye injuries within the United Kingdom fire service. *Eye* **9**: 54–58.

Pashby T. (1985) Eye injuries in Canadian amateur hockey. *Can J Ophthalmol* **20**: 2–4.

Pashby TJ, Pashby RC, Chisholm LD, Crawford JS. (1975) Eye injuries in Canadian hockey. *Can Med Assoc J* **113**: 663–674.

Peate WF. (2007) Work-related eye injuries and illnesses. *Am Fam Physician* **75**: 1017–1022.

Plestina-Borjan I, Klinger-Lasic M. (2007) Long-term exposure to solar ultraviolet radiation as a risk factor for age-related macular degeneration. *Coll Antropol* **31**(1): 33–38.

Quandt SA, Schulz MR, Talton JW, Verma A, Arcury TA. (2012) Occupational eye injuries experienced by migrant farmworkers. *J Agromedicine* **17**: 63–69.

Ramakrishnan T, Constantinou M, Jhanji V, Vajpayee RB. (2012) Corneal metallic foreign body injuries due to suboptimal ocular protection. *Arch Environ Occup Health* **67**: 48–50.

Randolph SA. (2017) Computer Vision Syndrome. *Workplace Health Saf* **65**(7): 328. Available from: doi: 10.1177/2165079917712727.

Saari KM, Parvi V. (1984) Occupational eye injuries in Finland. *Acta Ophthalmol Suppl* **161**: 17–28.

Schein OD, Hibberd PL, Shingleton BJ. (1988) The spectrum and burden of ocular injury. *Ophthalmology* **95**: 300–305.

Scott R. (2011) The injured eye. *Philos Trans R Soc Lond B Biol Sci* **366**: 251–260.

Serinken M, Turkcuer I, Cetin EN, Yilmaz A, Elicabuk H, Karcioglu O. (2013) Causes and characteristics of work-related eye injuries in western Turkey. *Indian J Ophthalmol* **61**: 497–501.

Simensen B, Thorud LO. (1994) Adult-onset myopia and occupation. *Acta Ophthalmol (Copenh)* **72**: 469–471.

Simmons ST, Krohel GB, Hay PB. (1984) Prevention of ocular gunshot injuries using polycarbonate lenses. *Ophthalmology* **91**: 977–983.

Smith GS, Lincoln AE, Wong TY. (2005) Does occupation explain gender and other differences in work-related eye injury hospitalization rates? *J Occup Environ Med* **47**(6): 640–648. Available from: doi: 10.1097/01.jom.0000165746.26873.d1.

Tang FC, Chen SC, Lee HS, Lin WF, Chou MC, Lee MC. (1999) Relationship between pterygium/pinguecula and sunlight exposure among postmen in central Taiwan. *Zhonghua Yi Xue Za Zhi (Taipei)* **62**: 496–502.

Taylor HR. (1982) Ultraviolet radiation and pterygium. *JAMA* **247**: 1698.

Taylor HR, West SK, Rosenthal FS, Munoz B, Newland HS, Emmett EA. (1989) Corneal changes associated with chronic UV irradiation. *Arch Ophthalmol* **107**: 1481–1484.

Tenkate T, Adam B, Al-Rifai RH, Chou BR, Gobba F, Ivanov ID, Leppink N, Loney T, Pega F, Peters CE, Prüss-Üstün AM, Silva Paulo M, Ujita Y, Wittlich M, Modenese A. (2019) WHO/ILO work-related burden of disease and injury: Protocol for systematic reviews of occupational exposure to solar ultraviolet radiation and of the effect of occupational exposure to solar ultraviolet radiation on cataract. *Environ Int* **125**: 542–553.

Tielsch JM, Parver L, Shankar B. (1989) Time trends in the incidence of hospitalized ocular trauma. *Arch Ophthalmol* **107**: 519–523.

Tielsch JM. (1995) Frequency and consequences of ocular trauma. A population perspective. *Ophthalmol Clin North Am* **8**: 559–567.

Thompson GJ, Mollan SP. (2009) Occupational eye injuries: A continuing problem. *Occup Med (Lond)* **59**: 123–125.

Vano E, Gonzalez L, Beneytez F, Moreno F. (1998) Lens injuries induced by occupational exposure in non-optimized interventional radiology laboratories. *Br J Radiol* **71**: 728–733.

Vinger PF, Vinger (1994) The eye and sports medicine. In: Tasman, W, Jaeger, EA. (eds.), *Duane's Clinical Ophthalmology*. Philadelphia, J.B. Lippincott, pp. 1–103.

Viso E, Gude F, Rodriguez-Ares MT. (2010) Prevalence of pinguecula and pterygium in a general population in Spain. *Eye (Lond)* **25**(3): 350–357.

Voon LW, Wong TY, See J, Tan DT. (1998) Epidemiology of eye trauma in Singapore: Perspective from a major eye casualty center. *Invest Ophthalmol Vis Sci* **39**: 637.

Wensor M, McCarty CA, Taylor HR. (1999) Prevalence and risk factors of myopia in Victoria, Australia. *Arch Ophthalmol* **117**: 658–663.

White MF, Morris R, Feist RM, Witherspoon CD, Helms HA, John GR. (1989) Eye injury: Prevalence and prognosis by setting. *South Med J* **82**: 151–158.

Wong TY, Tielsch JM. (2009) Epidemiology of ocular trauma. In: Tasman, W, Jaeger, EA. (eds.), *Duane's Foundations of Clinical Ophthalmology*. Philadelphia, J.B. Lippincott, pp. 1–13.

Wong TY, Tielsch JM. (1999) A population-based study on the incidence of severe ocular trauma in Singapore. *Am J Ophthalmol* **128**: 345–351.

Wong TY, Lincoln A, Tielsch JM, Baker SP. (1998) The epidemiology of ocular injury in a major US automobile corporation. *Eye* **12**: 870–874.

Wong TY, Seet B. (1997) A behavioral analysis of eye protection use by soldiers. *Mil Med* **162**: 744–748.

Wong TY, Foster PJ, Johnson GJ, Seah SK, Tan DT. (2001) The prevalence and risk factors for pterygium in an adult Chinese population in Singapore: The Tanjong Pagar survey. *Am J Ophthalmol* **131**: 176–183.

Wong TY, Foster PJ, Johnson GJ, Seah SK. (2002) Education, socioeconomic status, and ocular dimensions in Chinese adults: The Tanjong Pagar Survey. *Br J Ophthalmol* **86**: 963–968.

Yokota K, Johyama Y, Yamaguchi K, Takeshita T, Morimoto K. (1999) Exposure-response relationships in rhinitis and conjunctivitis caused by methyltetrahydrophthalic anhydride. *Int Arch Occup Environ Health* **72**: 14–18.

Zhang Y, Zhang MN, Qiu HY. (2009) Epidemiological characteristics of eye injury among soldiers in 15 military hospitals. *Zhonghua Liu Xing Bing Xue Za Zhi* **30**: 740–742.

Chapter 15

Metabolic and Endocrine Disorders

Eng Loon Tng and See Muah Lee*,†,‡*

Introduction

Obesity, diabetes mellitus (DM) and thyroid disorders are metabolic and endocrine conditions that the occupational physician will encounter frequently. Adrenal insufficiency (AI) is encountered less commonly but has important effects on work performance. This chapter discusses how work affect these conditions and vice versa. It describes the central role of the occupational physician in treating these conditions while integrating input from the employees, employers and other medical specialists.

Overweight and Obesity in the Workplace

The World Health Organization (WHO, 2020) defines overweight and obesity as states of abnormal or excessive fat accumulation that predispose to poor health. The body mass index (BMI) is a widely accepted indicator of weight. It is calculated by dividing weight in kilograms by the square of height in metres. The BMI is simple

* Ng Teng Fong General Hospital, National University Health System, Singapore.
† Saw Swee Hock School of Public Health, National University of Singapore, Singapore.
‡ Centre for Biomedical Ethics, National University of Singapore, Singapore.
Corresponding author: Eng Loon Tng (Eng_Loon_Tng@nuhs.edu.sg).

to calculate and it correlates well with fatness (Sun *et al.*, 2010). However, this correlation is imperfect and its association with adverse outcomes is weak (Flegal and Graubard, 2009). Moreover, Asians have higher fat mass for the same BMI when compared to Europids and Americans (WHO Expert Consultation, 2004). Table 1 shows the classification of overweight and obesity based on BMI (National Institutes of Health, 1998).

The waist circumference (WC) is another measure of weight. It is measured in a horizontal plane midway between the inferior margin of the ribs and the superior border of the iliac crest. WC is a good predictor of cardiovascular disease (CVD) (Yoshida *et al.*, 2009). The classification of overweight and obesity based on WC differs between ethnicities because body composition differs among races (Table 2) (Misra *et al.*, 2005).

Table 1. Classification of Overweight and Obesity Based on BMI

Classification	BMI Cut-off (Non-Asians) (kg/m^2)	BMI Cut-off (Asians) (kg/m^2)
Underweight	<18.5	<18.5
Normal	18.5–24.9	18.5–22.9
Overweight	25.0–29.9	23.0–27.4
Class 1 Obesity	30.0–34.9	≥27.5
Class 2 Obesity	35.0–39.9	—
Class 4 Obesity	50.0–59.9	—
Class 5 Obesity	≥60.0	—

Table 2. Ethnic-specific Values for Waist Circumference (adapted from Janssen *et al.*, 2004; Misra *et al.*, 2005; Wells, 2009)

Country/Ethnic Group	Waist Circumference
Europids (Caucasoids)	Females: ≥80 cm
	Males: ≥94 cm
South Asians (based on Chinese, Malay, and Asian-Indian population)	Females: ≥80 cm
	Males: ≥90 cm
Chinese	Females: ≥80 cm
	Males: ≥90 cm

Table 2. (*Continued*)

Country/Ethnic Group	Waist Circumference
Japanese	Females: ≥80 cm
	Males: ≥90 cm
Ethnic South and Central Americans	Use South Asian recommendations until more information is available
Sub-Saharan Africans	Use European recommendations until more information is available
Eastern Mediterranean and Middle East (Arab) populations	Use European recommendations until more information is available

General Facts on Obesity

The incidence of overweight and obesity is rising. 1.9 billion adults were overweight and 650 million adults were obese in 2016. More than 4 million people died from conditions related to excessive weight in 2017. The obesity epidemic occurs globally but the trend is concentrated in the urban areas of low- and middle-income countries (WHO, 2020). Body fat accumulates when energy consumption exceeds expenditure. Complex interactions between genes, behaviour and the environment facilitate fat accumulation under permissive conditions. Overweight and obesity increase the risk for many non-communicable diseases (Table 3).

Impact of Obesity on Work Performance and Stigmatisation

Obesity is associated with a higher frequency of absenteeism (Nexo *et al.*, 2018). Obese workers may have limited access to well-fitting personal protective equipment and be prone to musculoskeletal injuries or vibration-induced injuries (Walker-Bone *et al.*, 2003). Obese workers also have a higher frequency of compensation claims (Robroek *et al.*, 2013) and may require longer recovery periods following injuries (Bungum *et al.*, 2003). The loss of productivity and medical burden to employers can lead to discrimination of large-sized workers.

Table 3. Complications of Obesity

System	Examples
Cardiovascular System	CVD Varicose veins
Metabolic System	Dyslipidaemia Hypertension Type 2 DM
Respiratory System	Asthma Obesity Hypoventilation Syndrome Obstructive Sleep Apnoea
Gastrointestinal System	Gastro-oesophageal Reflux Disease Non-alcoholic Fatty Liver Disease Non-alcoholic Hepatic Steatohepatitis
Genitourinary System	Infertility Obstetric Complications Urinary Incontinence
Neuropsychiatric System	Depression Pseudotumour Cerebri
Musculoskeletal System	Osteoarthritis
Cancers	Breast Colon Endometrium

Obesity as a risk factor for occupational diseases

Pandalai *et al.* (2013) developed a series of models to describe the role of obesity as a risk factor for occupational diseases and the role of workplace factors in causing or aggravating obesity and its complications.

Model A: Obesity and occupational factors can act in conjunction to cause diseases.

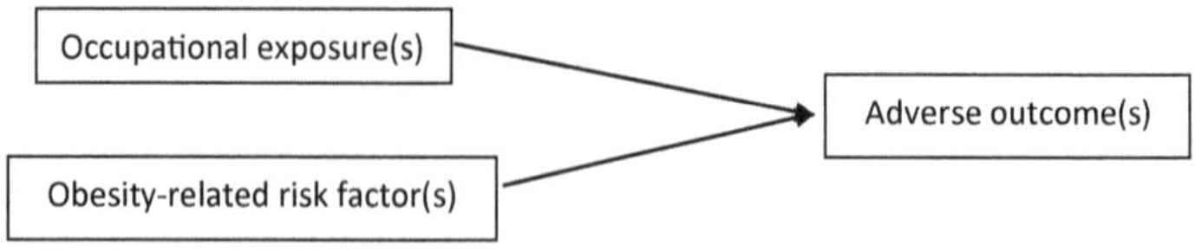

Increased soft tissue volume in obesity causes median nerve compression. Similarly, with poor ergonomics, carpal tunnel syndrome can arise. Obesity was reported to be a risk factor for accentuation of occupation-related carpal tunnel syndrome (Wieslander *et al.*, 1989; Tanaka *et al.*, 1997).

Model B: Obesity can exacerbate the risk for occupational diseases.

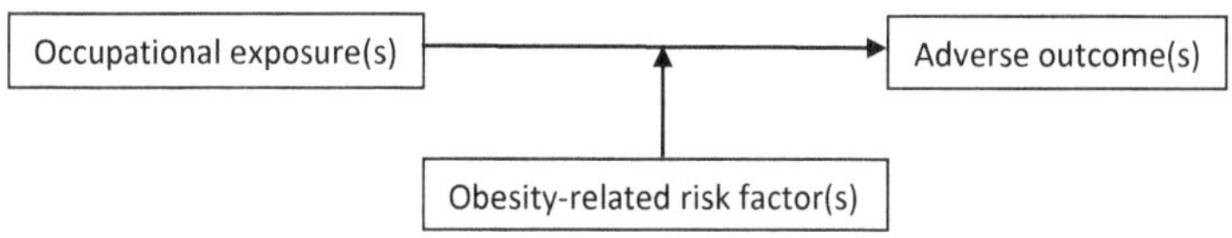

Nitrogen has higher solubility in fat so obese divers have more dissolved nitrogen in their bodies. They require longer periods of decompression when ascending from depths. The Norwegian Guidelines for Occupational Divers permit a maximum body fat content of 30% for vocational divers (Statens Helsetilsyn, 2000). Various naval authorities cap the body weight of divers at 20% above ideal weight while body fat content is limited at 22% in males and 28% in females. Obesity also increases the risk of biomagnification of xenobiotics and persistent organic pollutants in workers exposed to such substances (Li *et al.*, 2006).

Model C: Occupational factors can aggravate diseases arising from obesity.

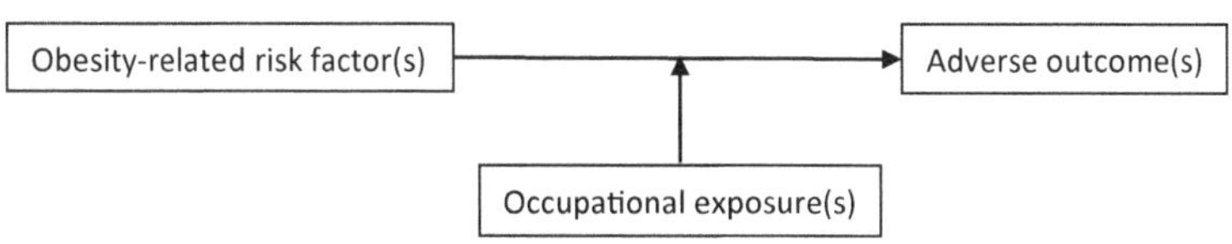

Asthma symptoms can be more severe in obese people due to heavier thoracic walls, weaker respiratory muscles and underlying obesity hypoventilation syndrome. Occupational exposure to triggers can cause occupational asthma or worsen the control of pre-existing asthma in obese people (Zammit *et al.*, 2010).

Model D: Occupational factors and obesity can each cause diseases that interact with each other.

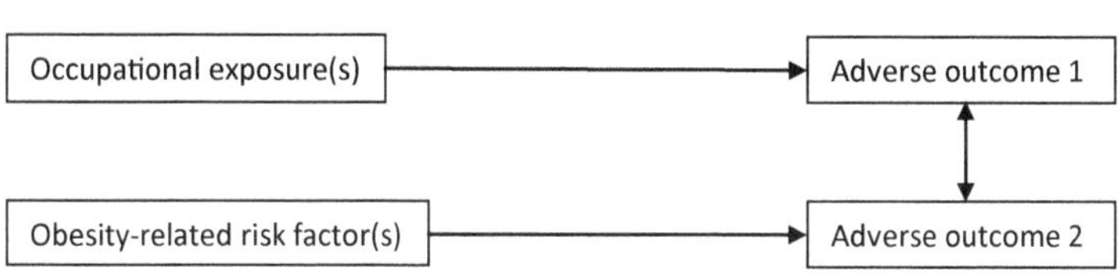

Chronic noise exposure was associated with CVD (Gan *et al.*, 2011) and hypertension (Attarchi *et al.*, 2013). The relationship between obesity, hypertension and CVD is well-established. It is plausible an occupational link between these conditions exist. Furthermore, obesity increases the risk for microvascular complications in DM, which may aggravate vibration-induced injuries in obese people (Fan *et al.*, 2015).

Assessing fitness to work in overweight and obese people

The assessment of job fitness is based on objective evaluation of the specific demands of the job and the suitability of the individual. Body weight should not be considered in the work assessment if it does not cause unacceptable added health risks or diminished work ability. Furthermore, overweight and obese workers who are fit and active may cope better with physically demanding jobs than slim but sedentary ones. Objective evaluations can be undertaken together with supervisors. A refinery recruiting operator has brought prospective applicants for onsite hands on testing of tasks, such as opening valves and handling stretchers and fire-fighting equipment. Some overweight workers have demonstrated acceptable agility and lifting strength.

Workplace adaptations for overweight and obese people

Workplace modifications should facilitate work for larger-sized workers. Simple measures include tailored uniform and personal protection equipment. Custom-made furniture may be costlier and complicated

Box 1. Sensitive Human Resource Management.

"I was extremely delighted to get the job, even more so when I reported for work, and noticed that my chair was extra large. That's what I call a good HR manager."

— A person with BMI of 40 kg/m^2

"Not to employ someone because of pre-conceived stereotyping about obesity might mean losing out on real talent. Some accommodations are really very simple to make."

— HR manager

to install. Altering the physical construct of the workplace is more challenging and older buildings may not be designed for the larger habitus of a new population. Consequently, employers may need to re-design certain areas such as escape hatches, ladders, elevators and confined spaces, which can be costly. Employers must bear in mind that adaptations for larger-sized workers may be non-ergonomic for smaller-sized ones. Having current and predicted anthropometric data of workers can facilitate such decisions.

Health promotion programmes in the workplace

Obesity is a common theme for health promotion programmes in the workplace as well as a popular subject for employee assistance programmes. Reasons to support health promotion programmes in the workplace include the significant amounts of time people spend at work, access to occupational health services and convenience in manipulating menus in staff canteens. Investments in health promotion programmes are aimed at lowering health care costs for companies.

Healthy lifestyle promotion campaigns, with their highly publicised nature, brings discomfiting attention to obese workers. Such campaigns may propagate the misconception that obesity is solely the outcome of indulgent lifestyle choices and often fail to highlight the complex pathophysiology of obesity that are beyond

Box 2. Quotable Quotes, What Works and What Does Not.

"We were given a half hour off to listen to an exercise trainer and a dietician. He told us to walk 10,000 steps a day. The dietician told us to eat less. I am already way beyond that. It was a total waste of time. Who are these people?"

"Leave me alone, I can take care of my health, and I am happy being fat. My unhappiness comes from you telling me to lose weight."

"I love the idea of the company gym. I do a half hour workout, bathe and change and am ready for a hard day's work. I wonder why so few people make use of it. It has always been there for as long as I can remember."

"I work in a hospital. I know it is bad for the image of a health care worker to be overweight."

(*Continued*)

Box 2. (***Continued***)

"The manager in my unit looks at me and I can sense her pity and contempt. There is a weight loss programme, where all the big-sized staff are encouraged to sign up. We have to attend work half an hour earlier in order to attend the gym class. I am still unable to lose weight. It is all so depressing."

"I eat all the fruits I need daily at the staff canteen. I am too lazy to shop for them. It is great."

"Strange, but I am getting used to the idea of fruits at meetings, rather than all the sticky sweet confectionery."

"My colleagues and managers were supportive. There was no pressure. I walk more, I try to diet, even though it is not successful all the time. I have not lost weight, but I have not lost hope."

"I am a marketing executive. I travel a lot to the Far East. There is a culture of eating and drinking in business entertainment. It is considered rude in certain places to refuse the offer of food. How you behave can affect client relations. Worst part is, I put on weight very easily."

individual control. Obese workers may feel targeted and stigmatised as a result.

Employers should be mindful of the ethical dimension of obesity intervention programmes. Compulsory or subtly coerced participation in health promotion programmes may not be justified if a worker does not desire to lose weight. Weight loss is holistically beneficial if it can be achieved voluntarily, safely and enthusiastically. Poorly planned and executed health promotion programmes can cause anxiety, depression and lowered self-esteem in the obese worker.

Summary Points

- Obesity is a risk factor for many morbid conditions.
- When assessing fitness to work, look for additional risks created for the obese worker at work, compared to when he is not at work, and propose appropriate risk reduction measures.
- Employers can help to promote a healthy lifestyle. However, this should be done in a supportive and sensitive manner.

Diabetes Mellitus in the Workplace

DM is defined by the American Diabetes Association as "a complex chronic illness requiring continuous medical care with multifactorial risk-reduction strategies beyond glycaemic control" (American Diabetes Association, 2020a).

Classification and Pathophysiology of Diabetes Mellitus

DM is classified by its aetiology and presentation into four main types (American Diabetes Association, 2020b):

1. Type 1 DM (T1DM)
2. Type 2 DM (T2DM)
3. Gestational DM
4. Specific types of DM due to other causes (Secondary DM)

The incidence of DM is rising rapidly. In 2000, 151 million adults have DM worldwide. In 2009, 285 million adults have DM, and in 2019, 463 million adults have DM. The rate of rise in prevalence of DM is faster in low- and middle-income countries. 4.2 million deaths were attributed to DM in 2019 (International Diabetes Federation, 2020).

Glycaemic Targets for Diabetes Mellitus

Strict glycaemic control is beneficial in DM. The Diabetes Control and Complications Trial Research Group (Diabetes Control and Complications Trial Research Group *et al.*, 1993; United Kingdom Prospective Diabetes Study, 1998) and Kumamoto Study (Ohkubo *et al.*, 1995) proved intensive glucose control reduced microvascular complications. The UKPDS in its follow-up study showed reduction in CVD in the intensive glucose control group (Holman *et al.*, 2008). The EMPA-REG OUTCOME trial showed that treatment of DM using sodium-glucose co-transporter type 2 inhibitors can prevent

CVD within 6 months, making it the first class of anti-diabetes medication that is proven to prevent CVD independent of HbA1c-lowering effect (Zinman *et al.*, 2015).

However, strict glycaemic control poses the risk for polypharmacy and hypoglycaemia. Some of the therapeutic agents, notably insulin and sulphonylureas can cause weight gain. The Action to Control Cardiovascular Risk in Diabetes study showed an increased rate of mortality in older patients with long-standing DM and multiple comorbidities (Action to Control Cardiovascular Risk in Diabetes Study Group Study Group *et al.*, 2008). Consequently, guidelines now recommend individualised glycaemic targets for people with DM based on shared-decision making processes. The main considerations in reaching mutually-agreed targets include:

- Age
- BMI
- Comorbidities, complications from medications and cost of medications
- Duration of DM

As a guide, younger patients with few comorbidities and shorter duration of DM may strive for intensive control (HbA1c at 6.5% or lower) while older patients with multiple diseases and whom are more sensitive to hypoglycaemia may aim for relaxed targets.

The Impact of Diabetes Mellitus on Occupational Diseases and Work Capacity

DM and its complications can affect work performance and predispose workers to workplace injuries. Workers with DM are more likely to be absent from work and experience work limitations compared to those without DM (Dray-Spira *et al.*, 2013; Nexo *et al.*, 2018). Blue collar workers with DM in the United States of America (USA) had a 17% increased risk for workplace injury (Kubo *et al.*, 2014).

Stigmatisation from Diabetes Mellitus

12% of workers with DM reported being stigmatised in a Singaporean study (Lee *et al.*, 2015). In a similar study in Switzerland, the rate of workplace discrimination was between 5% and 11% (Nebiker-Pedrotti *et al.*, 2009). Severe hypoglycaemia, DM complications, older age, certain ethnic groups and employment by small employers were risk factors for stigmatisation in people with DM (McMahon *et al.*, 2005). Interestingly, Lee *et al.* (2011) found that insulin injection was not a stigma marker, and postulated that modern insulin administration methods and increasing public knowledge on DM helped in reducing the stigma.

Diabetes Mellitus Causation and Aggravation by Occupational Factors

Occupational exposures can predispose people to T2DM. A meta-analysis of observational studies found a high odds ratio for DM in male shift workers (Gan *et al.*, 2015). This is possibly explained by food consumption during the night shift when there is increased insulin resistance (Knutsson and Kempe 2014; Suwazono *et al.*, 2009).

Workplace factors can also interfere with DM control. Irregular mealtimes from shift work is disruptive to timely insulin administration in people with T1DM. Shift work also interferes with circadian rhythm and worsens insulin resistance (Cappuccio *et al.*, 2010), which worsens glycaemic control in T2DM.

Assessing the Fitness to Work in People with Diabetes Mellitus

"Blanket bans" of people with DM from certain occupations are inappropriate because people with adequately controlled DM lead normal lives and can be gainfully employed. When deciding to employ people with DM, the decision should be based on the person's capabilities to meet the demands of the job. As the impact of DM and its management varies widely between people, the decision should be individualised. A well-motivated worker with optimally controlled DM should face little difficulties in performing the job while a worker with poor glycaemic control may compromise public safety. The provision of countermeasures for the latter may mitigate safety concerns.

The assessment of occupational fitness of people with DM should be performed by health care professionals experienced in treating DM and who are familiar with the demands of specific jobs. Multidisciplinary assessment involving the potential employee, worksite supervisor, occupational physician and diabetologist may be helpful. Independent assessment by an expert physician can be considered when there are conflicts of opinions between stakeholders.

When assessing occupational fitness of people with DM, up-to-date information on the DM status should be sought. Hyperglycaemia does not usually cause immediate incapacitation but cognitive performance can be compromised when blood glucose levels exceed 15 mmol/L (Cox *et al.*, 2005). A person's capacity to perform the specific job safely can be assessed based on the following (American Diabetes Association, 2009).

Glycaemic control

Regular HbA1c readings and blood glucose levels guide the treatment of DM. By themselves, the measurements do not determine the capacity to perform a job safely. In safety sensitive jobs or when control is not stable, self-monitoring of blood glucose is encouraged. Blood glucose records allow the patient and physician to detect hypoglycaemia and hyperglycaemia, understand the circumstances of each measurement, correlate with biological cues and adjust management.

Presence of diabetes complications

Diabetes complications may interfere with specific aspects of the job. The disabilities may be compensated by workplace accommodation. Employees with complications should be referred for evaluation by the relevant specialists.

Work environment and the specific task requirements of the job

Shift work patterns and their impact on timing of medications and meal times, and intensity of work activity should be ascertained. The availability of accompanying colleagues, accommodation of affected employees and access to medical help should be clarified. A task analysis of the job to examine which parts of a job are at high risk and therefore requiring special attention can be performed. There has to be a balance between what is seen as a recommendation over indulgence to the worker with DM against concerns of public safety, and the protection of the economic interests of employers.

Case Study 1: Copyeditor with Poorly Controlled Diabetes Mellitus

Miss Y is a copyeditor with poorly controlled DM. Her HbA1c was above 9% for several years. She is now 45 years old and has blurring of vision lately. She is worried about the impact of diabetic retinopathy on her career.

Discussion

Visual loss from diabetic retinopathy can clearly affect her job as a copyeditor. Early ophthalmological intervention and optimising glycaemic control will help to arrest deterioration of the diabetic retinopathy. Clinical trials have demonstrated that approximately eight years are needed before microvascular complications are prevented by strict glycaemic control. This emphasises the need for early diabetic eye screening and adherence to treatment. If Miss Y has significant visual impairment, she should be referred to specialised centers for visual rehabilitation.

Hypoglycaemia and its special challenges

Hypoglycaemia can occur suddenly in people with DM. When severe, neuroglycopaenia occurs and impairs cognition and work capacity (Nilsson *et al.*, 2019). The frequency and severity of hypoglycaemia must be evaluated during the job assessment for people with DM

(American Diabetes Association, 2005). The foremost concern is to determine if the worker can become incapacitated from severe hypoglycaemia and to examine its potential impact on public safety. Some countries mandatorily exclude people with DM from driving heavy goods vehicles and public transport, firefighting, flying aeroplanes or in combat military positions because of the concern of hypoglycaemia in employees with DM.

Fortunately, with education and awareness, most people with DM can manage their hypoglycaemia. When a worker has hypoglycaemia, the circumstances leading to the episode should be evaluated. A single episode of severe hypoglycaemia should not necessarily constitute a reason for termination of employment. However, recurrent severe

Table 4. American Diabetes Association Workgroup on Hypoglycaemia Classification

Classification	Definition
Severe Hypoglycaemia	An event requiring assistance of another person to actively administer carbohydrate, glucagon or other resuscitative actions. These episodes may be associated with sufficient neuroglycopaenia to induce seizure or coma. Plasma glucose measurements may not be available during such an event, but neurological recovery attributable to the restoration of plasma glucose to normal is considered sufficient evidence that the event was induced by a low plasma glucose concentration.
Documented Symptomatic Hypoglycaemia	An event during which typical symptoms of hypoglycaemia are accompanied by a measured plasma glucose concentration ≤3.9 mmol/L.
Asymptomatic Hypoglycaemia	An event not accompanied by typical symptoms of hypoglycaemia but with a measured plasma glucose concentration ≤3.9 mmol/L.
Probable Symptomatic Hypoglycaemia	An event during which symptoms of hypoglycaemia are not accompanied by a plasma glucose determination but was presumably caused by a plasma glucose concentration ≤3.9 mmol/L. Since many people with DM choose to treat symptoms with oral carbohydrate without a test of plasma glucose, it is important to recognise these events as "probable" hypoglycaemia.

Table 4. (*Continued*)

Classification	Definition
Relative Hypoglycaemia	An event during which the person with DM reports any of the typical symptoms of hypoglycaemia, and interprets those as indicative of hypoglycaemia, but with a measured plasma glucose concentration >3.9 mmol/L. This category reflects the fact that patients with chronically poor glycaemic control can experience symptoms of hypoglycaemia at plasma glucose levels >3.9 mmol/L as plasma glucose concentration decline toward that level. Though causing distress and interfering with the person's sense of well-being, and potentially limiting the achievement of optimal glycaemic control, such episodes probably pose no direct harm.

hypoglycaemia should render a person unsafe to work, at least until hypoglycaemia resolves. The occupational physician should, in conjunction with a diabetologist, evaluate the risk for recurrence of these episodes and examine ways to prevent hypoglycaemia. The risk assessment of the tasks specifically related to the intensity and nature of physical work involved should be evaluated. The availability of colleagues and accessibility to medical help are pertinent factors.

The meal times and medications of the worker should be checked to prevent further hypoglycaemia. Oral agents with low risks for hypoglycaemia can be chosen in this setting. These include metformin, incretin mimetics, incretin enhancers, glitazones, alpha-glucosidase inhibitors and sodium-glucose cotransporter type 2 inhibitors. The risks of hypoglycaemia associated with the use of sulphonylureas and insulin, their predicted onset, peak and duration of action, especially with the prandial insulins, should be explained to the worker. Insulin analogues (e.g. insulin aspart, lispro, glulisine, glargine, detemir, degludec or glargine U300) may be substituted for the conventional insulins because of their rapid onset, shorter duration of action or peakless action that may minimise the risk of hypoglycaemia. In highly motivated and educated workers with T1DM, continuous glucose monitoring and/or continuous subcutaneous insulin infusion pumps can be considered (Yeoh *et al.*, 2015).Workers with recurrent hypoglycaemia should have their glycaemic targets relaxed and assessed for hypoglycaemia unawareness. This is a condition where a person loses neurogenic perception of hypoglycaemia because of altered warning threshold from repeated uncorrected hypoglycaemia. People with hypoglycaemia unawareness can develop neuroglycopaenia without warning symptoms. Scrupulous avoidance of hypoglycaemia leads to recovery of hypoglycaemia awareness within weeks. The worker should perform monitoring of blood glucose levels and correlate the measurements to internal biological cues. Blood glucose awareness training has been proven effective in reducing driving mishaps (Cox *et al.*, 2001). It is reasonable to infer that such structured programmes would be helpful for the worker with DM performing safety sensitive tasks.

The affected worker and perhaps co-workers should be instructed on rescue measures for hypoglycaemia (Box 3). Cognitive recovery from hypoglycaemia may take up to an hour (Zammitt *et al.*, 2008) so the worker must not resume safety sensitive duties during this period.

The risk assessment and decision matrix for the employment of people with DM and hypoglycaemia is shown in Table 5 (Lee *et al.*, 2011).

The evaluation for hypoglycaemia should be customised to the context of the job duties. An example would be the condominium guard who is not expected to give chase to burglars but to call for help when needed. The resultant risks from hypoglycaemia is low. Any number of contentious job situations can be imagined: a croupier working in a casino, a clerk in a bank, an airport baggage handler, a dispatch driver or a safety inspector required to check on confined space; the list goes on. In all cases, an individualised risk assessment has to be applied.

Case Study 2: Diabetic Newly Started on Insulin

Mr. X is 32-year-old man with T2DM. He was newly started on twice-daily insulin injections. He works in a dispatch company and his duties include packing and transferring loads. He is required to do this for most of his working hours, although up to one quarter of his time may be spent

Table 5. Risk Assessment and Decision Matrix for Hypoglycaemia

		American Diabetes Association Classification of Hypoglycaemia		
			Documented Symptomatic Hypoglycaemia	Severe Hypoglycaemia
		Relative Hypoglycaemia	Probable Symptomatic Hypoglycaemia without Blood Glucose Determination	Hypoglycaemia Unawareness
Consequence to Others, Life and Property	Mild Consequences, e.g. Office Environment, Presence of Colleagues	A	A	B
	Moderate Consequences, e.g. Assembly Lines, Hot-Work and Crane Operation (with Colleagues)	A	A	C
	Moderate Consequences, e.g. Assembly Lines, Hot-work and Crane Operation (Alone)	A	B	C
	Severe Consequences, e.g. Firearm Handling	B	C	C

Notes:

A. Intensify medical intervention. Continuous improvement.

B. Intensify medical intervention. Urgent action — discuss with employer, may need to enhance work operations (including increased supervision and surveillance).

C. Intensify medical intervention. Immediate action — discuss with employer, may need temporary removal from task and job until remedial action has been taken and completed.

on sedentary work. Overtime work of two hours is required at least twice a week.

Since starting insulin, he has been experiencing late morning giddiness, sweating and tremors. His doctor however has insisted that he copes with it, because in the long run, a "low HbA1c is good for him."

Discussion

Mr. X needs advice and discussion on the management of hypoglycaemia. In the immediate short term, he must be instructed on how to respond appropriately to hypoglycaemia by consuming rapid-acting carbohydrate (Box 3). He appears to have hypoglycaemia awareness. If necessary, he should be referred to a diabetologist and adjustments made to his treatment. Meals, timing, dosage, choice of insulin and self-monitoring of blood glucose all have a role to play.

A further consideration is the operation of heavy machinery at work by Mr. X. Working at height is also contraindicated until hypoglycaemia is prevented. Depending on the severity and extent to which hypoglycaemia can be immediately remedied, his job may have to be modified in the interim. An individualised risk assessment, with periodic reviews, has to be made before establishing any opinion on his fitness for the job.

Box 3. Rescue for Hypoglycaemia.

Consume 15 grams of Simple Carbohydrate as Found in:

- Glucose tablets (follow package instructions)
- Glucose gel (follow package instructions)
- 2 tablespoons of raisins
- 4 ounces (1/2 cup) of fruit juice or regular soda (non-diet)
- 1 tablespoon of sugar, honey or corn syrup

It may be necessary to have a longer-acting carbohydrate, such as a few biscuits, a piece of fruit or a sandwich, especially if the next meal is some hours away.

Monitor Blood Sugar

Workplace Adaptations for Workers with Diabetes Mellitus

Workplace adaptations allow workers with DM to realise their full productivity. The USA and United Kingdom (UK) have legislation to ensure employers adopt reasonable modifications to provide fair workplace opportunities for workers with DM. The adaptations should be individualised and targeted at enhancing daily DM self-care and at preventing or alleviating diabetes complications. For example, food labelling can facilitate carbohydrate counting and promote adherence to dietetic advice.

Prior to employment, the employee with DM needs to negotiate with the employer on meal flexibility, breaks for blood glucose monitoring, facilities for safe disposal of insulin needles and safe storage of insulin vials. Employees with DM may need flexible working hours to attend diabetes clinics. Workers with poor glycaemic control may need to ask for fewer shift work to enhance glycaemic control. Visual aids for diabetic retinopathy may be needed.

Disclosure of Medical Information

Employees with DM should ideally have open relationships with their employers and colleagues so that their colleagues are aware of the chronic condition and accommodate it. However, employees with DM may not wish to disclose their condition for various reasons, particularly from fear of discrimination by employers and colleagues. Disclosure of the DM status is encouraged because colleagues can help to respond appropriately during emergencies. Veiling the condition in secrecy can aggravate the stigmatisation.

Disclosure of medical conditions, as a condition for employment, is a matter for negotiation between the employer and the employee. How the employer and the employee wish the physician to play a role in this has to be clarified and must not compromise the doctors' ethical position. Doctors are health advocates for workers. Employers have legitimate economic interests to protect. Disclosure by the physician in the absence of consent by the worker is a breach of patient confidentiality. It can be sanctioned only if legislatively driven or if the physician can show justification based on public interest, such as the case of a patient with erratic glycaemic control who has to handle firearms.

Summary Points

- DM is a chronic and progressive condition that requires a multi-faceted approach in its medical management. Risks associated with hypoglycaemia, hyperglycaemia, macrovascular and microvascular complications have to be regularly monitored and managed.
- The employment of people with DM may be regulated by legislation in specific industries.
- Consider the additional risk to the person with DM at work compared to when not at work. Consider how these risks can be reduced.
- Consider the risk created for other colleagues or the public when a worker with DM is employed.

Hyperthyroidism in the Workplace

Hyperthyroidism is a state of excess thyroid hormone production by the thyroid gland leading to thyrotoxicosis, a state of excess thyroid hormone action on the body. Overt hyperthyroidism is defined as a thyroid stimulating hormone (TSH) level below the reference interval with a concurrent thyroxine (FT4) level above the reference interval. Subclinical hyperthyroidism is defined as a TSH level below the reference interval with a concurrent FT4 level within the reference interval.

The prevalence of hyperthyroidism is between 0.23% and 2.7% based on data from South Korea, UK and USA. It is more common in females (Tunbridge *et al.*, 1977; Hollowell *et al.*, 2002; Chung, 2020). The incidence of hyperthyroidism is between 80 and 200 cases per 100,000 people per year (Tunbridge *et al.*, 1977; Vanderpump *et al.*, 1995) while the incidence of Graves' disease was 30 cases per 100,000 people per year for the Olmsted County in the USA between 1935 and 1967 (Furszyfer *et al.*, 1970).

Hyperthyroidism is most commonly due to Graves' disease (Taylor *et al.*, 2018; Nyström *et al.*, 2013). In Graves' disease, autoimmune antibodies bind TSH receptors and stimulate thyroid follicular growth and function, leading to goitre and hyperthyroidism. Another important cause is toxic nodular goitre, resulting from nodules undergoing gain-of-function mutations and producing thyroid hormone independent of physiologic feedback mechanisms.

Other causes of thyrotoxicosis include thyroiditis, where inflammation of the thyroid gland leads to leakage of thyroxine into the circulation. Thyrotoxicosis factitia can arise from intentional consumption of thyroid hormones when people take extracts and supplements. It can also occur from accidental consumption of meat products that are contaminated by thyroid hormones (Wartique *et al.*, 2017).

Drugs that can induce thyrotoxicosis include amiodarone, lithium, highly active anti-retroviral drugs, interferon alpha, tyrosine kinase inhibitors and immune checkpoint inhibitors (Martino *et al.*, 2001; Cukier *et al.*, 2017).

Hyperthyroidism can occur in pregnancy because human chorionic gonadotropin is structurally similar to TSH, and the markedly elevated levels in pregnancy allow it to act on TSH receptors to stimulate thyroid function. The same mechanism occurs in molar pregnancies. In struma ovarii, functional ectopic thyroid tissues in ovarian tumours cause hyperthyroidism.

People with hyperthyroidism may experience nervousness, irritability, increased alertness, sleeplessness, sweating, increased hair fall, palpitations, tremors, muscle weakness, hyperdefaecation and weight loss. Females may have reduced menstrual flow and reduced menstrual frequency.

Complications of Hyperthyroidism

Graves' disease can be complicated by inflammation of the retro-orbital and peri-orbital tissues which can lead to pain, photosensitivity, exposure keratitis, restrictive ophthalmoplegia, and optic nerve compression. This complication is more common in smokers and in White Caucasians (Tellez *et al.*, 1992). Fortunately, severe ophthalmopathy is uncommon and most cases tend to be mild and stable. Hyperthyroidism can also be complicated by thyrocardiac disease. High-output heart failure occurs when ventricular output cannot match the metabolic demands of body tissues during thyrotoxicosis. Tachycardia also leads to reduced ventricular relaxation time and further reduces cardiac output. Arrhythmias can occur from sinus node excitation, and intra-cardiac thrombus may form. Osteoclast stimulation leads to bone resorption and hypercalcaemia. Bone mineral density is reduced and this increases the risk for fragility fractures. Thyrotoxic periodic paralysis is a rare complication of hyperthyroidism. These are attacks of severe proximal muscle weakness. It is more common in Asian men and is secondary to enhanced intracellular potassium shift that is driven by heightened adrenergic sensitivity (Okinaka *et al.*, 1957; Kelley *et al.*, 1989).

Workplace Factors as Causative Factors of Hyperthyroidism

A cohort study in USA found the female spouses of private pesticide applicators were at risk for hyperthyroidism when the applicators sprayed insecticides (diazinon), fungicides (maneb/mancozeb) and herbicides (metolachlor). However, the study did not find increased risk for hyperthyroidism in the pesticide applicators (Shrestha *et al.*, 2018a, 2019).

Impact of Hyperthyroidism on Work Performance

Employees with hyperthyroidism may have poorer work performance and quality of life. The limitations can occur due to uncontrolled hyperthyroidism but may persist despite treatment (Fahrenfort *et al.*, 2000; Bianchi *et al.*, 2004). Hyperthyroidism is also a risk factor for absenteeism, lower rate of return to work, higher rate of unemployment and greater disability pensioning in a Danish cohort study (Nexo *et al.*, 2014).

Hyperthyroidism as a Risk Factor for Occupational Diseases

Poorly controlled hyperthyroidism may predispose employees to heat injuries and dehydration in environments with high ambient temperatures or those that are arid. Employees with Graves' ophthalmopathy may have aggravated xerophthalmia or photosensitivity in environments with dust and particle exposure or low humidity. Proximal weakness and reduced bone mineral density are risk factors for falls and fractures if the affected employee is deployed in areas that are slippery or require climbing.

Assessing Fitness to Work in People with Hyperthyroidism

People with active hyperthyroidism may experience varying degrees of work limitations. The main considerations in these employees are (Job Accommodation Network (JAN), 2020):

1. What are the current symptoms of the employee?
2. What specific job tasks are affected?
3. How do the limitations affect work performance?

The decision on fitness to work needs to be individualised. Often times, hyperthyroidism can be controlled quickly (within days to weeks) with anti-thyroid drugs and employees with mild symptoms can derive rapid symptom relieve with beta blockers. Most people with controlled hyperthyroidism and those in remission lead normal lives and should not have significant loss of productivity.

Workplace Adaptations for Employees with Hyperthyroidism

If treatment of hyperthyroidism effectively controls the symptoms, which is typically the case, permanent job modification is not needed. The exception is perhaps severe Graves' ophthalmopathy with proptosis and eye irritation, photosensitivity, restrictive ophthalmoplegia and optic nerve compression.

Workplace adaptations have to be discussed with the employee and individualised accordingly. These include job restructuring, teleworking and stand/lean stools for workers with decreased stamina or muscle weakness. The problem of tremor and sweaty palms may be alleviated with grip aids. Heat sensitivity is an issue that can be mitigated by portable air conditioners and avoidance of work in a heat stressed environment.

Case Study 3: Construction Worker with Graves' Disease

Mr. X is a 30-year-old man who has recently been diagnosed with Graves' disease. He is a construction worker who works under the sun for long hours. He is unable to tolerate the heat and frequently feels thirsty since he was afflicted with Graves' disease.

Discussion

Mr. X has heat intolerance and dehydration due to excessive sweating. He should be assessed for proximal myopathy and whether this impairs his job performance. His symptoms can be rapidly controlled with anti-thyroid drugs. He should be advised on measures to prevent heat injuries and be given opportunities to hydrate himself adequately.

Summary Points

- Hyperthyroidism is treatable.
- Workers with hyperthyroidism do not usually have permanent functional sequelae so permanent workplace adaptations are usually not needed.
- Most workplace adaptations for workers with hyperthyroidism can be effectively implemented if needed for persistent symptoms.

Hypothyroidism in the Workplace

Hypothyroidism is a state of inadequate thyroid hormone level or action in the body. Overt hypothyroidism is defined as a TSH level above the reference interval with a concurrent FT4 level below the reference interval. Subclinical hypothyroidism is defined as a TSH level above the reference interval with a concurrent FT4 level within the reference interval.

The prevalence of overt hypothyroidism in Europe was between 0.2% and 5.3% (Asvold *et al.*, 2013; McGrogan *et al.*, 2008), between 0.3% and 3.7% in the USA (Canaris *et al.*, 2000), 0.5% in Australia, 10% in India (Unnikrishnan *et al.*, 2013) and between 0.73% and 1.43% in South Korea (Chung, 2020). Subclinical hypothyroidism appears to be more common than overt hypothyroidism. The prevalence of subclinical hypothyroidism in Australia is 5.0% and 16.7% in China (Shan *et al.*, 2016).

The incidence of overt hypothyroidism was 35 cases per 10,000 surviving women and six cases per 10,000 surviving men in an English cohort (Vanderpump *et al.*, 1995). The incidence of overt hypothyroidism and subclinical hypothyroidism was 0.5% and 4.2%, respectively, in an Australian study. Hypothyroidism occurs ten times more commonly in females (Vanderpump, 2011).

The commonest cause of primary hypothyroidism in iodine-replete areas is Hashimoto's thyroiditis, an autoimmune disorder. Iodine is required for thyroxine synthesis and its dietary deficiency can lead to hypothyroidism. There is considerable geographic variation in iodine availability across the world. Less common causes of hypothyroidism include thyroidectomy, radioactive iodine ablation, congenital hypothyroidism and drug-induced hypothyroidism from amiodarone, lithium, tyrosine kinase inhibitors and immune checkpoint inhibitors.

Workplace Factors as Causative and Aggravating Factors of Hypothyroidism

Many industrial chemicals have been identified as potential endocrine disruptors that interrupt the thyroid hormone system via inhibition of iodine absorption, increased thyroxine clearance and decreased cellular uptake of thyroxine (Boas *et al.*, 2012; Crofton, 2008). The potential thyroid-disrupting chemicals include (Shrestha *et al.*, 2018b):

- Fungicides — benomyl, maneb/mancozeb and metalaxyl
- Herbicides — pendimethalin, dicamba, glyphosate and 2 4D
- Organochlorine insecticides — aldrin, chlordane, heptachlor and lindane
- Organophosphate insecticides — coumaphos, diazinon, dichlorvos and malathion

Occupational exposure to ionising radiation is another risk factor for hypothyroidism. Healthcare workers in Taiwan and Spain were found to have higher TSH and/or lower thyroxine levels following exposure to ionising radiation (Wong *et al.*, 2019; Luna-Sánchez *et al.*, 2019).

The complications of hypothyroidism can be aggravated by workplace factors. Hypothyroidism is a risk factor for carpal tunnel syndrome due to increased soft tissue volume in the carpal tunnel. Poor ergonomics or repetitive motion about the wrist may trigger carpal tunnel syndrome or aggravate it.

Impact of Hypothyroidism on Work Performance

Hypothyroidism is associated with absenteeism, lower rate of return to work and greater disability pensioning in a Danish cohort study (Nexo *et al.*, 2014).

Assessing Fitness to Work in People with Hypothyroidism

The manifestations of hypothyroidism are variable and employees with hypothyroidism will experience different degrees of workplace limitations. When assessing job fitness, the main considerations in these employees are (JAN, 2020):

1. What are the current symptoms of the employee?
2. What specific job tasks are affected?
3. How do the limitations affect work performance?

The decision on fitness to work needs to be individualised. The symptoms of hypothyroidism can usually be controlled within weeks and employees should not face significant or permanent workplace limitations after adequate thyroxine replacement is achieved.

Workplace Adaptations for Employees with Hypothyroidism

Workplace adaptations may be required for workers with persistent symptoms despite seemingly adequate thyroxine replacement therapy. Workplace adaptations have to be discussed with the employee and individualised accordingly. These may include teleworking and job restructuring to counter fatigue. Affected workers may find the use of workplace space heaters and avoidance of work in a cold stressed environment helpful to their condition (JAN, 2020).

Case Study 4: Secretary with Hashimoto's Thyroiditis

Ms. Y is a secretary who has Hashimoto's thyroiditis. She has not been adhering to her thyroxine tablets and now experiences pins and needles in her hands which are worse while typing emails and documents. She finds it difficult to focus on meetings.

Discussion

Ms. Y has carpal tunnel syndrome as a complication of hypothyroidism. Improving her workplace ergonomics will minimise compression on her median nerves. Her symptoms can be rapidly reversed with thyroxine therapy.

Summary Points

- Hypothyroidism is treatable.
- Workers with hypothyroidism do not usually have permanent functional sequelae so permanent workplace adaptations are usually not needed.
- Most workplace adaptations for workers with hypothyroidism can be effectively implemented if needed for persistent symptoms.

Adrenal Insufficiency in the Workplace

AI is not a common condition but it has significant impact on the work performance of employees. In Europe, the prevalence of primary AI was between 82 and 144 cases per million (Charmandari *et al.*, 2014). The prevalence of endogenous secondary AI was between 140 and 280 cases per million based on two studies from the UK and Spain. Endogenous secondary AI is more common in women and the peak age of incidence is around the sixth decade (Tomlinson *et al.*, 2001; Regal *et al.*, 2001). The prevalence of exogenous secondary AI is not well studied. Primary AI can occur from adrenal gland destruction from autoimmune disease (Addison's disease), infiltrative disease (metastases), haemorrhage (Waterhouse-Friderichsen syndrome) or infections (tuberculosis). Endogenous secondary AI can arise from pituitary apoplexy, lymphocytic hypophysitis, mass lesions in the para-sellar region or following cure from Cushing's syndrome. Exogenous secondary AI is due to corticotroph suppression by exogenous steroids.

Manifestations of Adrenal Insufficiency

Clinical features of AI include muscle weakness, joint pains, chronic fatigue, poor concentration and memory, abdominal pain, anorexia, weight loss, hypoglycaemia, orthostasis, salt craving and skin pigmentation.

Associated autoimmune conditions such as T1DM, Hashimoto's thyroiditis, coeliac disease or pernicious anaemia may also be present.

Adrenal crisis can occur in people with AI who are experiencing overwhelming physical stress and are unable to compensate with adequate cortisol production/administration. Adrenal crises occur in 8% of people with Addison's disease each year (White and Arlt, 2010). This is a life-threatening event and the commonest triggers are infections, fevers or severe injuries.

Impact of Adrenal Insufficiency on Work Performance

People with AI that are well-treated with timely cortisol replacement (to approximate circadian rhythm of cortisol secretion) can lead normal lives and should not face significant work limitations. Left untreated or poorly managed, people with AI may have impaired work performance, both physically and mentally.

When newly diagnosed with initial commencement of treatment, people with AI may require a period of time to return to their baseline health because it takes time to adjust to the medications. Once AI is optimally treated, the employee can resume usual duties and is not expected to require much accommodation at work.

Assessment of Fitness to Work in People with Adrenal Insufficiency

The role of the occupational physician is to help the employee with AI understand his condition and be acquainted with self-management.

Workplace Adaptations for Employees with Adrenal Insufficiency

Employees with AI do not usually need permanent workplace modification if there are no functional impairments. However, the manifestations of AI are variable and people with Addison's disease may experience weakness and fatigue despite cortisol replacement.

The employee and employer should communicate openly to discuss ways in which the employer can maximise the employee's productivity. Some examples include:

- Phased return to work in the initial period while the employee is getting used to living with AI, particularly for jobs requiring physical strength and prolonged standing.
- Later start in working hours so the employee can wait for the cortisol effect to kick-in before starting work.
- Fewer shift work so the employee does not need to adjust the cortisol timing frequently (higher cortisol demands may be required in times of increased physical activity as opposed to periods of rest).
- Identifying specific duties that may put the employee at risk for injuries and have an open discussion on whether the employee wishes to participate in such duties.

Case Study 5: Manager with Addison's Disease

Mr. X is a 42-year-old man with Addison's disease. He is a hospitality manager in a popular restaurant. He misses his afternoon dose of hydrocortisone frequently due to high customer volume at lunch time. As a consequence, he always feels exhausted in the early evenings and is unable to cope when the dinner crowd arrives.

Discussion

Mr. X needs to adhere to his medication to ensure he has sufficient energy to perform his job in the evenings and to avoid adrenal crises. He should be advised to carry hydrocortisone tablets with him so that he can take them at times of his convenience. If this is not practical, he may need to consult his endocrinologist on alternative glucocorticoid therapy with longer durations of action.

Summary Points

- Most workers with AI do not have permanent limitations and can regain full productivity with treatment.
- There could be some workers with persistent symptoms for whom individualised workplace adaptations may be helpful.

Conclusion

Obesity, DM, hyperthyroidism and hypothyroidism are prevalent conditions that do not impair work performance when controlled. AI is uncommon and does not usually cause long-term consequences once adequate glucocorticoid replacement therapy is started. In some cases, appropriate workplace modification may be needed to optimise work performance in people with such conditions.

References

Action to Control Cardiovascular Risk in Diabetes Study Group, Gerstein HC, Miller ME, Byington RP, Goff DC. Jr, Bigger JT, Buse JB, Cushman WC, Genuth S, Beigi FI, Grimm RH. Jr, Probstfeild JL, Simons DG, Friedewald WT. (2008) Effects of intensive glucose lowering in type 2 diabetes. *N Engl J Med* **358**(24): 2545–2559.

American Diabetes Association. (2005) Defining and reporting hypoglycemia in diabetes: A report from the American diabetes workgroup on hypoglycemia. *Diabetes Care* **28**(5): 1245–1249. Available from: https://doi.org/10.2337/diacare.28.5.1245.

American Diabetes Association. (2009) Diabetes and employment. *Diabetes Care* **32**(Suppl 1): 80–84. Available from: https://doi.org/10.2337/dc09-S080.

American Diabetes Association. (2020a) Introduction: Standards of medical care in diabetes — 2020. *Diabetes Care* **43**(Suppl 1): 1–2. Available from: https://doi.org/10.2337/dc20-Sint.

American Diabetes Association. (2020b) Classification and diagnosis of diabetes. *Diabetes Care* **43**(Suppl 1): 14–31. Available from: https://doi.org/10.2337/dc20-S002.

Asvold BO, Vatten LJ, Bjøro T. (2013) Changes in the prevalence of hypothyroidism: The HUNT study in Norway. *Eur J Endocrinol* **169**(5): 613–620.

Attarchi M, Golabadi M, Labbafinejad Y, Mohammadi S. (2013) Combined effects of exposure to occupational noise and mixed organic solvents on blood pressure in car manufacturing company workers. *Am J Ind Med* **56**(2): 243–251.

Bianchi GP, Zaccheroni V, Solaroli E, Vescini F, Cerutti R, Zoli M, Marchesini G. (2004) Health-related quality of life in patients with thyroid disorders. *Qual Life Res* **13**(1): 45–54. Available from: https://doi.org/10.1023/B:QURE.0000015315.35184.66.

Boas M, Feldt-Rasmussen U, Main KM. (2012) Thyroid effects of endocrine disrupting chemicals. *Mol Cell Endocrinol* **355**(2): 240–248. Available from: https://doi.org/10.1016/j.mce.2011.09.005.

Bungum T, Satterwhite M, Jackson AW, Morrow JR. (2003) The relationship of body mass index, medical costs, and job absenteeism. *Am J Health Behav* **27**(4): 456–62. Available from: https://doi.org/10.5993/ajhb.27.4.17.

Canaris GJ, Manowitz NR, Mayor G, Ridgway EC. (2000) The Colorado thyroid disease prevalence study. *Arch Intern Med* **160**(4): 526–534. Available from: https://doi.org/10.1001/archinte.160.4.526.

Cappuccio FP, D'Elia L, Strazzullo P, Miller MA. (2010) Quantity and quality of sleep and incidence of type 2 diabetes: A systematic review and meta-analysis. *Diabetes Care* **33**(2): 414–420. Available from: https://doi.org/10.2337/dc09-1124.

Cave M, Appana S, Patel M, Falkner KC, McClain CJ, Brock G. (2010) Polychlorinated biphenyls, lead, and mercury are associated with liver disease in American adults: NHANES 2003–2004. *Environ Health Perspect*

118 (12): 1735–1742. Available from: https://doi.org/10.1289/ehp.1002720.

Charmandari E, Nicolaides NC, Chrousos GP. (2014) Adrenal insufficiency. *Lancet* **383**(9935): 2152–2167. Available from: https://doi.org/10.1016/S0140-6736(13)61684-0.

Chung JH. (2020) Update on thyroid hormone levels and thyroid dysfunction in the Korean population based on data from the Korea national health and nutrition examination survey VI (2013 to 2015). *Endocrinol Metab* **35**(1): 7–13. Available from: https://doi.org/10.3803/EnM.2020.35.1.7.

Cox DJ, Gonder-Frederick L, Polonsky W, Schlundt D, Kovatchev B, Clarke W. (2001) Blood glucose awareness training (BGAT-2): Long-term benefits. *Diabetes Care* **24**(4): 637–642. Available from: https://care.diabetesjournals.org/content/24/4/637.

Cox DJ, Kovatchev BP, Gonder-Frederick LA, Summers KH, McCall A, Grimm KJ, Clarke WL. (2005) Relationships between hyperglycemia and cognitive performance among adults with type 1 and type 2 diabetes. *Diabetes Care* **28**(1): 71–77. Available from: https://doi.org/10.2337/diacare.28.1.71.

Crofton KM. (2008) Thyroid disrupting chemicals: Mechanisms and mixtures. *Int J Androl* **31**(2): 209–23. Available from: https://doi.org/10.1111/j.1365-2605.2007.00857.x.

Cukier P, Santini FC, Scaranti M, Hoff AO. (2017). Endocrine side effects of cancer immunotherapy. *Endocr-Relat Cancer* **24**(12): 331–347. Available from: https://doi.org/10.1530/ERC-17-0358.

Deierlein AL, Wolff MS, Pajak A, Pinney SM, Windham GC, Galvez MP, Rybak M, Calafat AM, Kushi LH, Biro FM, Teitelbaum SL. (2017) Phenol concentrations during childhood and subsequent measures of adiposity among young girls. *Am J Epidemiol* **186**(5): 581–592. Available from: https://doi.org/10.1093/aje/kwx136.

Diabetes Control and Complications Trial Research Group, Nathan DM, Genuth S, Lachin J, Cleary P, Crofford O, Davis M, Rand L, Siebert C. (1993) The effect of intensive treatment of diabetes on the development and progression of long-term complications in insulin-dependent diabetes mellitus. *N Engl J Med* **329**(14): 977–986.

Ding HB, Huang, JF, Xie, S., Wang, BY, Lin, T, Zhao, JM, Lin, QC. (2019) The association between glycometabolism and nonalcoholic fatty liver disease in patients with obstructive sleep apnea. *Sleep Breath* 23(1): 373–378. Available from: https://doi.org/10.1007/s11325-018-1744-1.

Dirinck E, Jorens PG, Covaci, A, Geens, T, Roosens, L, Neels, H, Mertens I, Van Gaal L. (2011) Obesity and persistent organic pollutants: Possible obesogenic effect of organochlorine pesticides and polychlorinated biphenyls. *Obesity* **19**(4): 709–714. Available from: https://doi.org/10.1038/oby.2010.133.

Dray-Spira R, Herquelot E, Bonenfant S, Guéguen A, Melchior M. (2013) Impact of diabetes mellitus onset on sickness absence from work: A 15-year follow-up of the GAZEL occupational cohort study. *Diabet Med* **30**(5): 549–556. Available from: https://doi.org/10.1111/dme.12076.

Elobeid MA, Padilla MA, Brock DW, Ruden DM, Allison DB. (2010) Endocrine disruptors and obesity: An examination of selected persistent organic pollutants in the NHANES 1999–2002 data. *Int J Environ Res Public Health* 7(7): 2988–3005. Available from: https://doi.org/10.3390/ijerph7072988.

Fahrenfort JJ, Wilterdink AM, van der Veen EA. (2000) Long-term residual complaints and psychosocial sequelae after remission of hyperthyroidism. *Psychoneuroendocrinology* **25**(2): 201–211. Available from: https://doi.org/10.1016/s0306-4530(99)00050-5.

Fan Z.J, Harris-Adamson C, Gerr, F, Eisen, EA, Hegmann, KT, Bao, S, Silverstein B, Evanoff B, Dalem AM, Thiesem AR, Kapellusch J, Burt S, Merlino L, Rempel D. (2015) Associations between workplace factors and carpal tunnel syndrome: A multi-site cross sectional study. *Am J Ind Med* **58**(5): 509–518. Available from: https://doi.org/10.1002/ajim.22443.

Flegal KM, Graubard BI. (2009) Estimates of excess deaths associated with body mass index and other anthropometric variables. *Am J Clin Nutr* **89**(4): 1213–1219. Available from: https://doi.org/10.3945/ajcn.2008.26698.

Furszyfer J, Kurland LT, McConahey WM, Elveback LR. (1970) Graves' disease in Olmsted County, Minnesota, 1935 through 1967. *Mayo Clin Proc* **45**(9): 636–644.

Gan WQ, Davies HW, Demers PA. (2011) Exposure to occupational noise and cardiovascular disease in the United States: The national health and nutrition examination survey 1999–2004. *Occup Environ Med* **68**(3): 183–90. Available from: https://doi.org/10.1136/oem.2010.055269.

Gan Y, Yang C, Tong X, Sun H, Cong Y, Yin X, Li L, Cao S, Dong X, Gong Y, Shi O, Deng J, Bi H, Lu Z. (2015) Shift work and diabetes mellitus: A meta-analysis of observational studies. *Occup Environ Med*

72(1): 72–78. Available from: https://doi.org/10.1136/oemed-2014-102150.

Hollowell JG, Staehling NW, Flanders DW, Hannon WH, Gunter EW, Spencer CA, Braverman LE. (2002) Serum TSH, T(4), and thyroid antibodies in the United States population (1988 to 1994): National health and nutrition examination survey (NHANES III). *J Clin Endocrinol Metab* **87**(2): 489–499. Available from: https://doi.org/10.1210/jcem.87.2.8182.

Holman RR, Paul SK, Bethel MA, Matthews DR, Neil HAW. (2008) 10-year follow-up of intensive glucose control in type 2 diabetes. *N Engl J Med* **359**(15): 1577–1589. Available from: https://doi.org/10.1056/NEJMoa0806470.

International Diabetes Federation. (2020) *Worldwide Toll of Diabetes.* Available from: https://diabetesatlas.org/en/sections/worldwide-toll-of-diabetes.html [Accessed on 19 August 2020].

Job Accommodation Network. (2020) *Accommodation and compliance: Thyroid disorders – about thyroid disorders.* Available from: https://askjan.org/disabilities/Thyroid-Disorders.cfm. [Accessed on 20 May 2020].

Karlsson B, Knutsson A, Lindahl B. (2001) Is there an association between shift work and having a metabolic syndrome? results from a population based study of 27,485 people. *Occup Environ Med* **58**(11): 747–752. Available from: https://doi.org/10.1136/oem.58.11.747.

Kelley DE, Gharib, H, Kennedy FP, Duda RJ, McManis PG. (1989) Thyrotoxic periodic paralysis: Report of 10 cases and review of electromyographic findings. *Arch Intern Med* **149**(11): 2597–2600. Available from: https://doi.org/10.1001/archinte.149.11.2597.

Knutsson A, Kempe A. (2014) 'Shift work and diabetes--a systematic review. *Chronobiol Int* **31**(10): 1146–1151. Available from: https://doi.org/10.3109/07420528.2014.957308.

Kubo J, Goldstein BA, Cantley LF, Tessier-Sherman B, Galusha D, Slade MD, Chu IM, Cullen MR. (2014) Contribution of health status and prevalent chronic disease to individual risk for workplace injury in the manufacturing environment. *Occup Environ Med* **71**(3): 159–166. Available from: https://doi.org/10.1136/oemed-2013-101653.

Lee SM, Koh D, Chui WKL, Sum CF. (2011) Diabetes management and hypoglycemia in safety sensitive jobs. *Saf Health Work* **2**(1): 9–16. Available from: https://doi.org/10.5491/SHAW.2011.2.1.9.

Lee SM, Lim LC, Koh D. (2015) Stigma among workers attending a hospital specialist diabetes clinic. *Occup Med* **65**(1): 67–71. Available from: https://doi.org/10.1093/occmed/kqu150.

Li QQ, Loganath A, Chong YS, Tan J, Obbard JP. (2006) Persistent organic pollutants and adverse health effects in humans. *J Toxicol Environ Health* **69**(21): 1987–2005. Available from: https://doi.org/10.1080/15287390600751447.

Lowden A, Moreno C, Holmbäck U, Lennernäs M, Tucker P. (2010) Eating and shift work - effects on habits, metabolism and performance. *Scand J Work Environ Health* **36**(2): 150–162. Available from: https://doi.org/10.5271/sjweh.2898.

Luna-Sánchez S, Del Campo MT, Morán JV, Fernández IM, Checa FJS, de la Hoz RE. (2019) Thyroid function in health care workers exposed to ionizing radiation. *Health Phys* **117**(4): 403–407. Available from: https://doi.org/10.1097/HP.0000000000001071.

Lundqvist G, Flodin U, Axelson O. (1999) A case-control study of fatty liver disease and organic solvent exposure. *Am J Ind Med* **35**(2): 132–136. Available from: https://doi.org/10.1002/(sici)1097-0274(199902)35:2<132::aid-ajim4>3.0.co;2-i.

Martino E, Bartalena L, Bogazzi F, Braverman LE. (2001) The effects of amiodarone on the thyroid. *Endocrine Rev* **22**(2): 240–254. Available from: https://doi.org/10.1210/edrv.22.2.0427.

McGrogan A, Seaman HE, Wright JW, de Vries CS. (2008) The incidence of autoimmune thyroid disease: A systematic review of the literature. *Clin Endocrinol* **69**(5): 687–696. Available from: https://doi.org/10.1111/j.1365-2265.2008.03338.x.

McMahon BT, West SL, Mansouri M, Belongia L. (2005) Workplace discrimination and diabetes: The EEOC Americans with disabilities act research project. *Work* **25**(1): 9–18.

Misra A, Wasir JS, Vikram NK. (2005) Waist circumference criteria for the diagnosis of abdominal obesity are not applicable uniformly to all populations and ethnic groups. *Nutrition* **21**(9): 969–976. Available from: https://doi.org/10.1016/j.nut.2005.01.007.

National Institutes of Health. (1998) Clinical guidelines on the identification, evaluation, and treatment of overweight and obesity in adults--the evidence report. *Obesity Res* **6**(Suppl 2): 51–209.

Nebiker-Pedrotti PM, Keller U, Hans-Ulrich I, Ruiz J, Pärli K, Caplazi A, Puder JJ. (2009) Perceived discrimination against diabetics in the workplace and in work-related insurances in Switzerland. *Swiss Med Wkly* **139**(7–8): 103–109. Available from: https://doi.org/smw-12432.

Newbold RR, Padilla-Banks E, Snyder RJ, Jefferson WN. (2007) Perinatal exposure to environmental estrogens and the development of obesity. *Mol Nutr Food Res* **51**(7): 912–917. Available from: https://doi.org/10.1002/mnfr.200600259.

Nexo MA, Watt T, Pedersen J, Bonnema SJ, Hegedüs L, Rasmussen AK, Feldt-Rasmussen U, Bjorner JB. (2014) Increased risk of long-term sickness absence, lower rate of return to work, and higher risk of unemployment and disability pensioning for thyroid patients: A Danish register-based cohort study. *J Clin Endocrinol Metab* **99**(9): 3184–3192. Available from: https://doi.org/10.1210/jc.2013-4468.

Nexo MA, Carlsen K, Pedersen J, Hetland ML, Watt T, Hansen SM, Bjorner JB. (2018) Long-term sickness absence of 32 chronic conditions: A Danish register-based longitudinal study with up to 17 Years of follow-up. *BMJ Open* **8**(6): e020874. Available from: https://doi.org/10.1136/bmjopen-2017-020874.

Nilsson M, Jensen N, Gejl M, Bergmann ML, Storgaard H, Zander M, Miskowiak K, Rungby J. (2019) Experimental non-severe hypoglycaemia substantially impairs cognitive function in type 2 diabetes: A randomised crossover trial. *Diabetologia* **62**(10): 1948–1958. Available from: https://doi.org/10.1007/s00125-019-4964-4.

Nyström HF, Jansson S, Berg G. (2013) Incidence rate and clinical features of hyperthyroidism in a long-term iodine sufficient area of Sweden (Gothenburg) 2003–2005. *Clin Endocrinol* **78**(5): 768–776. Available from: https://doi.org/10.1111/cen.12060.

Ohkubo Y, Kishikawa H, Araki E, Miyata T, Isami S, Motoyoshi S, Kojima Y, Furuyoshi N, Shichiri M. (1995) Intensive insulin therapy prevents the progression of diabetic microvascular complications in Japanese patients with non-insulin-dependent diabetes mellitus: A randomized prospective 6-year study. *Diabetes Res Clin Pract* **28**(2): 103–117. Available from: https://doi.org/10.1016/0168-8227(95)01064-k.

Okinaka S, Shizume K, Iino S, Watanabe A, Irie M, Noguchi A, Kuma S, Kuma K, Ito T. (1957) The association of periodic paralysis and hyperthyroidism in japan. *J Clin Endocrinol Metab* **17**(12): 1454–1459. Available from: https://doi.org/10.1210/jcem-17-12-1454.

Pandalai SP, Schulte PA, Miller DB. (2013) Conceptual heuristic models of the interrelationships between obesity and the occupational environment. *Scand J Work Environ Health* **39**(3): 221–232. Available from: https://doi.org/10.5271/sjweh.3363.

Regal M, Páramo C, Sierra SM, Garcia-Mayor RV. (2001) Prevalence and incidence of hypopituitarism in an adult caucasian population in northwestern Spain. *Clin Endocrinol* **55**(6): 735–740. Available from: https://doi.org/10.1046/j.1365-2265.2001.01406.x.

Robroek SJW, Reeuwijk KG, Hillier FC, Bambra CL, van Rijn RM, Burdorf A. (2013) The contribution of overweight, obesity, and lack of physical activity to exit from paid employment: A meta-analysis. *Scand J Work Environ Health* **39**(3): 233–240. Available from: https://doi.org/10.5271/sjweh.3354.

Rönn M, Lind L, van Bavel B, Salihovic S, Michaëlsson K, Lind PM. (2011) Circulating levels of persistent organic pollutants associate in divergent ways to fat mass measured by DXA in humans. *Chemosphere* **85**(3): 335–343. Available from: https://doi.org/10.1016/j.chemosphere.2011.06.095.

Shan Z, Chen L, Lian X, Liu C, Shi B, Shi L, Tong N, Wang S, Weng J, Zhao J, Teng X, Yu X, Lai Y, Wang W, Li C, Mao J, Li Y, Fan C, Teng W. (2016) Iodine status and prevalence of thyroid disorders after introduction of mandatory universal salt iodization for 16 years in China: A cross-sectional study in 10 cities. *Thyroid* **26**(8): 1125–1130. Available from: https://doi.org/10.1089/thy.2015.0613.

Shrestha S, Parks CG, Goldner WS, Kamel F, Umbach DM, Ward MH, Lerro CC, Koutros S, Hofmann JN, Freeman LEB, Sandler DP. (2018a) Incident thyroid disease in female spouses of private pesticide applicators. *Environ Int* **118**: 282–292. Available from: https://doi.org/10.1016/j.envint.2018.05.041.

Shrestha S, Parks CG, Goldner WS, Kamel F, Umbach DM, Ward MH, Lerro CC, Koutros S, Hofmann JN, Freeman LEB, Sandler DP. (2018b) Pesticide use and incident hypothyroidism in pesticide applicators in the agricultural health study. *Environ Health Perspect* **126**(9), 97008. Available from: https://doi.org/10.1289/EHP3194.

Shrestha S, Parks CG, Goldner WS, Kamel F, Umbach DM, Ward MH, Lerro CC, Koutros S, Hofmann JN, Freeman LEB, Sandler DP. (2019) Pesticide use and incident hyperthyroidism in farmers in the agricultural health study'. *Occup Environ Med* **76**(5): 332–335. Available from: https://doi.org/10.1136/oemed-2018-105518.

Statens Helsetilsyn. (2000) *Norwegian guidelines for medical examination of occupational divers.* Available from: https://www.yumpu.com/en/document/read/5728005/norwegian-guidelines-for-medical-examination-of-occupational-divers. [Accessed on 19 May 2020].

Sun Q, van Dam RM, Spiegelman D, Heymsfield SB, Willett WC, Hu FB. (2010) Comparison of dual-energy x-ray absorptiometric and anthropometric measures of adiposity in relation to adiposity-related biologic factors. *Am J Epidemiol* **172**(12): 1442–1454. Available from: https://doi.org/10.1093/aje/kwq306.

Suwazono Y, Dochi M, Oishi M, Tanaka K, Kobayashi E, Sakata K. (2009) Shiftwork and impaired glucose metabolism: A 14-year cohort study on 7104 male workers. *Chronobiol Int* **26**(5): 926–941. Available from: https://doi.org/10.1080/07420520903044422.

Tanaka S, Wild DK, Cameron LL, Freund E. (1997) Association of occupational and non-occupational risk factors with the prevalence of self-reported carpal tunnel syndrome in a national survey of the working population. *Am J Ind Med* **32**(5): 550–556. Available from: https://doi.org/10.1002/(sici)1097-0274(199711)32:5<550::aid-ajim18>3.0.co;2-1.

Taylor PN, Albrecht D, Scholz A, Gutierrez-Buey G, Lazarus JH, Dayan CM, Okosieme OE. (2018) Global epidemiology of hyperthyroidism and hypothyroidism. *Nature Rev Endocrinol* **14**(5): 301–316. Available from: https://doi.org/10.1038/nrendo.2018.18.

Tellez M, Cooper J, Edmonds C. (1992) Graves' ophthalmopathy in relation to cigarette smoking and ethnic origin. *Clin Endocrinol* **36**(3): 291–294. Available from: https://doi.org/10.1111/j.1365-2265.1992.tb01445.x.

Tomlinson JW, Holden N, Hills RK, Wheatley K, Clayton RN, Bates AS, Sheppard MC, Stewart PM. (2001) Association between premature mortality and hypopituitarism. *Lancet* **357**(9254): 425–431. Available from: https://doi.org/10.1016/s0140-6736(00)04006-x.

Tunbridge WM, Evered DC, Hall R, Appleton D, Brewis M, Clark F, Evans JG, Young E, Bird T, Smith PA. (1977) The spectrum of thyroid disease in a community: the Whickham survey. *Clin Endocrinol* 7(6): 481–493. Available from: https://doi.org/10.1111/j.1365-2265.1977.tb01340.x.

United Kingdom Prospective Diabetes Study Group. (1998) Effect of intensive blood-glucose control with metformin on complications in overweight patients with type 2 diabetes (UKPDS 34). *Lancet* **352**(9131): 854–865.

Unnikrishnan AG, Kalra S, Sahay RK, Bantwal G, John M, Tewari N. (2013) Prevalence of hypothyroidism in adults: an epidemiological study in eight cities of India. *Indian J Endocrinol Metab* **17**(4): 647–652. Available from: https://doi.org/10.4103/2230-8210.113755.

Vanderpump MP, Tunbridge WM, French JM, Appleton D, Bates D, Clark F, Evans JG, Hasan DM, Rodgers H, Tunbridge F. (1995) The incidence of thyroid disorders in the community: A twenty-year follow-up of the Whickham survey. *Clin Endocrinol* **43**(1): 55–68. Available from: https://doi.org/10.1111/j.1365-2265.1995.tb01894.x.

Vanderpump MPJ. (2011) The epidemiology of thyroid disease. *Br Med Bull* **99**: 39–51. Available from: https://doi.org/10.1093/bmb/ldr030.

Walker-Bone KE, Palmer KT, Reading I, Cooper C. (2003) Soft-tissue rheumatic disorders of the neck and upper limb: prevalence and risk factors. *Seminars in Arthritis Rheumatism* **33**(3): 185–203. Available from: https://doi.org/10.1016/s0049-0172(03)00128-8.

Wardle J, Steptoe A, Oliver G, Lipsey Z. (2000) Stress, dietary restraint and food intake. *J Psychosom Res* **48**(2): 195–202. Available from: https://doi.org/10.1016/s0022-3999(00)00076-3.

White K, Arlt W. (2010) Adrenal crisis in treated addison's disease: A predictable but under-managed event. *Eur J Endocrinol* **162**(1): 115–20. Available from: https://doi.org/10.1530/EJE-09-0559.

Wieslander G, Norbäck D, Göthe CJ, Juhlin L. (1989) Carpal tunnel syndrome (CTS) and exposure to vibration, repetitive wrist movements, and heavy manual work: A case-referent study. *Br J Ind Med* **46**(1): 43–47. Available from: https://doi.org/10.1136/oem.46.1.43.

Wong YS, Cheng YY, Cheng TJ, Huang CC, Yeh JJ, Guo HR. (2019) The relationship between occupational exposure to low-dose ionizing radiation and changes in thyroid hormones in hospital workers. *Epidemiology* **30**(Suppl 1): 32–38. Available from: https://doi.org/10.1097/EDE.0000000000001004.

World Health Organization Expert Consultation. (2004) Appropriate body-mass index for Asian populations and its implications for policy and intervention strategies. *Lancet* **363**(9403): 157–163. Available from: https://doi.org/10.1016/S0140-6736(03)15268-3.

World Health Organization. (2020) *Obesity and Overweight*. [Online] Available from: https://www.who.int/news-room/fact-sheets/detail/obesity-and-overweight [Accessed on 19 May 2020].

Yeoh E, Choudhary P, Nwokolo M, Ayis S, Amiel SA. (2015) Interventions that restore awareness of hypoglycemia in adults with type 1 diabetes: A systematic review and meta-analysis. *Diabetes Care* **38**(8): 1592–1609. Available from: https://doi.org/10.2337/dc15-0102.

Yoshida D, Toyomura K, Fukumoto J, Ueda N, Ohnaka K, Adachi M, Takayanagi R, Kono S. (2009) Waist circumference and cardiovascular risk factors in Japanese men and women. *J Atheroscler Thromb* **16**(4): 431–441. Available from: https://doi.org/10.5551/jat.no539.

Zammit C, Liddicoat H, Moonsie I, Makker H. (2010) Obesity and respiratory diseases. *Int J Gen Med* **3**: 335–43. Available from: https://doi.org/10.2147/IJGM.S11926.

Zammitt NN, Warren RE, Deary IJ, Frier BM. (2008) Delayed recovery of cognitive function following hypoglycemia in adults with type 1 diabetes: Effect of impaired awareness of hypoglycemia. *Diabetes* **57**(3): 732–736. Available from: https://doi.org/10.2337/db07-0695.

Zinman B, Wanner C, Lachin JM, Fitchett D, Bluhmki E, Hantel S, Mattheus M, Devins T, Johansen OD, Woerle HJ, Broedl UC, Inzucchi SE. (2015) Empagliflozin, cardiovascular outcomes, and mortality in type 2 diabetes. N Engl J Med **373**(22): 2117–2128. Available from: https://doi.org/10.1056/NEJMoa1504720.

Chapter 16

Reproductive Disorders

John Wah Lim[*,†] *and David Koh*[†,‡,§]

Introduction

Occupational exposure to various hazards can have adverse reproductive health impacts on both males and females. Generally, occupational hazards that affect reproductive health can be classified as chemical (e.g. solvents, pesticides), physical (e.g. heat, radiation), biological (e.g. viruses, parasites) and psychosocial (stress). Some occupational hazards may also affect pregnancy and the fetus. Prevention of the harmful effects of these occupational exposures requires assessment and management of reproductive risks in the workplace.

Reproductive Effects

Excessive occupational exposures can cause direct cell damage in the developing sperm and ovum, resulting in chromosomal abnormalities or gene mutations. It can also alter the sex hormone levels. This could

[*] Singapore General Hospital, Singapore.
[†] Saw Swee Hock School of Public Health, National University of Singapore, Singapore.
[‡] Yong Loo Lin School of Medicine, National University of Singapore, Singapore.
[§] PAPRSB Institute of Health Sciences, Universiti Brunei Darussalam, Brunei Darussalam.
Corresponding author: John Wah Lim (ephlimj@nus.edu.sg).

cause adverse effects on sexual function and reduced fertility in both genders. Adverse effects on both reproduction and development are most often due to exposures that happen during the vulnerable periods of ovulation, spermatogenesis and fetal organogenesis.

Toxicants such as antineoplastic agents may reduce of both male and female germ cells (sperms and ova), causing infertility and a shortened reproductive life span. Some effects seen in the offspring may only manifest years later. For example, lead (Pb) that is gradually accumulated in maternal tissue which is released during pregnancy or lactation could cause cognitive impairment in early childhood and beyond.

In males, occupational exposure can cause diminished libido and impotence, as well as infertility due to impairment of semen quality, including reduced sperm counts, morphologically abnormal sperm, and impaired stability of sperm chromatin or sperm DNA. Male reproductive disorders have well established causes related to the occupational environment, but are seldom recognised by work injury compensation authorities. This is possibly because the work ability is not affected by these disorders.

In females, occupational exposure can interfere with hormonal synthesis and secretion and result in menstrual disorders such as delayed menarche or premature menopause and ovarian dysfunction. Irregularities of the menstrual cycles are often caused by disturbances of follicular maturation or hormonal disturbances, whereas early onset of menopause has been interpreted as a marker of damage to the follicular pool.

Maternal exposure during pregnancy could potentially affect development of fetus, leading to an adverse pregnancy outcome. The exposure may affect the fetus directly or indirectly by interfering with the maternal, placental or fetal membrane functions. Most of the fetal toxicant exposures are concurrent with the pregnancy; however, others are the result of a previous exposure, but with ongoing maternal elimination of the toxicant, or by mobilisation of stored toxicants (e.g. Pb from bone stores, polychlorinated biphenyls from fat stores). Physiological changes during pregnancy may also alter quantity of toxins absorbed and delivered to the fetus, for example, increase tidal volume and minute ventilation increase absorption of respiratory toxin. Delayed in gastric emptying and reduced intestinal motility during pregnancy increase absorption of ingested toxins. Exposure during pregnancy can lead to spontaneous abortion, stillbirth, fetal death, intrauterine growth retardation, preterm birth, postnatal death, birth defects, and impairment of cognitive development or childhood cancer.

Time, duration and dose of exposure during pregnancy can lead to different outcomes. Exposures during first trimester of pregnancy may result in spontaneous abortion or birth defects. Exposure in the later trimesters of pregnancy could shorten the gestation period, resulting in preterm birth, low birth weight and may affect development of the brain. A lower dose of toxicant exposure may cause birth defects, but a high dose may cause spontaneous abortion or infertility. The fetal central nervous system, in particular the fetal brain, is very vulnerable to developmental injury throughout pregnancy due to the incomplete blood-brain barrier. Exposure to a neurotoxin (e.g. mercury or Pb) can adversely affect both structural and cognitive development throughout gestation.

A breastfeeding mother may secrete toxicants in her breast milk. Certain fat-soluble toxicants, such as dioxins and certain pesticides (e.g. organophosphate and organonochlorine pesticides) can diffuse into the mother's breast milk.

Endocrine disruptors are chemicals that can mimic the action of endogenous hormones. Many of these substances have oestrogenic and anti-androgenic effects and can produce adverse reproductive and developmental effects. It can cause maldevelopment of reproductive organs and poor semen quality in men. In women, it is linked to gynecological conditions such as endometriosis and benign tumors. Examples of chemicals that have been identified as possible endocrine disruptors include bisphenol A, pesticides, phthalates and polychlorinated organic compounds.

This chapter outlines the effects of occupational exposures to chemical, physical, biological and psychosocial hazards and their impacts on reproductive health in both genders. The role of occupational physicians in managing workers exposed to reproductive hazards as well as prevention of reproductive hazards at the workplace will also be discussed.

Chemical Hazards

There are many chemical agents which can have potential impacts on reproductive outcomes. However, to date, most chemical agents have not been studied for their potential hazards tothe human reproductive system.

Common chemical agents with adverse reproductive effects that have been reported in the human studies include metals, organic solvents, pesticides, pharmaceutical agents and carbon monoxide. This information is summarised in Table 1.

Table 1. Common Chemical Agents with Known Reproductive Effects on Humans

Agents	Industry/ Occupational Group at Risk	Effects on Male Workers	Effects on Female Workers
Metals			
Lead (Pb)	Battery, pigments, paints, smelting, soldering, foundries, pottery, ammunition industries	Reduced sperm quality, reduced fertility	Reduced fertility, fetal loss, birth defects, preterm birth, low birth weight, impaired cognitive development
Inorganic mercury (Hg)	Lamp industry, dental personnel	Decrease sperm count and quality	Reduced fertility, menstrual disorders, fetal loss
Organic solvents			
Benzene	Petrochemical industry, laboratory personnel	—	Reduced fertility, low birth weight, fetal loss
Carbon disulfide	Viscose rayon industry	Decreased libido and impotence	Menstrual disorders
Tetrachloroethylene	Dry cleaning, degreasing	—	Reduced fertility, fetal loss

Table 1. (*Continued*)

Agents	**Industry/ Occupational Group at Risk**	**Effects on Male Workers**	**Effects on Female Workers**
Toluene	Shoe industry, painting, laboratory personnel	Reduced semen quality	Reduced fertility, fetal loss
Pesticides	Agriculture, gardening	Reduced sperm quality, reduced fertility, fetal loss, birth defects	Reduced fertility, fetal loss, birth defects, preterm birth, reduced fetal growth, neurodevelopmental effects
Anaesthetic gases	Operating rooms, delivery suites, dental clinics	—	Fetal loss, reduced birth weight, preterm birth, birth defects, reduced fertility
Antineoplastic agents	Hospital workers, pharmaceutical industry	—	Menstrual disorders, reduced fertility, fetal loss, premature birth, low birth weight, birth defects
Carbon monoxide	Iron and steel foundries, welding, food industry, car repair	—	Preterm birth, intrauterine death

Metals

Inorganic lead

Occupational exposure to lead and lead compounds may occur in many industries, e.g. industries using lead based pigments, paints, lead battery accumulators, crystal glass containing lead, brass, soldering metals, bullets that contain lead, and lead based PVC plastics stabiliser. Lead exposure is also possible in the production, repair or demolishing of lead containing goods or materials.

Both environmental and occupational exposure of lead can adversely affect the hypothalamic–pituitary–testicular axis and therefore impair the induction of spermatogenesis which manifest as low sperm count (Ghandi *et al.*, 2017). Exposure to lead in women has been related to menstrual disorders among lead battery plant workers (Tang and Zhu, 2003). Low-level cumulative lead exposure is associated with an earlier age at menopause (Eum *et al.*, 2014). Lead is accumulated in bone and increased endogenous lead exposure has been demonstrated in women during periods of increased bone turnover, such as menopause. This may constitute a potential health issue to the woman during old age (Vahter *et al.*, 2002).

At low exposure levels during pregnancy, lead can cause spontaneous abortion (Borja-Aburto *et al.*, 1999), pregnancy-induced hypertension (Yazbeck *et al.*, 2009), preterm birth and low birth weight (Torres-Sánchez *et al.*, 1999; Jelliffe-Pawlowski *et al.*, 2006). Maternal exposure during first trimester is linked to impairment of neurodevelopment of the fetus and mental development of the child (Hu *et al.*, 2006; Bellinger, 2005). Lead is transferred across the placenta. At birth the blood lead concentration in the umbilical cord is close to that of the mother. The blood lead level of pregnant women should not exceed the level of the unexposed population. Women planning for pregnancy should ideally be withdrawn from excess exposure before the start of the pregnancy.

Mercury

Occupational exposure to inorganic mercury can occur in the chloralkali industry, in waste management and in recovery of mercury. Lesser exposures may occur in health care and in dental care. In males, exposure to mercury has been linked to a decrease in sperm count and quality (Wirth and Mijal, 2010). Inorganic mercury may cause menstrual disorders, delayed conception, and increase risk of spontaneous abortion in females (Lindbohm, 2007). Inorganic mercury is transferred to the fetus and also accumulates in the placenta. It is toxic to the nervous system and to the kidneys, thus exposure during pregnancy should be avoided.

Exposure to mercury may not cause clinical symptoms in the pregnant mother, but it can cause profound effects on the fetus, including intellectual impairment, persistence of primitive reflexes (sucking, rooting, grasping and crossed extension), cerebellar signs, and delayed physical development, as seen in congenital Minamata disease (Semionov, 2018).

Cadmium

Cadmium may act as an endocrine disruptor and consequently alter the function of the endocrine system and cause adverse reproductive effects, such as reducing semen volume, progressive motility, and altering sperm morphology in men (Li *et al.*, 2016) and pregnancy-related hypertension and pre-eclampsia in women (Pollack *et al.*, 2014).

Organic Solvents

Organic solvents have a wide range of applications across various industries, such as in auto repair, electronics, dry cleaning, health-care products, paints, glues and other industries. Workers may encounter high levels of exposure because of the high volatility of many organic solvents. The study findings on individual solvents must be interpreted with caution, because concomitant exposure to a mixture of solvents in the workplace is common, making it difficult to determine the exact contribution of one particular solvent to the adverse reproductive effects.

The impact of occupational exposure to organic solvents is more evident in women as compared to men. In men, volatile organic solvent exposure could have toxic effects on male sex steroids by directly affecting testicular function, especially in workers exposed for many years (Eldesouki *et al.*, 2013). It also has negative impact on ejaculate volume and sperm concentration (Ianos *et al.*, 2018).

In women, exposure to some solvents has been associated with oligomenorrhea (Cho *et al.*, 2001). Occupational exposure to solvents has also been associated with reduced fertility and increased risks of spontaneous abortion and congenital anomalies (Burdorf *et al.*, 2006). Exposure has also been associated with neural tube defects, orofacial clefts, and congenital heart anomalies in the offspring (Spinder *et al.*, 2019).

The most important routes of exposure to organic solvents are via inhalation, followed by dermal contact. Most solvents can pass through the placenta and can also be excreted into the breast milk. Therefore, it is prudent to minimise exposure to organic solvents during pregnancy and during breastfeeding.

Specific solvents

Specific solvents which have been found to be associated with adverse reproductive effects in human studies include carbon disulphide, tetrachloroethylene, toluene and benzene.

Carbon disulphide is used primarily in the manufacturing of viscose rayon fiber, in the production of carbon tetrachloride and in analytical chemistry. Exposure to carbon disulphide produces adverse reproductive effects in both males and females. Male workers exposed to carbon disulphide were found to have lower levels of testosterone and decrements in the sperm quality (Guo *et al.*, 2016). Menstrual disorders and early menopause have been reported in women who are chronically exposed to carbon disulphide in the viscose industry (Sieja *et al.*, 2018).

High levels of exposure to tetrachloroethylene (PER) in dry-cleaning work has been associated with an increased risk of spontaneous abortion (Doyle *et al.*, 1997). Effects of PER on sperm motility and morphology, and longer time to pregnancy were observed among exposed male workers (Eskenazi *et al.*, 1991; Eskenazi *et al.*, 1991).

Male workers who were exposed to toluene have been found to have decreased sperm motility and altered sperm morphology (Liu *et al.*, 1995). Exposure to toluene among shoe, audio speaker and laboratory workers was found to be associated with an increased risk of spontaneous abortion (Lindbohm, 1995). Reduced fertility has also been described for toluene exposure in women (Plenge-Bönig and Karmaus, 1999; Sallmén *et al.*, 2008).

Benzene exposure has been found to increase the risk of spontaneous abortion, low birth weight and shortened gestation in some studies (Xu *et al.*, 1998; Wang *et al.*, 2000; Zahran *et al.*, 2012). In males, occupational exposure to benzene was associated with increased incidence of chromosomally defective sperm (Marchetti *et al.*, 2012) and decrease in total sperm count and sperm motility (Katukam *et al.*, 2012).

Pesticides

Exposure to pesticides (which include herbicides, insecticides, fungicides and fumigants) can produce harmful reproductive effects in both men and women. The most common route of exposure to pesticide is via dermal contact, followed by inhalation and ingestion.

Certain pesticides, such as dichlorodiphenyltrichloroethane (DDT) and chlordecone, are persistent in the environment and can bioaccumulate in the food chain. As they also act as endocrine disruptors, their adverse effects on human reproduction may have far-reaching consequences.

Pesticides which have reproductive effects on males

Dibromochloropropane (DBCP), which was used as a soil fumigant and nematocide, is now banned after it was identified as a major testicular toxin. Long-term heavy exposure to DBCP has caused irreversible sterility due to azoospermia or severe oligospermia, damage of germinal epithelium, genetic alterations in the sperm, increased risk of spontaneous abortion among exposed workers' wives, hormonal imbalances, and altered sex ratio in offspring (Mehrpour *et al.*, 2014). Adverse effects on semen quality have also been found for exposure to other herbicides, e.g. 2, 4-dichlorophenoxyacetic acid (2, 4D), alachlor and atrazine, and three insecticides, i.e. chlordecone, carbaryl, and diazinon (Jensen *et al.*, 2006). Organophosphates (parathion and methyl parathion) can affect sperm concentration through damaging the seminiferous epithelium by affecting germ cell proliferation (Perry *et al.*, 2011).

Pesticides which have reproductive effects on females

Exposure to pesticides may increase the risk of birth defects, spontaneous abortion, or fetal death (Sallmén and Lindbohm, 2006). Similar to most studies of organic solvents, the risk could not be attributed to any individual pesticide.

DDT, its metabolite dichlorodiphenyldichloroethylene (DDE) and polychlorinated biphenyls (PCBs) are widespread organochlorines in the environment and human tissue. Menstrual disorders have been observed in women exposed to DDT and PCBs (Mendola *et al.*, 2008). Use of hormonally active pesticides (lindane, atrazine, mancozeb or maneb) has also been related to long menstrual cycles, intermenstrual bleeding and missed periods (Farr *et al.*, 2004). Several studies have found increased serum PCB levels among endometriosis patients (Mendola *et al.*, 2008).

Pharmaceuticals

Pharmaceutical agents, including anaesthetic gases and antineoplastic agents, have been found to have adverse reproductive effects, in particular among female workers.

Anaesthetic gases

Occupational exposure to anaesthetic gases has been associated with increase in genotoxic damage among operating room personnel (Yılmaz and Çalbayram, 2016). Female health care workers with occupational exposure to anaesthetic gases were found to have increased risk of spontaneous abortion, congenital malformation, low birth weight and a longer time to become pregnant in several studies, but these findings are limited by the studies were conducted before the introduction of waste gas scavenging devices and ventilation systems (Molina *et al.*, 2016). Efficient scavenging equipment, good ventilation and equipment for the administration of anaesthetics have been used to minimise the exposure to anaesthetic gases at the workplaces.

Antineoplastic agents

Health care workers can be exposed to antineoplastic agents used for cancer chemotherapy in hospitals when handling the concentrated drugs during the shipping, receiving and preparation processes, during administration and disconnection of infusion system in wards or clinics, and in cleaning and waste handling activities (Hon *et al.*, 2013). Exposure can also occur in laundries, pharmaceutical factories, veterinary clinics, home care and nursing homes (Meijster *et al.*, 2006).

Handling of antineoplastic agents has been associated with menstrual dysfunction, reduced fertility, spontaneous abortion, premature delivery, low birth weight, and birth defects of the offspring (Connor *et al.*, 2014).

Exposure to these agents should be minimised by engineering controls (such as closed infusion systems), good work practices, use of personal protective equipment and increasing awareness of workers of the potential hazards. Current prevention measures may not completely eliminate opportunities for exposure, and some countries have therefore adopted a policy of temporarily transferring pregnant workers who dilute and prepare antineoplastic drug solutions to other jobs.

Other Chemical Agents

Carbon monoxide is generated via incomplete combustion. It has an approximately 200 times greater affinity to bind haemoglobin compared to oxygen. Exposure to carbon monoxide may occur in smoke producing operations in various industries, e.g. welding work, iron and steel foundries, in producing smoked foods, as well as in car repair and service stations from car exhaust gases. There is some degree of exposure to carbon monoxide in the general outdoor environment in big cities with heavy traffic and in office with smokers (Rim, 2017). Carbon monoxide is transported through the placenta and in the fetus the concentration of blood carboxyhaemoglobin is 10–15% higher than in the mother's blood. Toxic effects of carbon monoxide on the developing fetus depend on chronicity of exposure and concentration as well as gestational age. Maternal carbon monoxide intoxication has been reported to be associated with decreased birth weight, premature birth, intrauterine deaths and brain injuries in the infant (Friedman *et al.*, 2015).

Phthalates, primarily used as plasticisers to induce the flexibility and workability of polymeric materials, are another group of endocrine-disrupters. Exposure to phthalates has been linked to hypospadias and anti-androgenic effects in newborns (Main *et al.*, 2010; Morales-Suárez-Varela *et al.*, 2011) and possible decrease in semen quality (Wang *et al.*, 2015).

Physical Hazards

Radiant Heat and Sedentary Body Posture

The testes are located outside the body to keep its temperature below the core body temperature. It is well established that elevation of the testis temperature impairs and even inhibits spermatogenesis. External heating for short periods of time may result in a significant but temporary decrease of semen quality (Mieusset and Bujan, 1995). Prolonged hours of sitting or exposure to radiant heat can lead to testicular heat stress, which can lead to spermatogenic arrest, germ cell apoptosis, oxidative stress, and sperm DNA damage (Durairajanayagam *et al.*, 2014; Gill *et al.*, 2019). Studies have showed reduced sperm count among men working in a hot environment (such as foundry workers, ceramic workers and bakers) due to radiant heat exposure of the testes (Thonneau *et al.*, 1998).

Radiation

Ionising radiation includes X-rays and radiation from radionuclides. Exposure to ionising radiation may occur at nuclear power plants, among health care professions and in flying aircraft (Grajewski *et al.*, 2015).

Ionising radiation at the work place is an established risk factor for testicular damage. The testis is one of the most radiosensitive tissues of the body and spermatogonia are the most radiosensitive cells of the spermatogenesis process. Chronic long-term exposure to low doses of ionising radiation could affect sperm motility, morphology, and the sperm DNA fragmentation index (Zhou *et al.*, 2016).

In women, small doses of radiation are not expected to increase the risk of congenital malformations, but it may have effects on fetal growth and increase the risk of childhood cancer. X-rays penetrate tissues and reach the fetus. Radionuclides vary in their ability to reach the fetal tissues and the exposure assessment may require analysing radioactivity secreted or excreted from the body from biological samples. There is weak evidence of an association between radiation exposure and primary infertility in women (Doyle *et al.*, 2000; Doyle *et al.*, 2001).

The advent of mobile phones has revolutionised communication trends across the globe. Exposure to radiofrequency electromagnetic waves radiation emitted by mobile phone use was found to be associated with reduced sperm motility and viability (Adams *et al.*, 2014).

Noise

Noise may cause adverse reproductive effects through a stress reaction induced by the increase of maternal catecholamine secretion, which may further stimulate or retard uterine contractions and affect utero-placental blood flow. Aircraft noise was found to be associated with preterm birth, low birth weight and congenital anomalies. There was also evidence for an association between road traffic noise and low birth weight, preterm birth and small for gestational age (Nieuwenhuijsen *et al.*, 2017). Occupational noise exposure during pregnancy is associated with hearing dysfunction in children, suggest that pregnant women should not be exposed to high levels of noise at work (Selander *et al.*, 2016).

Strenuous Physical Strain

Work entailing strenuous physical exertion may harmfully affect the reproductive health of women, although moderate physical activity is generally safe both for the mother and fetus. Strong physical effort may alter the hormonal balance and increase intrauterine pressure, and thus decrease the nutritional blood flow to the fetus. In later pregnancy it may also promote uterine contractions, and consequently increase the risk for preterm delivery.

Physically demanding work during pregnancy is associated with an increased risk of adverse pregnancy outcomes. Lifting objects is associated with an increased risk of miscarriage, pre-eclampsia, preterm delivery and low birth weight. Prolonged standing was associated with preterm delivery and having a small-for-age gestation (Cai *et al.*, 2020).

Strenuous physical exertion should be considered in the risk assessment and prevention of occupational reproductive hazards. During the second and third trimesters the physical work load may need to be decreased, opportunities for rest organised, and continuous standing and walking avoided. Where appropriate, work equipment and lifting gear should be adapted, storage arrangements altered, or workstations or job content redesigned. Long periods spent handling loads, or standing or sitting without regular movement to maintain healthy circulation should also be avoided.

Biological Hazards

Some infectious agents may have an impact on reproductive health, in particular on the pregnant mother and developing fetus. They can cause congenital anomalies, fetal growth retardation, low birth weight or systematic disease (Ekblad, 1995). Most observations of risk on reproduction are based on the general population studies rather than on specific occupational group. Examples of biological agents that can affect reproductive health include hepatitis B and C virus, rubella virus, varicella zoster virus, cytomegalovirus, human parvovirus B19, human immunodeficiency virus, Zika virus (ZIKV) and the severe acute respiratory syndrome coronavirus 2 (SARS-CoV-2).

Toxoplasmosis is a zoonosis due to exposure to cat faeces and uncooked meat containing the parasite *Toxoplasma gondii*. Veterinary staff and animal care workers may be exposed to toxoplasma. Listeriosis is a food-borne bacterial zoonotic disease worldwide caused by *Listeria spp*. It is an occupational hazard for veterinarians and ranchers who assist in delivery of infected and aborted calves. Both these zoonotic diseases can have adverse effects on pregnant women and their fetus.

Vaccine-Preventable Viral Diseases

Hepatitis B, rubella and varicella zoster viruses constitute a risk to reproductive health, particularly among health care workers.

Non-immune pregnant personnel should ideally avoid caring for patients with measles, rubella, varicella or herpes zoster, as these viruses may harm the fetus (Russi *et al.*, 2009). Most health care workers may already have natural immunity against the common viral diseases (e.g. varicella) via past infection or have been vaccinated against these viruses (e.g. measles, mumps, rubella, and varicella). Hepatitis B vaccination is recommended for all health care workers who are at risk of exposure to patients' blood and body fluids. Other than vaccinations, other ways to prevent infectious diseases include safe work practices and providing temporary job reassignment for non-immune pregnant workers.

Other viruses

Cytomegalovirus is a common cause of congenital infection. Most infected children are asymptomatic. However, a minority of affected children can suffer long-term complications including neurologic diseases, learning disability, deafness and blindness. Parvovirus B19 infection has been particularly prevalent among school teachers and women working with groups of children participating in after-school activities as compared with other pregnant women (Valeur-Jensen *et al.*, 1999). Maternal Parvovirus B19 infection during pregnancy can cause fetal anaemia, hydrops fetalis, spontaneous abortion and intrauterine fetal death (Xiong *et al.*, 2019). In the absence of effective vaccinations available against these viruses, the risk of both infections can be diminished by good basic hygiene, including hand washing (Buxmann *et al.*, 2017; American College of Obstetricians and Gynecologists, 2015).

ZIKV is an arthropod-borne flavivirus transmitted by *Aedes aegypti* mosquitoes. A widespread epidemic of ZIKV infection was reported in 2015 in South and Central America and the Caribbean. Other than mosquito bites, ZIKV can also be transmitted via maternal-to-fetal transmission, sexual contact, blood transfusion and organ transplantation. The United States (US) Centre for Disease Control and Prevention (CDC) reported one laboratory-acquired case of ZIKV infection via a needle stick while working with the Zika virus in a research laboratory in 2016. ZIKV can infect pregnant women in all three trimesters. Although pregnant women do not appear to be more susceptible to or more severely affected by ZIKV infection, maternal-fetal transmission has been documented and is associated with adverse neonatal outcomes, most notably microcephaly (Rasmussen *et al.*, 2016).

The outbreak of Coronavirus Disease 2019 (COVID-19) has become a major pandemic threat worldwide since it was first identified in December 2019. COVID-19 is caused by SARS-CoV-2. Health care workers are at risk of being infected by COVID-19 in the course of their work (Harrison *et al.*, 2020). A study revealed that male reproductive ability was affected in males infected with COVID-19 (Ling *et al.*, 2020).

Psychological Hazards

Job Stress

Occupational stress has been related to male infertility and reduced semen quality (Sheiner *et al.*, 2002; Clarke *et al.*, 1999). Men with high occupational stress were found to have higher level of sperm DNA damage (Radwan *et al.*, 2016).

For women in the workforce, psychosocial stress may lead to dysmenorrhoea, irregular menstrual cycle, spontaneous abortion, and other reproductive health problems due to fluctuations in female hormones (Cho *et al.*, 2014; Lawson *et al.*, 2015; Park and Moon, 2015).

Shift Work

Shift work is common in health care, manufacturing, transport and communication work. Shift work has been considered as a potential hazard for reproduction, because it may interfere with the circadian rhythm. This may lead to changes in hormonal concentrations that may affect reproductive capability. Working in shifts or during the night appears to increase the risk of menstrual cycle irregularity (Kang *et al.*, 2019) and endometriosis (Marino *et al.*, 2008). A meta-analysis showed that shift work significantly increased the risk of preterm delivery, abortion, low birth weight, small-for-gestational-age infants, menstrual disruption and infertility (Itani and Kaneita, 2016).

Case Study 1: Managing a Pregnant Shiftworker

A 39 year old pregnant nurse works full time at a hospital. She was referred during gestational week 7 in her 4th pregnancy. At the 8th week of gestation, she had a transient bleeding episode of a few days. She was feeling tired slightly, but was otherwise healthy. She works in a forward rotating three-shift schedule (0700–1500 hrs, 1500–2300 hrs and 2300–0700 hrs) and had on average four night duties per month. Job tasks included administration of pharmaceuticals, assisting doctors and manual tasks such as transfer of disabled patients from bed to chair and vice versa, in particular during evening and night shifts. There were about 15 patient transfers during a shift — usually performed by two persons.

What are the options that the occupational physician can suggest to the worker and employer?

1. *Can she be transferred to another department where she does not need to be on shift work, e.g. in the outpatient clinics?*
2. *She should be advised not to lift heavy burdens which in this case would include transfer of patients. Some job adjustment may be needed depending on her pregnancy status further into the gestation.*

The Role of Occupational Health Physician

Clinical Approach to Male Infertility

Suspicion of work related male infertility is raised when a hazardous work place exposure is present in a worker with reduced semen quality, that is not explained by a specific andrological disease (e.g. infection of the accessory sex glands, varicocele, congenital disorders etc.) or specific medical disorders (e.g. endocrine disease, kidney failure, liver cirrhosis).

In general, there are four criteria that must be fulfilled to establish that a case of infertility is most likely caused by a specific occupational exposure.

1. The adverse reproductive effect in terms of, e.g. reduced libido or reduced quantity or quality of semen, must fit with what is known about the adverse effect of the suspected hazardous exposure.

2. The exposure must be sufficient to cause the adverse effect. The occupational history is the main tool to obtain information on type, intensity and duration of an exposure. The mere presence of a toxic compound is not sufficient to cause damage. It is necessary to estimate the extent of exposure. Measurements of concentration in ambient air and/or by biological monitoring data may improve the validity of the exposure assessment.
3. It is important to consider the timing of exposure relative to the adverse effect. Irreversible effects of earlier exposure are difficult to document. Discontinuation of an ongoing exposure which is associated with an increased semen quality, e.g. in terms of increase in sperm count during subsequent weeks or months, is suggestive of a causal association. Chemical agents operating at the final stages of spermatogenesis (e.g. some pesticides) may have effects on sperm motility that may disappear several weeks after cessation of exposure. Chemical agents operating in the early stages of spermatogenesis may have effects lasting for several months after cessation of exposure, because the duration of human spermatogenesis is 3 months.
4. Other causes must be excluded. The occupational physician should consider alternative disorders that could explain the infertility. Sometimes, it may be necessary to consult an andrologist or urologist to ascertain other possible work-related factors that could have been contributory, for example stress, or lifestyle factors.

Occupational effects on male fertility depend critically on the timing of exposure. Men can often recover from testicular damage caused by temporary exposure at the work place. It is therefore important to keep in mind that a worker presenting with infertility may be exposed to reproductive hazards at the workplace. Infertility is not a prescribed occupational disorder in any country, and male infertility is not explicitly compensated by occupational health legislations. Nevertheless, identification of occupational reproductive disorders including male infertility is important for the individual worker who may be able to recover, if the exposure is eliminated.

In cases of couples being investigated for infertility, it would be necessary for the attending physician to ask an occupational history and consider if work factors could be a contributory factor. If indicated, it would be useful to refer the male or female to an occupational physician for further evaluation and management.

Recognition of individual cases of work related infertility may also promote general preventive measures at the work place.

Case Study 2: Male Subfertility

An unskilled 38 year old man (BMI 27 kg/m2) had been unsuccessful in trying to conceive with his wife (a 35 year old cleaner with a BMI of 31 kg/m2) for more than a year. Both were in general good health and are current smokers (10 cigarettes a day). The couple has a healthy child, aged 7 years. The previous preferred method of contraception was the oral contraceptive pills.

Following primary school, the man worked in agriculture for some years, then became a truck driver in various companies. Three years earlier, he started his current unskilled but well paid full time job in a car battery manufacturing company. His task in the clearing department entailed exposure to radiant heat and dust containing inorganic lead. His blood lead increased according to the statutory lead medical surveillance programme from less than 5 μg/dl blood to 45 μg/dl blood within the first half year of employment. It then declined to slightly lower levels around 35-40 μg/dl.

Lead is a possible main or contributing cause for the secondary infertility in this couple. Other established risk factors include female age of 35, male and female obesity and cigarette smoking, in particular in the woman. The infertility work-up did not reveal urogenital anomalies such as tubal occlusion or polycystic ovaries in the woman, while semen examination revealed low sperm counts (8 and 12 million/ml in two samples taken 2 weeks apart following 4 days of sexual abstinence). The follicle stimulating hormone (FSH) was slightly elevated pointing to a peripheral cause of hypogonadism. Serum testosterone and luteinizing hormone (LH) were in the normal range.

The man was transferred to the battery store department, and subsequently his blood lead declined to less than 10 μg/dl blood levels, and sperm counts increased to 65 million/ml semen after 1 year. Three months later, his wife became pregnant.

Pregnancy and Work

If a pregnant woman is not exposed to any known reproductive hazard it is generally not an issue for her to continue work throughout the pregnancy. Many countries have clauses in occupational health legislation that specifically relate to expectant and new mothers.

If a workplace risk to the pregnant employee has been identified, employers must take action to remove, reduce or control the risk. If the risk cannot be removed, measures such as temporary adjustment of her working conditions and/or hours of work or placement in suitable alternative work (if available) can be considered. As a last resort, employers can consider suspending her from work for as long as necessary, to protect her health and safety, and that of her child.

The occupational physician should appreciate the physiological changes and common complaints associated with each trimester of the pregnancy and relate it to the working conditions and possible agents that she may be exposed to (Table 2). For example, in the first

Table 2. Common Complains During Pregnancy that may Affect Work and Possible Job Modifications or Accommodations (Health and Safety Executive, 2004; Draper, 2006)

Common Complaints During Pregnancy	Impact of Work	Job Modification or Accommodation
Nausea and vomiting (Morning sickness) during early pregnancy	• Exposure to chemicals with strong, unpleasant smell • Early shift work	• Having frequent regular, healthy snacks • Later start, alternate duties or changes in the scheduling of their breaks • Extra time may be needed to complete required tasks, especially in the morning, when nausea and vomiting most frequently occur
Increase risk of back ache or injury caused by ligament laxity and shift in central gravity	• Back ache can be intensified by remaining in a specific position for a long period of time and by manual handling	• Pregnant women should avoid long periods spent handling loads • Provide the opportunity to alternate between standing and sitting

Table 2. (*Continued*)

Common Complaints During Pregnancy	Impact of Work	Job Modification or Accommodation
Shift in central gravity caused by the increased weight of the growing fetus and enlarged uterus results in difficulty in balancing	• Working at height • Problems of working on slippery, wet surfaces	• Work at heights and activities that require pregnant women to bend over constantly should be avoided or adjusted as necessary
Varicose veins from pressure of the growing uterus and fetus on pelvic vein	• Aggravated by prolonged standing/ sitting	• Alternate between standing and sitting tasks, with regular break If possible, have a chair or stool at the work station
Lower limb edema from pressure of the growing uterus and fetus on the lower limb vascular system	• Aggravated by prolonged sitting, standing, or walking • Unable to wear their regular shoe size by the end of pregnancy	• Alternate between standing and sitting • Regular rest breaks to elevate their feet and feet exercise to enhance venous return • Pregnant women should also be reminded not to wear tight, or constrictive, clothing on their hips or legs
Haemorrhoids caused by pressure of enlarged uterus obstruct venous return	• Aggravated by prolonged sitting in the workplace and working in hot conditions	• Alternate between standing and sitting • Advised to stay hydrated and monitor for problems related to constipation
Frequent micturition caused by compression of bladder by enlarging uterus	• Difficulty in leaving job/site of work	• Pregnant workers should be given ample time in and access to rest room facilities
Increasing in girth size from fetal growth with advance pregnancy	• Problems of working in tightly fitting work uniforms or use of protective equipment • Work in confined spaces may lead to strain or sprain injuries,	• Provide loosely fit uniform • Provide suitable alternative equipment to allow the work to be conducted safely and without risk to health to be conducted safely and without risk to health

(*Continued*)

Table 2. (*Continued*)

Common Complaints During Pregnancy	Impact of Work	Job Modification or Accommodation
	and increase risk of accident • Manual handling	• To alter the nature of the task to reduce risks from manual handling
Fatigue	• Aggravated by working overtime and shift work	• Adjustment to working hours, timing and frequency of rest breaks, and to change shift patterns and duration to avoid risks
Dizziness or faintness caused by peripheral vasodilatation	• Aggravated by continuous standing during the working day and hot environment	• Alternate between standing and sitting tasks, with regular break • If possible, have a chair or stool at the work station
Dyspnea from displaced diaphragm caused by expanding gravid uterus and growing fetus	• Aggravated by physical manual work	• Pregnant women who perform physical work should be given extra time to complete their tasks to compensate for the increased oxygen consumption of pregnancy
Heartburn caused by relaxation of pyloric sphincter and compressing of stomach by enlarging uterus	• Exacerbated by work requires frequent bending	• Avoid the work requires bending • Reminder to eat smaller and frequent meals

trimester of pregnancy, some women may experience morning sickness and nausea which could be aggravated by chemicals with strong, unpleasant odour. In the last trimester fatigue will increase which may pose a problem for the woman if the working conditions are inflexible or if she is doing shift work, especially the night shift. Frequency of micturition is another issue that needs to be considered, especially if the pregnant worker is involved in assembly line work, and may find difficulty in taking toilet breaks.

Breastfeeding and Work

Chemical contamination of breast milk through exposure of mothers at work has become a matter of concern in recent years among women who have followed the advice to breast-feed their infants. Maternal exposure at work to various chemicals may cause contamination of breast milk. Milk fat is excreted as a fat globule, and chemicals may be bound on the surface of the globule or trapped within the globule. The amount of chemicals in breast milk is determined by the extent of the exposure to the chemicals and the properties of the chemicals. Small lipophilic organic molecules, e.g. organic solvents and pesticides, are easily transferred from blood plasma to mammary gland cells, and concentrate in the fat globules.

The chemical exposure may be life-long exposure (accumulated chemicals) or due to periodic high exposure. A review on organic and inorganic chemicals in breast milk concludes that it is important to identify contaminant trends of highly exposed groups and take measures to improve the situation as far as possible (Massart *et al.*, 2008).

As a general guiding principle women who are breast feeding should not return to work with exposure to chemicals unless it can be ascertained that these chemicals are not excreted via the breast milk. They should only be returned to their original work when the child has been weaned. The employer, wherever possible, should make available facilities for the women to express her milk and keep it refrigerated so her child could continue to have breast milk. Some countries have legislation that require employers to provide suitable rest facilities for pregnant or breastfeeding workers. The facilities should be conveniently located (e.g. near to toilets) and allow the new or expectant mother to lie down.

Conclusion

Workplace hazards can adversely affect the reproductive system. However, many employers and employees are probably less aware of reproductive effects of workplace hazards compared to effects on other organ systems such as the skin, musculoskeletal or auditory systems.

The employer has a duty is to protect the safety and health of employees, including reproductive health of both male and female workers. Risk assessment at the workplace should also consider any specific reproductive risks to males as well as females of childbearing age who could become pregnant, and to new and expectant mothers. Any identified risk should be managed accordingly.

References

Adams JA, Galloway TS, Mondal D, Esteves SC, Mathews F. (2014) Effect of mobile telephones on sperm quality: A systematic review and meta-analysis. *Environ Int* **70**: 106–112.

American College of Obstetricians and Gynecologists. (2015) Practice bulletin no. 151: Cytomegalovirus, parvovirus B19, varicella zoster, and toxoplasmosis in pregnancy. *Obstet Gynecol* **125**(6): 1510–1525.

Bellinger DC. (2005) Teratogen update: Lead and pregnancy. *Birth Defects Res Part A Teratog Update* **73**(6): 409–420.

Borja-Aburto VH, Herz-Picciotto I, Rojas Lopes M, Farias P, Rios C Blanco J. (1999) Blood lead levels measured prospectively and risk of spontaneous abortion. *Am J Epidemiol* **150**: 590–597.

Burdorf A, Figa-TalamancaI, Jensen TK, Thulstrup AM. (2006) Effects of occupational exposure on the reproductive system: Core evidence and practical implications. *Occup Med* **8**: 516–520.

Buxmann H, Hamprecht K, Meyer-Wittkopf M, Friese K. (2017). Primary Human Cytomegalovirus (HCMV) Infection in Pregnancy. *Dtsch Arztebl Int* **114**(4): 45–52.

Cai C, Vandermeer B, Khurana R, Nerenberg K, Featherstone RSebastianski M, Davenport MH. (2020) The impact of occupational activities during pregnancy on pregnancy outcomes: A systematic review and meta-analysis. *Am J Obstet Gynecol* **222**(3): 224–238.

Cho IJ, Kim H, Lim S, Oh S-S, Park SY, Kang H-T. (2014) Emotional labor and dysmenorrhea in women working in sales and call centers. *Ann Occup Environ Med* **26**(1): 45–51.

Cho SI, Damokosh AI, Ryan LM, Chen D, Hu YA, Smith TJ, Christiani DC, Xu X. (2001) Effects of exposure to organic solvents on menstrual cycle length. *J Occup Environ Med* **43**: 567–575.

Clarke RN, Klock SC, Geoghegan A, Travassos DE. (1999) Relationship between psychological stress and semen quality among in-vitro fertilization patients. *Hum Reprod* **14**: 753–758.

Connor TH, Lawson CC, Polovich M, McDiarmid MA. (2014) Reproductive health risks associated with occupational exposures to antineoplastic drugs in health care settings: A review of the evidence. *J Occup Environ Med* **56**(9): 901–910.

Doyle P, Maconochie N, Roman E, Davies G, Smith PG, Beral V. (2000) Foetal death and congenital malformation in babies born to nuclear industry employees: Report from the nuclear industry family study. *Lancet* **356**:1293–1299.

Doyle P, Roman E, Beral V, Brookes M. (1997) Spontaneous abortion in dry cleaning workers potentially exposed to perchloroethylene. *Occup Environ Med* **54**: 848–853.

Doyle P, Roman E, Maconochie N, Davies G, Smith PG, Beral V. (2001). Primary infertility in nuclear industry employees: Report from the nuclear industry family study. *Occup Environ Med* **58**: 535–539.

Draper L. (2006) Pregnant women in the workplace: Distinguishing between normal and abnormal physiologic changes. *Workplace Health Saf* **54**(5): 217–225.

Durairajanayagam D, Sharma RK, du Plessis SS, Agarwal A. (2014) Testicular heat stress and sperm quality. *Male Infertil* 102–125.

Eldesouki MA, Sharaf NE, Shakour AAA, Mohamed MS, Hussein AS, Hasani IW. (2013) Study of the effect of occupational exposure to volatile organic compounds (VOC's) on male reproductive hormones. *World J Med Sci* **8**: 6–12.

Ekblad U. (1995) Biological agents and pregnancy. *J Occup Environ Med* **37**: 962–965.

Eskenazi B, Fenster L, Hudes M. (1991) A study of the effect of perchloroethylene exposure on the reproductive outcomes of wives of dry-cleaning workers. *Am J Ind Med* **20**: 593–600.

Eskenazi B, Wyrobek AJ, Fenster L. (1991) A study of the effect of perchloroethylene exposure on semen quality in dry cleaning workers. *Am J Ind Med* **20**: 575–591.

Eum K, Weisskopf MG, Nie LH, Hu H, Korrick SA. (2014) Cumulative lead exposure and age at menopause in the Nurses' Health Study Cohort. *Environ Health Perspect* **122**(3): 229–234.

Farr SL, Cooper GS, Cai J, Savitz DA, Sandler DP. (2004) Pesticide use and menstrual cycle characteristics among premenopausal women in the Agricultural Health Study. *Am J Epidemiol* **160**: 1194–1204.

Friedman P, Guo X, Stiller RJ, Laifer SA. (2015) Carbon monoxide exposure during pregnancy. *Obstet Gynecol Surv* **70**(11): 705–712.

Gandhi J, Hemandez R, Chen A, Smith N, Sheynkin Y, Joshi G, Khan S. (2017) Impaired hypothalamic-pituitary-testicular axis activity, spermatogenesis, and sperm function promote infertility in males with males with lead poisoning. *Zygote* **25**(2): 103–110.

Grajewski B, Whelan EA, Lawson CC, Hein MJ, Waters MA, Anderson JL, MacDonald LA, Mertens CJ, Tseng CY, Cassinelli RT, Luo L. (2015) Miscarriage among flight attendants. *Epidemiology* **26**(2): 192–203.

Gill K, Jakubik J, Kups M, Rosiak-Gill A, Kurzawa R, Kurpisz M, Fraczek M, Piasecka M. (2019) The impact of sedentary work on sperm nuclear DNA integrity. *Folia Histochem Cytobiol* **57**(1): 15–22.

Guo Y, Ma Y, Chen G, Cheng J. (2016) The effects of occupational exposure of carbon disulfide on sexual hormones and semen quality of male workers from a chemical fiber factory. *J Occup Environ Med* **58**(8): e294–e300.

Harrison D, Muradali K, El Sahly H, Bozkurt B, Jneid H. (2020) Impact of the SARS-CoV-2 pandemic on health-care workers. *Hosp Pract (1995)* 1–4.

Health and Safety Executive. (2004) *New and expectant mothers at work — A guide for employers* (2nd Ed). [Online] Available from: http://www.riskassessments.biz/guides/Booklets/pregnancy.pdf [Accessed on 4 April 2021].

Hon CY, Teschke K, Chu W, Demers P, Venners S. (2013) Antineoplastic drug contamination of surfaces throughout the hospital medication system in Canadian hospitals. *J Occup Environ Hygiene* **10**: 374–383.

Hu H, Tellez-Rojo MM, Bellinger D, Smith D, Ettinger AS, Lamadrid-Figueroa H, Schwartz J, Schnaas L, Mercado-Garcia A, Hernandez-Avila M. (2006) Foetal lead exposure at each stage of pregnancy as a predictor of infant mental development. *Environ Health Perspect* **114**: 1730–1735.

Ianos O, Sari-Minodier I, Villes V, Lehucher-Michel MP, Loundou A, Perrin J. (2018) Meta-analysis reveals the association between male occupational exposure to solvents and impairment of semen parameters. *J Occup Environ Med* **60**(10): e533–e542.

Itani O, Kaneita Y. (2016) The association between shift work and health: A review. *Sleep Biol Rhythms* **14**: 231–239.

Jelliffe-Pawlowski LL, Miles SQ, Courtney JG, Materna B, Charlton V. (2006) Effect of magnitude and timing of maternal pregnancy blood lead (Pb) levels on birth outcomes. *J Perinatol* **26**(3): 154–162.

Jensen TK, Bonde JP, Joffe M. (2006) The influence of occupational exposure on male reproductive function. *Occup Med* **56**: 544–553.

Kang W, Jang KH, Lim HM, Ahn JS, Park WJ. (2019) The menstrual cycle associated with insomnia in newly employed nurses performing shift work: A 12-month follow-up study. *Int Arch Occup Environ Health* **92**: 227–235.

Katukam V, Kulakarni M, Syed R, Alharbi K, Naik J. (2012) Effect of benzene exposure on fertility of male workers employed in bulk drug industries. *Genet Test Mol Biomark* **16**: 592–597.

Lawson CC, Johnson CY, Chavarro JE, Hibert ENL, Schernhammer ES. (2015) Work schedule and physically demanding work in relation to menstrual function: The Nurses' Health Study 3. *Scand J Work Environ Health* **41**(2): 194–203.

Li Y, Wu J, Zhou W, Gao E. (2016) Association between environmental exposure to cadmium and human semen quality. *Int J Environ Health Res* **26**(2): 175–186.

Lindbohm M-L. (1995) Effects of parental exposure to solvents on pregnancy outcome. *J Occup Environ Med* **37**: 908–914.

Lindbohm M-L, Ylöstalo P, Sallmén M, Henriks-Eckerman M-L, Nurminen T, Forss H, Taskinen H. (2007) Occupational exposure in dentistry and miscarriage. *Occup Environ Med* **64**: 127–133.

Ling M, Xie W, Li D, Shi L, Mao Y, Xiong Y, Zhang Y, Zhang M. (2020) Effect of SARS-CoV-2 infection upon male gonadal function: A single center-based study. *MedRxiv*.

Liu HX, Qin WH, Wang GR, Yang ZZ, Chang YX, Jiang QG. (1995) Some altered concentrations of elements in semen of workers exposed to trinitrotoluene. *Occup Environ Med* **52**: 842–845.

Main KM, Skakkebaek NE, Virtanen HE, Toppari J. (2010) Genital anomalies in boys and the environment. *Best Pract Res Clin Endocrinol Metab* **24**: 279–289.

Marchetti F, Eskenazi B, Weldon RH, Li G, Zhang L, Rappaport SM, Thomas ESchmid Xing C, Kurtovich E, Wyrobek AJ. (2012) Occupational exposure to benzene and chromosomal structural aberrations in the sperm of Chinese men. *Environ Health Perspect* **120**: 2.

Marino JL, Holt VL, Chen C, Davis S. (2008) Shift work, HCLOCK T3111C polymorphism, and endometriosis risk. *Epidemiology* **19**: 477–484.

Massart F, Gherarducci G, Marchi B, Saggese G. (2008) Chemical biomarkers of human breast milk pollution. *Biomark Insights* **3**: 159–169.

Mehrpour O, Karrari P, Zamani N, Tsatsakis AM, Abdollahi M. (2014) Occupational exposure to pesticides and consequences on male semen and fertility: A review. *Toxicol Lett* **230**(2): 146–156.

Mendola P, Messer LC, Rappazzo K. (2008) Science linking environmental contaminant exposures with fertility and reproductive health impacts in the adult female. *Fertil Steril* **89**: 81–94.

Meijster T, Fransman W, Veldhof R, Kromhout H. (2006) Exposure to antineoplastic drugs outside the hospital environment. *Ann Occup Hygiene* **50**: 657–664.

Mieusset R, Bujan L. (1995) Testicular heating and its possible contributions to male infertility: a review. *Int J Androl* **18**: 169–184.

Molina AJM, Ayora AA, Barbara RA, Gascó parici A, Medina LJA, Sol VJ, Sol L. (2016) Occupational exposure to volatile anaesthetics: A systematic review. *Occup Med* **66**(3): 202–207.

Morales-Suárez-Varela MM, Toft GV, Jensen MS, Ramlau-Hansen C, Kaerlev L, Thulstrup AM, Llopis-González A, Olsen J, Bonde JP. (2011) Parental occupational exposure to endocrine disrupting chemicals and male genital malformations: A study in the Danish National Birth Cohort study. *Environ Health* **14**: 3.

Nieuwenhuijsen MJ, Ristovska G, Dadvand P. (2017) WHO Environmental Noise Guidelines for the European Region: A Systematic Review on Environmental Noise and Adverse Birth Outcomes. *Int J Environ Res Public Health* **14**: 1252.

Park OI, Moon H. (2015) Effects of emotional labor on women's reproductive health of nurses. *J Korea Entertain Ind Assoc* **9**(2): 237–246.

Perry MJ, Venners SA, Chen X, Liu X, Tang G, Xing H, Barr DB, Xu X. (2011) Organophosphorous pesticide exposures and sperm quality. *Reprod Toxicol* **31**(1): 75–79.

Plenge-Bönig A, Karmau W. (1999) Exposure to toluene in the printing industry is associated with subfecundity in women but not in men. *Occup Environ Med* **56**: 443–448.

Pollack AZ, Ranasinghe S, Sjaarda LA, Mumford SL. (2014) Cadmium and reproductive health in women: A systematic review of the epidemiologic evidence. *Curr Environ Health Rep* **1**(2): 172–184.

Radwan M, Jurewicz J, Merecz-Kot D, Sobala W, Radwan P, Bochenek M, Janke W. (2016) Sperm DNA damage-the effect of stress and everyday life factors. *Int J Impot Res* **28**(4): 148–154.

Rasmussen SA, Jamieson DJ, Honein MA, Petersen LR. (2016) Zika virus and birth defects — Reviewing the evidence for causality. *N Engl J Med* **374**: 1981–1987.

Rim KT. (2017) Reproductive toxic chemicals at work and efforts to protect workers' health: A Literature Review. *Saf Health Work* **8**(2): 143–150.

Russi M, Buchta WG, Swift M, Budnick LD, Hodgson MJ, Berube D, Kelafant GA. (2009) Guidance for occupational health services in medical centers. *J Occup Environ Med* **51**: e1–e18.

Sallmén M, Lindbohm M-L. (2006) Pesticides, lead and solvents: Pregnancy outcome and fertility. *Tijdschrift voor Bedrijfs- en Verzekeringsgeneeskunde (TBV)* **14**: 396–400.

Sallmén M, Neto M, Mayan ON. (2008) Reduced fertility among shoe manufacturing workers. *Occup Environ Med* **65**: 518–524.

Selander J, Albin M, Rosenhall U, Rylander L, Lewné M, Per Gustavsson P. (2016) Maternal occupational exposure to noise during pregnancy and hearing dysfunction in children: A nationwide prospective cohort study in Sweden. *Environ Health Perspect* **124**: 6.

Semionov A. (2018) Minamata disease—Review. *World J Neurosci* **8**: 178–184.

Sheiner EK, Sheiner E, Carel R, Potashnik G, Shoham-Vardi I. (2002) Potential association between male infertility and occupational psychological stress. *J Occup Environ Med* **44**: 1093–1099.

Sieja K, Von MJ, Von MSJ. (2018) Health effect of chronic exposure to carbon disulfide (CS_2) on women employed in viscose industry. *Medycyna Pracy* **69**(3): 329–335.

Spinder N, Prins JR, Bergman J, Smidt N, Kromhout H, Boezen HM, de Walle, H. (2019) Congenital anomalies in the offspring of occupationally exposed mothers: A systematic review and meta-analysis of studies using expert assessment for occupational exposures. *Hum Reprod (Oxford, England)* **34**(5): 903–919.

Tang N, Zhu ZQ. (2003) Adverse reproductive effects in female workers of lead battery plants. *Int J Occup Med Environ Health* **16**: 359–361.

Thonneau P, Bujan L, Multigner L, Mieusset R. (1998) Occupational heat exposure and male fertility: A review. *Hum Reprod* **13**: 2122–2125.

Torres-Sánchez LE, Berkowitz G, López-Carrillo L, Torres-Arreola L, Ríos C, López-Cervantes M. (1999). Intrauterine lead exposure and preterm birth. *Environ Res* **81**: 297–301.

Vahter M, Berglund M, Akesson A, Lidén C. (2002) Metals and women's health. *Environ Res* **88**: 145–155.

Valeur-Jensen AK, Pedersen CB, Westergaard T, Jensen IP, Lebech M, Andersen PK, Aaby P, Pedersen BN, Melbye M. (1999) Risk factors for parvovirus B19 infection in pregnancy. *JAMA* **281**: 1099–1105.

Wang X, Chen D, Niu T, Wang Z, Wang L, Ryan L, Smith T, Christiani DC, Zuckerman B, Xu X. (2000) Genetic susceptibility to benzene and shortened gestation: Evidence of gene–environment interaction. *Am J Epidemiol* **152**: 693–700.

Wang Y, You L, Zeng Q, Sun Y, Huang Y, Wang C, Wang P, Cao W, Yang P, Li Y, Lu W. (2015) Phthalate exposure and human semen quality: Results from an infertility clinic in China. *Environ Res* **142**: 1–9.

Wirth JJ, Mijal RS. (2010) Adverse effects of low level heavy metal exposure on male reproductive function. *Syst Biol Reprod Med* **56**: 147–167.

Xiong Y, Tan J, Liu Y, He Q, Li L, Zou K, Sun X. (2019) The risk of maternal parvovirus B19 infection during pregnancy on fetal loss and fetal hydrops: A systematic review and meta-analysis. *J Clin Virol* **114**: 12–20.

Xu X, Cho S, Sammel M, You L, Cui S, Huang Y, Ma G, Padungtod C, Pothier L, Niu T, Christiani D, Smith T, Ryan L, Wang L. (1998) Association of petrochemical exposure with spontaneous abortion. *Occup Environ Med* **55**: 31–36.

Yazbeck C, Thiebaugeorges O, Moreau T, Goua V, Debotte G, Sahuquillo J, Forhan A, Foliguet B, Magnin G, Slama R, Charles M-A, Huel G. (2009) Maternal blood lead levels and the risk of pregnancy-induced hypertension: The EDEN Cohort Study. *Environ Health Perspect* **117**: 1526–1530.

Yılmaz S, Çalbayram NC. (2016) Exposure to anesthetic gases among operating room personnel and risk of genotoxicity: A systematic review of the human biomonitoring studies. *J Clin Anesthesia* **35**: 326–331.

Zahran S, Weiler S, Mielke HW, Pena AA. (2012) Maternal benzene exposure and low birth weight risk in the United States: A natural experiment in gasoline reformulation. *Environ Res* **112**: 139–146.

Zhou DD, Hao JL, Guo KM, Lu CW, Liu XD. (2016) Sperm quality and DNA damage in men from Jilin Province, China, who are occupationally exposed to ionising radiation. *Genet Mol Res* **15**: 1.

Chapter 17

Occupational Cancers

Lin Fritschi and Alison Reid**

Case Study 1: Bladder Cancer

A 64-year old man presents with a four-week history of painless haematuria. You have been seeing him occasionally for 15 years and his past history includes borderline hypertension, mild intermittent rosacea, and occasional acute bronchitis. He has never smoked and drinks 3–4 standard measures of alcoholic drinks a week. On questioning he states that he has noticed that he has increased frequency of urination including nocturia for the past year. He has some slight back pain but no other symptoms. Physical examination is unremarkable.

A mid-stream urine sample is grossly haematuric and so you refer him to an urologist. The urine sample is also sent for microscopy which is reported as 'no infection'. Urine cytology is reported as being positive for high-grade urinary carcinoma. The urologist diagnoses metastatic bladder cancer and despite treatment he dies two years later.

His wife is incapacitated with severe osteoarthritis in her hips and knees and he was her primary carer. They have no children. His death has severe ramifications for her, as she is unable to live at home alone, and they have virtually no savings and no assets.

* School of Public Health, Curtin University, Perth, Australia.
Corresponding author: Lin Fritschi (lin.fritschi@curtin.edu.au).

Could this situation have been averted if you had taken his comprehensive occupational history? Details of his job history are as follows:

- 1970: Labourer on various building sites, mainly assisting carpenters and bricklayers.
- 1971: Packer in chicken processing factory, wrapping, grinding and packing meat.
- 1978: Range of jobs in a rubber manufacturing plant including working in the vulcanisation area.
- 2000: Part-time cleaner in office blocks.
- 2017: Retired.

What could have been done in regards to:

- Screening?
- Early diagnosis?
- Advice on compensation?

The answers depend on obtaining an adequate occupational history, and available provisions of the healthcare system, manpower and facilities, and legislation of the country.

Introduction

An occupational cancer is a cancer which is caused wholly or partly by exposure to a carcinogen at work. There are a number of well-known occupational exposures which have been clearly established to cause cancer. For example, asbestos causes mesothelioma, vinyl chloride causes angiosarcoma of the liver, and wood dust causes sino-nasal cancer (International Agency for Research on Cancer (IARC), 2021a)

An occupational cause is relatively easy to prove if the carcinogenic effect of an agent is very strong and the cancer is rare. In this case, astute physicians may notice a “cluster” of cancers at a workplace (see later). It is more difficult to identify causes of common cancers where the effect of the carcinogen is not very strong. There are no pathological or clinical features which help distinguish occupational cancers from those arising from other non-occupational factors (e.g. smoking). In addition, there is often delay of many years or decades between the time of exposure and the diagnosis of cancer so the exposures may have been forgotten, or been poorly documented. Moreover, a person exposed to one carcinogen at work may have been exposed to multiple carcinogens in multiple workplaces, as well as being exposed to lifestyle factors which increase the risk of cancer.

There have been many attempts to estimate how many cancers are due to work. A review noted that the estimates of the fraction of all cancers attributable to occupation ranged between 2% and 8%, with higher estimates for men (range 3–14%) (Purdue *et al.*, 2015). The variation is due to the number of carcinogens included, the cancer sites included, the information available on the prevalence of exposure to each carcinogen and the relative risks chosen to estimate the strength of each carcinogen.

A comprehensive study of 41 carcinogens and 24 cancers estimated that 5.3% (95% confidence interval 4.6–6.6%) of cancer deaths in Great Britain in 2005 (8.2% in men and 2.3 in women) were attributable to occupational exposures (Rushton *et al.*, 2012). The number of incident cases of cancer per year was estimated to be over 13,500. In contrast, around 2,000 new cancer cases per year were granted compensation as being work related (Health and Safety Executive, 2020).

The type of cancer with the greatest number of cases due to work will differ according to the patterns of cancer in that country and the industry profile. In the Great Britain study the most common work-related cancers were: lung (from asbestos, silica, diesel exhaust and a range of other pulmonary carcinogens), non-melanoma skin cancer (from solar radiation, mineral oils and polynuclear aromatic hydrocarbons), mesothelioma (from asbestos), and female breast cancer (from shiftwork) (Rushton *et al.*, 2012).

From a physician's point of view, the attributable fraction may be more useful in practice. The attributable fraction estimates the proportion of a cancer type which is due to a particular exposure (in this case occupation). In the study above, among men, 97% of mesotheliomas, 43% of sino-nasal cancers, 21% of lung cancers, and 11% of nasopharyngeal cancers were due to occupation, meaning that if a physician sees these cases, it is important to think about an occupational cause (Rushton *et al.*, 2012).

Global Burden of Disease for Occupational Cancers

The only global study published so far included 14 carcinogens and eight resulting cancers and estimated that 3.9% (95% uncertainty interval 3.2–4.6%) of cancer deaths were due to exposure to occupational carcinogens in 2016 (GBD 2016 Occupational Carcinogens Collaborators, 2020). This equated to about 349,000 deaths (269,000–427,000) internationally. This is almost certainly an underestimate.

The estimates were derived using the population attributable fraction, and based on past population exposure prevalence and relative risks from the literature showed that:

- 349,000 deaths and 7.2 million DALYs in 2016 were due to exposure to 14 IARC Group 1 occupational carcinogens;
- These accounted for 3.9% of all cancer deaths and 3.4% of all cancer DALYs;
- 79% of deaths were in males and 88% in those aged 55–79 years.
- The commonest causes of death were lung cancer (86%), mesothelioma (7.9%) and laryngeal cancer (2.1%);
- Asbestos was responsible for the largest number of deaths due to occupational carcinogens (63%);
- Other important risk factors were secondhand smoke (14%), silica (14%) and diesel engine exhaust (5%).

The highest mortality rates were recorded in high-income regions, largely due to asbestos-related cancers. For the other regions, cancer deaths from secondhand smoke, silica and diesel engine exhaust were more prominent (GBD 2016 Occupational Carcinogens Collaborators, 2020).

Example of an Occupational Cancer: Mesothelioma

Mesothelioma initially occurred among workers involved in the mining or milling of asbestos, or those who worked with the raw product in asbestos cement or textile factories. Later cases of mesothelioma emerged among workers who used products that contained asbestos, e.g. insulators who sprayed asbestos onto pipes or inside structures as lagging or insulation. The "third wave" of mesothelioma cases are those that emerge among workers who received their exposure from the asbestos products in the buildings in which they renovate or maintain and service or demolish, for example, carpenters and plumbers.

Case Study 2: Mesothelioma

A 68-year-old man presents to his doctor with an eight-week history of shortness of breath on exertion or whilst lying down, and a dull pain in his shoulder and upper arm that did not improve with medication. He has never smoked, and until very recently was fit and active. On questioning he reports fatigue and weight loss. Chest examination reveals a pleural effusion.

Asking his occupational history uncovers that he had worked as a telecommunications technician and linesman for 41 years, commencing at age 15. In that role he installed and connected wires from structures and poles, towers or through trenches, tunnels, ducts, roof and crawl spaces, often lined with or constructed from asbestos cement. Telecommunications pits constructed before the 1990s were built with asbestos cement. He had to regularly drill through the pit wall to install or service the lines that ran into and out of the pit. He often drilled, cut, hammered or chiseled the asbestos cement, using power tools and raising dust in a confined environment. In addition, the older lines were lagged with asbestos as insulation.

The clinical presentation fits a case of respiratory system malignancy, which was subsequently confirmed following pleural biopsy as a mesothelioma. The occupational history highlights the work activities leading to exposure to asbestos — a recognised cause of mesothelioma. This case stresses the importance of clinical features and the taking of a work history to determine occupational exposure in confirming a case of occupational disease.

Mechanisms of Occupational Carcinogenesis

Cancer is a very diverse condition, and different cancers may have a range of different molecular capabilities compared to healthy non-cancerous cells. In 2000, Hannahan and Weinberg suggested a set of properties of cancer cells which could be used as a logical framework for understanding this diversity and named them the "hallmarks of cancer" (Hanahan and Weinberg, 2000). The original six hallmarks, were: "sustaining proliferative signaling, evading growth suppressors, resisting cell death, enabling replicative immortality, inducing angiogenesis, and activating invasion and metastasis." Other related factors were added in 2011: genome instability, inflammation, reprogramming of energy metabolism and evading immune destruction (Hanahan and Weinberg, 2011). These hallmarks describe the changes in the behaviour of the cells within a cancer which allow it to grow and spread.

There are many different mechanisms by which cells in the body can develop these hallmarks. Different carcinogenic agents may have different actions which lead to the hallmark changes in cells along the pathway to cancer. The features of the carcinogenic agents which are relevant to the causation of cancer have been categorised into 10 "Key Characteristics of Carcinogens" (Smith *et al.*, 2015). Carcinogens are likely to have more than one of these characteristics. The 10 characteristics are given below with examples of occupational carcinogens which have each characteristic (Smith *et al.*, 2015):

1. Is electrophilic or can be metabolically activated (ethylene oxide, polycyclic aromatic hydrocarbons, benzene);
2. Is genotoxic (e.g. glyphosate, trichloroethylene);
3. Alters DNA repair or causes genomic instability (e.g. cadmium, solar radiation);
4. Induces epigenetic alterations (e.g. ionising radiation, nickel);

5. Induces oxidative stress (e.g. asbestos, ionising radiation);
6. Induces chronic inflammation (e.g. silica, asbestos);
7. Is immunosuppressive (e.g. cyclosporine);
8. Modulates receptor-mediated effects (e.g. dioxin, PCBs);
9. Causes immortalisation (e.g. viruses such as hepatitis C virus);
10. Alters cell proliferation, cell death or nutrient supply (e.g. diesel engine exhaust, arsenic).

Identifying Occupational Carcinogens

Diagnosis and prevention of occupational carcinogenesis depends on physicians and occupational health and safety professionals knowing which chemicals are carcinogenic. There are many thousands of chemicals which are in use in industry today and new ones are being introduced every year. For each chemical there is a vast literature of *in vitro*, animal, and epidemiological studies examining the risk of cancer. Major challenges arise in even reading the literature, let alone being able to synthesise the findings into an overall conclusion which can be acted upon.

There are several organisations which review and synthesise the literature. These include organisations which: (a) undertake hazard assessments and classify agents as carcinogenic or not; and (b) undertake risk assessments and classify agents as to the degree of risk or provide occupational exposure limits (OELs).

Hazard Assessments

Case Study 3: Shiftwork and Breast Cancer

The manufacturing company has heard that shiftwork causes breast cancer and is concerned for his workforce. They produce sterile injectable products in an aseptic environment and have about 500 workers who work a 24 hour, 7 days a week roster. The shift roster consists of four 9-hour night-shifts, followed by four 9-hour day shifts and then four days off. They work in bright, white light, with three half-hour breaks during their shift. The manager is wondering if the company should change rosters or provide anything else to reduce the risk of breast cancer.

In this case you would need to consider the factors which influence how well someone adapts to night work and resets their body clock. These include the direction of the roster rotation, the time each worker has to recuperate, the lighting at work, and the availability of healthy food which is easy to digest.

The IARC is the specialised cancer agency of the World Health Organization and it undertakes regular reviews of the literature to classify agents as carcinogenic or not. The IARC Monographs (IARC, 2021b) report the findings of interdisciplinary working groups of expert scientists who review the evidence on the carcinogenicity of chemicals, complex mixtures, occupational exposures, physical agents, biological agents, and lifestyle factors. Agents are classified based on animal, human and mechanistic data into one of five groups:

- Group 1: Carcinogenic to humans;
- Group 2A: Probably carcinogenic to humans;
- Group 2B: Possibly carcinogenic to humans;
- Group 3: Not classifiable as to its carcinogenicity to humans;
- Group 4: Probably not carcinogenic to humans.

As an example of a recent assessment that resulted in a Group 2A classification, "night shift work" was classified as probably carcinogenic to humans (IARC, 2020).

This was based on limited evidence from human data and sufficient evidence in animal experiments as well as strong mechanistic evidence in experimental systems, based on effects consistent with immunosuppression, chronic inflammation, and cell proliferation. A challenge in occupational medicine practice with this assessment is what practical measures can be recommended to reduce the risk of breast cancer in workers involved in shift work, since up to a quarter of the workforce in many countries do shift work including night work, e.g. nurses, drivers, and assembly line workers.

Assessment of carcinogenicity of other newly introduced agents, such as various nanomaterials, may have to wait for years until data is accumulated. In such instances, prevention using the precautionary principle may be warranted.

Table 1. Occupational Agents and Circumstances Classified as Carcinogenic (Group 1) by the International Agency for Research on Cancer and the Cancer Types Known to be Caused by Each Agent as of 2020 (IARC, 2021a)

1,2-Dichloropropane	Liver and bile duct
1,3-Butadiene	Leukaemia and/or lymphoma
2,3,7,8-Tetrachlorodibenzo-para-dioxin	All cancer sites (combined)
2-Naphthylamine	Urinary bladder
4-Aminobiphenyl	Urinary bladder
Acheson process, occupational exposures associated with	Lung
Acid mists, strong inorganic	Larynx
Aluminum production	Lung, Urinary bladder
Arsenic and inorganic arsenic compounds	Lung, Skin (other malignant neoplasms), Urinary bladder
Asbestos (all forms)	Larynx, Lung, Mesothelium (pleura and peritoneum), Ovary
Auramine production	Urinary bladder
Benzene	Leukaemia and/or lymphoma
Benzidine	Urinary bladder
Beryllium and beryllium compounds	Lung
Bis(chloromethyl)ether; chloromethyl methyl ether (technical grade)	Lung
Cadmium and cadmium compounds	Lung
Chromium(VI) compounds	Lung
Coal gasification	Lung
Coal-tar distillation	Skin (other malignant neoplasms)
Coal-tar pitch	Lung, Skin (other malignant neoplasms)
Coke production	Lung
Engine exhaust, diesel	Lung
Erionite	Mesothelium (pleura and peritoneum)
Fluoro-edenite	Mesothelium (pleura and peritoneum)
Formaldehyde	Nasopharynx, Leukaemia and/or lymphoma
Haematite mining (underground)	Lung

(*Continued*)

Table 1. (*Continued*)

Ionising radiation (various types)	Salivary gland, Oesophagus, Stomach, Colon and rectum, Liver and bile duct, Gall bladder, Nasal cavity and paranasal sinus, Lung, Bone, Skin (other malignant neoplasms), Breast, Kidney, Urinary bladder, Brain and central nervous system, Thyroid, Leukaemia and/or lymphoma, Multiple sites (unspecified)
Iron and steel founding	Lung
Isopropyl alcohol production	Nasal cavity and paranasal sinus
Leather dust	Nasal cavity and paranasal sinus
Lindane	Leukaemia and/or lymphoma
Magenta production	Urinary bladder
Mineral oils, untreated or mildly treated	Skin (other malignant neoplasms)
Nickel compounds	Nasal cavity and paranasal sinus, Lung
ortho-Toluidine	Urinary bladder
Outdoor air pollution	Lung
Painting	Lung, Mesothelium (pleura and peritoneum), Urinary bladder
Particulate matter in outdoor air pollution	Lung
Pentachlorophenol	Leukaemia and/or lymphoma
Polychlorinated biphenyls	Skin (melanoma)
Rubber production industry	Stomach, Lung, Urinary bladder, Leukaemia and/or lymphoma
Shale oils	Skin (other malignant neoplasms)
Silica dust, crystalline	Lung
Solar radiation	Skin (melanoma), Skin (other malignant neoplasms)
Soot	Lung, Skin (other malignant neoplasms)
Tobacco smoke, second-hand	Lung
Trichloroethylene	Kidney

Table 1. (*Continued*)

Ultraviolet emissions from welding	Eye
Vinyl chloride	Liver and bile duct
Welding fumes	Lung
Wood dust	Nasopharynx, Nasal cavity and paranasal sinus

Many national bodies undertake similar hazard assessments, e.g. the Chemicals Evaluation and Research Institute (Japan), and the European Chemicals Agency. The American Conference of Governmental Industrial Hygienists (ACGIH) uses a similar set of classifications for their hazard assessments with carcinogenicity of an agent indicated by A1–A5 based on the weight of evidence:

- A1 Confirmed human carcinogen;
- A2 Suspected human carcinogen;
- A3 Animal carcinogen. "Available evidence suggests that the agent is not likely to cause cancer in humans except under uncommon or unlikely routes or levels of exposure";
- A4 Not classifiable as a human carcinogen. "There are inadequate data on which to classify the agent in terms of its carcinogenicity in humans and/or animals";
- A5 Not suspected as a human carcinogen.

Often the various bodies come to different decisions despite all relying on the same body of evidence (Nilsson *et al.*, 1993). This is because of the different criteria used to select included data and the different emphasis placed on the human, animal and mechanistic data as well as the non-scientific considerations which influence policy decisions. As a practitioner, it is often difficult to determine which voices to listen to, given that there is often not the time and the expertise to review the original sources. When the agent first comes to attention as a possible carcinogen, there may not be enough information to convince all review bodies. However, over time, as evidence accumulates, it is eventually clear that an agent is or isn't a carcinogen (for example asbestos — which clearly is a carcinogen (Loomis *et al.*, 2018), or coffee — which now clearly is not (Loomis *et al.*, 2016). However, the evidence may take years or even decades to accumulate and during the phase of uncertainty it is important to consider the processes used by the different bodies and any conflicts of interest that the members of the panels or the organisations might have had (if known).

Labelling of Carcinogens

Under the United Nations Globally Harmonised System of Classification and Labelling of Chemicals (United Nations Economic Commission for Europe, 2019), chemicals or a mixture of chemical substances are classified as carcinogenic if they induce cancer or increase its incidence. Substances and mixtures in this hazard class are assigned to one of two hazard categories based mainly on strength of evidence. Category 1 agents are known or presumed human carcinogens which are divided into Category 1A agents which are known to have carcinogenic potential for humans based largely on human evidence and Category 1B which are presumed to have carcinogenic potential for humans based largely on animal evidence. Category 2 agents are suspected human carcinogens where there is some evidence of carcinogenicity but it is not sufficiently convincing to place the substance in Category 1. This system was operational globally in 2008 and for the first time there was one system for the classification of chemical hazards (Winder *et al.*, 2005). The pictogram for carcinogenic agents (Fig. 1) is also used for

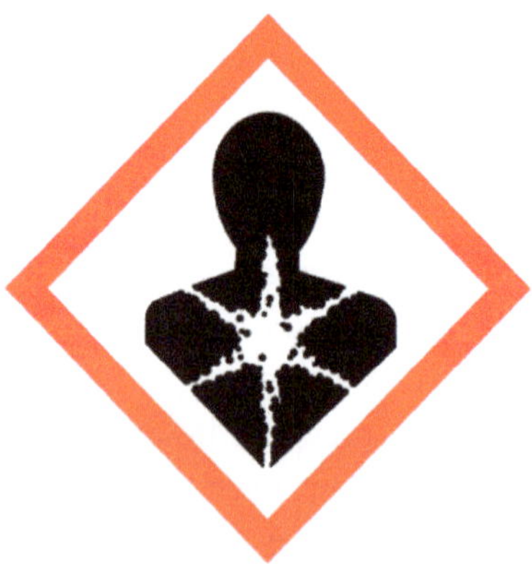

Fig. 1. Pictogram for carcinogenic agent.

respiratory sensitisation, germ cell mutagenicity, reproductive toxicity, and specific target organ toxicity and aspiration hazard.

Risk Assessments

Some bodies, such as the Scientific Committee on OELs at the European Commission and the United States (US) Environmental Protection Agency (EPA), also undertake risk assessments which estimate the nature and magnitude of health risks to humans from agents. Processes at different organisations tend to differ in the specifics, but usually involve four steps: hazard identification, dose-response assessment, exposure assessment and risk characterisation.

During the hazard identification, the risk assessors need to develop a clear definition of the agent of interest. For example, a specific chemical will be easy to define using a CAS number, whereas a mixture (such as diesel engine exhaust) is more difficult to define clearly. They also need to determine how the agent enters the body (e.g. inhalation, ingestion, dermal) and the Absorption, Distribution, Metabolism and Excretion of the agent within the body. In addition, the decision on which outcome will be used is made. For carcinogenicity, this is usually the site of cancer.

Once this essential information is collated, the risk assessors need to determine the association between how much of an agent a person is exposed to and the risk of developing a disease. When clear dose-response data is not available from the published studies on humans

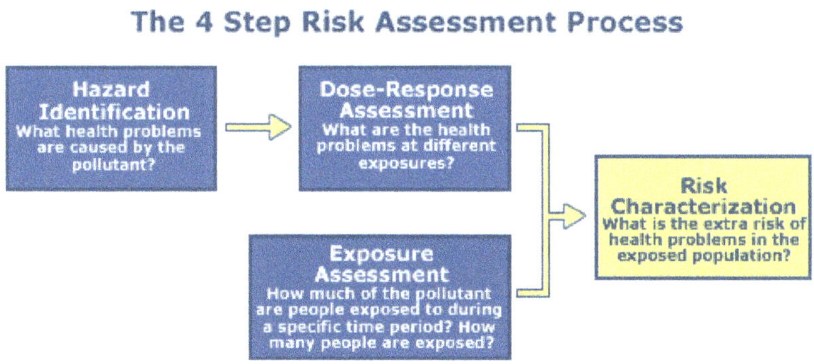

Fig. 2. Risk assessment process.

or animals, this step may depend on less reliable data such as in vitro studies, or case reports (Laszcz-Davis *et al.*, 2014).

The exposure assessment phase depends on finding information on the population groups who are exposed to that agent and the levels of exposure that they are usually subjected to.

Finally, the data are combined to determine the risk of the outcome at each level of exposure.

Occupational Exposure Limits for Carcinogens

Carcinogenicity risk assessments are used to develop OELs for carcinogens. OELs are set by a number of organisations. One of the best known organisations is the ACGIH which sets guideline threshold limit values (TLVs).

OELs for other countries include Workplace Exposure Levels (WELs) in the United Kingdom (UK); Maximum Workplace Concentration (MAK) in Germany, and Occupational Exposure Standards (OES) in Australia. The OELs often differ between countries due to different processes to establish these limits. The GESTIS database collates OELs for some countries (Gestis, 2020).

It is important to note that TLVs and other OELs take into account all health effects not just cancer. If a small amount of the agent causes a non-carcinogenic condition, then the OEL may be low, even when that level of the agent is not known to cause cancer.

Occupational exposure limits in Asia

Globalisation has seen the movement of manufacturing from developed countries to developing countries. This included the transfer of hazardous industries and processes from countries with regulated occupational health and safety to countries with less stringent regulation, large labour forces and lower labour costs (Sim and Boffetta, 2009). For example, when the asbestos industry moved from developed countries to Asia, their health and safety measures did not (Choi *et al.*, 2013). Industrialisation occurred rapidly in these developing countries. For example, China was a largely agrarian economy in the

1960s but by the 2000s it was the manufacturing powerhouse of the world. In order to accommodate this rapid transition, vast numbers of untrained farmers moved into industries such as coal mining, construction and manufacturing with subsequent implications for occupational health and safety and for worker protection (Liang *et al.*, 2006). Agricultural intensification emerged with the need to feed these larger urbanised populations alongside a reduced farm labour workforce. Pesticide use in Vietnam increased annually by 7.6% between 1990 and 2003 (Khanh *et al.*, 2006). Two compounds being sold to Vietnamese farmers in 2009 (endosulfan and DDT) had been earlier banned by the Stockholm Convention, which Vietnam ratified in 2006, but weak regulatory enforcement permitted their use (Hoi *et al.*, 2009).

The setting of OELs has been a relatively recent phenomenon in Asia: 1985 in Korea (Jeong *et al.*, 2010), 1980 in China (Liang *et al.*, 2006), 1984 in Malaysia (Rampal *et al.*, 2006), compared with 1946 in the United States (Schenk *et al.*, 2008). However, the value assigned as the OEL depends on more than just the health risk assessments from the scientific literature. Technological and socioeconomic factors relevant for each country are also considered, in addition to "acceptable risk" and political considerations. Therefore, the OEL values often differ widely between countries, even when based on the same data and methods (Ding *et al.*, 2011). For example, China has higher OELs for asbestos (0.8f/cc) and silica compared with that of the ACGIH (0.1f/cc for all types of asbestos) (Liang *et al.*, 2006). Moreover, a recent comparison of OELs in the European Union and Asia did not show any obvious evidence of harmonisation and in general Asian OELs were less protective than European OELs (Ding *et al.*, 2011).

Despite the variation in values, within country improvements in exposure to carcinogens among workers have been observed. Historically, workers in the shoemaking industry in China were exposed to excessive levels of benzene, from their use of glues and solvents. A search of the Chinese medical literature showed case reports of benzene poisoning and results of industrial hygiene surveys between 1978 (beginning of economic growth) and 2002–2004 (introduction of new OEL for benzene). Between 1978 and 1990 the average reported benzene concentration was 405.3 mg/m^3, 10 times above the maximum allowable concentration of 40 mg/m^3. By 2004, the reported average was 69.7 mg/m^3, which although markedly lower was still seven times higher than the new short-term exposure limit (STEL) introduced in 2002 (10 mg/m^3) (Wang *et al.*, 2006).

Migrant Workers and Exposure to Occupational Carcinogens

Migrant workers, who tend to work in the "3 D jobs" (i.e. dirty, dangerous and difficult), may also be at increased risk of exposure to occupational carcinogens, although little work has examined exposure to carcinogens among this group of workers (Ahonen *et al.*, 2007).

Work from Australia showed that exposure to occupational carcinogens differed by ethnicity (Boyle *et al.*, 2015a). Overall, the prevalence of exposure between all ethnic minority workers (31.6%) and Australian-born workers (29.7%) was similar. However, differences emerged when comparing between ethnic groups. A higher proportion of workers of Arabic background were exposed to one or more carcinogens compared with either workers of Chinese or Vietnamese background. Similarly, Arabic workers had a higher prevalence of exposure to silica than Australian-born workers and this difference remained after adjusting for occupational group. This suggests that the Arabic and Australian-born workers are doing different tasks in the same jobs (Boyle *et al.*, 2015b). Further, those workers who responded to the telephone interview in Arabic, Cantonese, Mandarin or Vietnamese were significantly more likely to be exposed to a carcinogen at work than those who responded in English (Boyle *et al.*, 2015b). This work highlights that exposure to carcinogens is not homogenous in the population and the importance of addressing occupational health and safety among sub groups of the population.

Case Study 4: Migrant Workers and E-Waste Recycling

E-waste recycling has become an important source of employment for many workers in developing countries. E-waste recycling in China has emerged as a major industry (Wang et al., 2020) In many instances, informal processes such as burning, melting and using acid chemical baths, without any use of worker protection, are used to extract gold and valuable metals from the e-waste. Because of these practices, workers are exposed to high levels of a range of carcinogens including heavy metals (e.g. cadmium, lead and mercury), and polychlorinated biphenyls (PCBs).

In China, much of this work is undertaken by migrant workers, those workers who leave their homes to live and work in other cities. As at 2019, there were 291 million internal migrants in China (China Labour Bulletin, 2020). These workers tend to do the more labour intensive jobs and have few work or social rights. A comparison of occupational exposure to PCBs between native and migrant workers in the e-waste industry in China found higher levels of occupational exposure to PCB gas and dust among migrant than locally born workers. Furthermore, levels of PCB were higher in the houses of migrant workers compared with local residents. Moreover, migrant workers were estimated to have a health risk from exposure to PCBs 3.8 times higher than that of local residents (Wang et al., 2016).

Case Study 5: Cholangiocarcinoma Cluster

In 2012, five cases of cholangiocarcinoma were reported from a small printing company in Japan. The Japanese National Institute of Occupational Safety and Health investigated the cases and found a further six cases of cholangiocarcinoma in the same company and eventually a total of 17 cases were detected (Kumagai et al., 2013; Kubo et al., 2014). Cholangiocarcinoma is a rare cancer and in Japan; the lifetime risk to age 75 is about 0.6% (Global Cancer Observatory, 2021).

The printing company had been in operation since 1969, and had moved into a new building in 1991. The cases were all men who had worked in the offset color proof-printing department of the company. About 111 former or current workers had worked in this department sometime between 1981 and 2012.

The proof-printing room was located in the basement and had very poor ventilation. There were seven single-color printing machines.

A series of proofs were printed for each print job with each proof consisting of one color — red, blue, black or yellow. After printing a small number of sheets with one color, the workers removed ink from the ink-roller using kerosene, and from a rubber roller (known as the 'blanket') using organic solvents including 1,2-dichloropropane (1,2-DCP) and/or dichloromethane (DCM). During a day, several hundred ink-removal operations took place. Both 1, 2-DCP and DCM are highly volatile but while workers wore plastic gloves for ink-removal, they did not use respiratory protection.

The case study above is an example of a cancer cluster. A cluster is defined as "the occurrence of a greater than expected number of cancer cases among a group of people in a defined geographic area over a specific time period" (National Cancer Institute, 2018). Cancer clusters have been responsible for the identification of a number of well-known occupational carcinogens such as angiosarcoma among vinyl chloride workers (Waxweiler *et al.*, 1976)

Generally, there are three features which determine whether investigating a potential cluster is likely to lead to the identification of a cause (National Health and Medical Council, 2012).

- Firstly, the cancers should be of the same or related types. Because different types of cancer are caused by different risk factors, and cancer is a relatively common disease, when a proposed "cluster" consists of a number of different, common cancers, it is likely that they have different underlying causes and the clustering arose by chance.
- Secondly, there should be more cancers than would be expected by chance in that population. It is easier to determine this for rare cancers or for cancers occurring in an age group in which that cancer is rare (e.g. children). In Case Study 5 it was obvious that the occurrence of 17 cases of a very rare cancer in a population of 110 people was very unusual. This criterion is often difficult to determine as it is not always easy to identify the population from where the cases arise. If the printing factory above had employed hundreds of staff at a time over many different sites, identifying the cases may have been relatively easy relying on medical records or word of mouth. However, identifying everyone who had ever

worked at any of the sites would have been more difficult to determine accurately. Employment records potentially could be used, but in the real world these are often lost when systems, management, or ownership of the company changes.
- Thirdly, initial investigation suggests that the population from which the cases arise have some factor in common which might be responsible. This is often the workplace where unusual agents may be present or exposure to more common agents may be of a very high level.

In the US, a group of investigators reviewed environmental cancer cluster investigations over 20 years to determine whether they had "improved our understanding of cancer aetiology, or informed cancer prevention and control" (Goodman *et al.*, 2012). Of 567 investigations, there were only 72 (12.7%) in which the number of cancer clusters was greater than expected and a common environmental exposure was found in only three investigations. Most investigations are environmental, and evidence on how many occupational clusters lead to important public health outcomes is not available. The US Centers for Disease Control and Prevention (CDC) guidelines for cluster investigations reported that the only one positive finding in over 500 cluster investigations in Minnesota was in an occupational setting (CDC, 1990).

It seems clear that very few cluster investigations find a definitive cause for a proposed cluster of cancers. Despite the findings of the experts, once a local community or workplace has become concerned, the belief that "something" must have caused the cancers often persists, with one study suggesting that the refusal to accept the experts' determinations is due to the innate human tendency to see patterns, and a lack of social trust in experts (Siegrist *et al.*, 2001). The community often have expectations that the "something" will be identified and removed and this can lead to frustration and a deepening of the divisions between the community and the "experts." Studies have suggested that many factors influence the way that experts' determinations are received including belief that the affected community had some control in the process and the feeling that they had been treated fairly (McComas *et al.*, 2007).

It is important that any perceived cluster is dealt with appropriately from the beginning. Poor management from the start can lead to months or years of frustration and conflict, and these issues almost always end up unsatisfactorily.

Prevention of Occupational Cancer

The primary prevention of occupational cancer follows the same process as for other occupational injuries and diseases. Firstly, there must be an awareness of the hazard, and then the hierarchy of controls must be implemented to control the hazard.

Many large companies, particularly in the developed world have good understanding of the carcinogens used or produced in their sites. However, little is known about the prevalence of exposure to occupational carcinogens on a national scale. This is important in order for regulatory and enforcement bodies to concentrate on the most common and important exposures. Surveys of exposure can help to identify areas where exposure is most common. For example, in Australia, about 40% of the working population were estimated to be exposed to at least one of 38 known carcinogens at work (Carey *et al.*, 2014). The most common carcinogens among male workers were solar ultraviolet, diesel engine exhaust, and environmental tobacco smoke. The occupations with the highest prevalence of exposure in men were farmers, heavy vehicle drivers and miners.

In many countries the regulatory approach is piecemeal with different rules for different carcinogens. In Massachusetts, US, a different approach was taken (Roelofs *et al.*, 2000). The Toxics Use Reduction Act (TURA) applies to all Massachusetts companies that use large quantities of specified chemicals to report on their use annually and to develop a plan to reduce use. TURA has resulted in a reduction of generation of toxic waste by 50%, has changed the culture towards reduction of use as the preferred means for achieving compliance, and has reduced costs for many employers.

Secondary prevention, which aims to reduce the impact of occupational cancer, can include surveillance or screening programmes. Any surveillance programme needs to be suited to the exposures within the industry. For example, a French group of experts reviewed the literature and determined the worker categories with increased risk of bladder cancer (including rubber and plastics industry workers, workers in dye manufacturing, textile dyeing, leatherworking and tanning, and pesticide manufacturing workers) (Clin *et al.*, 2014). They recommended that urine cytology was the only current suitable screening technique, and developed an algorithm for medical follow-up for workers currently or previously exposed to bladder carcinogens. Surveillance for exposure to occupational carcinogens is only useful if there are good methods for early detection with high sensitivity and specificity, and if early detection enables successful clinical intervention.

Compensation for occupational cancer can be difficult, especially if a worker with cancer is required to demonstrate clear evidence of occupational exposure to a known carcinogen, with a time interval that fits in with the known latent period between initial exposure and development of the malignancy. A major limitation is that there may be many years or decades between the exposure and the development of cancer. For example, the risk of mesothelioma continues to increase until at least 45 years after first exposure (Reid *et al.*, 2014). There may also be a time limitation for the affected worker to claim for compensation, and/or that his state of health after diagnosis may make the claims process onerous or difficult. In addition, there are often other risk factors. For example, for lung cancer in a smoker who was also exposed to asbestos compensation systems can have difficulty awarding benefits proportionate to the extent of contribution by different aetiological agents (Guidotti, 2002).

Conclusion

Occupational cancers are quite common, with between 2% and 8% of all cancers attributable to occupational exposure to a variety of agents. However, identifying an occupational cause in an individual case is often difficult, and requires the physician to be alert to the possibility of an occupational cause, to take a comprehensive occupational history, and to have the knowledge of which jobs involve exposure to which agents. Since there are so many different agents, and the literature is changing all the time, it is important that physicians are aware of the international bodies which review and classify agents as to their carcinogenicity.

Prevention of occupational cancer is important, especially as many of the cancers caused by occupational agents have low survival rates (e.g. mesothelioma, liver cancer or lung cancer). Primary prevention of occupational cancer involves recognising the hazard, identifying the determinants of exposure and implementing the hierarchy of control. Secondary prevention (such as chest X-rays or urine cytology) can be implemented in order to detect cancers early. As a last resort, it is important that physicians are aware of the compensation schemes in their own country to ensure that workers who do develop cancer receives at least some monetary recompense.

References

Ahonen EQ, Benavides FG, Benach J. (2007) Immigrant populations, work and health — a systematic literature review. *Scand J Work Environ Health* **33**(2): 96–104.

Boyle T, Carey RN, Peters S, Glass DC, Fritschi L, Reid A. (2015a) Demographic and occupational differences between ethnic minority workers who did and did not complete the telephone survey in English. *Ann Occup Hygiene* **59**(7): 862–871. Available from: doi: 10.1093/annhyg/mev021.

Boyle T, Carey RN, Glass DC, Peters S, Fritschi L, Reid A. (2015b) Prevalence of occupational exposure to carcinogens among workers of Arabic, Chinese and Vietnamese ancestry in Australia. *Am J Ind Med* **58**(9): 923–932.

Carey RN, Driscoll TR, Peters S, Glass DC, Reid A, Benke G, Fritschi L. (2014) Estimated prevalence of exposure to occupational carcinogens in Australia (2011–2012). *Occup Environ Med* **71**: 55–62.

CDC. (1990) Guidelines for investigating clusters of health events. *Morb Mortal Wkly Rep* **39**(RR-11): 1–16.

China Labour Bulletin. (2020) *Migrant Workers and Their Children*. [Online] Available from: https://clb.org.hk/content/migrant-workers-and-their-children. [Accessed on 28 March 2021].

Choi Y, Lim S, Paek D. (2013) Trades of dangers: A study of asbestos industry transfer cases in Asia. *Am J Ind Med* **56**(3): 335–346. Available from: doi: 10.1002/ajim.22144.

Clin B, RecoCancerProf Working Group, Pairon J. (2014) Medical follow-up for workers exposed to bladder carcinogens: The French evidence-based and pragmatic statement. *BMC Public Health* **14**: 1155.

Ding Q, Schenk L, Malkiewicz K, Hansson SO. (2011) Occupational exposure limits in Europe and Asia — Continued divergence or global harmonisation? *Regul Toxicol Pharmacol* **61**(3): 296–309.

GBD 2016 Occupational Carcinogens Collaborators. (2020) Global and regional burden of cancer in 2016 arising from occupational exposure to carcinogens: A systematic analysis for the Global Burden of Disease Study 2016. *Occup Environ Med* 77(3): 151–159. Available from: doi:10.1136/oemed-2019-106012.Gestis. (2020)

GESTIS International Limit Values. [Online] Available from: https://limitvalue.ifa.dguv.de. [Accessed on 28 March 2021].

Global Cancer Observatory. (2021) *Cancer Today.* [Online] Available from: http://globocan.iarc.fr/Default.aspx. [Accessed on 28 March 2021].

Goodman M, Naiman JS, Goodman D, LaKind JS. (2012) Cancer clusters in the USA: What do the last twenty years of state and federal investigations tell us? *Crit Rev Toxicol* **42**(6): 474–490.

Guidotti TL. (2002) Apportionment in asbestos-related disease for purposes of compensation. *Ind Health* **40**(4): 295–311.

Hanahan D, Weinberg RA. (2011) Hallmarks of cancer: The next generation. *Cell* **144**(5): 646–74.

Hanahan D, Weinberg RA. (2000) The hallmarks of cancer. *Cell* **100**(1): 57–70.

Hoi PV, Mol A, Oosterveer P, van den Brink PJ. (2009) Pesticide distribution and use in vegetable production in the Red River Delta of Vietnam. *Renewable Agric Food Syst* **24**: 174–185.

Health and Safety Executive (HSE). (2020) *Occupational cancer statistics in Great Britain, 2020.* [Online] Available from: https://www.hse.gov.uk/statistics/causdis/cancer.pdf. [Accessed on 28 March 2021].

IARC. (2021a) *Agents Classified by the IARC Monographs, Volumes 1–129.* [Online] Available from: https://monographs.iarc.who.int/agents-classified-by-the-iarc/. [Accessed on 19 April 2021].

IARC. (2021b) *IARC Monographs on the Identification of Carcinogenic Hazards to Humans.* [Online] Available from: https://publications.iarc.fr/Book-And-Report-Series/Iarc-Monographs-On-The-Identification-Of-Carcinogenic-Hazards-To-Humans. [Accessed on 28 March 2021].

IARC. (2020) *Night shift work.* IARC Monographs on the Identification of Carcinogenic Hazards to Human Volume 124. [Online] Lyon, France,

IARC. Available from: https://publications.iarc.fr/Book-And-Report-Series/Iarc-Monographs-On-The-Identification-Of-Carcinogenic-Hazards-To-Humans/Night-Shift-Work-2020. [Accessed on 28 March 2021].

Jeong JY, Choi S, Young LK, Kim PG. (2010) Extensive changes to occupational exposure limits in Korea. *Regul Toxicol Pharmacol* **58**(2): 345–348.

Khanh TD, Xuan TD, Chin DV, Chung IM, Abdelghany EA, Tawata S. (2006) Current status of biological control of paddy weeds in Vietnam. *Weed Biol Manage* **6**(1): 1–9.

Kubo S, Nakanuma Y, Takemura S, Sakata C, Urata Y, Nozawa A, Nishioka T, Kinoshita M, Hamano G, Terajima H, Tachiyama G, Matsumura Y, Yamada T, Tanaka H, Nakamori S, Arimoto A, Kawada N, Fujikawa M, Fujishima H, Sugawara Y, Tanaka S, Toyokawa H, Kuwae Y, Ohsawa M, Uehara S, Sato KK, Hayashi T, Endo G. (2014) Case series of 17 patients with cholangiocarcinoma among young adult workers of a printing company in Japan. *J Hepatobiliary Pancreat Sci* **21**(7): 479–88.

Kumagai S, Kurumatani N, Arimoto A, Ichihara G. (2013) Cholangiocarcinoma among offset colour proof-printing workers exposed to 1, 2-dichloropropane and/or dichloromethane. *Occup Environ Med* **70**(7): 508–510.

Laszcz-Davis C, Maier A, Perkins J. (2014) The hierarchy of OELs: A new organizing principle for occupational risk assessment. *Synergist* 26–30.

Liang Y, Wong O, Yang L, Li T. (2006) The development and regulation of occupational exposure limits in China. *Regul Toxicol Pharmacol* **46**(2): 107–113.

Loomis D, Guyton KZ, Grosse Y, Lauby-Secretan B, El Ghissassi F, Bouvard V, Benbrahim-Tallaa L, Guha N, Mattock H, Straif K, International Agency for Research on Cancer Monograph Working Group. (2016) Carcinogenicity of drinking coffee, mate, and very hot beverages. *Lancet Oncol* **17**(7): 877–878. Available from: doi: 10.1016/S1470-2045(16)30239-X.

Loomis D, Guha N, Hall AL, Straif K. (2018) Identifying occupational carcinogens: An update from the IARC Monographs. *Occup Environ Med* **75**(8): 593–603. Available from: doi: 10.1136/oemed-2017-104944.

McComas KA, Trumbo CW, Besley JC. (2007) Public meetings about suspected cancer clusters: The impact of voice, interactional justice, and risk perception on attendees' attitudes in six communities. *J Health Commun* **12**(6): 527–549.

National Cancer Institute. (2018) *Cancer clusters.* [Online] Available from: http://www.cancer.gov/about-cancer/causes-prevention/risk/substances/cancer-clusters-fact-sheet. [Accessed on 28 March 2021].

National Health and Medical Council. (2012) *NHMRC statement on cancer clusters.* [Online] Available from: https://www.nhmrc.gov.au/about-us/publications/nhmrc-statement-cancer-clusters. [Accessed on 28 March 2021].

Nilsson R, Tasheva M, Jaeger B. (1993) Why different regulatory decisions when the scientific information base is similar? — Human risk assessment. *Regul Toxicol Pharmacol* **17**(3): 292–332.

Purdue MP, Hutchings SJ, Rushton L, Silverman DT. (2015) The proportion of cancer attributable to occupational exposures. *Ann Epidemiol* **25**(3): 188–192. Available from: doi:10.1016/j.annepidem.2014.11.009.

Rampal KG, Mohd Nizam J. (2006) Developing regulations for occupational exposures to health hazards in Malaysia. *Regul Toxicol Pharmacol* **46**(2): 131–135.

Reid A, de Klerk NH, Magnani C, Ferrante D, Berry G, Musk AW, Merler E. (2014) Mesothelioma risk after 40 years since first exposure to asbestos: A pooled analysis. *Thorax* **69**(9): 843–50.

Roelofs CR, Moure-Eraso R, Ellenbecker MJ. (2000) Pollution prevention and the work environment: The Massachusetts experience. *App Occup Environ Hygiene* **15**(11): 843–850.

Rushton L, Hutchings SJ, Fortunato L, Young C, Evans GS, Brown T, Bevan R, Slack R, Holmes P, Bagga S, Cherrie JW, Van Tongeren M. (2012) Occupational cancer burden in Great Britain. *Br J Cancer* **107**(1): 3–7.

Schenk L, Hansson SO, Rudén C, Gilek M. (2008) Occupational exposure limits: A comparative study. *Regul Toxicol Pharmacol* **50**(2): 261–270.

Siegrist M, Cvetkovich GT, Gutscher H. (2001) Shared values, social trust, and the perception of geographic cancer clusters. *Risk Anal* **21**(6): 1047–1053.

Sim MR, Boffetta P. (2009) Occupational cancer: An emerging problem in newly industrializing countries. *Asia-Pac J Public Health* **21**(3): 241–243. Available from: doi: 10.1177/1010539509341404.

Smith MT, Guyton KZ, Gibbons CF, Fritz JM, Portier CJ, Rusyn I, DeMarini DM, Caldwell JC, Kavlock RJ, Lambert P, Hecht SS, Bucher JR, Stewart BW, Baan R, Cogliano VJ, Straif K. (2015) Key characteristics of carcinogens as a basis for organizing data on mechanisms of carcinogenesis. *Environ Health Perspect* **124**(6): 713–721. Available from: doi: 10.1289/ehp.1509912.

United Nations Economic Commission for Europe. (2019) *Globally Harmonised System of Classification and Labelling of Chemicals (GHS)*. [Online] Available from: https://unece.org/about-ghs. [Accessed on 28 March 2021].

Wang K, Qian J, Liu L. (2020) Understanding environmental pollutions of informal e-waste clustering in global south via multi-scalar regulatory frameworks: A case study of Guiyu town, China. *Int J Environ Res Public Health* **17**(8): 2802. Available from: doi: 10.3390/ijerph17082802.

Wang L, Zhou Y, Liang Y, Wong O, Armstrong T, Schnatter AR, Wu Q, Fang J, Ye X, Fu H, Irons RD. (2006) Benzene exposure in the shoemaking industry in China, a literature survey, 1978–2004. *Regul Toxicol Pharmacol* **46**(2): 149–156.

Wang Y, Hu J, Lin W, Wang N, Li C, Peng L, Hashmi MZ, Wang W, Su X, Chen C, Liu Y, Huang R, Shen C. (2016) Health risk assessment of migrant workers' exposure to polychlorinated biphenyls in air and dust in an e-waste recycling area in China: Indication for a new wealth gap in environmental rights. *Environ Int* **87**: 33–41.

Waxweiler RJ, Stringer W, Wagoner JK, Jones J, Falk H, Carter C. (1976) Neoplastic risk among workers exposed to vinyl chloride. *Ann N Y Acad Sci* **271**: 40–48.

Winder C, Azzi R, Wagner D. (2005) The development of the globally harmonised system (GHS) of classification and labeling of hazardous chemicals. *J Hazard Mater* **125**(1–3): 29–44.

Section 2 —

Special Issues in Occupational Medicine

Chapter 18

Aviation Medicine

Brian See,[*,†,‡] *Dominic Tan*[*] *and Wee Hoe Gan*[§,¶,||]

Introduction

Aviation Medicine, also known as Aerospace Medicine or Flight Medicine, is a sub-specialised field of Occupational Medicine that addresses the unique physical, physiological and psychological challenges of flight and the flight environment. It encompasses the wide spectrum of aviation — from piloting light aircraft, gliders and unpowered balloons; to flying commercial airliners, military jets, unmanned aerial vehicles and spacecraft; to air traffic control. In many air forces and civil aviation regulatory bodies, Aviation Medicine physicians are also involved in the development of aviation medical standards as well as the subsequent medical selection and certification of aircrew and air traffic control officers. In the aviation industry, even seemingly minor

[*] Air Force Medical Service, Republic of Singapore Air Force, Singapore.
[†] Occupational Health Service, Changi General Hospital, Singapore.
[‡] Saw Swee Hock School of Public Health, National University of Singapore, Singapore.
[§] Department of Occupational and Environmental Medicine, Singapore General Hospital, Singapore.
[¶] Changi Aviation Medicine Centre, Changi General Hospital, Singapore.
[||] Duke-NUS Medical School, National University of Singapore, Singapore.
Corresponding author: Brian See (see_cheong_yan_brian@defence.gov.sg).

functional physical or mental limitations can potentially result in catastrophic outcomes.

Aviation Medicine traces its history to high altitude physiology (Gan *et al.*, 2011). As early as the 16th century, the Spanish army had documented discomfort with mountain travel during the wars to conquer Mexico and neighboring territories in the New World. Throughout the 17th and 18th centuries, scientists ranging from Otto von Guericke (1602–1686) to Robert Boyle (1627–1691) experimented and made discoveries in the laws of Physics and Physiology, which were to form the fundamentals of our understanding and practice of Aviation Medicine today. In the 19th century, Paul Bert (1833–1886), acknowledged by some to be the Father of Aviation Medicine, performed hundreds of experiments to study the physiological effects of pressure change in an altitude chamber, many with himself as the subject.

The success of the first powered flight by the Wright brothers in 1903 was a milestone event that paved the way for rapid development of the aviation industry. The exceedingly high fatality rates from aviation accidents during World Wars (WW) I and II further catalysed significant progress in Aviation Medicine. For example, 90% of British military pilot deaths in the first year of WWI resulted from human factors, of which two-thirds were reportedly due to physical defects in pilots (Jones, 2008). This prompted the Royal Flying Corps to institute selection medical standards for pilots, which contributed to a drastic reduction in physical defect-related deaths to "20% during the second year and 12% during the third year" of WWI (Gibson and Harrison, 2005).

The rapid growth of global commercial air travel and major strides in military aviation technology in the second half of the 20th century have further pushed the frontier of Aviation Medicine. From the humble beginnings of one route and one passenger in 1914, the commercial aviation industry today serves almost four billion passenger journeys per annum (International Air Transport Association, 2019). This has raised public expectations of the safety standards of air travel, not least the medical fitness of the airline transport pilots who are responsible for transporting hundreds of individuals from one destination to another. In the area of military aviation, modern day military jets are not only capable of pulling high gravitational (G) forces; their speed and network-centricity also shorten the OODA (observe, orient, decide and act) loop and place stringent cognitive demands on their aircrew.

Looking ahead, technological advancements will continue to push the boundaries of Aviation Medicine practice from the conventional practice of protecting the aviator from the hazards of the flight environment to encompass aircrew performance maximisation in the ever-growing flight and task envelopes. The adage "Man is the weakness link" is now more evident than ever.

The Aviation Environment

Man is a terrestrial being; the aviation environment is foreign to the evolution of normal human physiology. In the air, aviators (especially military aviators) will often have their visual, vestibular and proprioceptive systems challenged in-flight by virtue of their changing orientation relative to the Earth's surface and the normal gravitational axis (i.e. vertical). Aircraft-induced factors, such as high G forces and vibration, also affect human physiology and performance. Together with the challenges of atmospheric conditions, flight conditions and the flight environment pose significant challenges to the human physiology. It is therefore essential that the practice of Aviation Medicine be built upon a good understanding of the aviation environment and the spectrum of job and task requirements, as these factors interplay to influence the outcomes of health and performance of the aviator.

The Atmosphere

Aircraft operate within a medium known as the atmosphere, and an understanding of the atmospheric properties is necessary to understand the physiological challenges faced by the aviator. The nature of the atmosphere varies with altitude and latitude, and is not a medium with uniform characteristics. It comprises five layers, each with distinctive characteristics: (1) troposphere, (2) stratosphere, (3) mesosphere, (4) thermosphere and (5) exosphere. The troposphere is the layer proximate to the Earth's surface and the most important in conventional aviation, although certain military aircraft may operate within the stratosphere. The troposphere extends from the Earth's surface to approximately 58,000 feet (17,678 m) at the Equator and at slightly lower altitudes at the Poles as a result of reduced solar heating and, therefore, less gaseous expansion. The exosphere represents the beginning of true space.

Temperature

The ambient temperature decreases by 1.98°C per 1,000 feet ascent in the troposphere. Hence, at the typical cruising altitude of an airliner at 33,000 feet and assuming a ground temperature of 30°C, the exterior atmospheric temperature can be expected to approximate –35°C. Modern aircraft are equipped with environmental control systems to regulate temperature (in addition to air supply and aircraft cabin pressurisation) in the cabin or cockpit. Thus, the main at-risk groups are high-altitude ballooning enthusiasts and parachutists, who require appropriate clothing to protect against hypothermia.

Pressure

Atmospheric pressure decreases as altitude increases. This is primarily due to gravitational force exerting a stronger influence closer to the Earth's surface whereas with altitude, the force of gravity is increasingly opposed by the expansion of gases into the near zero gravity space environment. At sea level, the pressure exerted by the weight of the atmosphere is 760 mmHg. As atmospheric pressure exponentially decreases with altitude, the ambient pressure is halved (380 mmHg) at an altitude of 18,000 feet, and one-quarter (190 mmHg) that of sea level at 33,700 feet.

Gaseous Composition

The gaseous composition of the atmosphere is fairly constant up to an altitude of about 300,000 feet (91,440 m), mainly comprising ~78.1% of nitrogen and ~20.9% of oxygen by volume. Hence, hypoxia occurs in an aviator as a direct consequence of a *decrease in atmospheric pressure* and therefore oxygen tension, rather than a decrease in oxygen concentration at altitude.

Ozone

Ozone is a triatomic form of oxygen which is formed by the sun's ultraviolet radiation of molecular oxygen. It is found in the highest concentration in the ozonosphere (within the stratosphere), which stretches from 40,000 feet (12,192 m) to 140,000 feet (42,672 m). The ozonosphere protects the Earth from ultraviolet radiation. However, ozone is a strong oxidant and, when inhaled at sufficiently high concentrations, may cause pulmonary oedema. With the drawdown of the Concorde — which routinely flew at supersonic speeds at altitudes of 50,000–60,000 feet (15.2–18.3 km) — in 2003, there are no commercial aircraft in this present day that fly within the ozonosphere. Certain military aircraft have high cruising altitudes at the lower ozonosphere, but they are equipped with special filters to break down ozone and prevent its harmful effects on military aircrew.

Ionising Radiation

Occupational exposure to ionising radiation in aviation is mainly due to the galactic cosmic radiation at commercial cruise altitudes. At sea level, the effect of ionising radiation is mitigated due to collision and degradation of protons, electrons and neutrons with atmospheric molecules. At higher altitudes, this degradation effect is lessened and the levels of ionising radiation are higher. The aircraft fuselage provides little shielding and the dose received by the crew and passengers during flights depend on the altitude, latitude and flight time.

Ionising radiation is classified as a Group 1 carcinogen by the International Agency for Research on Cancer (IARC) (IARC, 2012). Exposure monitoring and assessments have shown that the radiation doses due to individual commercial flight segments typically range from 0.3 to >60 µSv per flight (depending on altitude, latitude and duration), and annual doses range from 0.2 to 5 mSv (Waters *et al.*, 2000). Hence, while the International Commission on Radiological Protection has identified aircraft crew as an occupationally exposed group (International Commission on Radiological Protection, 2016), the prevailing evidence shows that the typical commercial aircrew's exposure does not exceed the recommended occupational exposure limit for ionising radiation of a 5-year average effective dose of 20 mSv per year.

A meta-analysis on the risk of melanoma in airline pilots and cabin crew found that they had twice the incidence of melanoma compared to the general population (Miura *et al.*, 2018). On the other hand, another study among Australian commercial pilots from 2011 to 2016 suggested that the risk of invasive melanoma among Australian commercial pilots was comparable to the general population (Olsen *et al.*, 2019). Overall, the general consensus remains that the likelihood of developing cancer due to occupational exposure to galactic cosmic radiation is a small addition to health risks experienced by the general population, but it is not possible to establish that an abnormality or disease in a particular individual resulted from exposure to galactic cosmic radiation at the doses likely to be received while flying (Federal Aviation Administration, 2014).

For the general public and pregnant women (including aircrew), the recommended exposure limits are 1 mSv per annum and 1 mSv over the course of a 40-week pregnancy, respectively (AOCG Committee on Obstetric Practice, 2009). The latter limit for pregnant crewmembers may easily be exceeded within 1–2 months of regular long-haul flying (Lim, 2002). The potential extent of the effects of ionising radiation exposure on the pregnant flight crew and on the risk of cancers will continue to remain a concern in aviation, principle of “as low as reasonably achievable (ALARA)” in radiation protection also applying to the aerospace industry.

Stressors of Flight

Hypoxia

Hypobaric hypoxia is one of the most serious hazard of flight. In the aviation context, the main causes of hypoxia in-flight are due to either failure of the breathing apparatus or cockpit/aircraft cabin depressurisation. The ensuing reduction in alveolar oxygen tension results in a deficiency of oxygen supply to the tissues. However, many of the clinically significant and even life-threatening symptoms of hypoxia only manifest when alveolar oxygen tension falls below 60 mmHg, which is equivalent to ascent up to 8,000–10,000 feet without supplemental oxygen. This is the reason why in the event of an onboard oxygen system malfunction or aircraft cabin depressurisation, pilots are taught to descend the aircraft to below 10,000 feet.

The effects of acute hypoxia can be insidious, manifesting at lower altitudes (below 10,000 feet, or 3,048 m) as milder, but nonetheless significant, symptoms of impairment of night vision, narrowing of peripheral vision, and mild psychomotor and memory impairment. At higher altitudes, the physical, psychological and cognitive effects are more marked, resulting in personality changes, loss of judgement and decision-making capabilities, euphoria, sensory loss and muscular incoordination. There are also physiological effects of concurrent hyperventilation due to hypoxia, resulting in dizziness, neuromuscular irritability, paraesthesia and carpopedal spasms. When the hypoxia becomes severe, loss of consciousness and death will result.

Case Study 1: Hypoxia

On 14 August 2005, a commercial airliner operated by Helios Airways was put back in service with the cabin pressurisation setting at manual. This went unrecognised by the flight crew during their pre-flight procedures. Despite system warnings after take-off, the flight crew were unable to identify the cause of the warnings and reasons for the activation of the warnings. The flight crew and passengers then lost consciousness due to hypoxia, resulting in the continuation of the flight via the autopilot until depletion of fuel. After fuel exhaustion, the engines flamed out and the aircraft impacted terrain, killing all crew and passengers (Air Accident Investigation and Aviation Safety Board, 2006).

The Time of Useful Consciousness (TUC) describes the interval between a reduction in inspired oxygen tension to a specified degree of performance impairment, usually taken to be the state where the aviator is no longer able to make appropriate flight inputs. TUC is variable between individuals and is dependent on various factors such as provision of supplemental oxygen, rate of decompression and individual fitness. The concept of TUC highlights the importance of recognising hypoxic symptoms early so as to institute prompt corrective actions before incapacitation sets in. The TUC may be as short as 2 min at 30,000 feet cruising altitude.

Hypoxia is prevented by aircraft cabin pressurisation or the provision of oxygen via a well-fitted mask, utilised singularly or in combination. Commercial airliners employ cabin pressurisation as the primary approach against hypoxia. Robust airframes and advanced aviation systems allow airliners to maintain and withstand large pressure differentials, with aircraft cabins pressurised to the equivalent of 5,000–8,000 feet (1,524–2,438 m) when the true cruise altitude is over 30,000 feet (9,144 m). This allows passengers and crew to travel in relative comfort without being exposed to hypoxic, hypobaric or hypothermic conditions. Oxygen is available to both crew and passengers through emergency oxygen masks should the cabin pressurisation be compromised.

Military fighter aircraft cannot be pressurised to this extent without significantly trading off their combat manoeuvring performance. As such, most fighter aircraft have a cockpit pressure equivalent to an altitude of 8,000 feet below 24,000 feet cruising altitude, and 18,000–20,000 feet at a cruising altitude above 30,000 feet. Military fighter pilots will don oxygen masks at all times to increase the oxygen concentration, and therefore oxygen tension, at the point of inspiration. Helicopters are usually unpressurised and hence, maintain an operational ceiling of 10,000 feet (3,048 m) to minimise the effects of hypoxia unless supplemental oxygen systems are employed for specific operational missions.

The effects and symptomatology of hypoxia may vary between individuals. To this end, many air forces put their pilots and aircrew through training in a hypobaric chamber or using reduced oxygen breathing devices to experience and recognise their individual symptoms that indicate the onset of hypoxia (commonly termed "hypoxia signature").

Pressure Changes

Boyle's Law states that at a constant temperature, the volume of a fixed mass of gas is inversely proportional to the pressure to which it is subjected. Hence, as aircraft ascend and atmospheric pressure falls, the air volume of the human body will increase.

The physiological implication of Boyle's Law is very relevant in the context of Aviation Medicine. Our human body comprises closed and semi-closed cavities such as the lungs, middle ear, paranasal sinuses, gastrointestinal tract and even dental cavities. Consideration of even small pockets of gas post-surgery (e.g. eye surgery) is also important when certifying fitness for flying.

The effects of Eustachian tube dysfunction during or over the recovering phase of an upper respiratory tract infection is a manifestation of pressure changes in flight. The middle ear communicates with the external atmosphere by way of the Eustachian tube, which act as a one-way passive valve and opens into the nasopharyngeal space. During ascent and increasing altitude, the air in the middle ear expands; pressure between the middle ear and the ambient environment is equalised through venting of air through the Eustachian tube. However, during descent, as the air volume in the middle ear decreases, the Eustachian tube remains closed and does not passively allow air to flow back to the middle ear. Therefore, the Eustachian tube must be actively forced open through swallowing, yawning or other active manoeuvres such as the Valsalva manoeuvre. Upper respiratory tract infections or inflammation can cause congestion and mucosal oedema of the Eustachian tube, resulting in an inability to equalise middle ear pressure. This may lead to injury of the tympanic membrane, which is known as otitic barotrauma.

Case Study 2: Barotrauma

An airline flight attendant working onboard a return flight to Singapore was recovering from a bad bout of allergic rhinitis flare up while on layover. During the last half an hour of flight on the descent phase, she felt fullness over the left ear, which worsened rapidly to sharp ear pain. This persisted despite manoeuvres such as swallowing and yawning. The pain became increasingly unbearable and she was about to call for assistance from her fellow cabin crew when she experienced a 'pop' sensation over the left ear, with resolution of pain. After landing, she consulted a doc-

tor at the airport clinic, who confirmed that she sustained perforation of her left tympanic membrane.

Paranasal sinuses are small cavities that drain into the nose either via ducts or ostia. Similar to otitic barotrauma, sinus barotrauma occurs more often during descent, usually due to mucosal inflammation secondary to illness or infection, which results in blockage of the ducts or ostia. The resulting inability to equilibrate air volumes during descent leads to intense facial pain and may cause tearing and damage of the mucosal lining of the sinuses with consequent haemorrhage into the sinus cavities. In both otitic and sinus barotrauma, the symptoms may sometimes be so severe that they distract or even incapacitate the aircrew.

Sub-atmospheric Decompression Sickness

Sub-atmospheric decompression sickness (DCS), also known as Caisson Disease, may arise with hypobaria. The first documented cases of DCS were among miners in 1841 who used air-pressurised mine shafts.

The occurrence of DCS follows Henry's Law which states that the mass of gas that will dissolve in a liquid at a given volume is directly proportional to the partial pressure of the gas above the liquid and its solubility coefficient at a given temperature. At ground level, the tissues and blood of the human body contain dissolved nitrogen, wherein the partial pressure is equal to that of the nitrogen in inspired air. During ascent, the fall in partial pressure causes the body tissues to release the nitrogen into the blood for excretion via the lungs. However, as the solubility of nitrogen in blood is low, the rate of fall of the *absolute pressure* in the tissues is greater than the rate of fall of the *partial pressure* of nitrogen in those tissues. The tissues become supersaturated with nitrogen, which leads to the formation of nitrogen bubbles within the tissues. Nitrogen bubbles, either within the tissues where they are formed or carried by the circulation to another organ, result in the clinical syndrome of DCS.

Sub-atmospheric DCS rarely occurs below an altitude of 18,000 feet (5,486 m). The incidence below 25,000 feet (7,620 m) is relatively low, with DCS becoming a significant threat only above this altitude.

The risk of DCS for passengers in commercial airliners is non-existent as the cabin pressure is kept at 5,000–8,000 feet, but for one important exception; a passenger with recent exposure to pressures greater than one bar (such as diving or undertaking compressed air works). In this regard, the United Kingdom (UK) Diving Medical Advisory Committee provides recommendations on the minimum surface time based on the preceding dive profile (ranging from 2 to 48 h) before embarking on a flight (Diving Medical Advisory Committee, 2017). Other risk factors for DCS include increasing age, obesity, recent joint injury, infection, inter-current illness and a previous episode of DCS.

DCS can manifest as joint pain ("bends"), skin disturbances (itching, tingling, "creeps") respiratory disturbances (chest tightness, sense of chest constriction, "chokes"), neurological disturbances (paraesthesia, convulsions, "staggers"), visual disturbances (blurring of vision, scotomata, hemianopia) and cardiovascular collapse. Symptoms may occur during or after high altitude exposure, which makes it important to advise exposed crew to stay vigilant of symptoms and seek timely medical attention.

DCS is prevented primarily through aircraft cabin pressurisation. However, if prolonged exposure to high altitudes is unavoidable, the principal method of prevention is through pre-oxygenation (also known as de-nitrogenation). This involves the breathing of 100% oxygen for at least 30 min pre-flight to wash out the body's nitrogen. The duration of pre-oxygenation depends on the altitude and duration of the intended exposure. This strategy is commonly employed for high-altitude parachutists, pilots of special military aircraft and astronauts.

Should DCS symptoms occur during altitude exposure, a decrease in altitude and administration of 100% oxygen will usually result in rapid recovery and amelioration of symptoms. Severe cases may require hyperbaric compression treatment.

High G_z Forces Exposure and G-induced Loss of Consciousness

High performance aircraft, such as military fighter aircraft, function in a 3-dimensional space. Therefore, during high performance flights, the aircrew will experience acceleration in all three axes. By convention, this acceleration is termed "G," which is a multiple of the acceleration due to the force of gravity ("g"), the latter being equals 9.8 ms^{-2}. The direction in which this acceleration or inertial force acts on the human is conventionally denoted by G_x (chest-back axis), G_y (left-right lateral axis) and G_z (head-foot axis), with a plus or minus sign in front describing the direction of the acceleration.

In aviation, the accelerative force of concern is usually $+G_z$. The direction of this accelerative force (head to foot) imposes increased weight of the head, neck, trunk and limbs. For example, at $+3G_z$, the pilot will feel that his limbs weigh three times heavier compared to under normal gravity, and may experience difficulty in elevating them. Another important effect of $+G_z$ is the pooling of blood away from the head and towards the lower limbs. Therefore, when the $+G_z$ forces are high enough to reduce blood flow to the eyes and brain, the aviator will experience visual symptoms (e.g. grey out, tunneling of vision) and eventually become incapacitated due to G-Induced Loss of Consciousness (G-LOC).

Case Study 3: G-Induced Loss of Consciousness (G-LOC)

During an aerial demonstration training flight involving six F-16 aircraft, a fighter pilot executed an aerial manoeuvre which involved an initial −2.0 G_z exposure. He then transited to a +8.5 G_z exposure within 5 seconds and experienced a G-LOC. He was incapacitated for approximately 4 seconds and only recovered consciousness just prior to impact. Based on the aircraft's dive angle and altitude, any attempts by the pilot to recover the aircraft would be futile. The pilot died on impact, and the air accident investigation attributed the preceding −G_z exposure (which reduced the pilot's subsequent tolerance to +G_z) and the pilot's ineffective Anti-G Straining Manoeuvre (AGSM) as the main contributory factors (Metzler, 2020).

There are four strategies for combating G-LOC. The first and most important method is by a combination of sustained muscle-tensing and the rhythmic execution of a modified Valsalva manoeuvre every 3 s. Known as the Anti-G Straining Manoeuvere (AGSM), this combination effort reduces venous pooling and increases the intrathoracic pressure, which in turn supports the increase in blood flow to the brain. If well executed, it can provide approximately $+3G_Z$ improvement in G-tolerance. The second is by donning an anti-G suit, comprising multiple circumferential air bladders that auto-inflate as $+G_Z$ increases during combat air manoeuvres. This prevents pooling of blood in the lower limbs and improves venous return to the thorax under increased $+G_Z$ acceleration and afford the aviator up to 2.5 $+G_Z$ protection. Thirdly, the AGSM may be augmented by the employment of a positive pressure breathing apparatus for G-protection to increase intrathoracic pressure and increase blood pressure directly on the heart and great vessels. Finally, some fighter aircraft incorporate the engineering measure of integrating the pilot seat at an optimal seat angle to reduce the hydrostatic effect of $+G_Z$ acceleration. For example, the F-16 fighter aircraft has a 30-degree seat angle, which provides an estimated $+1G_Z$ added protection due to a corresponding reduction in head-heart vertical height.

Spatial Disorientation

Spatial disorientation is a significant factor in a large percentage of serious military aviation mishaps, with the United States (US) Air Force reporting 72 spatial disorientation-related mishaps from 1993 to 2013 that resulted in the loss of 101 lives and 65 aircraft (Poisson and Miller, 2014). The human system of orientation depends on inputs from three organ systems, namely visual, vestibular and proprioceptive (Fig. 1). Of these, the visual system is the most powerful and visual cues can override conflicting vestibular and proprioceptive cues. However, the flight environment has the potential to degrade, confuse and mislead the human special senses. With night, fog or snow, visual references may be obscured, resulting in inadequate visual cues to the pilot for the perception of orientation, such as the altitude and attitude of the aircraft.

The vestibular and proprioceptive systems are conditioned to function at normal gravity. Under the influence of G forces across three axes, these two systems may mislead the brain regarding the

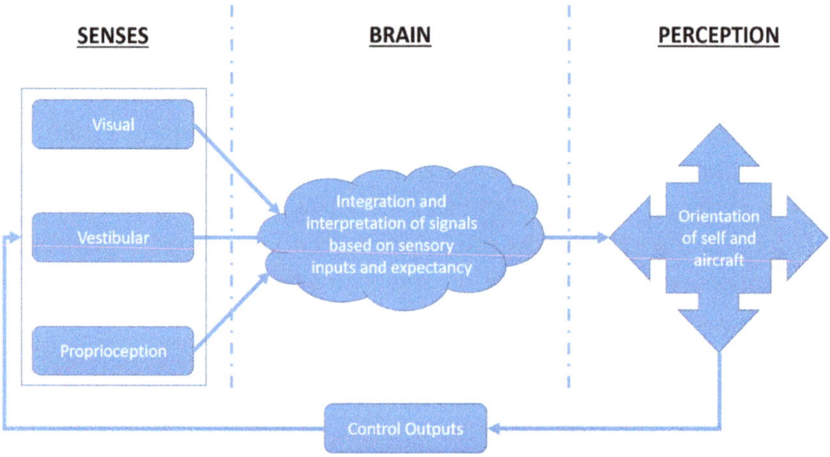

Fig. 1. Overview of human spatial orientation.

body's true orientation in the air. Examples of such illusions common in aviation include the Coriolis Effect, somatogravic or somatogyral illusions, and the leans.

Spatial disorientation is prevented primarily through education and training of aircrew. Pilots are instructed regarding the limitations of their bodily orientation systems, the risk factors in the flight environment and flight profiles that can predispose them to spatial disorientation, and the mechanics of various common illusions. This may be followed by training in a spatial disorientation trainer, a simulator that is capable of replicating common illusions and allows pilots to not only experience them, but also take the appropriate in-flight corrective actions.

Aeromedical Fitness

The bidirectional relationship between work and health underpins all fitness for flying evaluations. Specifically, the medical examiner is required to make a professional assessment of: (1) whether the individual has any medical condition that may be aggravated by the stressors of flight; and (2) whether the individual has any medical condition or treatment that may pose a threat to flight safety. The former aims to safeguard the health of the aviator against the hazards presented by his or her work environment, while the latter is a regulatory requirement that seeks to protect both the individual and the general public from aircraft accidents that may result from in-flight pilot medical incidents.

Medical Conditions that may be Aggravated by Flight

As described in the previous section, the flight environment is fraught with numerous physical, physiological and psychological stressors that may affect the aircrew's ability to operate safely and effectively. Consequently, individuals with certain illnesses or physiological states are unsuitable for flying duties as exposure to such an environment may adversely affect their conditions. This may be either temporary or permanent. For instance, individuals with severe spinal scoliosis are *permanently* disqualified from flying fighter jets, which involves exposure to high $+G_z$ forces that may worsen their spinal pathology. On the other hand, based on the ALARA principle adopted by some operators, a pregnant aviator should be *temporarily* removed from flying duties for the duration of her pregnancy to minimise the exposure of her foetus to flight-related cosmic radiation (Bagshaw, 2000), and may subsequently be returned to normal flying after her puerperium.

In determining whether a medical condition will be aggravated by flight, it is essential that the medical examiner understand the aircrew's workplace environment and job demands. For example, the physiological stressors experienced by the aircrew on a commercial airliner are quite different from those that military aviators are subjected to. Even so, civil aviation medical examiners need to differentiate the differing job demands on pilots *vis-à-vis* cabin crew, while military flight surgeons must be familiar with the flying environments peculiar to fighter jets, helicopters and transport aircraft.

Case Study 4: Pre-Employment Medical Screening

A 20-year-old military pilot trainee applicant was found to have a haemoglobin level of 11.8 g/dL on complete blood count performed during pre-employment medical screening. As the blood film revealed microcytic red cells and serum ferritin level was normal, a haemoglobin electrophoresis was ordered. This suggested a diagnosis of alpha-thalassaemia trait. In view of this, the air force medical authority rejected his application as it was of the opinion that he was at an increased risk of hypoxia in the low cabin pressure environment of military jets. He subsequently applied to be a pilot cadet with an airline company. Despite self-declaring his history of alpha-thalassaemia trait and a repeat complete blood count showing that his haemoglobin level was borderline abnormal at 11.7 g/dL, he was accepted into pilot cadet training on the basis of him being asymptomatic and likely to possess full functional capability in the pressurised aircraft cabins of commercial airliners.

Medical Conditions that may Threaten Flight Safety

Incapacitation is a central concept in Aviation Medicine that directly influences the aeromedical disposition of an aircrew. The International Civil Aviation Organization (ICAO) defines incapacitation as any decrease in medical fitness to a degree or of a nature that is likely to jeopardise flight safety (ICAO, 2012). This not only encompasses diseased states, but also extreme physiological conditions which may result in an inability of the aviator to respond in accordance with his or her training. In assessing the medical fitness of an individual for pilot duties, the medical examiner must evaluate his or her risk of in-flight incapacitation. Such incapacitation can occur across the spectrum of disease presentation, from acutely incapacitation events that lead to complete loss of function, to distracting symptoms, to an insidious or partial loss of function.

For license applicants who have known medical conditions, an objective assessment of whether he or she is of acceptable aeromedical risk can be performed. In this regard, many regulatory authorities have adopted the "1% Rule" and accept a maximum pilot incapacitation risk of 1% per annum. Employers and militaries may adopt stricter aeromedical risk thresholds, particularly at the recruitment stage as pilot training represents a substantial investment.

First introduced in the 1980s for cardiac conditions, the 1% Rule was derived based on an objective risk assessment approach to human

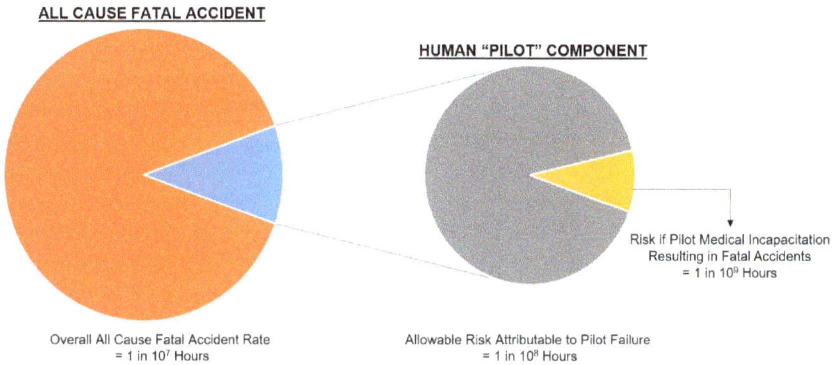

Fig. 2. Medical incapacitation as a proportion of all-cause fatal accident risk.

failure (Turnstall-Pedoe, 1988). This rule is based on a target all-cause fatal accident rate (FAR) of 1 per 10^7 flying hours. Each aircraft component (e.g. pilot) should not contribute more than 10% ($1/10^8$ h) to the overall FAR and within each component, the component subsystem (e.g. pilot medical condition) should similarly not contribute more than 10% ($1/10^9$ h) to overall risk of the component failing (Fig. 2).

The derivation of "1% Rule" is based on two pilot operations and several assumptions: (1) the average length of each flight sector is 1 hour; (2) only 10% of the time ($1/10^8$ h) in each flight sector is critical (i.e. takeoff, climb out, descent, approach, landing) (Fig. 3); and (3) based on simulator studies, in less than 1 in 100 events during the critical periods ($1/10^6$ h) would a second pilot not be able to take control in time to avoid a fatal accident (Chapman, 1984). *Therefore, in order to achieve the target medical-cause FAR of not more than* $1/10^9$ *h, neither pilot in a 2-pilot aircraft should have a medical incapacitation risk in excess of* 1 *in* 10^6 *h*. This translates to an acceptable pilot incapacitation risk of 1% (0.01) per annum, as each year has approximately 10,000 (10^4) h (1% per annum = 0.01 medical incapacitation per 10^4 h = 1 medical incapacitation per 10^6 h).

The 1% Rule is considered by some to be excessively restrictive as some of the assumptions may no longer hold true. A less stringent aeromedical risk threshold has therefore been proposed for civil aviation to take into account the increase in average flight sector duration

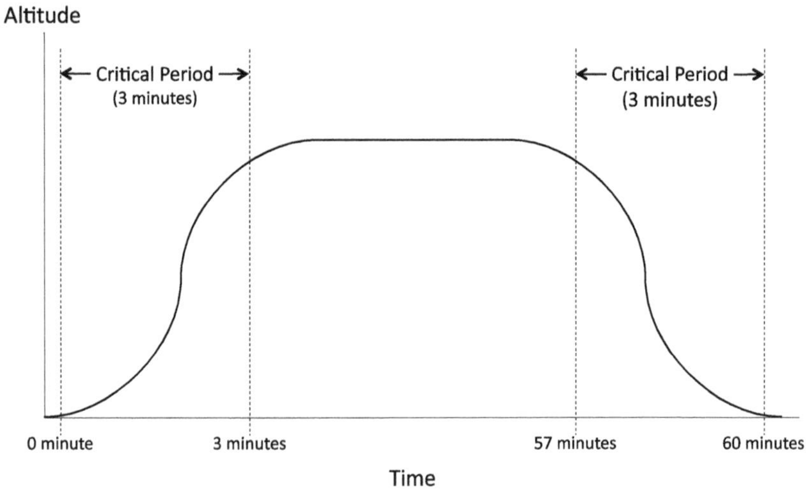

Fig. 3. Critical periods of the average flight sector of 1 h.

and decrease in proportion of flight time deemed critical, with at least one licensing authority of a major ICAO Contracting State adopting 2% as its acceptable aeromedical risk limit (Mitchell and Evans, 2004).

Case Study 5: Aeromedical Fitness for Flying Duties

The key concerns with diabetes mellitus in pilots are hypoglycaemia from treatment, as well as longer-term cardiovascular and visual complications. A 35-year-old military helicopter pilot was diagnosed with uncomplicated type 2 diabetes mellitus by his family physician, and was treated initially through dietary control and exercise. His unrestricted flying status was left unchanged, as there was no risk of hypoglycaemia with such lifestyle risk factor modifications. Despite good compliance, his HbA1c remained high at 7.8% after 6 months, and he was started on metformin. He duly informed his flight surgeon, who restricted him to "as-or-with co-pilot" status in view of the small but theoretical risk of lactic acidosis. Over the next 6 years, he was maintained on this flying status as he consistently attained reasonable glycaemic control on this single agent and did not develop any complications of diabetes. In the 7th year, his family physician added gliclazide to his drug regimen in response to his *worsening HbA1c trend. As gliclazide is associated with a hypoglycaemic attack risk of more than 1% per annum (Staa et al., 1997), he was certified unfit for flying duties by the air force medical authority.*

While cardiovascular events and epileptic seizures are the common dramatic causes of acute incapacitation (DeJohn *et al.*, 2006; McCormick and Lyons, 1991), in-flight incapacitations from inter-current illnesses are considerably more frequent. In a survey conducted among airline pilots, 29% of 4,345 respondents reported at least one incident of in-flight incapacitation severe enough to require another crewmember to assume their duties, with the most common causes being gastrointestinal symptoms (58.4%), earache due to a nasal or sinus congestion (13.9%), and faintness or general weakness (8.5%) (James and Green, 1991). This was corroborated by more recent data reported by the Australian Transport Safety Bureau (ATSB), which showed that gastrointestinal illness was by far the commonest cause of in-flight incapacitation (ATSB, 2016). Despite this being so, it is not possible for regulatory authorities to monitor license holders on a daily basis, and pilots are required to not exercise the privileges of their licenses when they are aware of any decrease in their medical fitness to do so safely. Pilots are also required to seek clarification from a medical examiner or the regulatory authority when they develop any major health issues, such as being diagnosed with a chronic disease or started on medications for long-term use, sustaining injuries that result in functional incapacity, or becoming pregnant.

Conditions that cause insidious or subtle incapacitation pose a specific challenge to regulatory authorities, as the signs and symptoms of incapacitation may not be easily detectable and their incapacitation risks are difficult to quantify. For instance, while a pilot with subtle mental incapacitation from a neuropsychiatric disorder or its treatment may function normally under normal circumstances, he or she may be unable to respond appropriately or in a timely fashion during an aircraft emergency. However, based on present medical evidence, it is difficult to quantity the aeromedical risk posed by his or her condition. More importantly, despite psychiatric causes being an important cause of in-flight incapacitation (Evans and Radcliffe, 2012), most of such conditions are not easy to elucidate on routine pre-employment or periodic medical examinations. The current expert consensus is that while rapid screening questionnaires (e.g. CAGE questionnaire to screening for alcoholism, PHQ-4 to screen for anxiety and depression) may be useful in the context of the licensing medical examination, extensive psychiatric evaluations as part of such routine aeromedical assessments of pilots are neither productive nor cost effective (Aerospace Medical Association Working Group on Pilot Mental Health, 2016).

Case Study 6: Depression

On 24 March 2015, air traffic control lost contact with an Airbus A320 operated by Germanwings on a scheduled passenger flight from Barcelona to Dusseldorf. The aircraft wreckage was subsequently found scattered in a remote region of the French Alps. All 144 passengers and six crewmembers were killed. Evidence recovered from the cockpit voice recorder showed that the co-pilot, who had locked out the pilot-in-command and was alone in the cockpit during the cruise phase of the flight, intentionally modified the autopilot instructions to order the aircraft to descend until it collided with the terrain. A review of the co-pilot's medical records found that he had a significant past history of major depressive disorder and had been under treatment for the condition (Bureau d'Enquêtes et d'Analyses, 2016).

Current Issues in Aviation Medicine

Aircrew Fatigue

Fatigue is defined by ICAO as "a physiological state of reduced mental or physical performance capability resulting from sleep loss, extended wakefulness, circadian phase, and/or workload (mental and/or physical activity) than can impair a person's alertness and ability to perform safety related operational duties" (Fig. 4). It arises due to an imbalance between the physical and mental exertion from all wake activities (including non-flying related activities) and recovery from such exertion, which requires sleep.

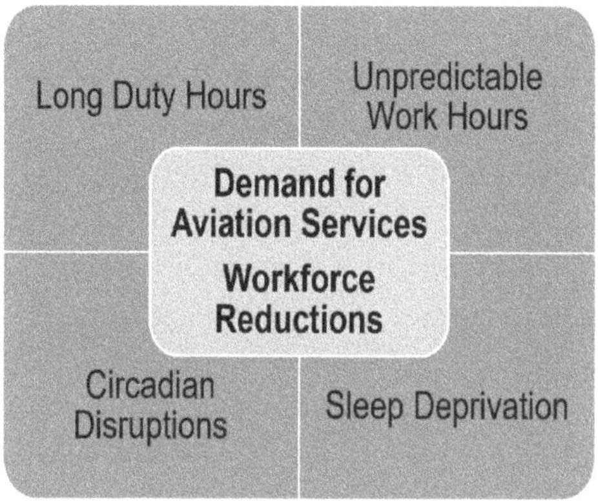

Fig. 4. Factors contributing to aircrew fatigue.

Fatigue is a flight safety hazard as it affects most aspects of a crewmember's ability to do his or her job. It is both common and under-reported, and must therefore be properly managed at all levels — by the regulator, the employer, and the individual aircrew. A self-assessment conducted by the European Cockpit Association on over 6,000 pilots found that over 50% experienced fatigue in the cockpit, with more than three out of every five pilots in Sweden, Norway and Denmark admitting to mistakes due to fatigue (European Cockpit Association, 2012). In a more recent survey of 625 pilots conducted by the ATSB, 17% reported obtaining less than 12 h of sleep in the preceding 48 hours, which was determined to be the threshold consistent with impaired performance due to fatigue (ATSB, 2019).

Traditionally, the regulatory approach to fatigue management is to prescribe limits on the maximum daily, monthly and yearly flight and duty hours, as well as the required minimum breaks within and between duty periods. This approach reflects early understanding that prolonged and continuous periods of duty ("*time-on-task*") produce fatigue, and that sufficient time is required to recover from work demands. However, this approach fails to take into account two other key aspects that determine fatigue levels, which are: (1) the impact of inadequate or poor quality sleep for restoring and maintaining waking functions ("*time awake*"); and (2) the human circadian rhythms ("*time-of-day*"). The former causes an accumulation of sleep debt with concomitant dose-dependent decrements in performance and buildup of homeostatic sleep pressure, while the latter drives the daily cycle of the circadian body clock and strongly influence rhythms in subjective fatigue, performance levels and sleep propensity.

The ICAO described two approaches for crew fatigue management, namely: (1) a prescriptive approach based on scheduling and safety management processes; and (2) a performance-based approach that utilises a Fatigue Risk Management System (FRMS) (ICAO, 2016). Unlike the prescriptive approach that addresses fatigue through duty and flight time limits, the FRMS approach uses data to proactively identify and predict sectors with higher fatigue risk so that fatigue mitigation strategies can be implemented.

Fatigue management can be broadly divided into non-pharmacological and pharmacological means. The most common non-pharmacological measure used to mitigate fatigue in aviation is the augmentation of the two-pilot flight deck crew with an additional pilot, or additional set of pilots, to provide sleep opportunities during long- and ultra-long-haul flights. The quality of rest facilities, which can range from normal seats to lie-flat seats to crew bunks, are also important considerations as they determine the sleep quality of the crewmembers during in-flight rest periods.

Case Study 7: Fatigue Management

Ultra-long-range (ULR) flights are flights that have planned flight-sector lengths of 16 hours or more and flight duty periods of 18–22 hours. In February 2004, Singapore Airlines (SIA) launched its inaugural scheduled ULR flights between the Singapore-Los Angeles city pair, which required a flight duty period of almost 20.5 hours. Prior to this, the Civil Aviation Authority of Singapore (CAAS) had reviewed the scientific basis for the flight time and duty time limits worldwide, as well as conducted mathematical modeling of anticipated crew alertness levels. Data was also collected from SIA flight crew during long-haul flights with planned flight-sector lengths of between 12 and 16 hours (Ho et al., 2005). In its provisional regulations governing flights between these two cities, a four-pilot flight crew, with two crewmembers possessing pilot-in-command qualifications, was mandated. Additionally, CAAS required that the flights depart at specific times; that the aircraft had rest facilities conducive to sleep; and that each pilot had two in-flight rest periods. SIA was also required to establish guidelines and conduct ULR training programmes for the flight crew on topics such as in-flight rest and sleep management, alertness management and fatigue countermeasures.

Individual crewmembers can minimise their fatigue levels through good sleep hygiene. To this end, crewmembers should maintain their pre-sleep "rituals" while away from home, and should avoid caffeine, heavy exercise and large meals in the few hours prior to sleep opportunities. Although alcohol reduces sleep latency and may therefore appear to be useful for sleep initiation, the onset of the first rapid eye movement (REM) sleep period is significantly delayed at all doses, and consumption of more than one to two standard drinks of alcohol is generally associated with a reduction in total night REM sleep and early awakening (Ebrahim *et al.*, 2013). As such, alcohol should not be used as a hypnotic as it is more likely than not to increase the risk of fatigue.

Medications such as hypnotics, including "over-the-counter" hypnotics, should not be routinely used by crewmembers, and all relevant non-pharmacological methods of improving sleep initiation and maintenance should be exhausted before the use of hypnotics is considered. However, in instances when the sleep environment is suboptimal (e.g. noisy or physically uncomfortable ground accommodations) or when the sleep opportunity occurs at a time that is not in synchrony with the body's circadian body clock (e.g. jet lag), they may be prescribed to crewmembers under strict usage guidelines, including the stipulation of a minimum interval between ingestion of the medication and return to duty. In this regard, temazepam, zolpidem and zaleplon are short-acting hypnotics that have been found to be useful in the aviation context (Caldwell *et al.*, 2009). Alertness enhancers such as Modafinil may also be employed although its usage is usually limited to militaries to maintain an operational edge (Ooi *et al.*, 2019).

Apart from causing fatigue, circadian disruptions following transmeridian air travel may cause jet lag and result in neuroendocrine disruptions similar to those experienced by those who engage in night shift work. The IARC has classified "shift work that involves circadian disruptions" as a Group 2A carcinogen since 2007 (Straif *et al.*, 2007), and had updated the exposure nomenclature to "night shift work" in 2019 to better reflect the main evidence base for its updated evaluation. Of note, transmeridian air travel was specifically included in the definition of night shift work by the IARC Working Group (IARC Monograph Vol 124 group, 2019). Although large cohort studies within the general population did not find a significant association between night shift work and breast cancer (Travis *et al.*, 2016), a prospective cohort study of almost 115,000 subjects followed-up for 14 years in the Nurses' Health Study II found that the risk of breast cancer was significantly higher in women with 20 or more years of shift work at baseline (Wegrzyn *et al.*, 2017). To address the heterogenous exposure assessment of exposure to night work, data from five population-based case control studies across different countries were pooled using a common definition of night work (Cordina-Duverger *et al.*, 2018). This found that breast cancer risk in pre-menopausal women was higher among current or recent night workers, compared to those who had stopped night work for at least 2 years. Some studies also suggested that night shift work was positively associated with the risk of prostate and colorectal cancer, but chance and bias could not be excluded by the IARC Working Group as they were fewer in number (IARC Monograph Vol 124 group, 2019).

Case Study 8: Transmeridian Air Travel and Cancer

A 40-year-old flight attendant presented to the airline company doctor with concerns that her job increased her risk of developing breast cancer. She is a 10 pack-year smoker, and her late mother was diagnosed with late-stage breast cancer 5 years ago at the age of 62. She cited a recent newspaper report that mentioned the classification of long haul air travel as a risk factor for developing breast cancer.

The airline company doctor confirmed that night shift work (including transmeridian air travel) was recently classified as a probable carcinogen by the International Agency for Research on Cancer in 2019.

However, she was also counselled that there were other modifiable (e.g. insufficient physical activity, drinking alcohol) and non-modifiable (e.g. age, family history) risk factors that have been shown to have stronger epidemiological associations with breast cancer. The doctor explained that while the suspected mechanism for the increased risk among night shift workers was the suppression of melatonin secretion due to nighttime light exposure, it was also plausible that such individuals had less opportunities to make lifestyle choices that would reduce their modifiable lifestyle risk factors for cancer.

As such, he encouraged her to maintain sufficient physical activity, eat a healthy and balanced diet, moderate her alcohol intake, and stop smoking, as well as to undertake regular breast self-examinations and periodic mammography based on prevailing breast cancer screening guidelines. Finally, he shared that even in jurisdictions that offered compensation to shift workers who developed breast cancer, only those with prolonged night shift work exposure of 20 years or more and had no other risk factors qualified for compensation (Wise, 2009).

The Ageing Pilot

The incidence and prevalence of many diseases increases with age. While this also applies to pilots, the healthy worker effect is pronounced within this selective occupational group whose members undergo stringent pre-employment medical screening and regular periodic medical re-certifications thereafter. This is supported by a study of a cohort of retired airline pilots which found that they had a median life expectancy advantage of more than 5 years over the general US white male population (Besco *et al.*, 1995). Nevertheless, ageing remains a safety and performance concern in aviation in view of its clear associations with cardiovascular diseases, deterioration of the special senses, and cognitive decline.

While the prevalence of lifestyle risk factors such as smoking and obesity tend to be lower among pilots *vis-à-vis* the general population (Pizzi *et al.*, 2008), age remains a non-modifiable risk factor for coronary heart disease and other chronic conditions that increase a pilot's overall cardiac risk. A cross-sectional study of 2,979 CAAS license holders who underwent medical assessment in 2013 found that the prevalence of hypertension among those in the 60–64 age group was 31.5%, compared to 14.0% in the 50–59 age group and 2.9% in the 40–49 age group (Anbalagan *et al.*, 2015). A similar pattern was observed for hyperlipidaemia, with the proportions reported as 22.4%, 9.2% and 2.7% in the 60–64, 50–59 and 40–49 age groups, respectively. It was this age-associated increase in cardiovascular disease risk that served as the primary basis for the implementation of the "Age 60 Rule" — a rule that required airline pilots to retire upon reaching their 60th birthday — in the 1960s.

The human special senses that are important in flying, namely vision and hearing, generally also decline with age. Presbyopia and presbycusis are almost universal conditions that accompany the ageing process, while more serious ophthalmic and auditory conditions have higher incidences among older people. Some of these are treatable through surgery or the wearing of spectacles or hearing aids, while others (e.g. severe macular degeneration or Menière's disease) may not be as amenable to treatment and could result in a loss of medical certification of fitness for flying.

Pilot performance and cognitive skills have been found to decline with increasing age. In general, studies have found that increased pilot experience does not appear to alter the typical age-related deterioration in cognitive skills (Hardy and Parasuraman, 1997; Taylor *et al.*, 2007) although the decline might be slower in more experienced pilots. On the other hand, there had been growing concern in recent decades that the Age 60 Rule might result in an opposite of the desired effect, as increased pilot flight experience is associated with reduced crash risk (Li *et al.*, 2003). The overall consensus based on the current body of scientific evidence is that experience gained by a pilot reduces but does not eliminate the expected age-related decline in his or her flying performance (Aerospace Medical Association Aviation Safety Committee Civil Aviation Safety Subcommittee, 2004).

The Age 60 Rule continued as the international standard for many years and generated much debate within the aviation community (Huster *et al.*, 2014). Many also felt that it condoned age discrimination

(Wilkening, 2002), particularly at a time when life expectancy and national retirement ages were increasing, and contributed to a growing shortage of air transport pilots. More importantly, it was exceedingly broad in its approach towards risk management and did not take into account the higher flight experience levels of older pilots. From the late 20th century, some national regulatory authorities started to relax their upper age limits for pilots, and ICAO formally extended the age limit to 65 years for multi-pilot operations in 2006 (Cornell *et al.*, 2007). To mitigate the age-related increase in cardiovascular risk, older pilots must undergo more frequent regulatory medical examinations from the ages of 40 and 60 years in order to be certified fit to fly single and multi-crew aircraft, respectively.

Antidepressant Use and Flying

Depression is a common mood disorder associated with low mood, decreased interest or pleasure in most activities, insomnia or hypersomnia, agitation or psychomotor retardation, fatigue, diminished ability to think or concentrate, and recurrent thoughts of death. The condition is often of an insidious onset and may persist for many months if left untreated. Mild cases of depression may be treated non-pharmacologically through programmes based on cognitive-behavioural therapy (Gloaguen *et al.*, 1998), while moderate to severe depression will require antidepressant medication, with Selective Serotonin Reuptake Inhibitors (SSRIs) generally recommended as the first line. To reduce the risk of recurrence, the current recommendation is for patients with first episode depression to continue taking antidepressants at full treatment dosage for 6–9 months following remission of symptoms (Geddes *et al.*, 2003), and for those with a second episode of depression to do so for up to 2 years after remission of symptoms (Loonen *et al.*, 1991). All individuals diagnosed with depression must be assessed for their risk of suicide.

Mood disorders, and their pharmacological treatment, are often associated with cognitive and neurophysiological disturbances that can impair performance and safety in safety-critical tasks. However, concerns have been raised that such stringent certification policies might, paradoxically, be detrimental to flight safety as afflicted aircrew would withhold information from the regulatory authorities and continue flying with a diagnosis of depression, treated or not (Jones and Ireland, 2004). Australia's Civil Aviation Safety Authority (CASA) was the first national regulatory authority to recognise this paradox and has, since 1987, allowed aircrew to return to flying duties after they had been effectively treated and were stable on antidepressants. A subsequent study comparing CASA licensees on antidepressants at some point over a 10-year period *vis-à-vis* age-sex matched pilots serving as the control group found no difference in pilot-attributable accidents between the two groups (Ross *et al.*, 2007).

In 2009, ICAO introduced a new recommendation stating that "an applicant with depression, being treated with antidepressant medication, should be assessed as unfit unless the medical assessor, having access to the details of the case concerned, considers the application's condition as unlikely to interfere with the safe exercise of the applicant's license and rating privileges." Since then, some regulatory authorities have adopted a more permissive position on the compatibility of antidepressant use with a pilot's medical certification for flying duties. For example, the US Federal Aviation Administration, Transport Canada, UK Civil Aviation Authority, and Australia's CASA now permit aircrew with depression and who have been stabilised on an approved SSRI to return to flying following a period of symptom stability.

Among military forces worldwide, the Canadian Forces was a forerunner in allowing select military aircrew to fly while on approved antidepressants (i.e. sertraline, citalopram, escitalopram and bupropion). All four approved antidepressants had been previously assessed by Defense Research and Development Canada to not cause significant decrements in aviation-relevant psychomotor tests (i.e. serial reaction time, logical reasoning, serial subtraction, and multitask performance) (Paul *et al.*, 2007; Paul *et al.*, 2002a; Paul *et al.*, 2002b), and aircrew being treated for depression may be returned to restricted flying status while on these medication after a 6-month observation period following the resolution of symptoms. The US Air Force has implemented an almost identical antidepressant use policy for its trained aircrew

(Aeromedical Consultation Service Neuropsychiatry Branch and Van Syoc, 2015).

Infectious Diseases and Air Travel

Infectious diseases may be transmitted through various routes, viz droplet, airborne, faecal-oral, blood, contact and vector-borne. In regard to air travel, the greatest public health concerns are directed towards infectious diseases that are spread via airborne and droplet transmission, as they have the highest propensity to rapidly propagate beyond international borders. Examples of such diseases include Tuberculosis (TB), influenza, meningococcal disease and coronaviruses. The Severe Acute Respiratory Syndrome (SARS) coronavirus outbreak in 2003 (Olsen *et al.*, 2003) and the COVID-19 pandemic in 2020 (Koh, 2020) are prime examples of how rapidly an infectious disease can spread via air travel in modern times. These two events brought to the fore the need for international public health collaboration, given the high degree of interconnectedness between countries.

Case Study 9: Severe Acute Respiratory Syndrome (SARS)

The first cases of SARS surfaced in Guangdong, China towards the end of 2002, and the disease was imported into other countries via commercial air travel. The first case of documented in-flight transmission of SARS was onboard a Singapore Airlines flight between New York and Singapore, with a transit stop in Frankfurt. During the New York to Frankfurt flight sector, a previously well 22-year-old flight attendant had brief contact (only meal service, with minimal verbal communications) with an infected passenger. Four days after the flight, the flight attendant was diagnosed with SARS and was hospitalised. The flight attendant made a full recovery (Wilder-Smith, 2003).

Understanding aircraft ventilation provides the basis for the conventional recommendation of tracing passengers seated within two rows from an infected case (Schenkel *et al.*, 2009). Air movement in modern aircraft is generally transverse with air supplied into the cabin from overhead and flowing downwards towards outflow valves near the floor. Fore to aft air movement is no longer employed in modern commercial airliners. While 50% or more of the air may be re-circulated, it is passed through High-Efficiency Particulate Air (HEPA) filter systems at aircraft cabin air exchange rates of between 15 and 20 air changes per hour. Nonetheless, it is important to realise that the two-row transmission zone rule is affected by many factors, and recent experiences with COVID-19 (Shen, 2020), SARS and influenza (Hertzberg and Weiss, 2016) has shown that this rule does not always hold true. Failure to consider other factors, such as interactions between passengers/aircrew, fomites and deplaning processes, may result in incomplete contact tracing.

The European Centre for Disease Prevention and Control provides useful guidelines for management of infectious disease transmission and investigation of potential disease outbreaks onboard airliners (Schenkel, 2009). The risk assessment for disease transmission should take into account factors that affect the likelihood for disease transmission within the enclosed cabin space and factors that have an impact on human health. In light of the COVID-19 pandemic, the International Air Transport Association (IATA) has also proposed measures including wearing of face masks and modification of cabin operations to reduce the risk of transmission (IATA, 2020). Under the International Health Regulations, member states are obliged to notify the World Health Organization of all events that may constitute a public health emergency of international concern within its territory, including events of disease transmission on international flights.

Conclusion

In keeping with good occupational medicine practice, sufficient understanding of the aviation environment and the attendant stressors of flight is essential for the Aviation Medicine practitioner to competently determine an aviator's aeromedical fitness for his work. Current issues in Aviation Medicine have also been discussed in this chapter to provide the reader with contemporary perspectives on these matters of topical interest.

References

Aeromedical Consultation Service Neuropsychiatry Branch, Van Syoc D. (2015) Mood disorders: Depressive, bipolar and related disorders (Mar 15). In: *Air Force Waiver Guide*. United States Air Force, pp. 567–578.

Aerospace Medical Association Working Group on Pilot Mental Health. (2016) Pilot mental health: Expert working group recommendations — revised 2015. *Aviat Space Environ Med* **87**(5): 505–507.

Aerospace Medical Association Aviation Safety Committee Civil Aviation Safety Subcommittee. (2004) The age 60 rule. *Aviat Space Environ Med* **75**: 708–715.

Air Accident Investigation & Aviation Safety Board. (2006) *Aircraft Accident Report: Helios Airways Flight HCY522 Boeing 737-31S at Grammatiko, Hellas on 14 August 2005*. Athens, AAIASB.

Anbalagan G, Chia SE, Chong CH. (2015) Analysis of medical examination data of commercial pilots in Singapore. In: *10th Public Health and Occupational Medicine Conference*. Singapore.

AOCG Committee on Obstetric Practice. (2009) AOCG Committee Opinion No. 443: Air travel during pregnancy. *Obstet Gynecol* **114**(4): 954–955.

Australian Transport Safety Bureau. (2016) *Pilot Incapacitation Occurrences 2010–2014*. Canberra, ATSB (Report No. AR-2015-096).

Australian Transport Safety Bureau. (2019) *Fatigue Experiences and Culture in Australian Commercial Air Transport Pilots*. Canberra, ATSB (Report No. AR-2015-095).

Bagshaw M. (2000) Perspectives of those affected: An airline's perspective. *Health Phys* **79**: 608–609.

Besco RO, Sangal SP, Nesthus TE, Veronneau SJ. (1995) *A Longevity and Survival Analysis for a Cohort of Retired Airline Pilots*. Washington DC, US Department of Transportation (DOT/FAA/AM-95/5).

Bureau d'Enquêtes et d'Analyses. (2016) *Final Report: Accident on 24 March 2015 at Prads-Haute-Bléone (Alpes-de-Haute-Provence, France) to the Airbus A320-211registered D-AIPX operated by Germanwings*. Paris, BEA (D-AIPX – 24 March 2015).

Caldwell JA, Mallis MM, Caldwell JL, Paul MA, Miller JC, Neri DF. (2009) Fatigue countermeasures in aviation. *Aviat Space Environ Med* **80**(1): 29–59.

Chapman PJ. (1984) The consequences of in-flight incapacitation in civil aviation. *Aviat Space Environ Med* **55**(6): 497–500.

Cordina-Duverger E, Menegaux F, Popa A, Rabstein S, Harth V, Pesch B. (2018) Night shift work and breast cancer: A pooled analysis of population-based case-control studies with complete work history. *Eur J Epidemiol* **33**(4): 369–379.

Cornell A, Parker SP, Li G. (2007) Age-60 rule: The end is in sight. *Aviat Space Environ Med* **78**(6): 624–626.

DeJohn CA, Wolbrink AM, Larcher JL. (2006) In-flight medical incapacitation and impairment of airline pilots. *Aviat Space Environ Med* 77(10): 1077–1079.

Diving Medical Advisory Committee. (2017) *Flying After Diving: Recommendations.* London, DMAC (DMAC 07 Rev. 2).

Ebrahim IO, Shapiro CM, Williams AJ, Fenwick PB. (2013) Alcohol and sleep I: Effects on normal sleep. *Alcoholism Clin Exp Res* **37**(4): 539–549.

European Cockpit Association. (2012) *Pilot Fatigue Barometer.* Brussels, ECA.

Evans S, Radcliffe SA. (2012) The annual incapacitation rate of commercial pilots. *Aviat Space Environ Med* **83**(1): 42–49.

Federal Aviation Administration. (2014) *Advisory Circular: In-flight Radiation Exposure.* Washington DC, US Department of Transportation (120-61B).

Gan WH, Low R, Singh J. (2011) Aviation medicine: Global historical perspectives and the development of aviation medicine alongside the growth of Singapore's aviation landscape. *Singapore Med J* **52**(5): 324–329.

Geddes JR, Carney SM, Davies C, Furukawa TA, Kupfer DJ, Frank E. (2003) Relapse prevention with antidepressant drug treatment in depressive disorders: A systematic review. *Lancet* **361**(9358): 653–661.

Gibson TM, Harrison MH. (2005) Aviation medicine in the United Kingdom: Early years, 1911–1918. *Aviat Space Environ Med* **76**(6): 599–600.

Gloaguen V, Cottraux J, Cucherat M, Blackburn IM. (1998) A meta-analysis of the effects of cognitive therapy in depressed patients. *J Affect Disord* **49**(1): 59–72.

Hardy DJ, Parasuraman R. (1997) Cognition and flight performance in older pilots. *J Exp Psychol* **3**(4): 313–348.

Hertzberg VS, Weiss H. (2016) On the 2-row Rule for Infectious Disease Transmission on Aircraft. *Ann Glob Health* **82**(5): 819–823.

Ho P, Landberger S, Singh J, Stone B. (2005) The Singapore experience: Task force studies scientific data to assess flights. *Flight Saf Dig* **24**: 20–40.

Huster KM, Müller A, Prohn MJ, Nowak D, Herbig B. (2014) Medical risks in older pilots: A systematic review on incapacitation and age. *Int Arch Occup Environ Health* **87**(6): 567–578.

IARC Monograph Vol 124 group. (2019) Carcinogenicity of night shift work. *Lancet Oncol* **20**(8): 1058–1059.

International Agency for Research on Cancer. (2012) A review of human carcinogens: Radiation. In: *IARC Monographs on the Evaulation of Carcinogenic Risks to Humans, v. 100D*. Lyon, IARC.

International Air Transport Association. (2019) *World Air Transport Statistics 2019*. Montréal, IATA.

International Air Transport Association. (2020) *Guidance for Cabin Operations During and Post Pandemic* (4th Ed). Montréal, IATA.

International Civil Aviation Organization. (2012) Flight crew incapacitation. In: *Manual of Civil Aviation Medicine* (3rd Ed). Montréal, ICAO (Doc 8984).

International Civil Aviation Organization. (2016) *Manual for the Oversight of Fatigue Management Approaches* (2nd Ed). Montréal. ICAO (Doc 9966).

International Commission on Radiological Protection. (2016) Radiological protection from cosmic radiation in aviation (ICRP Publication 132). *Ann ICRP* **45**(1): 1–48.

James M, Green R. (1991) Airline pilot incapacitation survey. *Aviat Space Environ Med* **62**(11): 1068–1072.

Jones DR. (2008) Flying and dying in WWI: British aircrew losses and the origins of US military aviation medicine. *Aviat Space Environ Med* **79**(2): 139–146.

Jones DR, Ireland RR. (2004) Aeromedical regulation of aviators using selective serotonin reuptake inhibitors for depressive disorders. *Aviat Space Environ Med* **75**(5): 461–470.

Koh D. (2020) Occupational risks for COVID-19 infection. *Occup Med (Lond)* **70**(1): 3–5.

Li G, Baker SP, Grabowski JG, Qiang Y, McCarthy ML, Rebok GW. (2003) Age, flight experience, and risk of crash involvement in a cohort of professional pilots. *Am J Epidemiol* **157**(10): 874–880.

Lim MK. (2002) Cosmic rays: Are aircrew at risk? *Occup Environ Med* **59**(7): 428–433.

Loonen AJ, Peer PG, Zwanikken GJ. (1991) Continuation and maintenance therapy with antidepressive agents. Meta-analysis of research. *Pharm Weekbl Sci* **13**(4): 167–175.

McCormick TJ, Lyons TJ. (1991) Medical causes of in-flight incapacitation: USAF experience 1978–1987. *Aviat Space Environ Med* **62**(9 Pt 1): 884–887.

Metzler MM. (2020) G-LOC due to push-pull effect in a fatal F-16 mishap. *Aerosp Med Hum Perform* **91**(1): 51–55.

Mitchell SJ, Evans AD. (2004) Flight safety and medical incapacitation risk of airline pilots. *Aviat Space Environ Med* **75**(3): 260–268.

Miura K, Olsen CM, Rea S, Marsden J, Green AC. (2019) Do airline pilots and cabin crew have raised risks of melanoma and other skin cancers? Systematic review and meta-analysis. *Br J Dermatol* **181**(1): 55–64.

Olsen CM, Miura K, Dusingize JC, Hosegood I, Brown R, Drane M. (2019) Melanoma incidence in Australian commercial pilots, 2011–2016. *Occup Environ Med* **76**(7): 462–466.

Olsen SJ, Chang HL, Cheung T, Tang A, Fisk TL, Ooi S. (2003) Transmission of the severe acute respiratory syndrome on aircraft. *N Engl J Med* **349**(25): 2416–2422.

Ooi T, Wong SH, See B. (2019) Modafinil as a stimulant for military aviators. *Aerosp Med Hum Perform* **90**(5): 480–483.

Paul MA, Gray G, Kenny G, Lange M. (2002a) The impact of bupropion on psychomotor performance. *Aviat Space Environ Med* **73**(11): 1094–1099.

Paul MA, Gray G, Lange M. (2002b) The impact of sertraline on psychomotor performance. *Aviat Space Environ Med* **73**(10): 964–970.

Paul MA, Gray G, Love RJ, Lange M. (2007) SSRI effects on pyschomotor performance: Assessment of citalopram and escitalopram on normal subjects. *Aviat Space Environ Med* **78**(7): 693–697.

Pizzi C, Evans SA, De Stavola BL, Evans A, Clemens F, dos Santos SI. (2008) Lifestyle of UK commercial aircrews relative to air traffic controllers and the general population. *Aviat Space Environ Med* **79**(10): 964–974.

Poisson RJ, Miller ME. (2014) Spatial disorientation mishap trends in the US Air Force 1993–2013. *Aviat Space Environ Med* **85**(9): 919–924.

Ross J, Griffiths K, Dear K, Emonson D, Lambeth L. (2007) Antidepressant use and safety in civil aviation: A case-control study of 10 years of Australian data. *Aviat Space Environ Med* **78**(8): 749–755.

Schenkel K, Amorosa R, Mücke I, Dias-Ferrao V, Diercke M, Leitmeyer K. (2009) *ECDC Technical Report: Risk Assessment Guidelines for Infectious Diseases Transmitted on Aircraft*. Stockholm, ECDC.

Shen Y, Li C, Dong H, Wang Z, Martinez L, Sun Z. (2020) Community outbreak of SARS-CoV-2 transmission among bus riders in eastern China. *JAMA Intern Med* **180**(12): 1665–1671.

Staa VT, Abenhaim L, Monette J. (1997) Rates of hypoglycemia in users of sulfonylureas. *J Clin Epidemiol* **50**(6): 735–741.

Straif K, Baan R, Grosse Y, Secretan B, El GF, Bouvard V. (2007) Carcinogencity of shift-work, painting, and fire-fighting. *Lancet Oncol* **8**(12): 1065–1066.

Taylor JL, Kennedy Q, Noda A, Yesavage JA. (2007) Pilot age and expertise predict flight simulator performance: 3-year longitudinal study. *Neurology* **68**(9): 648–654.

Travis RC, Balkwill A, Fensom GK, Appleby PN, Reeves GK, Wang X-S. (2016) Night shift work and breast cancer incidence: Three prospective studies and meta-analysis of published studies. *J Nation Cancer Institute* **108**(12).

Turnstall-Pedoe H. (1988) Acceptable cardiovascular risk in aircrew. *Eur Heart J* **9**(Suppl G): 9–11.

Waters M, Bloom TF, Grajewski B. (2000) The NIOSH/FAA Working Women's Health Study: Evaluation of the cosmic radiation exposures of flight attendants. *Health Phys* **79**(5): 553–559.

Wegrzyn LR, Tamimi RM, Rosner BA, Brown SB, Stevens RG, Eliassen AH. (2017) Rotating night-shift work and the risk of breast cancer in the Nurses' Health Studies. *Am J Epidemiol* **186**(5): 532–540.

Wilder-Smith A, Leong HN, Villacian JS. (2003) In-flight transmission of Severe Acute Respiratory Syndrome (SARS): A case report. *J Travel Med* **10**(5): 299–300.

Wilkening R. (2002) The age 60 rule: Age discrimination in commercial aviation. *Aviat Space Environ Med* **73**(3): 194–202.

Wise J. (2009) Danish night shift workers with breast cancer awarded compensation. *BMJ* **388**: b1152.

Chapter 19

Diving Medicine

Jeremiah Chng and Gregory C.T. Chan*[†,‡,§]

Introduction

Man's first historical forays into the sea were apparently driven by work — beginning with breath-hold diving for seafood, pearls, and shells from about 4,500 BC. It was said that the navies of Greece and Rome were among the first to militarise diving around 1,190 BC by using breath-hold divers to sabotage wooden enemy ships by drilling holes in their hulls, cutting anchor lines and constructing submerged port defences. Diving has evolved since then from the use of primitive diving bells which trap air in inverted containers for divers to breath, followed by the use of rudimentary breathing tubes that pump air from the surface to the diver working below, to the modern Surface Supplied Breathing Apparatus (SSBA) and Self-contained Underwater Breathing Apparatus (SCUBA) diving sets.

* Woodlands Health Campus, Singapore and Saw Swee Hock School of Public Health, National University of Singapore, Singapore.

† Occupational and Diving Medicine Centre, Singapore.

‡ Singapore General Hospital and Sengkang Health.

§ Saw Swee Hock School of Public Health, National University of Singapore, Singapore.

Corresponding author: Jeremiah Chng (jeremiah_chng@whc.sg).

Self-contained Underwater Breathing Apparatus Diving

In SCUBA diving, the diver carries one or more gas tanks strapped to his back which allows him the freedom of movement underwater. Pressurised gas is supplied from the tanks through regulators which reduce the pressure and control the flow of the gas so that it is delivered safely to the diver to breathe underwater. Most SCUBA diving sets commonly seen today are open circuit breathing apparatus in which the gas, usually air, is inhaled from the gas tanks and exhaled into the surrounding sea. These are usually used for recreational and some types of commercial diving. More complex diving sets such as semi-closed- and closed-circuit breathing apparatus which automatically clean the exhaled breathing gas and recirculate it back to the diver are commonly used in military and scientific diving as they produce less bubbles and noise while allowing the diver to stay underwater longer.

Surface Supplied Breathing Apparatus Diving

In SSBA diving, the diver wears a diving suit and is connected to the surface via a diver's umbilical. This umbilical incorporates a standard group of components that include a breathing gas hose, pneumofathometer hose (which informs the dive supervisor at the surface of the diver's depth) and a diver communications cable. Depending on the type of work done underwater, it may also include other cables such as a video cable, fibre-optic light cable, electrical cable to operate underwater tools and a hot water hose that pumps hot water down to the diver to keep him warm when diving in cold water. The umbilical components are twisted into a multistrand single-unit cable which is then securely connected to the diver's harness. The umbilical is strong enough for dive attendants to use to haul the diver back to the surface, saving him from having to swim back after completion of his task. As part of the SSBA gear, the diver can either wear a metal or reinforced-plastic dive helmet which is securely attached to the diver and offers head protection, or a full-face mask which is lighter, more comfortable to wear underwater, provides a greater field of vision but does not protect the head and may be dislodged more easily. SSBA divers commonly carry a "bail-out bottle" when underwater, which provides sufficient breathing gas for the diver to use to return to the surface in emergency scenarios, such as should the air compressor fail, or the umbilical is accidentally severed. Due to the high equipment cost and complexity of SSBA diver operations, this set up is mainly used in commercial and military diving. Because of the mobility restrictions imposed by the umbilical, it is best used in operations where the diver has to stay underwater for prolonged periods but only has to operate within a small area. Although SSBA diving requires more equipment than SCUBA diving, having almost unlimited quantities of breathing air, clear visual and audio communications between the diver and the surface team, and a secured line attaching the diver to the surface all ensure a safer, more efficient and better controlled dive compared to commercial SCUBA diving. SSBA is also the preferred choice for diving in contaminated water as the full dive suit and dive helmet isolates the diver from the contaminated environment that he is in.

A low-technology, bare-bones version of SSBA, commonly called hookah diving or compressor diving also uses surface supplied air for diving. This type of diving looks almost like SCUBA diving except that instead of drawing air from gas tanks, the diver breathes his air through a hose that is connected to a fuel-powered air compressor on the surface. Because of the ability to move around underwater easily without the encumbrance of a scuba suit and tanks, hookah diving is increasing in popularity among recreational divers. Hookah diving is usually done in shallow waters of less than 12 m of water and is commonly used in low-hazard work such as underwater research, aquaculture, aquarium and boat maintenance, lobster fishing and pearl harvesting (Abalone Victoria (Central Zone), 2014). However, there are advanced commercial systems that can support a diver up to 40 m of water. Because recreational hookah diving, unlike SCUBA diving, does not require a certification, many recreational hookah divers may not have received adequate training and may not be able to handle emergencies underwater — they often forget that they are breathing pressurised air underwater and hence suffer pressure-related injuries should they panic and forget to exhale when ascending to the surface. Also, without a SCUBA tank on their back, these divers may forget their dive safety training and neglect the time that they spend at depth and increase their risk of decompression sickness (DCS). Because of the relatively inexpensive cost of a hookah dive set up, it has been used in many developing countries for aquaculture activities with dangerous consequences. With poor legislation, insufficient training and inadequate medical support, many of these divers suffer diving-related injuries and are not able to get access to the necessary recompression treatment. In studies of divers in Mexico (Oswaldo *et al.*, 2018), the Galapagos Islands (Westin *et al.*, 2005), China and South Korea (Cha *et al.*, 2019), it was found that many of the pearl, abalone and lobster harvesters frequently exceeded their no-decompression dive limits and the number of dives allowed daily in order to maximise their earnings. It was therefore not surprising that hookah divers had up to three times the rate of DCS compared to standard commercial divers (Workplace Health and Safety Queensland, 2005).

Beyond the standard diving-related health hazards, one of the unique risks of surface-supplied diving is carbon monoxide contamination of the diver's air supply by exhaust fumes. If the air compressor's air inlet is downwind of a boat exhaust or any other nearby engine, the air supply delivered to the diver may become contaminated with carbon monoxide and other dangerous particulates from the exhaust fumes. Carbon monoxide is an odourless, colourless and tasteless gas which preferentially binds to the oxygen-carrying portions of red blood cells. With prolonged exposure to air contaminated with carbon monoxide, the diver's oxygen carrying capacity will drop over time and he may develop carbon monoxide poisoning. Often, carbon monoxide poisoning presents first as a dull headache, dizziness and breathlessness with exertion. As the carbon monoxide accumulates in the body, it can rapidly cause confusion, loss of consciousness and death. As the initial signs and symptoms are often insidious, the diver may not be aware that he is suffering from carbon monoxide poisoning until it is too late. This is compounded by the fact that diving at depth increases the toxic effect of carbon monoxide.

Case Study 1: Carbon Monoxide Poisoning during Surface Supplied Diving

A 40-year-old commercial diver was working underwater inspecting boat hulls, using an airline from a surface compressor. After diving for 45 minutes at a depth of 7 metres, he made an uneventful return to the surface. On return to the quayside, he complained of a dull headache and lethargy and his co-workers noted that he was coughing frequently. After a 3-hour break, he still had a slight headache but resumed his dive work. After 15 minutes at a depth of 10 metres, he swam rapidly to the surface and was noted to be acting strangely and appeared confused. He then slowly sank back down into the water. When his co-workers hauled him back to the surface, he was found to be unconscious with a weak and rapid pulse. At the hospital, his toxicology report showed that he had 45% carbon monoxide in his red blood cells and he required treatment in an intensive care unit. The diagnosis was carbon monoxide poisoning. In the ensuing investigation, it was found that the air intake of the compressor was not only downwind of a nearby boat that had its engine running, but was also situated in a poorly ventilated space. It was also highlighted that the diver should not have commenced the second dive as he was still feeling unwell. The dive supervisor should also have sent the diver for a medical check, halted the dive job and conducted a check to ensure that there were no potential safety and health issues.

Saturation Diving

Saturation diving is one of the most advanced forms of commercial diving. Due to the heavy technical, logistical and safety requirements, as well as the requirements for highly trained and specialised divers, it is usually used when great depths and long work hours are required to complete the task, such as the laying of undersea pipelines and cables and the maintenance of offshore oil rig platforms. Commercial saturation diving took hold with the emergence of the offshore oil and gas industry in the 1960s and can be found in the North Sea and Brazil where water depths extend from 100 to 180 m deep. In the military, it can be used for submarine rescue and salvage of sunken aircraft and ships. During saturation diving, the amount of inert gas (in this case, nitrogen) that the diver absorbs into his tissues reaches an equilibrium with the underwater ambient pressure due to the long time he spends at depth, and this "saturation" usually occurs within 24 hours of him being at this depth. Thereafter, no more extra inert gas can be absorbed by the tissues unless the diver descends deeper. Once a diver's body is saturated with the inert gas, he can theoretically have unlimited time at that working depth as his body will not be able to absorb extra inert gas beyond what he has already absorbed. Therefore, his decompression time requirements will not increase even with further exposure. Saturation divers usually work for a maximum of 28 days under such conditions. Contrary to common belief, most saturation divers do not stay underwater when they are on the job. While it is possible to stay in underwater saturation habitats, they are incredibly expensive and technically challenging to maintain in the seawater environment. Therefore, most commercial saturation divers live onboard on-site dive support vessels that provide hyperbaric living quarters that are pressurised to the depths that the divers are working at. The divers will stay in these hyperbaric chambers for their entire work duration. Food and supplies are delivered to them through small airlocks and they are transferred daily into a diving bell which will transport the diver down to the work site and back. When the entire saturation dive is finally completed, the divers are then decompressed very slowly to allow for all the inert gases in their tissues to diffuse out and prevent DCS. The rate of decompression is approximately 30 metres a day so a decompression from a depth of 200 m will take about 8 days to complete. Saturation diving allows for a more efficient use of the divers' time as it eliminates the need for daily decompression and limits their risk of DCS. However, because of the obvious difficulty in accessing and evacuating the divers once they are in the hyperbaric chamber, a saturation diving operation requires the preparation of comprehensive dive, safety and medical contingency plans, very stringent diver fitness standards, careful monitoring of the divers' physiological and psychological parametres and strict management of the chamber's environmental conditions (Naval Sea Systems Command, 2016).

Free Diving

Although considered a dying trade now as diving equipment becomes more accessible, free diving was once used regularly to harvest items such as abalone, shellfish, and pearls. In fact, the *Ama* divers in Japan who have harvested pearls and seafood through free diving since 927 AD, are now a tourist attraction at Japan's Mikimoto Pearl island (McCurry, 2006). Free divers rely on breath holding while underwater instead of the use of breathing apparatus. While they are less likely to suffer from diving-related injuries such as DCS, these divers still face pressure-related risks such as lung squeeze due to the compression of the lungs by the surrounding water pressure, as well as asphyxia and drowning if they run out of air and are unable to reach the surface in time.

Type of Breathing Gases

The types of breathing gases used in diving have also become more varied over time to overcome diving depth limitations and some of the side effects of the common breathing gases. Some of the commonly available breathing gases are described here. *Nitrox*, which contains air with a higher oxygen concentration relative to nitrogen, can be used to prolong a dive and reduce the accumulation of high amounts of nitrogen in the body's tissues and hence lower the risk of DCS. Other than causing DCS, use of a breathing gas that contains nitrogen at depths below 40–50 ms can also cause nitrogen narcosis, which can be dangerous and has been implicated in drowning cases among divers. Nitrogen narcosis is further discussed later on. To prevent nitrogen narcosis, *Heliox* (where nitrogen is replaced with helium) is commonly used in deep commercial dives as helium is four times less narcotic than nitrogen. However, *heliox* too, has problems of its own. At depths deeper than 150 m, a diver breathing *heliox* can suffer from a helium-associated side effect called High Pressure Neurological Syndrome (HPNS). HPNS presents as muscle tremors, nausea, dizziness, fatigue, stomach cramps, vomiting, myoclonic jerking and decreased mental performance. Similar to nitrogen narcosis, these symptoms resolve when the diver ascends to a shallower depth. Other gas mixtures such as *Trimix* (helium, nitrogen and oxygen mixes) can be used at deep depths as it limits the effects of nitrogen narcosis and oxygen toxicity. However, such dives are usually highly technical and require complex dive planning. Pure oxygen, too, can be used in diving and is commonly used in the military for stealth diving. However, because of the risk of acute oxygen toxicity and convulsions at depth, divers are not allowed to dive deeper than 6 msw when breathing pure oxygen. Other gas blends that use hydrogen and neon have been explored but are still mainly under research and have not been mainstreamed for use in diving.

Occupational Diving

Occupational divers work in a unique and hostile environment. Not only do they have to possess the technical skills for the job that they are employed to do, they also need to master the ability to complete this task underwater. These workers not only face the work-related hazards that arise from operating heavy equipment, manual handling of materials and usage of power tools. They are also subjected to a number of challenging health and environmental hazards which their land-based counterparts do not face, such as the risk of pressure-related illnesses, drowning, injuries from underwater currents, encounters with dangerous marine animals and the underwater effects of sound and temperature on the human body. In 2019, the United States Bureau of Labor Statistics reported that from the estimated 3,380 commercial divers in the United States, there were 460 nonfatal occupational injuries and illnesses among commercial divers from 2011 to 2017 and an additional 39 fatal occupational injuries during that period (U.S. Department of Labor, Bureau of Labor Statistics, 2019). Based on findings by the United Kingdom (UK) Health and Safety Executive (HSE), the UK commercial diver fatality rate ranges from 20–40 per 100,000, which is up to 24 times higher than that of their construction sector counterparts (Health and Safety Executive, 2020). In a 2016 global analysis of fatal accidents in commercial diving, 53% of the fatalities were attributed to pressure-related injuries and drowning, while the rest were contributed by work-related causes such as crush injuries, underwater explosions and other accidents (Hermans, 2016). It is no wonder that occupational diving is therefore considered highly hazardous work and is subject to strict occupational health and safety legislations in many countries.

Types of Occupational Divers

There are several branches of occupational diving, of which the commonly known ones are commercial diving, scientific diving, military/police diving and recreational dive instructors.

Commercial diving

Commercial diving is an occupation in which a diver is engaged to undertake an engineering, construction, maintenance or any other commercially related task which is similar to work that is done on land except that the operating environment is underwater. Commercial diving is commonly divided into offshore and inshore diving (Association of Diving Contractors International, 2016).

Offshore diving is commonly done in oceans, gulfs and seas, and is usually done in support of the oil and gas industries in places such as the North Sea, Norway, Gulf of Mexico and Gulf of Thailand. The main work of offshore divers involves the building, inspection and maintenance of the underwater structures that are essential to the process of oil production. The depth of diving is normally deep. Divers use either surface-supplied or SCUBA gear for depths up to 90 m. For depths deeper than that, saturation diving would usually be conducted (International Marine Contractors Association, 2019). The difficult and dangerous work conditions, long working hours and exposure to rapid weather changes make offshore diving the most hazardous employment for occupational divers.

Inshore diving is another form of commercial diving. The diver is usually employed in civil engineering projects such as underwater inspection of bridges and dams, construction, and repair work. The dive sites involved can be very diverse; inshore divers can be found working in canals, harbors, dams, drainage systems, pipelines, and reservoirs. Due to the close proximity to shore, inshore divers don't need to stay onboard a dive support vessel for weeks on end and are able to go home daily. The equipment that these divers use can be SSBA or SCUBA and this choice usually depends on the type of tasks they are assigned, the time required to complete their work and the dive environment that they will be working in.

Military and police divers

Military divers specialise in in-water tasks such as explosive ordinance disposal, underwater demolition, reconnaissance, and ships husbandry. They may also be called upon to provide diving support in civilian contingencies such as search and rescue missions arising from sea or airplane disasters. In the military, they are usually also the first responders in the rescue of distressed submarines. A subset of military divers are combat divers, who are trained to dive in a tactical manner and almost exclusively use rebreather dive sets to prevent the release of bubbles that would reveal their location.

Police divers are police officers who are trained to conduct rescue diving as well as search and recovery diving for contraband items, crime evidence and corpses. Due to the conditions in which accidents often happen or places where criminal evidence may be disposed of, police divers are trained to dive in contaminated and hostile conditions such as poor underwater visibility, fast currents and water contaminated with toxins and bacteria. These divers need to be vaccinated against diseases such as Hepatitis B and tetanus, wear protective dive gear, undergo extensive post-dive decontamination and have comprehensive safety procedures in place in case of emergencies (Singapore Standards Council, 2018).

Scientific divers

Scientific diving is undertaken by researchers who conduct scientific activities pertaining to the marine environment. The spectrum of scientific diving activities includes inspection and deployment of scientific equipment, collection of underwater specimens, archeological and geological work. Research divers usually work for a research, educational or government agency. For example, the United States Environmental Protection Agency as well as the UK Environment Agency employ divers to recover water samples and marine organisms and conduct regular inspection of sea, lake or riverbed material to examine for signs of pollution. Majority of scientific dives are in shallow waters and use SCUBA dive techniques. In general, scientific diving does not require the heavy physical exertions required of commercial diving. The diving depths are usually shallow and almost exclusively do not require decompression stops — the majority of US scientific diving is done shallower than 10 m depth and UK diving is commonly done between 10 and 19 m deep. Finally, majority of scientific diving is performed at the undergraduate and postgraduate levels, with the predominant age group between 18 and 34 years old, which makes them less prone to some of the common diving-related illnesses and injuries, of which increasing age is a recognised risk factor. All these factors make scientific diving one of the safer types of occupational diving. In a 2005 survey of 508,771 scientific dives, it was found that that there were only 28 serious diving-related incidents (seven fatalities and 21 cases of decompression illness). This rate of 0.06 incidents per 1,000 dives is far lower than those previously reported for military dives (0.14 incidents per 1,000 dives) and recreational dives globally (ranges from 0.07 to 0.12 incidents per 1,000 dives) (Sayer, 2005).

Recreational dive instructors and dive leaders

These divers instruct and supervise recreational divers as well as bring tourists on underwater guided tours. They are equipped to teach a wide variety of diving-related skills, from the use of SCUBA and rebreather dive sets, to technical skills such as rescue, night, deep water and cave diving. Dive instructors are also responsible for the safety of novice recreational divers who are under their instruction and are trained to be able to rescue divers in distress.

Future of Occupational Diving

Remotely operated vehicles (ROV) were invented in the 1950s and since then the technology has advanced considerably such that their use in commercial diving has become widespread. ROVs are able to explore depths and confined spaces which may be beyond the reach of divers, and at a cheaper cost with less safety risks. Divers working underwater need to juggle a multitude of activities, which only increase as the complexity of the task and the depth of the dive increases. At a bare minimum, they need to complete their tasks, report progress updates, watch out for safety hazards and monitor their gas supply. Also, due to the limited endurance of the human body, divers have a finite amount of time they can spend underwater every day before their risk of DCS and other dive-related illnesses increase. ROVs are able to operate continuously without rest, air or risk of diving illnesses. They improve the way work can be done underwater and have gradually replaced some of the tasks that are currently done by divers. That being said, divers are still needed. Unlike ROVs, they are able to enter small spaces, are more versatile than machines and possess the dexterity needed for work that requires fine motor skills. While ROVs will not herald the obsolesce of occupational divers, it may however reduce the frequency of deep dives conducted by divers. While this reduces the exposure risk of the divers, it also reduces the amount of experience such divers will accumulate. Whether this will increase the overall risk to deep sea divers remains to be studied. However, what is clear is that this technology offers the opportunity for man and machine to be used together to improve safety at work, reduce costs and explore new methods of underwater work.

Hazards of the Underwater Environment

Humans function normally within the narrow atmospheric envelope on the earth's surface. Once outside the boundaries of this envelope, the environment turns hostile and being able to survive underwater is dependent on our bodies' ability to adapt to the new environment and utilise techniques to mitigate its adverse effects on our bodies. While diving-related injuries can and do occur, more often than not, the failure of a diver to follow underwater safety guidelines and his subsequent panicked actions during an accident are major contributory factors. Unexpected events can happen underwater, such as the malfunctioning of equipment, failure of the air supply and occurrence of a non-diving related health problem. Understanding the effects of the underwater environment and its hazards and following underwater work safety regulations will go a long way in ensuring that a well-trained diver does not panic, is able to assess and resolve the situation calmly and return to the surface safely (Department of Justice and Attorney-General, 2018).

Effects of water on light, sound and pressure

When a diver views objects underwater, light passes through the water, the facemask lens, and the air in the facemask before it reaches his eyes. Light rays are refracted at each of these interfaces and the resulting distortion makes objects appear longer and closer by a factor of about 25%. Also, visibility is markedly reduced in water compared to on land. Only about 12.5% of light reaches a water depth of 30 m; light rays are also scattered by particles in the water, making shadows less pronounced. Restricted visibility is a common hazard in occupational diving, often made worse by the disturbance of sediments from the seabed by the dive operation and the deep depths the diver may be working at.

Sound waves in air usually get reflected at the air-water interface. Underwater, sound waves travel much faster than in air, hence making localisation of the source more difficult as the sound reaches our ears simultaneously. Furthermore, it has been shown that divers are more susceptible to the effects of noise underwater because acoustic energy underwater does not dissipate as quickly as in air. Divers working close to seismic operations, sonar transmissions or piling operations may be exposed to dangerously high levels of noise. The type of dive equipment that the diver uses also plays a part. For example, a diver who uses a SSBA dive helmet will be less tolerable of high noise levels compared to a diver who wears a wetsuit hood. This is because the helmeted diver's head is surrounded by air and he will hear the noise by air conduction whereas the wetsuit diver, whose head is surrounded by water, hears by bone conduction which is less sensitive to high noise levels. Work done underwater, such as high-pressure water jets and rock drilling may give rise to high noise levels of 90–105 dB and long-term occupational exposure to such high levels of noise will lead to hearing impairment.

Should an explosion occur on land, the air absorbs most of the energy of the pressure wave. Water is practically incompressible, which means that the energy of a pressure wave created by an explosion passes through water largely unchanged and travels for a much greater distance than in air (Colicchio *et al.*, 2015). Commercial divers use explosives in underwater salvage and demolition; accidental explosions can also occur when divers carry out underwater welding and cutting. Military divers also use explosives for underwater mine clearance. When an explosion occurs underwater, a high-pressure gas bubble is created, followed by the propagation of pressure waves that travel outward from the center and pass through the water. Should a diver be in the vicinity of the explosion, these waves will pass into his body. Because the human body is largely comprised of water and incompressible, the pressure waves pass through the body with little or no damage to the solid tissues. However, because of the difference between the transmission of pressure waves in air and water, tissues that line the air spaces in the body are subjected to a violent shearing force at the interface between the tissues and air. This can cause severe damage to the organs involved. Divers who experience an underwater blast injury may present with severe damage to the ears, lung contusions and severe alveolar damage and intestinal perforation.

Changes in temperature

Normal body temperature is 37°C, and oceanic water temperature is commonly 12–20°C in temperate climates and 25–28°C in tropical climates. Hence the diver is almost always immersed in water at a lower temperature than his body. Water also has much higher heat conductivity than air, thus conducting thermal energy from the diver. The body attempts to maintain a steady temperature by reducing heat loss and increasing heat production and shunts blood flow from the peripheries to the core via peripheral vasoconstriction so as to maintain body core temperature.

Hypothermia is a medical condition in which the body loses significant heat which results in disruption of normal bodily functions, and can occur when divers dive in waters cooler than our body temperatures for an extended time period. Hypothermia can present as shivering, slurred speech, lack of muscular coordination, confusion, and in severe cases, loss of consciousness and death. The effects of hypothermia vary between divers and are influenced by individual factors (such as body fat, cold adaptability and type of insulation used) and the work environment (type of activity, water temperature and duration of exposure). Prevention of hypothermia during diving is possible with appropriate insulation, such as wearing of a wetsuit or drysuit and drinking adequate fluids to ensure good hydration.

Hypothermia is more common in divers than hyperthermia. Conversely, is less common. However, this does not mean it is not seen. Divers who are working in the tropics can be at risk of hyperthermia, which occurs when the body's core temperature rises above its normal level and overheats. This can lead to conditions such as heat cramps, heat exhaustion, and in severe cases, heat stroke. Common causes of hyperthermia are prolonged exposure to warm and sunny surface conditions, while wearing wetsuits performing strenuous pre-dive preparatory work. This may cause significant dehydration, further putting the diver at risk before he even enters the water. Hyperthermia should be considered a potential risk any time the air temperature exceeds 32°C and the water temperature is above 27°C. It is important to ensure that divers at the work site be maintained in thermal balance as either excessive heat or cold will affect their health and safety.

Currents and sea states

Currents are flowing masses of water within a body of water and can be divided into major ocean currents and tidal currents. Currents produce forces that affect the diver and his activities and equipment. A diver facing such underwater currents will need to expend significant energy to overcome these forces. Prolonged exposure to currents will cause fatigue, reduce productivity, and increase the risk of a diving incident.

The sea state refers to how "rough" the sea is, and can impact all stages of the diving operation. During rough sea states, it may be necessary to stop the dive operation.

Medical Issues Related to Diving

Near drowning

Drowning during occupational diving is a fatality caused by the filling of the lungs by water, rendering breathing ineffective and leading to death due to asphyxia. Near drowning is initial survival (for at least 24 h) following a drowning incident with the possibility of serious secondary complications occurring later. Hypoxaemia can develop and may result in acute respiratory distress syndrome, hypoxic brain damage, cardiac arrhythmias, electrolyte disturbances and multi-organ failure. The early clinical presentation includes dyspnea, blood-stained frothy sputum, tachypnea and cyanosis. Recovery is usually complete, and there have been some cases known to have survived even after 15–45 min immersion. Thus, resuscitation for drowning cases must always be attempted. Secondary drowning is death due to physiological changes in the lungs in response to an irritant. Inhaled fluid, even small amounts, can act as an irritant inside the lungs. Pulmonary edema can develop subsequently, leading to impaired gas exchange in the alveoli and cause respiratory failure. This has been described as a person "drowning in his own body fluid." This reaction can also take place up to 72 h after a near drowning incident.

Construction and offshore divers can encounter accidents while underwater that can contribute to drowning incidents. This may arise from safety violations or accidents that result in the diver being trapped underwater, such as a collapsed construction piling that traps a diver underwater or a diver being sucked into a sluice gate and getting trapped due to the suction pressure. Divers also can get entangled by their umbilical lines or trapped in a confined space.

Case Study 2: Drowning of a Commercial Diver

A 40-year-old diver, Mr H, who was part of a 2-man dive team, was cleaning the hull and gratings for a container vessel anchored in an anchorage. As the two divers were working on the underside of the hull, there was a lack of natural light and visibility was very poor. After 30 minutes, Mr H's dive buddy signaled that that he was returning to the surface as he had suffered some cuts on his hands and his air sup-

ply was running low. Mr H decided to continue to work underwater alone. 25 minutes later, the diving supervisor noticed that Mr H had not surfaced and sent the standby diver into the water to look for him. The standby diver could not locate Mr H and a subsequent search operation was similarly unsuccessful. Mr H's body was recovered two days later and the autopsy showed evidence of a heart attack as well as drowning. The investigation findings revealed several safety issues. No diver should work underwater alone. A replacement dive buddy should have been sent down to assist Mr H or both Mr H and his dive buddy should have surfaced together. Also, the divers should have been provided with two-way communication with the dive supervisor who was on the surface. This would allow the divers to sound the alarm if they encountered trouble. The divers should also have been provided with a lifeline so that they could be evacuated from underwater in an emergency. Finally, it was noted that the use of SCUBA dive gear is normally recommended for underwater inspections or for light work of short durations. In this case, surface-supplied diving equipment, which provides divers with an unlimited supply of air and communications would have been a better choice of dive gear.

Barotrauma (pressure-related) injuries

When a diver is in the water, he is weightless. However, there is still pressure acting on him — there is the weight of the water column that exerts pressure upon him in addition to the weight of the atmosphere. The pressure exerted by the atmosphere's weight is known as 1 atmospheric pressure (or 1 bar) at sea level. As a diver descends deeper into the water, the amount of water above him increases and hence the pressure exerted on his body, also known as hydrostatic pressure, increases. The pressure increases by approximately 1 bar for every 10 m depth of water. The pressure exerted on a diver at a certain water depth is the sum of the water and air pressures above him. To function safely, a diver must attain a pressure balance between his body and the water pressure at his depth. Otherwise, he may experience pressure-related injuries, otherwise known as barotrauma, due to the pressure disequilibrium.

Our air-filled organs within our bodies are affected by changes in pressure (in accordance to one of the Laws of Physics known as *Boyle's*

Law). As pressure increases within the air-filled organ (as the diver descends into the water with increasing depth), the volume of the air within the organ decreases in the presence of constant temperature. Conversely, as pressure decreases within the air-filled organ (as the diver ascends towards the surface), the volume of air within the organ increases. Simply put:

$$\textit{Pressure } 1 \times \textit{Volume } 1 = \textit{Pressure } 2 \times \textit{Volume } 2$$

Hence, barotrauma can occur when a diver ascends or descends the water column. Usually, air can vent freely to and from the environment and pressure equalisation will naturally take place between the air-filled organ and the environment. However, should there be an obstruction that prevents the venting of air, the build up of pressure may cause trauma to the surrounding tissues. The types of air-filled organs in the body include the lungs, external and middle ear, sinuses, and intestines. Depending on the depth and pressure that the barotrauma occurs at and the part of the body that is affected, barotrauma can be mild, severe or even life threatening. The incidence and severity of barotrauma is especially high near the water surface due to the greater pressure and volume changes at shallow depths. To illustrate this, the volume of a gas bubble shrinks by 50% when it travels down 10 m from the water surface. However, after travelling another 10 m deeper, the volume of the gas bubble at 20 m depth has now shrunk to 33% of the original size at the water surface.

The most common barotrauma in diving occurs in the ear. There are three sections in the ear: the external, middle and inner ear and each section can be affected by barotrauma. The outer ear leads from the ear canal to the ear drum; the middle ear is a small air-filled space behind the ear drum that is connected to the upper throat via a short tube called the Eustachian tube; the inner ear contains the organs for hearing and balance. There are three types of aural barotrauma: external, middle and inner ear barotrauma with the most commonly occurring one being middle ear barotrauma. Middle ear barotrauma usually occurs when a diver descends into water and the difference between the pressure in the middle ear (lower pressure) and the external ear (which has the same pressure as the surrounding water) is not equalised. As the pressure differential increases, either the ear drum ruptures, thereby allowing water to enter the middle ear to equalise the pressure, or blood vessels around the middle ear rupture will rupture to allow bleeding into the middle ear to equalise the pressure between the external and middle ear. The most common reason for middle ear barotrauma is due to blockage of the Eustachian tube, which prevents the pressure in the middle ear from being equalised with that of the surrounding environment. This can occur due to a mechanical obstruction of the tube, congestion of the tube due to an upper respiratory tract infection, or natural anatomical variations in the Eustachian tube's size and shape that hinders pressure equalisation.

Barotrauma can also occur in the sinuses, which are cavities in the forehead and cheekbones that are connected to the back of the nose. These spaces are normally open to the atmosphere and hence pressure equalisation during diving and flying can take place automatically. Should these cavities be blocked, the pressure in the sinuses would not be equalised with the pressure of the surrounding environment during a diver's descent or ascent. The difference in pressure may cause the blood vessels in the sinuses to rupture, causing a "tearing" sensation in the sinuses, pain and bleeding from the nose.

The most dangerous form of barotrauma occurs in the lungs due to the severe damage that pressure injuries can cause to delicate lung tissue, as well as the resultant complications that may occur as air escapes from torn lung tissue into the bloodstream. The most common occurrence of pulmonary trauma occurs during ascent from a deeper to a shallower water depth (also known as pulmonary overinflation syndrome). As mentioned in Boyle's Law, the volume of a gas will increase when pressure decreases. When a diver who is at depth takes a breath of gas from his SCUBA cylinder and ascends to the surface, the gas in his lungs will expand as the pressure drops. If he holds his breath while ascending, the gas will continue to expand in the lungs until the lungs have expanded to their maximum volume. The lungs comprise of extremely delicate tissue and a transpulmonary pressures of more than 60–70 mmHg is sufficient to cause lung tissue to rupture. This pressure can be caused by an ascent of

0.7–1.2 m in the water! Once the gas pressure in the lungs exceed the limits of the lungs, the alveoli will start to rupture. Because the alveoli are almost completely surrounded by blood vessels, most of the escaped air will enter the arterial blood circulation and get pumped out to the body.

Barotrauma of the lungs can have three complications: arterial gas embolism, subcutaneous/mediastinal emphysema and pneumothorax. Arterial gas embolism occurs when gas escaping from ruptured lung tissues enters the circulatory system and these gas bubbles are transported via the arteries to other parts of the body. As the first major branches of the aorta after it leaves the heart supply blood to the brain, a large amount of this gas therefore is transported to the brain. There, these bubbles block blood flow in the small arteries, causing hypoxic damage to the brain tissues these arteries supply. The signs and symptoms of arterial gas embolism depend on the area of the brain that is affected and can present in a wide variety of ways such as headache, localised muscle weakness, loss of sensation, inability to speak, visual disturbances, confusion, paralysis or loss of consciousness. The brain cannot function for more than a few minutes without oxygen. Therefore, should a diver suffer from arterial gas embolism, the signs and symptoms usually occur within a few minutes of him reaching the surface. Arterial gas embolism is a life-threatening condition, and the treatment is oxygen and immediate recompression in a hyperbaric chamber to reduce the size of the bubbles and restore oxygenation to affected tissues. With rapid treatment, a diver may recover rapidly but usually severe arterial gas embolism leads to shock and death.

Occasionally, air that escapes from the alveoli does not enter the arterial circulation but escapes into the potential spaces that surround the lungs. When the escaped air moves centrally outside of the airways and blood vessels into the mediastinum (the space between the lungs), it can cause subcutaneous or mediastinal emphysema. This can be symptomless if the amount of gas is small, or present as chest discomfort, neck fullness, voice changes or difficulty in swallowing if there is a substantial amount of gas stretching the tissues. If the gas tracks upwards into the subcutaneous tissues in the neck, it may cause slight swelling and a crackling sensation when the skin is palpated.

More rarely, both the alveoli and the tough membrane that surrounds the lung, called the pleura, rupture. Usually this scenario occurs in divers who have an underlying lung pathology, such as pulmonary blebs, which are air sacs found on the surface on the lungs that cause weakening of the pleura in that area. These air sacs communicate with the bronchi, often through very small openings and are prone to rupture either spontaneously or from an inability to keep up with the pressure changes associated with diving. When this happens, air enters the pleura and reduces the lung's ability to inflate. This is called a pneumothorax and can present as pain in the chest, difficulty in breathing and shock. Should air continue to escape from the ruptured lung, the pressure buildup may cause both lungs to collapse and death may ensue.

Case Study 3: Mild Case of Barotrauma

A 21-year-old military diver did a series of four training divers in one day, each lasting 1 hour to a maximum depth of 12 metres. The first three dives were uneventful. During the fourth dive, he experienced an increasing tightness and heaviness in his chest and neck. He ignored the symptoms as he thought it was due to fatigue and continued with the dive. Near the end of the dive, he felt a sudden sharp pain in his throat and decided to abort the dive. On reaching the surface, his chest tightness had worsened and he developed increasing difficulty in breathing. He also noticed that his neck was swollen with a crackly feel to the skin, his voice was hoarse and his throat felt sore. He was immediately evacuated to hospital, where X-rays confirmed emphysema both in the mediastinum and neck regions. He was started on 100% oxygen to help absorb the subcutaneous air more quickly and given medication to control the pain. He recovered and was discharged from hospital after three days. Subsequent investigations of the incident revealed that the diver had been holding his breath intermittently throughout his dives to try and conserve his air and had occasional difficulty controlling his buoyancy during his dives. Such 'skip breathing' techniques and breath-holding are not safe and increase the risk of pulmonary barotrauma. Also, the diver should have aborted his dive when he first started feeling unwell and sought medical treatment promptly. Not doing so increased the risk of an incident occurring underwater and put both him and his dive buddy in unnecessary danger.

Case Study 4: Severe Case of Barotrauma

A 30-year-old dive instructor had been showing some diving tourists the marine life at the diving resort when one of the tourists dropped her camera during her ascent. The tourist had gone back down to retrieve her camera but had gotten entangled in debris at the sea bed and was running out of air and panicking. The dive instructor managed to cut the tourist free. Once the tourist saw that she was free, she immediately inflated her buoyancy compensator and shot to the surface, dragging the dive instructor along with her. The dive instructor lost consciousness at the surface and was evacuated immediately to the nearby hospital. At the hospital, he awoke with the right-sided hemiplegia and had slurred speech. His chest X-ray showed a left-sided pneumothorax. He was diagnosed with pulmonary barotrauma and cerebral air-gas embolism. A chest tube was inserted and he immediately underwent recompression therapy in the hyperbaric chamber. His slurred speech resolved at depth and there was improved sensation and muscle strength in the right side of his body. He underwent a total of five recompression treatments before his recovery plateaued. He was left with permanent residual weakness and numbness in both his right upper and lower limbs and had to use a cane for walking.

Decompression sickness

DCS is a term given to a collection of signs and symptoms that arise during and after decompression from a higher to a lower pressure. The clinical presentation of this disease is widely varied and the severity can range from mild to life-threatening. It is not only a risk factor in occupations such as diving and underground tunneling but can also affect aviators and astronauts when they ascend from the ground into the sky (going from a normobaric environment on land to a low pressure environment). Decompression sickness is also commonly referred to as the bends or caisson disease.

As DCS is brought about by gases, knowledge of the properties and behaviour of gases, especially breathing gases, is vitally important to understanding its pathophysiology. Based on Henry's Law of Solubility, the amount of any given gas dissolved in a liquid is directly proportional to the partial pressure of the gas over the liquid. Air is made up of about 79% nitrogen and 21% oxygen and hence at the surface, the partial pressure of nitrogen in the tissues of our bodies will be about 0.8 atmospheres. When a diver who is breathing air descends into water to 10 m depth, he is exposed to increased pressure. The partial pressure of nitrogen at 10 m depth will be 1.6 atmospheres and hence more nitrogen will dissolve into his body tissues. This amount of nitrogen dissolved in the diver's tissues is referred to as nitrogen load, and the nitrogen loading is higher for dives of greater depths and longer duration. Nitrogen loading will continue until the diver is saturated with nitrogen, which usually requires him being at a specific depth for 24 h. When the diver returns to the surface, the extra nitrogen will gradually come out from its dissolved state into the gaseous state in accordance to *Henry's Law*, and will normally leave the body during gas exchange in the lungs. However, should the elimination of the excess nitrogen via gaseous exchange fail to keep up with the reduction in the external pressure, the diver will then reach a state of supersaturation in which the nitrogen can no longer remain in its dissolved state. Nitrogen bubbles may then form *in-situ* in intravascular and extravascular areas such as the skin, blood vessels, joints or solid tissues within the body. These bubbles may press on and cause mechanical injury of the surrounding tissues, obstruct blood flow to vital organs or be perceived by the body to be a foreign body and cause the activation of secondary inflammatory pathways. In some cases, DCS is mild and may resolve spontaneously. In other cases, serious injury may occur and cause permanent damage.

DCS is classically described as Type 1 (tends to be mild and results in painful joints or skin manifestations) or Type 2 (may be life-threatening and often causes central and peripheral nerve disorders such as numbness, arm or leg weaknesses, vertigo, and cardiorespiratory symptoms such as difficulty breathing and chest pain). Usually, symptoms of DCS occur soon after the last dive, but more slowly than that of arterial gas embolism and pulmonary barotrauma. 99% of DCS symptoms occur within 24 h of the dive. There may also be a delayed presentation of DCS, known as dysbaric osteonecrosis, which can present at least 6 months to a year later. Dysbaric osteonecrosis causes damage to the long bones of the body, especially in the shoulder and hip. If the damage is close to a joint, it can lead to persistent pain, long term damage and severe disability. It rarely occurs in recreational divers but is an occupational risk among workers who work in a compressed air environment and deep-sea divers due to their frequent exposure to high pressures.

The risk factors for DCS include that pertaining to the dive profile (such as repetitiveness, depth, duration, dive pattern), violation of the diving table limits, flying shortly after diving, the type of gas used (enriched air, associated with lower nitrogen loading has a theoretical reduced DCS risk for the same dive compared to using air) and the individual's medical status (gross obesity, dehydration, previous injuries, previous DCS have all been described to promote risk).

The treatment of DCS and arterial gas embolism is by recompression and hyperbaric oxygen therapy (Figs. 1 and 2). This involves bringing the patient under pressure again and providing him oxygen at depth. This treatment helps to shrink the size of nitrogen bubbles, restore normal blood flow and increase the amount of oxygen delivered to affected tissues. The pressure is then gradually reduced, which allows sufficient time for the excess nitrogen gases in the body to diffuse out of the tissues and be exhaled. Recompression therapy may be repeated over several days as DCS symptoms may reappear or worsen during the acute phase of injury.

Case Study 5: Decompression Sickness

A young researcher presented with fatigue, lapses in memory and inability to concentrate. She had just completed an intensive week of diving collecting coral samples and recording data as she rushed to meet her research project timelines. She did not consider the possibility of decompression sickness as her dives were shallow (less than 15 metres). Upon evaluation, the dive profile was consistently between 2 to 10 m deep and she would stay in excess of two hours at a go. She also made multiple ascents during the dive to bring samples or equipment, and she had repetitive dives averaging 4

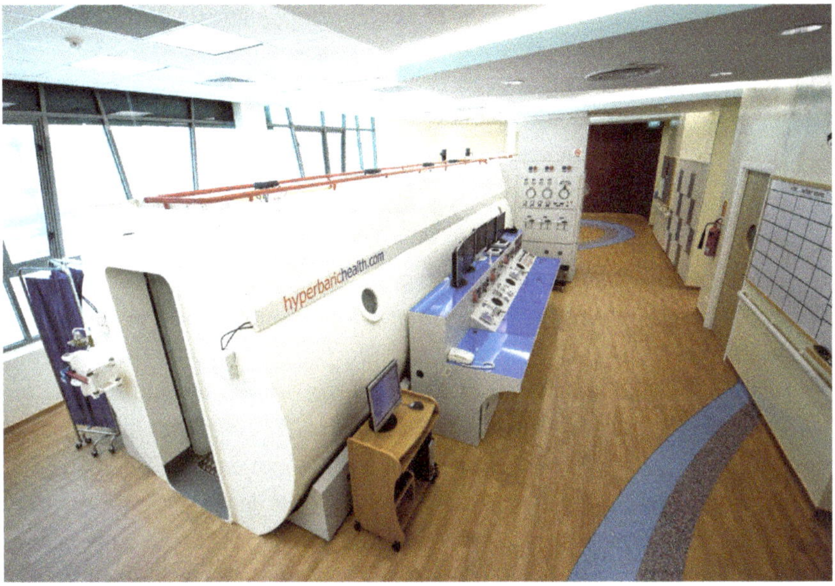

Fig. 1. Large recompression chamber facility in a hospital. (Photo courtesy of Singapore General Hospital.)

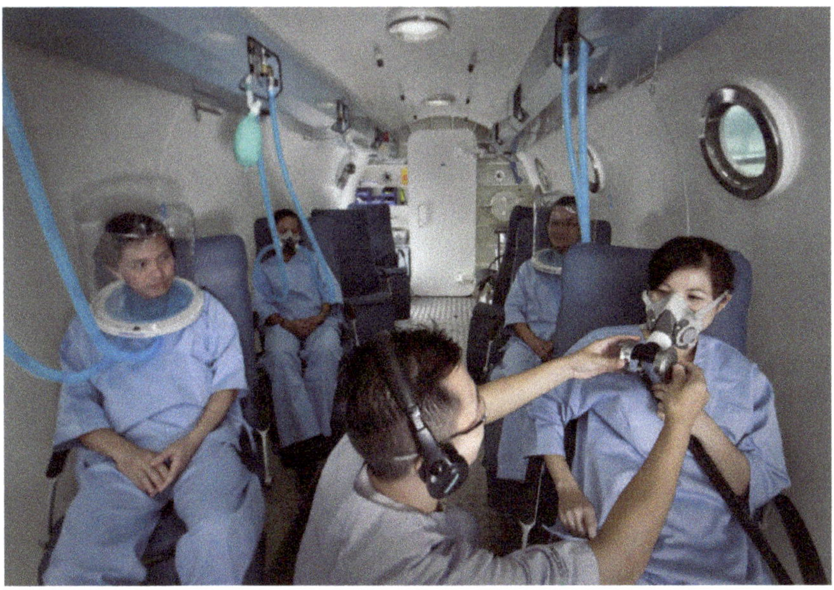

Fig. 2. Hyperbaric nurse in the recompression chamber during hyperbaric oxygen therapy. (Photo courtesy of Singapore General Hospital.)

dives per day. She was also noted to be overweight with a BMI of 31. In view of the risk factors, a diagnosis of decompression sickness was made. She was treated with hyperbaric oxygen therapy and made a complete recovery.

Case Study 6: Decompression Sickness

A 45-year-old scientific diver did a SCUBA air dive to a depth of 30 metres with a total bottom time of 45 minutes. However, as he was preparing to ascend, his dive regulator malfunctioned and started leaking air. He made an emergency ascent to the surface and missed all his required decompression stops. On the surface, he only complained of a mild headache and the dive supervisor placed him on 100% oxygen. His headache resolved after 20 minutes of oxygen and he was keen to go home. However, his dive supervisor insisted that he be brought to the nearest hospital for a checkup. On examination by the doctor, he was found to have a patch of numbness over his left leg with brisk left lower limb reflexes. He also started to feel fatigued and giddy and the doctor immediately started recompression therapy for the diver. Four recompression treatments later, the diver made a complete recovery and was discharged from hospital. In this case, while immediate breathing of 100% oxygen is an appropriate first aid measure, it may also mask the early signs and symptoms of decompression sickness and hence such divers should not be allowed to go home even if they claim to be well — more serious symptoms could occur when they are home at night and some distance from the nearest recompression facility. Based on the dive profile and the missed decompression stops, this diver was clearly at high risk of decompression sickness and so recompression therapy was an appropriate treatment as it would quickly resolve any symptoms present and also prevent the occurrence of more serious ones.

Immersion pulmonary edema

IPE is an accumulation of fluid in the lung tissues, which disrupts the gaseous exchange that takes place. It has become more commonly reported over the years and has occurred in both divers and open-water swimmers. The exact mechanism of this condition is not known well but is probably related to immersion at depth and the resultant shift of fluid from the peripheral to the central circulatory system. This results in the excessive increase of pressure in the pulmonary blood vessels which causes the leakage of tissue plasma into the pulmonary air spaces. Some risk factors of IPE include diving in cold water as it causes peripheral vasoconstriction, heavy exercise while underwater, overhydration by divers prior to dives, a medical history of hypertension and other cardiovascular disorders as well as poor physical fitness levels. IPE can occur early during a dive, at depth or upon reaching surface with affected divers commonly reporting symptoms such as chest pain, difficulty breathing, wheezing and blood-tinged sputum. Treatment of the affected diver includes supplemental oxygen, diuretics to reduce intravascular fluid and mechanical ventilation if necessary. While this condition usually resolves quickly in a healthy diver, occurrence of such signs and symptoms at depth may precipitate other diving-related injuries such as barotrauma and arterial gas embolism should the diver panic and make an uncontrolled ascent to the surface (McFall *et al.*, 2017).

Gas toxicities in a pressurised environment

Divers can face problems during diving that arise from the toxic effect of gases that they are breathing while under pressure. While these gases, such as nitrogen and oxygen, may not cause problems at normal atmospheric pressure, they may cause toxicity in higher concentrations and increased partial pressures in the underwater or pressurised environment. Some of these problems also affect people who work in pressurised environments on land, such as caisson workers. *Dalton's Law* states that the total pressure exerted by a mixture of gases is equal to the sum of the pressures that would be exerted by each of the gases if it alone were present and occupied the total volume.

$$P_{\text{Total}} = P_{pl} + P_{p2} + \cdots + P_{pn}$$

where P_p denotes the partial pressure of the particular gas component.

In a gas mixture, the portion of the total pressure contributed by a single gas is called the partial pressure of that gas. The two components of air are primarily nitrogen and oxygen.

Nitrogen narcosis

A high concentration of nitrogen present in our bodies has a narcotic effect on our central nervous system. This clinical syndrome becomes noticeable at depths beyond 35 m when breathing air and is usually incapacitating beyond 90–100 m. The symptoms of nitrogen narcosis are akin to that of alcohol intoxication and include impairment of reasoning, poor judgment, memory, concentration, attention, loss of coordination and hallucination. A number of diving fatalities have been attributed to nitrogen narcosis. It may start to appear within a few minutes of reaching the given depth and its effects increases as the depth increases. However, it is readily reversible as a diver ascends to shallower depths. A diver can suffer nitrogen narcosis on a dive even though he had previously dived to the same depth without problems. Some individual factors increase the likelihood of nitrogen narcosis including anxiety, inexperience, alcohol consumption, fatigue, cold water and carbon dioxide retention. One can develop tolerance with frequent exposure to a particular depth. To minimise the effects of nitrogen narcosis, divers who dive to deep depths often do not breath air, but replace it with special breathing gas blends such as *Heliox*, that comprises oxygen that is diluted with helium instead of nitrogen as helium does not cause narcosis.

Oxygen toxicity

Some divers use enriched air (with higher partial pressures of oxygen) or even pure oxygen along the course of their work. However, oxygen too can be toxic to the human body under certain conditions. Oxygen breathed at a partial pressure of more than 1.6 atmospheric pressure places the diver at risk of central nervous system oxygen toxicity. This is akin to diving at 6 m depth with 100% oxygen, or diving at 70 m depth with air. The symptoms of oxygen toxicity are wide-ranging and include dizziness, nausea, twitching, agitation, disorientation, hearing loss and convulsion. These symptoms resolve once the oxygen supply is removed. Sometimes, the early recognition of oxygen toxicity symptoms may provide sufficient warning to the diver so that he can reduce the oxygen partial pressure of his gas mixture timely and prevent the onset of more dangerous symptoms. However, a convulsion, the most serious direct consequence of oxygen toxicity, has also been known to occur suddenly without any warning signs. It is believed that the risk of oxygen toxicity increases as the oxygen partial pressure and exposure time increase, and when a diver dives in cold water, does heavy while underwater and retains carbon dioxide.

Carbon dioxide toxicity

Carbon dioxide toxicity (hypercarbia) occurs when there is a build-up of carbon dioxide in the body and may occur with or without a drop in oxygen in the body. Breathing compressed air at depth requires greater respiratory effort as the air is denser. Hence a diver working underwater may accumulate carbon dioxide in the body due to inadequate lung ventilation. It can also be caused by inadequate ventilation of surface supplied diving helmets. Also, in an effort to conserve air and lengthen bottom time, some divers also consciously reduce their breathing rate (this is known as skip breathing) which causes carbon dioxide to build up over time. A diver with elevated carbon dioxide in the body can present with a throbbing headache, increased pulse and respiratory rate and at very high concentrations, cause loss of consciousness. A high carbon dioxide level in the bloodstream signals the body to breathe. Breath-hold divers often circumvent this by hyperventilating before a dive so as to breathe out as much carbon dioxide from the body as possible, which allows them to stay underwater longer without feeling the urge to breathe. However, this is dangerous as a breath-hold diver may run out of oxygen and lose consciousness underwater before his carbon dioxide level reaches a level that signals him to return to the surface. This is known as shallow water blackout and is often a cause of drowning among commercial and professional breath-hold divers.

Carbon monoxide poisoning

Carbon monoxide is a byproduct of incomplete fuel combustion and is commonly found in the exhaust of internal combustion engines. It is a colorless, odorless and tasteless gas and can easily contaminate a diver's air supply if the air intake of the compressor used to provide the diver his air is placed too close to an engine exhaust. The exhaust gases are sucked in with the fresh air when these compressors are charging SCUBA bottles or delivering air directly to divers. Symptoms of carbon monoxide poisoning include headache, dizziness, nausea, confusion and clumsiness. In severe cases, it can cause seizure, loss of consciousness and death. Because carbon monoxide has a very high affinity for haemoglobin, treatment requires the delivery of high concentration of oxygen, and if necessary, high-pressure oxygen therapy in a hyperbaric chamber. Carbon monoxide poisoning is avoidable and it is a good practice for all divers, be it recreational or commercial, to do a portable air analysis of their SCUBA tanks prior to a dive.

High pressure nervous syndrome

In deep diving using helium mixes, divers sometimes suffer from a phenomenon known as High Pressure Nervous Syndrome (HPNS). The signs and symptoms are worsened by a fast rate of compression and deep diving depths. HPNS is characterised by dizziness, nausea, vomiting, postural and intention tremors, fatigue, somnolence, myoclonic jerking, stomach cramps, and confusion. This syndrome resolves spontaneously when the diver ascends or when he slows down his rate of descent. While the underlying mechanisms of HPNS are not well understood, the addition of nitrogen in the breathing mixture, staged compressions, and warming have been useful in ameliorating HPNS in deep diving using helium/oxygen mixtures.

Prevention of Diving Related Disorders

Dive and Safety Plans

Fortunately, the health risks in diving can be reduced significantly through stringent pre-dive, dive and post-dive health and safety protocols (Workplace Safety and Health Council, 2010). For instance, prior to the actual dive, a comprehensive dive plan with a thorough risk assessment and reasonable safety measures should be prepared. The dive plan should also include the control measures to mitigate potential environmental hazards such as foul or sudden changes in the weather, bad sea state, poor underwater visibility, strong underwater currents and water temperature. It is also important to consider and mitigate the specific occupational hazards that the diver may face in the dive environment that he will be working in, which includes the health risks from diving in contaminated water, loud noises produced by underwater tools, sonar, underwater piling and other construction work, and possible accidents while working underwater. Finally, the decompression procedures for the diver and the contingency response plans in the event of emergencies should be prepared beforehand and briefed to the entire dive team.

It is also essential that the diver who is engaged for the work is medically fit to dive, adequately trained in the diving apparatus and breathing gas that he is using and technically competent in doing the work required. Any diver who wishes to become a commercial diver normally requires specific competency training for the type of diving he will participate in, and must satisfy the dive medical standards that the country-specific regulatory agencies require (Workplace Safety and Health Council, 2009).

Once the diving commences, the dive team that is supporting the dive operations should be alert, maintain regular communications with the diver and be ready to respond to any dive emergencies. In most dive operations, the dive team will minimally comprise a dive supervisor, the commercial divers, a dive attendant and a standby diver. This number may be increased depending on the risk assessment of the dive operation and the number of divers deployed. Once the diving operation is completed, it is also good practice for the dive team to conduct a post-operation debriefing and go through the events of the day, capture feedback and discuss the learning points so as to improve future operations.

Medical Fitness to Dive

Occupational diving is a very demanding job, both in terms of physical as well as psychological demands. The diver works in an unpredictable and irrespirable work environment, often in poorly lit and confined spaces. The type of work that an occupational diver does underwater can vary widely and the various work environments and dive tasks all have their own unique hazards. That being said, it is universally accepted that all types of occupational diving are hazardous, and a high standard of medical fitness is necessary for the diver to minimise his job risk as well as ensure he can respond to any underwater emergency. The list of medical contraindications to diving is long and can be divided into absolute and relative contraindications. However, it is too simplistic to measure the diver against these criteria and automatically disqualify all divers who have abnormal examination findings or test results. While it would be ideal to only accept perfectly healthy people to train as occupational divers, this will probably exclude a lot of potential candidates who probably would be able to dive and work underwater safely despite having a minor medical condition. Furthermore, in reality, only allowing perfectly healthy people to do commercial diving is not feasible in the long run as even healthy occupational divers will eventually age and develop medical conditions over time while it takes years to fully train a replacement.

Hence, pre-employment, periodic and fitness-to-return-to-work medical examinations are important tools to help divers maximise their safety underwater. Such medical examinations should ideally be done by a qualified doctor who is trained in diving and occupational medicine. Being able to understand the complex interactions between the effects of the underwater environment, the demands of a diver's specific diving duties and the ability of the human body to tolerate these stressors puts this doctor in the well-placed position to identify the diving-related medical issues and provide the medical recommendations in accordance to the specific requirements of the individual diver. For instance, the medical standards would be comparatively more stringent for an offshore and saturation diver when compared with a scientific diver due to the fact that the former are usually working offshore for months on end, may not have ready access to advanced medical care and have to undertake strenuous underwater work regularly while the latter are usually shore-based and the work is relatively less physically demanding.

The conduct of medical examinations to assess fitness to dive in the occupational diver has the following objectives:

- To meet the country's legislative requirements and relevant commercial diving medical standards (Standards Australia Limited/ Standards New Zealand, 2015).
- To ensure that the diver is able to conduct the diving activities safely without injury to self or others.
- To ensure that diving does not aggravate any underlying medical condition in the diver.

The outcomes of the diving medical examination would fall into one of these groups:

- Fit to dive with no restriction.
- Fit to dive with restriction, e.g. on the type of diving, depth, time, and diving environment.
- Temporary unfit to dive.
- Permanently unfit to dive.

Conduct of the Medical Review

Occupational fitness to dive examinations are usually done prior to the start of the diving operation, annually during the employment and on an ad hoc basis following an extended period of non-diving due to a medical event (such as hospitalisation or prolonged sick leave). This forms part of the medical surveillance programme for occupational divers. The scope of the diving medical examination usually comprises of a health questionnaire with a signed declaration by the diver, a series of investigations, and a medical review by a doctor. The routine investigations could comprise of audiometry, spirometry and a chest X-ray. Where indicated, further tests may be done to evaluate the severity of an underlying medical condition such as a hypertonic saline challenge tests for potential divers who have a history of asthma and an exercise stress test for a diver who has recovered from ischaemic heart disease and is reviewed for his fitness to return to work (Urick *et al.*, 2021).

As part of the medical examination, there are general and specific considerations that the doctor should take into account when ascertaining a diver's fitness to dive. While some of them are described here, it is recommended that a medical examiner of occupational divers should at least have attended a basic diving medicine course that covers the different types of diving that commercial divers do, the physiological aspects of working underwater, the common dive and work-related hazards and illnesses in occupational divers, and the management of such conditions. Such courses are regularly conducted by institutions such as the Undersea & Hyperbaric Medical Society (UHMS) and the National Oceanic and Atmospheric Administration (NOAA) in the United States, the Institute of Naval Medicine and the Royal College of Surgeons of Edinburgh in the UK, and the Singapore General Hospital Hyperbaric and Diving Medicine Centre in Singapore.

Age

The international consensus for the minimum age limit of an occupational diver is that he be at least 18 years of age as a degree of physical and emotional maturity is required for working safely underwater. There is no upper age limit for occupational diving as long as the diver can maintain a high health and fitness level. Therefore, it is more important to assess a diver's physiological, rather than chronological age when determining his physical fitness levels. Physical fitness levels normally peak in the late 20s and steadily decline thereafter, therefore an older diver may find it increasingly challenging to maintain a high fitness level as he ages. Diving is very hard work — studies have shown that recreational diving uses between 3 and 5 metabolic equivalents (METs) of energy (Buzzacott *et al.*, 2014). This could easily rise to between 10 and 12 METs as the demands from the work, sea state and underwater environmental conditions intensify, and it still has not included a fitness reserve to meet the near-maximal physical efforts required should a life-threatening emergency situation arise while a diver is underwater. Functional fitness testing can be done to assess the fitness of a diver. As part of the standards required for working divers, the UK HSE mandates that a diver must have a minimum fitness level of 13 METs, independent of age or sex (Health and Safety Executive, 2015). Beyond physical fitness, a diver's lung function, vision and hearing similarly decline with age and these should be assessed regularly during the diver's routine medical review to ensure that the diver can continue to function underwater safely.

Gender

There is no restriction on gender in occupational diving as long as the diver's medical and fitness requirements are met. However, a diver who is pregnant or suspects that she is pregnant is strongly recommended not to undertake diving. Given the obvious ethical challenges of conducting research on diving during pregnancy, much of the research in humans are observational studies and prone to bias. However, studies that have been conducted on animals in hyperbaric chambers suggest that a range of developmental abnormalities such as low birth weight, fetal abortion, malformed limbs, abnormal development of the heart and severe fetal decompression illness are associated with hyperbaric exposure. In addition to the possible risk to the fetus, changes in a woman's body during pregnancy may increase the safety risks — the changes in body habitus will affect equipment fitting and a diver's underwater buoyancy, swelling of the mucous membranes may make ear clearing difficult and pregnancy-related nausea and vomiting may make diving not only uncomfortable but dangerous (Reid and Lorenzo, 2018). Therefore, while it cannot be conclusively proven that diving causes adverse outcomes to a human fetus, there is enough associated evidence and safety risks to recommend that a commercial diver who is pregnant or suspects that she might be pregnant should not dive. After a female diver delivers, she should also wait at least six weeks to give her body time to heal and reduce the risk of intrauterine complications before she resumes her dive career.

Obesity

An obese diver usually has a lower level of fitness, is less mobile and agile underwater, and due to his increased cross-sectional area, often has to work harder to overcome the water resistance. Also, obesity is associated with an increased risk of chronic diseases like diabetes and cardiovascular disease. In terms of diving-related risks, an obese diver is at increased risk of DCS. Fat absorbs five times as much nitrogen as water. As fat has a relatively poor blood supply, there will be relatively little nitrogen absorption and health impact on a recreational diver who does relatively few and short dives. However, in an occupational diver who does multiple long dives or saturation dives, the long amount of time spent underwater will result in a significant amount of nitrogen being stored in his fat tissues. Again because of the poor blood supply to fat tissues, the nitrogen will not be able to be removed timely, thus increases a diver's risk of DCS with bubbles forming in his fat tissue. The risk in an obese diver is higher than that of a fit diver — an obese diver is usually less fit and hence works (and breathes) harder during a dive and takes up more nitrogen.

The body mass index (BMI) is traditionally used to identify a person most likely to be obese and high BMI values generally indicate excessive body fat. Most international guidelines for occupational divers recommend a BMI cutoff between 33 and 35. However, should the high BMI be potentially due to high muscle mass, a bioimpedance test or waist circumference check may be used to predict body fat percentage. Some commercial organisations accept divers who do not meet the weight limits but have less than 23% body fat for males and 34% body fat for females.

Smoking and alcohol

Everybody should be discouraged from smoking due to the considerable negative health effects of smoking on the body. However, there are several effects of smoking that are of particular concern to divers. Cigarette smoke contains significant amounts of carbon monoxide, which has 250 times more affinity for haemoglobin than oxygen and forms carboxyhaemoglobin (COHb) which reduces the oxygen-carrying capacity of blood. The maximum level of carbon monoxide allowed in breathing gas is 0.001% whereas studies have shown that smokers can have COHb levels of between 3% and 15% (Schimmel *et al.*, 2018). Such high COHb levels reduce exercise tolerance and a diver's physical ability to respond in an emergency. Smoking also constricts the airways in the lungs, thereby increasing breathing resistance and the overall work of breathing. The smoke also irritates the lung tissue and results in an increased mucus production in the lungs, nose and sinuses while impairing its drainage. In the lungs, this can cause mucous plug blockages that trap air and result in pulmonary barotrauma. In the ears and sinuses, this increases the risk of middle ear and sinus barotrauma. Finally, chronic smoking damages the delicate tissues in the lungs and break down lung alveolar walls, causing the formation of air sacs called bullae. These bullae can trap gas during a dive and increase a smoker's risk of pulmonary barotrauma and arterial gas embolism.

Alcohol is a common cause of drowning and has been associated with up to 80% of all drownings in adult males (Sean and Pollock, 2012). The most obvious impact of sending an inebriated diver underwater to work is the impairment of his physical and cognitive abilities. The acute effects of alcohol also cause an increase in heat loss and a resultant risk of hypothermia, dehydration and an increased risk of DCS and disturbance of a diver's balance and equilibrium which may cause him to vomit and aspirate while underwater. Long term alcohol abuse can also lead to learning and memory problems as well as mental health issues such as depression and anxiety (Perrine *et al.*, 1994). An occupational diver should not have any form of alcohol, drug or substance abuse.

Medication use

An occupational diver may get medication from his family physician for common acute conditions such as the common cold, muscle sprains etc, and long-term medications for chronic illnesses. A detailed medication history during the diving medical review is an important part of the process. However, the challenge that a diving medicine specialist will face after attaining this information is how to determine the safety of these medication at work. There are very few studies conducted on the effects of medications in an underwater or hyperbaric environment. As a guide, should a diver dive under the influence of acute or chronic medication, the attending doctor should consider the underlying illness which requires the use of the medication, whether this illness affects diving, the effect of the medication on a diver's physiology, the potential effect of such medications during emergencies or strenuous work activities, and the effect of abrupt cessation of this medication on the diver. For example, some anti-hypertensives such as beta-blockers reduce blood pressure but also limits a person's heart rate and his response to exercise. This will cause fatigue and a reduced exercise capacity in a diver. Diuretics control high blood pressure through increasing fluid loss, but it also increases the risk of dehydration, electrolytic imbalance and DCS in a diver. Angiotensin-converting enzyme (ACE) inhibitors are another commonly-used anti-hypertensive medication. Some patients develop a dry cough, which is a side effect of ACE inhibitors. While the medication does not affect diving per se, coughing while a diver ascends in the water column is a risk factor for pulmonary barotrauma. Other common medications such as bronchodilators, used in the long-term treatment of asthma, may cause tachycardia and central nervous system impairment.

Another area of particular concern is over-the-counter (OTC) medication, which most people will automatically assume are completely safe both on surface and underwater, given that they do not need a doctor's prescription. While it is true that OTC medications have lower risk and a greater margin of safety than prescription medications, all medications can have side effects, and even untoward effects when used underwater. One of the common OTC medication used by divers is decongestants, which divers use to relieve ear and sinus congestions and help improve pressure equalisation. However, decongestants also may cause a mild central nervous system stimulation which can present as nervousness, dizziness, restlessness and tachycardia. Another common medication used is antihistamines, which provide symptomatic relief from allergies and the common cold but also causes dryness of the mouth and throat, drowsiness and decreased mental acuity — all of which can affect a diver's ability to think clearly, complete his work tasks safely and react appropriately should an emergency arise.

Doctors should be aware of the potential effects of medications used by occupational divers and observe caution when prescribing acute or chronic medications to divers. As far as possible, an occupational diver having medical problems should seek the attention of a doctor trained in diving medicine and who is familiar with the specific occupational hazards that the diver is exposed to. For the use of OTC medication, it is advisable that a diver read and understand the warnings, precautions and potential side effects it may have on him, and then do a trial course of the medication for at least two days prior to diving to assess his individual reaction to the drugs. For prescription and chronic medications, it is recommended that the diver take the medication for at least one month prior to diving to ensure that the dosage is correct and to reveal any side effects the diver is likely to experience. When in doubt, the diver should seek advice from both his medical specialist as well as a doctor trained in diving medicine.

Systematic Review

The systematic medical examination of prospective and current divers should include the pertinent aspects of their present and past history to detection conditions that may place them at increased risk for decompression illness, barotrauma, loss of consciousness and an inability to mentally or physically handle the underwater environment. One of the challenges faced by the doctor is that while there are clear absolute medical contraindications to dive that most diving medicine specialists have agreed on and that almost all national guidelines abide by, there is also a wide spectrum of medical conditions that doctors and national authorities up until today do not have a uniform agreement on regarding fitness to dive. Another challenge the doctor faces is the recurrent need to consider both the interests of the employer and the working diver without compromising professional and ethical standards. In the occupational setting, the employer is primarily responsible for the occupational diver and oversees the nature of diving activities; in contrast the recreational diver is solely responsible for his decision whether to dive or not.

Cardiorespiratory systems

The cardiovascular and respiratory systems are important areas to cover in a diver's medical assessment. The key focus of this system review is to ensure that the occupational diver has sufficient cardiovascular and respiratory capacities to cope with the intense physical requirements for working underwater, and to exclude any medical conditions that could cause an in-water emergency. Therefore, any conditions such as organic heart disease, symptomatic ischaemic heart disease, abnormal cardiac rhythms, presence of lung bullae and a history of spontaneous pneumothorax that could incapacitate a diver while underwater should be absolute contraindications to occupational diving. However, there are medical conditions that need further assessments before a decision can be made. For example, while coronary artery bypass surgery will likely render a diver unfit to dive, percutaneous transluminal coronary angioplasty with revascularisation and a recovery of cardiac function may not necessarily be a contraindication to diving. Similarly, while uncontrolled hypertension increases the risk of a heart attack and stroke and is an absolute contraindication to diving, once it is controlled with medication, a diver's fitness to dive status can be reviewed. A cardiologist's opinion on the diver's prognosis and fitness level may be more important then, rather than basing the diver's fitness purely on a blood pressure threshold. A history of asthma is also a controversial topic in fitness to dive. Traditionally, divers with any history of asthma have been excluded from diving due to the risk of an asthma attack while underwater, which can be precipitated by exercise and the inhalation of cold, dry air. However, some organisations such as the UK HSE do allow occupational divers with a history of asthma to dive, subject to these divers meeting stringent medical criteria and passing of respiratory investigations such as spirometry and exercise challenge tests.

Endocrine system

Diving is an inherently stressful occupation both mentally and physiologically. Sources of physiological stress include pressure, cold, hypoxia, and physical activity. A diver with an unstable or uncontrolled endocrine disease that affects hormonal responses and causes impaired thermoregulation, cardiac or muscular insufficiency would unlikely be fit to dive. However, advances in medicine have made it possible for treatments that can control or actually eliminate the disease, rendering the diver fit to dive again. For example, a diver who is initially diagnosed with hyperthyroidism or hypothyroidism would not be fit to dive. However, once he is treated and the condition is stabilised, there is no reason why he cannot be certified fit to dive as long as he did not develop any permanent complications of the disease. This is one of the reasons why regular medical assessments and health surveillance of divers are very important. A diver may not notice the early signs and symptoms of an endocrine disease — early diagnosis and intervention may prevent complications and a permanent impact on a diver's health and possibly, his career.

Regarding diabetes, a persistently high blood sugar level will increase the likelihood of a person to suffer from complications such as stroke, ischaemic heart disease and vascular problems. However, in the acute setting, it is actually low blood sugar (hypoglycaemia) that is more dangerous to the diver than hyperglycaemia. The brain is very sensitive to fluctuations in blood glucose levels. A drop in blood sugar levels can lead to a lack of concentration, impaired judgement and unconsciousness in a diver who is working underwater. If a potential occupational diver is found to have diabetes during his pre-employment screening, he should not undergo professional diver training due to the high likelihood of later disqualification due to diabetic complications. However, the challenge arises when an existing commercial diver develops diabetes. A straightforward disqualification from diving is logical, but is not always an acceptable option to the diver, who may find a mid-career switch challenging to say the least, and to the employer, who has invested time and effort in training the diver. Suffice to say, the diver will need to manage his blood sugar level pristinely for the rest of his diving career — any evidence of poor diabetes control (be it hypoglycaemia or hyperglycaemia) or development of diabetic complications such as retinal changes, vascular disease, nephropathy and neuropathy should automatically disqualify the diver permanently from diving. However, should his diabetes be well controlled, a detailed and individualised medical assessment may be warranted where the nature of the diver's work, the diving environment he is in, the onsite medical support available and the diver's motivation as well as knowledge of his medical condition are taken into account. Certain measures could be put in place to ensure the safety of the diver, such as assigning a mandatory dive buddy, carrying oral glucose for dives, limiting the dive duration and depth and frequent blood glucose monitoring.

Mental health

Mental health is an important part of the diver's fitness to work, especially when one takes into account the various stresses that are associated with the type of work he does, remote location he works in and the attendant risks involved. An occupational diver must be able to think clearly, make sound decisions, conduct his work safely, maintain good situational awareness and be ready for any emergencies that may happen while underwater. All these are contingent on him being in a good physical and mental state prior to and during the dive. There are three areas to consider when assessing fitness for diving from a mental health perspective — disorders that are unrelated to diving but can affect the safety of the diver underwater, disorders that are related to or arise from diving, and the effects of the medications used to treat these disorders. Particular emphasis should be placed on anxiety-related disorders due to the clear link between anxiety, panic and diving-related injuries. Some conditions such as schizophrenia and bipolar affective disorder would be absolute contraindications to diving, whereas other disorders should as depression, acute stress reaction and adjustment reactions would likely necessitate a psychiatrist's report on the diagnosis, prognosis, treatment and suitability of the diver to continue functioning underwater safely.

As part of the complete medical assessment, the doctor should also do an examination of the diver, including checks of the nervous, musculoskeletal, gastrointestinal, genitourinary systems, skin, vision and ear, nose and throat, keeping a look out for any conditions that are contraindicated to diving.

A non-exhaustive general list of medical contraindications is shown in Table 1 (Edmonds *et al.*, 2015).

Table 1. Selected Medical Contraindications to Diving

Risk of Sudden Death	Asthma, Coronary Artery Disease, Intracranial Aneurysm or Atrioventricular Malformation, Other Cerebrovascular Disease, Cardiac Arrhythmia, Severe Hypertension, Congestive Heart Failure
Impaired Consciousness	Drugs/Medication, Epilepsy, Diabetes Mellitus, Cardiac Arrhythmia, Transient ischaemic Attacks
Impaired Judgment	Drugs, Psychosis, Severe Anxiety, Severe Depression, Claustrophobia
Risk of Disorientation	Tympanic Membrane Perforation, Inner Ear Disease, Uncorrected Poor Visual Acuity
Impaired Mobility	Spinal Cord Disease or Injury, Neuromuscular Disease, Obesity, Poor Physical Fitness, Pregnancy
Risk of Barotraumas	Asthma, Spontaneous Pneumothorax, Pulmonary Cysts, Fibrosis, Scars, Bronchitis, Chronic Obstructive Airway Disease, Blocked Eustachian tubes, Acute or Chronic Respiratory Infections
Risk of Decompression Sickness	Obesity, Acute Physical Injury, Spinal Cord Disease or Injury, Intracardiac Shunts, Pregnancy

Complex medical conditions do arise during the fitness to dive assessment. For such cases, the doctor doing the medical assessment of the occupational diver should reach out to the medical specialist responsible for the diver's clinical care, especially if this is the first time he is seeing that diver. Having a discussion with the medical specialist will help the doctor understand the state of the diver's medical condition better as well as help him make a more complete assessment on the impact that working underwater may have on the diver's health, and the potential that the medical condition could affect his safety underwater.

Fitness to Return to Diving Work

An injury, surgery, new illness or change in a diver's medical condition may affect his ability to dive and function underwater safely. A return-to-work assessment by a doctor is important to determine any new factors or impairments that may affect the diver's health, his ability to work underwater safely, as well as his capacity to manage underwater emergencies such as the evacuation of a fellow diver. For example, a diver who has undergone leg surgery will need time to regain lower limb mobility and strength and should recover fully before he can safely return to water. Likewise, if a diver was recently diagnosed with hypertension, he would need to stabilise his condition before he can be certified fit to return to dive work. Similar to a regular diving medical review, the doctor conducting the return-to-work assessment should also be aware of the diver's specific underwater work environment, potential hazards, and the work tasks he is to perform. This is so that he can make an objective and well-informed assessment of the diver, and recommend the appropriate work restrictions, if any.

A return to work following DCS and arterial gas embolism requires very careful and deliberate considerations. Beyond the assessment of residual signs and symptoms and permanent damage to organs that may predispose to future life-threatening complications, the doctor should also look at the contributory factors to the decompression injury such as the dive profile and environmental factors the diver experienced during his underwater work. If it was assessed that this was an "undeserved" hit, i.e. the diver developed manifestations after a relatively safe dive, further investigations such as a patent foramen ovale test and an assessment by a cardiologist, as well as a review by a respiratory physician for an underlying respiratory pathology may be pertinent towards assessing the overall fitness of a diver to continue diving.

Case Study 7: Fitness to Return to Diving

Mr J, a 25-year-old scientific diver did a 30-minutes dive in the sea with a fellow scientific diver to collect water samples and study the underwater ecosystem in that area. He did a SCUBA air dive and the maximum depth he reached was 15 metres. It was an easy dive with no strenuous physical exertion needed and no decompression stops required. After surfacing, both divers returned to shore. 45 minutes later, Mr J started complaining of headache, nausea and an unusual feeling in his right leg. He was put on 100% oxygen immediately and attended to by a medic. On examination, he was found to have a rapid pulse, poor hand-eye coordination, decreased strength in his right lower limb and numbness over his right calf. He was immediately evacuated to a nearby recompression chamber and successfully treated with recompression therapy. He made a full recovery with all symptoms resolved. He was thereafter referred to a diving medicine specialist for an assessment as he had suffered serious decompression illness despite it being a relatively safe dive with no obvious dive-related risk factors. Investigations revealed that the diver had a large Patent Foramen Ovale (PFO), which is a known risk factor for serious decompression illness (Smart et al., 2015). A PFO allows some blood from the right side of the heart to flow into the left heart, bypassing the lungs. In a diver with a PFO, intravascular bubbles that form in the venous system after a dive will therefore flow into the arterial circulation without being filtered out by the pulmonary circulation. These bubbles may then travel to the brain, spinal cord and other organs and cause damage. Mr J was referred to a cardiologist for closure of his PFO. The procedure was successfully completed and a bubble contrast echocardiogram conducted 3 months later showed that the PFO remained closed. Mr J was certified fit to return to diving thereafter with no restrictions.

Whether, or how soon a diver returns to occupational diving after suffering from DCS and arterial gas embolism depends on the severity of the symptoms he experienced, his response to recompression treatment, the type of diving that he will undertake in the future and the risk of serious injury from a future decompression injury (Diving Medical Advisory Committee, 2017). About 70% of divers experience an immediate and complete recovery after recompression treatment whereas other divers may take weeks to months after treatment to recover fully, or unfortunately, have permanent residual deficits. The advice on return to diving after DCS varies in the literature and among doctors. Based on the United States Navy guidelines, divers with uncomplicated, pain-only DCI who make a complete recovery may return to diving after 48 h of symptom relief while divers who had cardiorespiratory or neurological symptoms and make a complete recovery should wait at least four weeks. The UK Diving Medical Advisory Committee recommends that divers who experienced limb pain or non-specific manifestations abstain from diving between 7 and 14 days while those who experienced neurological or pulmonary symptoms wait between 1 and 3 months and return to diving only after review by a diving medicine specialist.

If a diver has suffered permanent neurological injuries, not only will he be a potential safety hazard to himself and other divers in the water, his likelihood of a future decompression illness episode will be higher and the ability to recover also impaired. Unfortunately, such a diver should be considered unfit for any form of occupational diving.

Compressed Air Works

There are a group of workers who are exposed to hyperbaric work environments without the water, commonly known as compressed air workers. They include tunneling workers, caisson workers and hyperbaric medical facility healthcare workers.

In tunneling, compressed air is usually used during the construction of a tunnel to prevent ground water from entering into the freshly bored space. Up to the early 1980s, tunnels were excavated by hand or conventional tunnel boring machines (TBMs) and the tunnel was filled with compressed air to prevent flooding by ground water and the entrance of toxic gases such as methane gas. The prolonged hours in the compressed air environment and intense manual labour unsurprisingly led to a high incidence of DCS among these workers. The modern TBMs have largely eliminated the need to pressurise the entire tunnel and relieved the need for large numbers of workers working at high pressures. However, some workers may still be exposed to a pressurised environment occasionally as the cutting face of the TBM is still pressurised. This area is directly in front of the machine and is pressurised to prevent ground water and toxic gases from entering. Workers need to enter this space periodically for inspection, maintenance and repair of the cutting head and hence face the concomitant risks of a pressurised environment. These workers enter the pressurised environment through a chamber called a man-lock. Once inside, the man-lock is pressurised to the requisite pressure so that the workers can enter the pressurised space. When they are ready to come out, they will enter the man-lock again where the air pressure would be slowly reduced to atmospheric pressure in accordance with a decompression table. On top of the hyperbaric-associated health risks, the tunneling and caisson workers are also exposed to a number of construction-related health risks (physical, chemical and biological hazards) that can produce acute or chronic adverse health effects (Table 2). These effects need to be considered when excluding pressure-related injuries such as DCI. For instance, it can sometimes be a challenge differentiating musculoskeletal injuries from the joint pains arising from DCS.

Table 2. Construction Related Health Risks for Tunneling and Caisson Workers

Physical Hazards	Chemical Hazards	Biological Hazards
Mechanical injuries, noise related injuries or noise induced deafness, heat stress, nuisance dust, fire	Gas toxicities from soil contaminants (e.g. hydrogen sulphide, methane) or from gas supply (e.g. carbon monoxide), chemicals used in grouting	Infectious diseases such as influenza, foodborne diseases and tetanus

Case Study 8: Decompression Illness in a Compressed Air Worker

During tunneling works on an underground sewer construction project, 3 workers were required to enter the working space in front of the Tunnel Boring Machine to remove some large rock debris. The 3 workers were in the compressed air environment for a total of 5 hours at 1 bar (equivalent to a depth of 10 metres in water), where they had to manually clear the areas of heavy rocks. The temperature was about 30 degrees Centigrade and humidity was about 85%. The work was uneventful, and the workers were decompressed in accordance with the appropriate schedules. After completion of their work that day, two of the workers flew back to their hometown that same night. During the flight, one of them developed pains in both his elbows while the other worker developed pain in his right knee. There was no joint swelling, skin rashes or any neurological symptoms. The pains were deep seated but not debilitating and resolved when the airplane landed in their country. They were brought to their local hyperbaric facility where they underwent recompression therapy. The third worker did not report any signs or symptoms of decompression illness. The three compressed air workers had done heavy manual work in a compressed air environment; dehydration was also a likely contributory factor due to the hot and humid work conditions. While one worker did not develop decompression sickness, it is likely that all three workers had a significant nitrogen load in their tissues and the low cabin pressure in the airplane precipitated decompression sickness at altitude in the two workers. Similar to diving, compressed air workers should have a minimum surface interval before they fly.

Control of DCS Risk

The risk of DCS depends largely on the working pressure of the worker. In general, there is a low risk for DCS if the working pressure is less than 0.7 bar; moderate risk from 0.7 to 1.0 bar; and high risk when it is more than 1.0 bar. The other factors contributing to the risk of DCS depends on the decompression profile (riskier profiles include longer work duration and repetitive dives) and individual factors (such as obesity, heat stress and dehydration).

However, there are various control measures that can ameliorate the DCS risk. The one that has had the largest health and safety impact is the aforementioned advent of TBMs that eliminated the need for manual and labour-intensive mining works. These days, the number of workers that need to enter the pressurised areas of tunneling works have dropped significantly, and the amount of time that they need to stay under pressure has reduced too. The strict compliance to decompression schedules to remove the inert gases from the miners' bodies has also contributed to the low DCS at the worksite. In Singapore, the incidence of DCS when it first started tunneling work in the 1980s was an impressive 0.087% (164 cases out of 188,538 man-decompressions with a working pressure of up to 2.5 bar) (How *et al.*, 1990). In India, there were only three workers who presented with pain-only DCS, out of the 35,000 man-hours of work that was carried out in the compressed air environment during the construction of the Chennai underground metro rail system between 2009 and 2015 (Kulkarni, 2017).

Medical selection during the pre-placement and periodic examinations were also useful to identify health risk factors. Surveillance for symptoms at the end of the work shift facilitated early detection of DCS symptoms and hence more effective treatment (Ong, 2002). Health education of the workers also helped them to understand the pressure risks and recognise DCS and barotrauma symptoms, and the need for adequate hydration and rest before, during and after each work shift.

Conclusion

Occupational diving and working in a compressed air environment expose workers to both common workplace hazards, as well as short and long-term hazards unique to the underwater and pressurised environment. To ensure that these workers' health and lives are protected requires a concerted effort between legislators, employers, medical professionals and the workers themselves. There is a need to ensure standards of practice in diving and compressed air works that are regulated and enforced. Employers must put in place strong operating and emergency procedures as well as training standards to ensure that the dive and work environment is safe for their employees and that their health and safety are looked after. Medical professionals must ensure that they are kept up to date with the latest medical knowledge in diving and hyperbaric medicine and conduct pre-employment and periodic medical examinations for commercial diving in accordance to industry standards. Lastly, this is a physically and mentally demanding industry that places the workers in an austere and unforgiving environment. Individual divers have a responsibility to maintain their fitness, take charge of their equipment and safety, and exercise judgment to suspend or abort a dive if they find conditions that are unsafe. By working together, all stakeholders can ensure the safety and health of diving and compressed air workers.

References

Abalone Victoria (Central Zone). (2014) *Industrial Standard for Abalone Diving Victoria V1.2.* [Online] Available from: https://abalonevictoria.com.au/members-area/2014-industry-standard-for-abalone-diving. [Accessed on 9 Dec 2020].

Association of Diving Contractors International. (2016) *International Consensus Standards for Commercial Diving and Underwater Operations* (6th Ed). Houston, TX, Association of Diving Contractors International.

Buzzacott P, Pollock NW, Rosenburg M. (2014) Exercise intensity inferred from air consumption during recreational scuba diving. *SPUMS J* **44**(2): 74–78.

Cha SG, Byun YS, Jeon MJ, Sakong J. (2019) Diving patterns and decompression sickness among South Korean fishery divers. *J Occup Health* **61**(1): 143–153. Available from: doi:10.1002/1348-9585.12035.

Colicchio G, Greco M, Brocchini M, Faltinsen OM. (2015) Hydroelastic behaviour of a structure exposed to an underwater explosion. *Philos Trans Royal Soc A* **373**(2033). Available from: doi:10.1098/rsta.2014.0103.

Department of Justice and Attorney-General. (2018) Inquest into the death of Andrew John Thwaites. *Coroners Court of Queensland Findings of Inquest.* 2016/3336. [Online] Available from: https://www.courts.qld.gov.au/__data/assets/pdf_file/0004/577093/cif-thwaites-aj-20180724.pdf. [Accessed on 9 Dec 2020].

Diving Medical Advisory Committee. (2017) *Fitness to Return to Diving after Decompression Illness.* DMAC Guidance. [Online] Available from: https://www.dmac-diving.org/guidance. [Accessed on 9 Dec 2020].

Edmonds C, Bennett M, Lippmann J, Mitchell S. (2020) *Diving and Subaquatic Medicine.* Boca Raton, Florida, CRC Press.

Health and Safety Executive. (2015). MA1. *The Medical Examination and Assessment of Commercial Divers.* United Kingdom, HSE.

Health and Safety Executive. (2020) *Construction Statistics in Great Britain, 2020.* [Online] Available from: https://www.hse.gov.uk/statistics/industry/. [Accessed on 9 Dec 2020].

Hermans F. (2016) *Survey and Analysis of Fatal Accidents in the Commercial Diving Sector.* [Online] Available from: https://www.academia.edu/27691526/survey_and_analysis_of_fatal_accidents_in_the_commercial_diving_sector. [Accessed on 9 Dec 2020].

How J, Vijayan A, Wong TM. (1990) Acute decompression sickness in compressed air workers exposed to pressures below 1 bar in the Singapore Mass Rapid Transit project. *Singapore Med J* **31**(2): 104–110.

International Marine Contractors Association. (2019) *IMCA International Code of Practice for Offshore Diving.* [Online] Available from: https://www.imca-int.com/product/imca-international-code-of-practice-for-offshore-diving/. [Accessed on 9 Dec 2020].

Kulkarni A. (2017) Compressed air working in Chennai during metro tunnel construction: Occupational health problems. *Indian J Occup Environ Med* **21**(3): 105. Available from: doi:10.4103/ijoem.ijoem_38_17.

McCurry J. (2006) *Ancient Art of Pearl Diving Breathes its Last. The Guardian.* [Online] Available from: https://www.theguardian.com/world/2006/aug/24/japan.justinmccurry. [Accessed on 9 Dec 2020].

McFall GB, Heine JN, Bozanic JE. (2017) *NOAA Diving Manual Diving for Science and Technology.* North Palm Beach, Florida, Best Publishing Company.

Naval Sea Systems Command. (2016) SS521-AG-PRO-010. *US Navy Diving Manual Revision 7.* United States of America, NSSC.

Ong MCC. (2002) Medical Support for the North East Line Mass Rapid Transit Project by the Republic of Singapore Navy's Naval Medicine Hyperbaric Centre. *Singapore Med J* **43**(9): 463–466.

Oswaldo HL, Alvaro HF, Raúl VP, Eduardo G. (2018) The cost of decompression illness: The case of lobster and sea cucumber fishery in Yucatan, Mexico. *Undersea Hyperb Med* **45**(5): 531–539.

Perrine MW, Mundt JC, Weiner RI. (1994) When alcohol and water don't mix: Diving under the influence. *J Stud Alcohol Drugs* **55**(5): 517–524. Available from: doi: 10.15288/jsa.1994.55.517.

Reid RL, Lorenzo M. (2018) SCUBA diving in pregnancy. *J Obstet Gynaecol Canada* **40**(11): 1490–1496. Available from: doi: 10.1016/j.jogc.2017.11.024.

Sayer DJM. (2005) The international safety record for scientific diving. *SPUMS J* **35**(3): 117–119.

Schimmel J, George N, Schwarz J, Yousif S, Suner S, Hack JB. (2017) Carboxyhemoglobin Levels induced by cigarette smoking outdoors in smokers. *J Med Toxicol* **14**(1): 68–73. Available from: doi: 10.1007/s13181-017-0645-1.

Sean S, Pollock NW. (2012) Alcohol and diving. In: Steller, D., Lobel, L. (eds.), *Diving for Science 2012. Proceedings of the American Academy of Underwater Sciences 31st Symposium.* Dauphin Island, Alabama, AAUS.

Smart D, Mitchell S, Wilmshurst P, Turner M. (2015) Joint position statement on persistent foramen ovale (PFO) and diving. South Pacific Underwater Medicine Society (SPUMS) and the United Kingdom Sports Diving Medical Committee (UKSDMC). *SPUMS J* **45**(2): 129–131.

Standards Australia Limited/Standards New Zealand. (2015) AS/NZS 2299.1-2015. *Occupational Diving Operations, Part 1: Standard Operational Practice.* New Zealand, Standards Australia Limited/Standards New Zealand.

Singapore Standards Council. (2018) SS 511. *Code of Practice for Diving at Work.* Singapore, Spring Singapore.

U.S. Department of Labor, Bureau of Labor Statistics. (2019) *Databases, Tables & Calculators by Subject.* U.S. Bureau of Labor Statistics. [Online] Available from: https://www.bls.gov/data/. [Accessed on 9 Dec 2020].

U.S. Department of Labor, Bureau of Labor Statistics. (2019) *Fatal Occupational Injuries by Selected Worker Characteristics and Selected Occupation, all U.S., All Ownerships, 2011–2017, Commercial Divers.* U.S. Bureau of Labor Statistics. [Online] Available from: https://www.bls.gov/iif/oshcfoi1.htm. [Accessed on 9 Dec 2020].

Urick S, Schleiger D, Tartt M, Jara A. (2021) *NOAA Diving Standards and Safety Manual (NDSSM).* 12 February 2020. NOAA Diving Standards and Safety Manual (NDSSM) | Office of Marine and Aviation Operations. [Online] Available from: https://www.omao.noaa.gov/find/media/documents/noaa-diving-standards-and-safety-manual-ndssm. [Accessed on 9 Dec 2020].

Westin AA, Asvall J, Idrovo G, Denoble P, Brubakk AO. (2005) Diving behaviour and decompression sickness among Galapagos underwater harvesters. *J Undersea Hyperb Med Soc* **32**(3): 175–184.

Workplace Health and Safety Queensland. (2005) *Carbon Monoxide Poisoning, Hookah Compressors and Diving.* [Online] Available from: https://www.worksafe.qld.gov.au/news-and-events/alerts/workplace-health-and-safety-alerts/2005/carbon-monoxide-poisoning-hookah-compressors-and-diving. [Accessed on 9 Dec 2020].

Workplace Safety and Health Council. (2009) *Technical Advisory for inland/Inshore Commercial Diving Safety and Health.* [Online] Available from: https://www.wshc.sg/files/wshc/upload/infostop/attachments/2014/IS2010012500122/WSH_Commercial_Diving_TA_26_Oct_09.pdf. [Accessed on 9 Dec 2020].

Workplace Safety and Health Council. (2010) *Prevention of Compressed Air Illness and Barotrauma.* [Online] Available from: https://www.wshc.sg/files/wshc/upload/cms/file/2014/Compressed%20Air%20Work_A5%20Final.pdf. [Accessed on 9 Dec 2020].

Chapter 20

Remote Health Care

*John Nelson Norman**

Introduction

The global coronavirus disease 2019 (COVID-19) pandemic has brought many of the principles of remote healthcare into sharp focus in 2020. Indeed, it is doubtful whether the practice of medicine will ever return to the prior concepts held before the virus struck the world. Yet remote healthcare has been practised since time immemorial in times of war and many important advances were made by military requirements. Resuscitation on the battlefield during the war in Vietnam added much knowledge on the principles of shock management and much new knowledge was added to plastic surgery following the horrendous burns suffered by aircrew in the Second World War. It is equally possible that army catering corps practices developed after Napoleon observed that, "An army marches on its stomach" or the importance of teeth and the establishment of the dental corps when Earl Haig developed severe toothache during the first war.

Remote medicine, however, only began its emergence and recognition as a specialty of medicine in the mid-1970s when the inter-

* Environmental Medicine, University of Aberdeen, Aberdeen, Scotland, United Kingdom *and* Institute of Remote Healthcare, United Kingdom.
Corresponding author: John Nelson Norman (jnorman.nelson@gmail.com).

national oil industry arrived in the middle of the North Sea and began drilling for oil. This required new and advanced engineering techniques and the construction of huge offshore structures which needed to be fixed to the sea bed some 400 to 600 feet below the surface. That in turn required divers using the new technique of saturation diving which was barely out of the experimental laboratories of the Royal and United States (US) Navies. The morbidity and mortality figures were not acceptable and both the industry and its doctors were inexperienced in working in such an inclement environment.

The University of Aberdeen established an Institute of Environmental and Offshore Medicine as a joint venture with industry and both groups set about devising a system of healthcare for the offshore personnel. This system, which consisted of five elements or priorities, worked well and has survived the passage of time. It is now known as Remote Medicine and has emerged as a specialty in its own right. The first textbook on Remote Medicine for trainee specialists was published in 2020 (Normal and Valentine, 2020).

The five priorities in the system of remote healthcare (Norman and Brebner, 1985) are as follows:

1. Training of the whole population at risk in immediate care to cover the vital interval of time before the casualty can be delivered to definitive care.
2. The development of increasingly sophisticated systems of communication.
3. The establishment of a medical co-ordinating centre.
4. The availability of appropriate means of evacuation.
5. Audit and research.

The research base of the system followed rather than preceded its establishment but it was validated by duplication for the very different population of scientists working for the British Antarctic Survey in the most remote and hostile conditions on the planet.

The following case studies from the medical archives of the British Antarctic Survey Medical Unit illustrate some of the special problems of remote healthcare and their solutions.

Case Study 1: Cardiac Arrest at Sea

An expedition ship was being anchored to the sea ice a few hundred miles from the South Pole by digging a hole in the sea ice and placing a massive sea anchor within it when a senior crewman (the 'bosun' or 'boatswain') suffered a cardiac arrest. He was given cardio-pulmonary resuscitation (CPR) since all the personnel sailing under the Survey's flag at that time had been trained in CPR before departure. He was returned to the ship in sinus rhythm. In the sick bay, he was attached to an electrocardiogram (ECG) monitor and cared for by the resident practitioner who was a recently qualified doctor. Contact was made with the United Kingdom (UK) headquarters and arrangements were made to land an aircraft on the ice to transport the patient to New Zealand. The distant supervising consultant, however advised the alternative procedure not to evacuate the casualty, but to keep him warm in the sickbay under the care of the resident practitioner, and decreed that an ECG should be telemetered to Aberdeen where a consultant cardiologist could advise on the further clinical management of the case from a distance, until the patient was deemed fit enough to be transferred to the Falkland Islands and after assessment, back to Aberdeen where after angioplasty he was considered fit to return to work.

Case Study 2: Evacuation During Extended Trip to Remote Area

This case concerns a senior officer on board another ship while it was moored in South Georgia preparing to go for an extended trip to the Antarctic. He sought advice from the resident doctor about a small lump on his arm. The lump looked insignificant but the doctor was suspicious since there seemed to be some nerve involvement, and he advised his patient to be evacuated for investigation before the ship sailed. The patient rejected the advice and invoked the support of the Captain who supported him. The doctor then contacted his consultant in Aberdeen and after discussion, it was advised that the casualty should be evacuated. This took place and after biopsy, the patient needed treatment for a rare but aggressive sarcoma. All this occurred within 10 days after his first consultation on the expedition ship in South Georgia.

These two cases illustrate the importance of using the range of facilities and manpower available in extreme remote situations. They highlight the value of having of a senior consultant back at a co-ordinating centre and the possibility of providing care at least as good in a remote situation as in any on-shore location with modern clinical support and staff. This requires careful planning, preparation and provision that caters for each situation at risk (Norman and Laws, 1988).

Priority Areas for Remote Healthcare

Components of Training for Remote Healthcare

The term "First Aid" conjures up a variety of images in the mind of various training organisations. It can be limited to a mother applying a plaster to the cut finger of a child to the immediate care provided by a doctor for a life-threatening injury at a remote site. The term is used by the UK Health and Safety Executive (HSE) in describing the statutory training schedules of "rig medics" (Health and Safety Executive, 2016). The basic course for Offshore personnel provided by the Institute of Environmental and Offshore Medicine in Aberdeen provided a theoretical understanding of the reasons for the various actions advised rather than a purely didactic protocol. For example, though normal first-aid teaching states that nothing should be given to drink in trauma or burns cases, it is necessary to explain that the reason is that it may delay the administration of an anaesthetic when the casualty arrives in hospital. Even if an anaesthetic is needed and the journey to hospital may take several hours, the casualty could be in a poor dehydrated state when he arrives, especially in hot weather, unless he is given oral fluids.

Other important aspects of training are as follows:

- The importance of communication (see section on "Communication" below) in terms relevant to a doctor so that useful advice can be given to cover the vital time interval. The first aider should be able to communicate the urgency of the situation and whether the

casualty is deteriorating or improving so that the medical authorities can organise appropriate speed and priority of evacuation.
- An understanding of "shock" and proper measuring and recording of vital signs over time (Norman *et al.*, 2004; Cox, 1987).
- Frequent short refresher courses are the best way to maintain clinical skills, but interest can also be sustained by initiating frequent different exercises with appropriate scenarios.

Training for remote locations for the oil and gas industry

The oil and gas industry is a good example where workers can be located in remote worksites, e.g. on offshore rigs, or in isolated desert locations. The North Sea oil and gas industry initially preferred to hire military medics to provide first aid care for remote locations because they were used to working on their own initiative and most problems were related to trauma. Subsequently state registered nurses took on some of these roles, although this created a divide between the perceived and required skills and responsibilities of the practitioners from different backgrounds. In common, many identified similar problems with professional isolation, lack of professional identity, poorly co-ordinated and very variable educational facilities, and lack of regulation and registration. (Horsley, 2005).

In 1988, a study of remote healthcare in the North Sea oil and gas industry examined the indications for evacuation and those related to trauma were considered separately from illness. Since evacuation by the unscheduled, emergency system was much more expensive than using a routine helicopter flight, routine versus emergency evacuation were considered separately. By 1980, there were about equal numbers of cases of trauma and illness warranting emergency evacuation. The trend since then has been towards more cases of illnesses than trauma. This may be due to better training on safety to reduce accidents or the ageing of the workforce increasing the occurrence of cardiovascular and cerebrovascular incidents. Dental problems are now becoming a common reason for evacuation, although cardiovascular conditions still predominate (Norman *et al.*, 1988; Cheesman, 2008; Thibodeax *et al.*, 2014; Berg *et al.*, 2015).

Institute of Remote Healthcare

An Institute of Remote Healthcare was established in 2007 as an independent academic unit designed to improve healthcare for those who live and work in remote places, through education and research. A conference of oil companies, providers of remote medical services and universities met in Bergen in 2013 to provide a consensus opinion and guidance on the educational requirements for training remote healthcare practitioners for the oil and gas industry (Klein and Mohammed, 2016). Following a Delphi study, which measured the extent of consensus for components of a syllabus for training, a definitive document was released as the educational requirements to produce competent, international remote healthcare practitioners. The Institute also formed an association with the Royal College of Surgeons of Edinburgh and had established a Faculty of Remote Healthcare within the college. An examination process was proposed for attaining membership. This would give the practitioners a professional home, end professional isolation, and promote recognition of their status (Klein and Mohammed, 2016).

Communications

Communications is stated as second priority in remote healthcare but is probably the most important since distant care could not be provided without some form of communication. The revolution in medical communication technology is truly mind boggling since their initial use in caring for the first explorers on their way to the moon. For example, Max House was previously the only neurologist in the provinces of Newfoundland and Labrador. He used aspects of the new technology to transmit electroencephalograms (EEGs) from the whole area for him to report from his base in Memorial University, St John's. The huge technological leap in communication technology has allowed enormous progress to be made towards the ultimate aim of remote healthcare — namely to provide equally effective healthcare for those who work in remote and hazardous areas as those who are close to sophisticated medical facilities.

Problems which had to be considered and solved were the need for good audio-visual links, maintenance of medical confidentiality (particularly since there is now a requirement to transmit patient data across international boundaries), comprehensive record keeping and practitioner confidence in the use of the technology. The distortion in speech caused by helium in saturation divers affected communication, but this is now overcome by the use of electronic facilities. In particular, the use of e-mail and videoconferencing has been a major advance in communication and advantages include allowing time for interpretation of difficult messages in foreign languages.

For diagnosis, good results can be obtained by the use of standard techniques and video facilities add to the accuracy of the operation. For example, in the diagnosis of the acute abdomen, it is vital that the camera should be placed so that the distant doctor can see both the face and the abdomen together with the actions of the remote practitioner. The history will normally have been transmitted and discussed by phone or e-mail prior to the event but the occasional additional point of clarification may help to provide relaxation and confidence in the patient. During the examination, it is now possible for the distant doctor or specialist to pick up familiar body language signs and to guide the remote practitioner's hands, say, over the abdomen as almost an extension of his own. By the end of the procedure he should have as much confidence in the result of the history and examination as if he had performed it himself and in his own consulting room. Much of this is of course dependent on the prior training of the remote practitioner and the rapport developed between him and the remote specialist. It can be a great advantage for the remote specialist to have been directly involved in clinical training of developing remote practitioners in much the same way as consultants are involved in training their registrars.

Telemedicine

Telemedicine has developed at a rapid pace in the last few years and at present, workers in remote areas can benefit from telemedicine applications for many health conditions. Among these include chronic disease management, e.g. diabetes (Begenstal *et al.*, 2020), mental health disorders (Howland *et al.*, 2020), remote assessment of vertigo (Green *et al.*, 2020), ophthalmic conditions (Gensheimer *et al.*, 2020), remote management of sleep (Chapoutout et al., 2020), or gastrointestinal disorders (Lim *et al.*, 2020). The COVID-19 pandemic has accelerated the use of telemedicine applications. For example, virtual occupational skin health clinics have been offered for healthcare workers (Chowdhury *et al.*, 2020).

In a simulator-based prospective study using a simulated offshore wind power plant (Landgraf *et al.*, 2019), performance of teams of offshore engineers ($n = 38$) and teams of paramedics ($n = 34$) who conducted the primary survey of a simulated patient were studied. Teams were supported by transmission technology and a remote emergency physician in Berlin. They found that first response to medical emergencies in offshore wind farms with substantially delayed professional care were improved by tele-medical support.

Another innovation is the use of a jet suit for paramedics to "fly" to remote areas inaccessible to conventional transport. Such a service has been tested by the Great North Air Ambulance Service in the UK (Barbour, 2020). The flying paramedic could carry a medical kit with strong pain relief and even a defibrillator.

With the advent of new communication technologies such as 5G networks, improvements in health care in areas such as telerobotic surgery are already appearing and are expected to develop further (Tian *et al.*, 2020).

Case Study 3: Diagnostic Aids at a Distance

Accurate diagnosis will help determine the management of the condition with some confidence no matter where the patient is located. Recent advances in diagnostic equipment have made it possible to provide almost the whole range of diagnostic aids at a distance. An early example was dealing with chest pain in saturation divers, when pneumothorax was a differential diagnosis and a real problem. A technique was developed to take X-rays through the port of a pressure chamber and by plumbing an electric stethoscope across the hull of the chamber so that the chest could be auscultated from without.

Case Study 4: Tele-Diagnosis in Histology

It is the difficult to view histological slides on a remotely located microscope. While it was always reasonably easy to transmit histological slides from one site to another, it was more difficult for the remote consultant to move the slide on the stage of a remote microscope which is essential for histological diagnosis. Such diagnostic consultations can now take place routinely as modern equipment with facilities for transmission of histological information is now available. Colonoscopy with biopsy and histology with visualisation from a distant site can now be performed. While almost any remote visualisation is now possible it must be accompanied by training of the equipment operators at both ends, as advanced communication technology is not usually part of the routine training of doctors and nurses.

Medical Co-ordinating Centres

This third priority is as important as the first and second since there is little point in developing sophisticated communications if there is no-one to communicate with. Individuals and teams at coordinating centres should avoid the use of technical terms and medical jargon when advising the remote healthcare practitioner. Consultants and advisers at these coordinating centres should appreciate the level of training, knowledge, and expertise of the healthcare provider/s at the remote site so that complex manoeuvres and procedures beyond the experience and capability of the remote healthcare providers are not advised. The coordinating centres must also be aware of where to contact appropriate specialists for special situations and areas requiring unique expertise, e.g. in industrial poisoning cases, or if an unusual undersea problem occurs. An important consideration is for the clinical staff at the co-ordinating centres also to be fully trained remote healthcare practitioners themselves and have preferably served for a time in a remote location.

Evacuation

Evacuation is a necessary universal option for the sick and injured in all situations and has led to the development of ambulances and ambulance services to a high degree of efficiency and the development of professional ambulance personnel. Remote places, however, pose certain special problems. Some of these problems have been solved by the use of lifeboats, helicopters and fixed wing ambulances and there has been the unique hyperbaric, titanium capsule designed to transfer a saturation diver from an offshore pressure chamber to a large operating pressure chamber in an on-shore medical support facility, without altering the atmospheric pressure. This has not been deemed practical and was probably not the best solution for the management of illness in deep diving casualties. Nevertheless, in dealing with much lower pressure levels, a modification of the concept is coming into use for sport divers and harbour divers.

In the development of remote healthcare, the clinical management of the casualty being transported over a long distance and time is an important aspect. The same five priority headings apply. Training of ambulance personnel on this aspect of care is already well developed but special circumstances may apply in transport from remote places over considerable time such as casualties with epilepsy in helicopters from offshore structures, or workers experiencing acute psychiatric episodes. The development of the intensive care ambulance service in Glasgow for moving a critically ill patient undergoing intensive care from one hospital to another with additional equipment is worthy of consideration when considering extending the need from intercity situations to greater distances (Wright *et al.*, 1988). A similar development is taking place in India where intensive care is being practiced in ambulances.

Communications from the ambulance to a supporting hospital are key considerations. Miniaturisation of measuring equipment now allows many physiological measurements, including 12 lead ECGs, to be transmitted and thus allowing scope for early intervention, e.g. for initiating thrombolysis for acute myocardial infarction. Video cameras allowing visualisation by hospital and medical centre staff of the casualty being transported, e.g. by aircraft is another development in facilitating care during evacuation. This is a major concern for the air industry since diversion of an aircraft to an unscheduled destination when a passenger becomes ill results in very considerable financial consequences.

Researchers have recently compiled travel times from remote areas to health facilities with and without access to motorised transport in unprecedented detail, by combining data from available databases such as OpenStreetMap and Google Maps (Weiss *et al.*, 2020). They estimate that 8.9% of the global population (646 million people) are unable to reach healthcare within an hour if they have access to motorised transport, while 43.3% (3.16 billion people) cannot reach a healthcare facility by foot within 1 hour.

The need for rapid intervention in acute illness has been underlined by the realisation of the urgency of diagnosis of stroke and the requirement to distinguish between cerebral thrombosis and haemorrhage since in cerebral thrombosis, thrombolysis within an hour or so can result in cure. Combined transcranial ultrasound and clinical assessment ("TUCA" model) could accurately triage these patients and improve access to thrombectomy (Antipova *et al.*, 2020). It is equally important that ambulance personnel should be trained not only to use the technology but also to be able to apply the treatment recommended by the hospital. This requires much further consideration since there are local laws to be considered and different systems apply worldwide.

The huge development of mobile phone technology is relevant to the development of transportation of the sick and in education in remote areas of Africa where there is currently no availability of sophisticated communication equipment. This is an area where the advance of such communication technology opens up major opportunities for healthcare in small, very remote communities in a variety of impoverished locations worldwide.

Research and Audit

The new category of healthcare specialists (the remote healthcare professional) is closely related to occupational medicine but nevertheless sufficiently different in emphasis and direction to warrant its existence as a separate independent entity. Research and audit are essential priority areas for continuing development of the specialty in its own right. There are certain general areas which need to be maintained in a new developing specialty and these are continuing audit of innovations. Research through or together with academic institutions can provide the evidence base for sound practice. Audit will determine the extent of compliance with suggested standards.

There have been several academic manifestations since the Institute of Environmental and Offshore Medicine was established in the mid-1970s which have added to the development of the specialty and the emergence of the remote healthcare practitioner as a specialist in his own right. The Institute of Remote Healthcare (IRHC), established in 2007, attempted to define the educational and skill requirements to produce fully competent remote healthcare practitioner at the Bergen conference. The provisions were largely confined to the oil and gas industry and Europe, however, and these were extended to the international scene by the International Remote Medicine Association (IRHCA), established in 2017 in Tomsk, Siberia to take account of the divergent world scene including extreme remote locations and both extreme heat and extreme cold climates. A Faculty of Remote and Rural Health has also been established by the Royal College of Surgeons of Edinburgh and this will allow members to obtain international recognition as with existing specialists and also provide a professional home for the new practitioners. These latter two developments have been delayed by the COVID-19 crisis.

The Hostile Environment of Remote Locations

An important consideration for the provision of remote health care is a good understanding of the often hostile environment in which some workers are placed. Some illnesses related to these environments include those resulting from working in underwater environments, exposure to extremes of temperature, and working in conflict-torn regions.

The following are examples of clinical conditions that may need to be managed by a remote healthcare practitioner.

Heat Illnesses

There are two basic types of heat illness based on the ambient relative humidity.

1. Heat accompanied by high humidity — as in offshore or coastal areas. In such environments, heat illness leading to collapse is relatively common but fairly easy to manage since there have been no major compensatory fluid shifts before the collapse. Removal of the casualty into a cool place with free access to fluids will soon establish recovery and there are no circulatory or electrolyte changes of note.
2. Heat in low humidity areas — as in an inland hot, dry environment. This is an entirely different situation which can result in heat stroke which is a very serious, life-threatening medical emergency which requires urgent attention.

The spectrum of effects (Norman *et al.*, 2004; Clarke and Edholm, 1985) resulting from these two basic types of heat illness include the following in the next few sections.

Heat cramps

Heat cramps occur in people who sweat profusely, and do not have adequate salt replacement. The onset occurs when the salt level falls below a critical value and is manifest by severe cramps affecting various muscle groups including the abdominal muscles. The condition was initially recognised in mines at the beginning of the 20th Century and was prevented when the miners added salt to their diet. In more recent times, salt tablets have been provided at tropical work-sites.

The condition re-appeared and was recognised in the field areas of the Abu Dhabi oil companies in the 1980s when salt tablets were removed from the mess tables in the field areas during summer. This was due to the concern about the relationship between salt and hypertension and it was prevented when 300g salt tablets were re-instated for daily consumption by the work-force during the summer months. Individuals working in high degrees of environmental heat require extra salt if heat cramps are to be avoided. In the study conducted by Al-Ahwal and Norman, heat cramps were eliminated in all workers except two. When the reason was sought, it was found that they were nurses reading the current literature, who did not take the salt tablets for fear of hypertension and they succumbed to heat cramps. This is an example of research which has been carried out in a temperate zone and applied to a tropical area without taking account of the different environmental factors which may apply (Al-Ahwal *et al.*, 2000; Al-Ahwal, 1996; Brebner, 1990).

Heat exhaustion

Heat exhaustion results from a fluid and electrolyte disturbance. It occurs in people who have been working strenuously in the heat for some time and the massive fluid shifts required in association with this has resulted in an imbalance of the concentrations of salts and water. During maximal sweating, it is possible to lose (and to require to replace) about 30 L of fluid over 24 hours. Heat exhaustion is sometimes difficult to recognise; the symptoms are vague and include weakness, giddiness and general malaise. The temperature and pulse rate are usually normal and sweating still occurs freely. The condition is managed by resting in a cool place for a day or so and administering fluids.

Heat stroke

Heat stroke is not particularly common in well organised industrial environments where the medical and safety departments supervise the work shifts and the fluid and salt replacement regimes. It does, however, occur in accident situations when an injured man in an isolated location is unable to obtain hydration.

In desert environments with very high environmental temperatures especially in summer, and at worksites without sun shelter, collapsed individuals can be subject to an additional source of heat from the terrain. A rapid rise in core body temperature leads to mental confusion and disorientation (at about 41°C), and unconsciousness and death occurs from irreversible brain damage at core temperatures of about 44°C or 45°C. In general, individuals with pre-existing cardiac conditions have poorer prospects for recovery when suffering from heat stroke. Cardiac health is thus an important factor in selecting and advising personnel for work in extremely hot environments. The main principles in the management of casualties with heat stroke are removal from further sources of heat, provision of adequate shade and cooling, and prompt hydration. Transport involving rough passage over uneven ground is not the best management for a patient with heat stroke and pre-existing cardiac conditions; nor is the use of ice baths which at one time were advised and often resulted in cardiac arrest (Norman *et al.*, 2004; Al-Ahwal *et al.*, 2000; Clarke and Edholm, 1985; Al-Ahwal, 1996; Brebner, 1990).

Exposure to Environmental Cold

Attention on the problems of cold in the past have largely been related to urban hypothermia in the elderly living in poorly heated houses or the use of induced hypothermia as an aid to cardiac and neurosurgery. The establishment of the offshore oil industry in the cold waters and low temperatures of the North Sea brought the problems of environmental cold into focus since a large workforce was exposed to such extreme conditions. New facts emerged which were also of value to a wide spectrum of occupational and recreational groups such as soldiers, polar explorers, hill walkers and sport divers.

Hypothermia can be induced as an aid in some types of cardiac or neurosurgery, or it can be accidental as occurs in occupational groups working in cold surroundings. Safety at work in cold climates thus demands a higher margin of cardiac health than in temperate zones and this has implications on medical selection for those who work in cold climates and on the ongoing medical surveillance with an ageing workforce, or following rehabilitation after a cardiac event. Cardiac fitness is thus an important factor in considering workers for postings to both extremely hot as well as cold environments (Norman, 1986).

The subjective appreciation of thermal comfort can cause special problems particularly in deep saturation diving where due to the greatly enhanced thermal conductivity of oxygen-helium mixtures (helium conducts heat many times faster than air), small increases or decreases in temperature can cause hypo- or hyperthermia. The temperature within diving chambers is therefore controlled with precision. Saturation divers are also not always able to determine whether the environmental temperature is too warm or too cold. Antarctic divers were studied by Light who used a subjective scoring method of thermal comfort when the divers performed diving in icy surroundings. He found such a spread of scores that he concluded that individuals are unable to determine accurately their thermal status with any degree of accuracy on the basis of a perception of thermal comfort (Light *et al.*, 1980).

Immersion hypothermia

Hypothermia occurs when the body temperature falls below 35°C. It is not a common occurrence in well-regulated industrial situations and is usually the result of an accident, as when an individual falls into very cold water. Symptoms develop quickly following immersion since water is a good conductor of heat. The casualty should be advised to move as little as possible so as to avoid displacing pockets of water around him which are partially heated by the body. Immersion hypothermia is common in marine and offshore worksites and should be treated as an emergency.

The phenomenon of post-rescue death is well recognised and was extensively studied by the Royal Navy in survivors of 448 merchant ships sunk during 1940–1944. The casualty is recovered from the water and seems in reasonable health but dies suddenly at a variable period thereafter — even up to 24 hours later. Immersion in cold water puts a great strain on the heart due to the sudden increase in oxygen requirements to supply the shivering muscles. There is added strain when the casualty attempts to get out of the water. The best treatment is immediate re-immersion in a bath of warm water (40–42°C), handling the casualty as gently as possible with no urgency to remove clothing as the effort is likely to compound the problem. Following the restoration of body temperature to normal levels, the patient should rest quietly in bed for 48 hours, to allow for cardiac recovery and the restoration of the fluid and electrolyte shifts which may have taken place (Burton and Edholm, 1955; Keatinge, 1969; Adam, 1981).

Exposure to dry cold

Fatal hypothermia due to dry cold conditions is very rare in industrial settings but minor degrees occur in cold weather or where a casualty is lying exposed to the elements before being moved to warmer surroundings. In exposure to dry cold, the temperature fall is gradual and if not halted, will cause extreme fatigue and exhaustion. As this can adversely affect the victim's judgement, it is important to be able to recognise the symptoms and to manage the condition urgently since what may seem to be a minor problem can deteriorate into a serious life-threatening situation.

The warning signs include the following:

- A change of personality, where the normally aggressive person can become withdrawn and apathetic, while the introvert loses his temper and becomes aggressive;
- Increasing slowness in physical and mental responses;
- Slurring of speech;
- Stumbling and shivering;
- Blurred vision.

The following pieces of advice on care of the affected individual include:

- Handle gently and do not move unnecessarily until ready to evacuate;
- Protect from wind and rain and insulate from direct contact with wet terrain;

- Wrap in dry clothing, blankets or sleeping bag;
- Provide warm drinks.

Recovery usually takes place uneventfully in a few hours when in bed in a warm room but judgement may be impaired for 24–48 hours so the individual should not return to the work-site for that time.

Local cold injury

Local cold injury occurs in two main situations:

1. Freezing cold injury — when parts of the body are exposed to extreme cold.
2. Non-freezing cold injury — when parts of the body are exposed to temperatures close to freezing and are damp or wet for prolonged periods.

Freezing cold injury

Frostnip: This develops suddenly (often within seconds) in exposed tissues over the cheek or earlobe. It appears as a waxy, white patch of skin and is painless. It is easily treated by re-warming with a gloved hand and no permanent injury occurs if the skin is rapidly rewarmed. However, if not recognised and rapidly treated, it will proceed to frostbite. There is much value during prolonged cold exposure in using the "buddy system" in observing the exposed skin of colleagues since frostnip is painless.

Frostbite: In this injury, both the skin and underlying tissues are frozen. The area is white and numb and may also be discoloured. In less serious cases, the affected tissue may remain soft but in serious cases it will be hard. Those who have had previous cold injury appear more susceptible during further work in cold climates.

Re-warming of frozen tissue is best undertaken by immersing the affected part in warm water (38–40°C). Initially, this can cause discomfort and pain. Analgesia is indicated and the temperature of the water can gradually be increased. The speed and timing of re-warming of frozen tissue is subject to some debate and controversy, so if in doubt it will be best to await rescue instead of attempting rewarming (Milne *et al.*, 1988).

Recommendations on stopping work because of adverse weather conditions include situations of excessive heat and cold. However, much depends on not just ambient temperature, but also on wind speed and relative humidity. Potential effects on individuals also depend on a vast array of human factors such as body composition, ability to shiver and sweat, and cardiac fitness. It is therefore difficult to produce a general index to cover all these areas, and is therefore probably best to rely on the local knowledge of an experienced and well-trained healthcare practitioner who is familiar with the levels of work and the environment (Tipton, 2013).

It may thus seem surprising that man has been able to reach the summit of the highest mountain or plumb the depths of the sea but this is only achieved by taking his required environment with him by the use of clothing, heating and shelter. In a study of the responses of man to life and work in the Antarctic it was found that when the mean annual temperature of the station was minus 19.6°C, the sub-clothing temperature did not vary with the seasons or the work shift provided an acceptable degree of thermal comfort was maintained. In cold weather, the subjects did not leave the living quarters for longer than necessary and when time spent out of doors was graphed against the ambient temperature of the station, there was a direct, straight line relationship (Norman, 1961; Clarke and Edholm, 1985; Burton and Edholm, 1955).

Non-freezing cold injury

An example of a non-freezing cold injury includes trench foot. This occurs when feet are cold and wet for prolonged periods. Small arteries become constricted, limiting the availability of blood supply to the tissues. If allowed to persist, nerves and other tissues may be permanently damaged. The affected toes and feet become waxy and mottled and this leads to swollen, red and discoloured feet with easily damaged skin. In addition to warming, dryness is important in the management of this form of cold injury.

Underwater Environments

Diving medicine was a dominant medical problem in the North Sea industry since the water depth required saturation diving techniques which had not been practiced previous to the 1970s. There were very few doctors outside the British and American navies who had experience in hyperbaric medicine and this resulted in serious problems since the industry had little experience of functioning in such hazardous environmental conditions. Indeed, it was concentration on the problem of access to the sick saturation diver which resulted in the development of the system of remote healthcare in use today.

An attempt was made to determine whether a sick diver could be evacuated to a shore based facility without reducing the pressure, and a titanium chamber was developed which could be transported by helicopter from an offshore chamber to an operating hyperbaric system in Aberdeen.

The alternative proposal was to establish a group of medical specialists to proceed offshore and be prepared to enter an offshore chamber to carry out the necessary treatment. There were problems with both proposals including a) the possibility of deterioration of the evacuee in the mobile chamber during transport when it would not be possible to provide the emergency care necessary, and b) the undoubted hazards of administering care — particularly operative surgery — in a cramped offshore chamber. These arguments were shadowed by strong economic pressures from the industry, since the presence of a sick man in an offshore chamber which prevented its use for other purposes was very expensive. There were strong pressures to clear the chamber as soon as possible. The companies therefore preferred the transfer — under-pressure option — though not always in the best interests of the casualty. In fact, the transfer capsule in Scotland was only employed once and that was for a case of mediastinal emphysema and from a pipe-laying barge in Peterhead to the operating chamber in Aberdeen.

The importance and dominance of diving medicine in the 1970s and 80s resulted in the establishment of introductory and advanced diving medical courses together with appropriate research so that by the turn of the century, diving medicine had become almost routine and this did much for sport diving also which became more safe since the medical profession is now in a position to manage its hazards effectively (Norman and Brebner, 1985; Cox, 1987; Bennet and Elliott, 1975; Hayward and Keatinge, 1979).

The emergence of remotely operated vehicles and the progressive decline in the need for saturation divers have now resulted in diving medicine being consigned to the back-burner in remote practitioner training and consigned to the area of specialist training in such other areas as aviation medicine. That further emphasises the dynamic nature of remote healthcare and the need to review training requirements constantly with the passage of time. As the offshore industry matures and the need to remove offshore structures gains momentum, there may be a resurgence in diving activity to detach the platform jackets from the sea bed. If that only involves separation of the legs low enough to avoid marine fouling, however, it seems possible that saturation techniques may not be used unless the operational depth exceeds 150 feet (Bennet and Elliott, 1975). Remotely operated vehicles are likely to be the technology of choice. Even in depths less than 150 feet where air range diving is possible, saturation technology is generally considered to be more safe nowadays.

Conclusion

In regard to provisions for delivery of remote healthcare, the location and conditions at the remote site are key considerations. If the worksite is onshore and close to a standard medical centre, all that may be needed is a telephone and availability of a general practitioner with special training. If the worksite means that the casualty cannot be evacuated for 48 hours or more or even cannot be evacuated at all as in the Antarctic winter, high quality medical care can still be provided but it requires up-grading of all five elements of the system. There is a special need for increased training of the resident practitioners, much more sophisticated communications, and fully trained and selected consultants at the co-ordinating centre.

Training of remote healthcare practitioners requires an understanding of the basic nature of clinical emergencies, with a need for modifying clinical care depending on the circumstances at the remote location. Thus, provision of special training and experience would advance the development of a specialist remote healthcare professional. This could range from special courses for laymen through training of various grades of remote healthcare practitioners, to specialists and consultants.

References

Adam JM. (1981) *Hypothermia — Ashore and afloat.* Aberdeen, Aberdeen University Press.

Al-Ahwal SH. (1996) *The Pattern of Occupational Illness in Desert Oil Industry Worksite.* MSc thesis, University of Aberdeen.

Al-Ahwal SH, Norman JN, Brebner JA. (2000) Heat cramps in a hot desert work-site. *Kuwait Med J* **32**: 382–386.

Antipova D, Eadie L, Makin S, Shannon H, Wilson P, Macaden A. (2020) The use of transcranial ultrasound and clinical assessment to diagnose ischaemic stroke due to large vessel occlusion in remote and rural areas. *PLOS One* **5**(10). Available from: doi: 10.1371/journal.pone.0239653.

Barbour S. (2020) Jet suit paramedic tested in the Lake District 'could save lives'. [Online] Available from: https://www.bbc.com/news/uk-england-54331994. [Accessed on 4 April 2021].

Bennet PB, Elliott DH. (1975) *The Physiology and Medicine of Diving and Compressed Air Work.* London, Bailliere Tindall.

Berg J, Toner S, Stiltz R, Klein S, Williams H, Pearson J, Fraser A, Norman N. (2015) Remote health care: A game changer for the Arctic. *OTC Arctic Technology Conference.*

Bergenstal RM, Layne JE, Zisser H, Gabbay RA, Barleen NA, Armento LA, Majithia AR, Parkin CG, Dixon RF. (2020) Remote application and use of real-time continuous glucose monitoring by adults with type 2 diabetes in a virtual diabetes clinic. *Diabetes Technol Ther* **23**(2): 128–132. Available from: doi:10.1089/dia.2020.0396.

Brebner JA. (1990) *The Provision of Healthcare in Remote Hostile Environments.* [Online] Available from: https://rgu-repository.worktribe.com/output/248885/the-provision-of-health-care-in-remote-hostile-environments. [Accessed on 4 April 2021].

Burton AC, Edholm OG. (1955) *Man in a Cold Environment.* London, Edward Arnold Ltd.

Chapoutot M, Peter-Derex L, Schoendorff B, Faivre T, Bastuji H, Putois B. (2020) Telehealth-delivered CBT-I programme enhanced by acceptance and commitment therapy for insomnia and hypnotic dependence: A pilot randomized controlled trial. *J Sleep Res* **30**(4). Available from: doi: 10.1111/jsr.13199.

Cheesman M. (2008) *Medical Evacuation and the UK Offshore Oil Industry.* MFOM dissertation, Faculty of Occupational Medicine, Royal College of Physicians, London.

Chowdhury MM, Bevan N, Ryan K. (2020) Covid-19: Virtual occupational skin health clinics for healthcare workers. *BMJ.* Available from: doi: 10.1136/bmj.m2281.

Clarke RP, Edholm OG. (1985) *Man and His Thermal Environment.* London, Edward Arnold Ltd.

Cox RAF. (1987) *Offshore Medicine.* London, Springer-Verlag.

Gensheimer WG, Miller KE, Stowe J, Little J, Legault GL. (2020) Military Teleophthalmology in Afghanistan using mobile phone application. *JAMA Ophthalmol* **138**(10): 1053–1060. Available from: doi: 10.1001/jamaophthalmol.2020.3090.

Green KE, Pogson JM, Otero-Millan J, Gold DR, Tevzadze N, Saber TAS, Zee DS, Newman-Toker DE, Kheradmand A. (2020) Opinion and Special Articles: Remote evaluation of acute vertigo: Strategies and technological considerations. *Neurology* **96**(1). Available from: doi: 10.1212/WNL.0000000000010980.

Hayward M.G, Keatinge WR. (1979) Progressive symptomless hypothermia in water: Possible cause of diving accidents. *BMJ* **1**(6172). Available from: doi: 10.1136/bmj.1.6172.1182.

Health and Safety Executive. (2016) *Health Care and First Aid on Offshore Installations and Pipeline Works. Offshore Installations and Pipeline Works (first-aid) Regulations 1989. Approved Code of Practice and Guidance* (3rd Ed). [Online] United Kingdom, Crown. Available from: https://www.hse.gov.uk/pubns/priced/l123.pdf. [Accessed on 4 April 2021].

Horsley HD. (2005) *An Exploration of the Role, Practice and Educational Needs of Offshore Medics in the United Kingdom Continental Shelf.* MSc dissertation, University of Aberdeen.

Howland M, Tennant M, Bowen DJ, Bauer AM, Fortney JC, Pyne JM, Shore J, Cerimele JM. (2020) Psychiatrist and psychologist experiences with telehealth and remote collaborative care in primary care: A qualitative study. *J Rural Health.* Available from: doi: 10.1111/jrh.12523.

Keatinge WR. (1969) *Survival in Cold Water*. Oxford, Blackwell Scientific Publications.

Klein S, Mohammed H. (2016) Reaching a consensus on the competency and training for healthcare practitioners working in remote oil and gas operations: A collaborative approach. *J Inst Remote Healthc* 7: 8–11.

Landgraf P, Spies C, Lawatscheck R, Luz M, Wernecke KD, Schröder T. (2020) Does Telemedical Support of First Responders Improve Guideline Adherence in an Offshore Emergency Scenario? A Simulator-Based Prospective Study. *BMJ Open* **9**(8). Available from: doi: 10.1136/bmjopen-2018-027563.

Lim MH, McMahon A, Radford-Smith GL. (2020) Telehealth in inflammatory bowel disease. *Intern Med J*. Available from: doi: 10.1111/imj.15068.

Light IM, White MA, Allan D, Norman JN. (1980) Thermal balance in divers. *Lancet* **1**: 1362.

Milne AH, Norman JN, Brebner JA, Johnson IWB. (1988) *British Antarctic Survey Medical Manual*. Swindon, North American Electric Reliability Corporation.

Norman JN. (1961) *Man in the Antarctic* [Online]. Available from: http://theses.gla.ac.uk/79370/. [Accessed on 4 April 2021].

Norman JN, Brebner JA. (1985) *The Offshore Health Handbook*. London, Martin Dunitz Ltd.

Norman JN. (1986) Work in cold climates. *Int J Environ Stud* **26**: 329–340.

Norman JN, Laws RM. (1988) Remote health care for Antarctica: The BAS medical unit. *Polar Record*. **24**: 317–320.

Norman JN, Ballantine BN, Brebner JA, Brown B, Gauld SJ, Mawdsley J, Roythorne C, Valentine MJ, Wilcock SE. (1988) Medical evacuations from offshore structures. *Br J Ind Med* **45**: 619–623

Norman JN, Al-Mesaabi SH, El-Sadig Haj Ahmed M. (2004) *Emergency First-aid for Industrial and Remote Settings*. Trafford Publishing, Victoria, Canada.

Norman JN, Valentine M. (2020) *Remote Medicine. A Textbook for Trainee and Established Remote Healthcare Practitioners*. London, World Scientific Publishing.

Tian W, Fan M, Zeng C, Liu Y, He D, Zhang Q. (2020) Telerobotic spinal surgery based on 5G network: The first 12 cases. *Neurospine* **17**(1): 114–120. Available from: https://doi.org/10.14245/ns.1938454.227.

Tipton M. (2013) *The Influence of Climatic Factors on Work Performance in the Oil and Gas Industry*. London, Energy Institute publication.

Thibodeax DP, Bourgeois RM, Loeppke RR, Konicki DL, Hymel PA, Dreger M. (2014) Medical evacuations from oil rigs off the Gulf Coast of the United States from 2008 to 2012. *J Occup Environ Med* **56**(7): 681–685.

Weiss DJ, Nelson A, Vargas-Ruiz CA, Gligorić K, Bavadekar S, Gabrilovich E, Bertozzi-Villa A, Rozier J, Gibson HS, Shekel T, Kamath C, Lieber A, Schulman K, Shao Y, Qarkaxhija V, Nandi AK, Keddie SH, Rumisha S, Amratia P, Arambepola R, Chestnutt EG, Millar JJ, Symons TL, Cameron E, Battle KE, Bhatt S, Gething PW. (2020) Global maps of travel time to healthcare facilities. *Nature Med* **26**(12): 1835–1838. Available from: doi: 10.1038/s41591-020-1059-1.

Wright IH, McDonald JC, Rogers PN, Ledingham IM. (1988) Provision of facilities for secondary transport of seriously ill patients in the United Kingdom. *BMJ* **296**(6621): 543–545.

Chapter 21

Medical Disasters Planning and Response

Halim Mohamed and Abu Hasan Samad†*

Introduction

Major industrial accidents or "industrial disasters" are sudden, unexpected industrial events with significant impact to people, the environment and infrastructure. These catastrophic events are commonly associated with a major chemical release, nuclear emissions, and/or fires and explosions resulting in multiple casualties and loss of lives in a way that overwhelms the day-to-day medical resources available at the workplace. Examples include the poisonous gas leak from the Union Carbide insecticide plant in Bhopal, India in 1984 (Case Study 1), the Chernobyl nuclear disaster, Ukraine in 1986 (Case Study 2), the Texas City Refinery explosion, United States of America (USA) in 2005 (Case Study 3), the Deepwater Horizon oil spill, USA in 2010 (Ramesh and Kumar, 2010) (Case Study 4) and Fukushima Daaichi Nuclear Plant disaster, Japan in 2011 (Case Study 5).

Between January 1901 and October 2020, there have been 1,525 major industrial accidents causing 60,262 direct deaths and 230,976 direct injuries worldwide.

*Shell Malaysia, Kuala Lumpur, Malaysia.
†Twin Towers Medical Centre KLCC Sdn Bhd, Malaysia and Academy of Occupational and Environmental Medicine, Malaysia.
Corresponding author: Abu Hasan Samad (abuhasan.samad@gmail.com).

There is no single universally accepted definition of an industrial disaster, its true overall incidence is not known. The Centre for Research on the Epidemiology of Disasters (an independent research collaboration under the support of World Health Organization (WHO) and Belgian government) maintains an Emergency Events Database (EM-DAT), from which this data was derived (Centre for Research on the Epidemiology of Disasters, 2020). This illustrates the fact that the risk of major industrial accidents cannot be totally eliminated, even with the best controls. As such, when they do occur, the effects must be minimised as much as possible.

This chapter aims at assisting the occupational physician and the management in planning and organising the necessary medical emergency response (MER) and recovery, in order to mitigate the medical impact of major industrial accidents (McEntire, 2015).

Case Study 1: Poisonous Gas Leak, Bhopal, 1984

3 December 1984: Over 30 tons of methyl isocyanate, a chemical intermediate in the production of carbaryl, a commonly used pesticide, was acci-

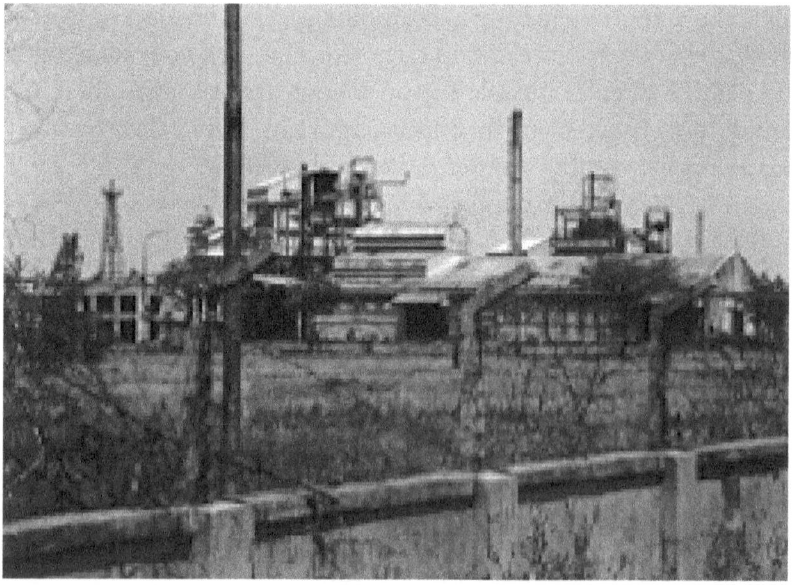

Fig. 1. The Union Carbide Plant, Bhopal, India, site of a chemical gas leak which killed and injured thousands.

dentally released from a Union Carbide plant in Bhopal, India (Fig. 1). The incident occurred in the middle of the night. The nearby residents had no knowledge of effective evacuation plans or procedures. Between 50,000 and 100,000 people were affected enough to seek some form of medical care. India's Supreme Court put the death toll at 3,800 in 1991 when it awarded US$480 million in damages against U.S.-based Union Carbide Corp and its Indian subsidiary. By 1994, ten years to the day after the disaster, official government records showed 6,495 people had died as a result of exposure to the toxic methyl isocyanate.

Case Study 2: Chernobyl Nuclear Disaster, 1986

26 April 1986: The overheating of a water-cooled nuclear reactor in Chernobyl (in present-day Ukraine) led to explosions in its reactor core. Thirty-one deaths were directly attributed to the accident, all among the reactor staff and emergency workers. An estimated 150–200 million curies (Ci) of radioactive material were released into the environment within the first 10 days. The highest concentrations of radionuclides fell over the Ukraine, Belarus, and Russia, and raised levels were found as far away as North America. The UNSCEAR (United Nations Scientific Committee on the Effects of Atomic Radiation) found that, as of 2005, some 6,000 thyroid cancers and 15 thyroid cancer deaths are attributable to the accident (Reiners, 2009) (Fig. 2).

Case Study 3: Texas City Refinery Explosion, 2005

23 March 2005: Hydrocarbon vapour was accidentally released from an isomerisation unit at BP's Texas City refinery, Texas, and was ignited by a running vehicle parked nearby (Fig. 3). The resulting explosion caused blunt force trauma and killed 15 people working on-site. The pressure wave was so powerful it shattered windows of buildings up to a distance of 1.2 km away. Another 180 plant workers and residents of nearby neighbourhoods were injured. Medical emergency response personnel from several government and private agencies worked hand-in-hand and rushed victims to three hospitals in the area. Subsequent investigations revealed that operator fatigue was a likely contributing factor (amongst many others). The United States Occupational Safety and Health Administra-

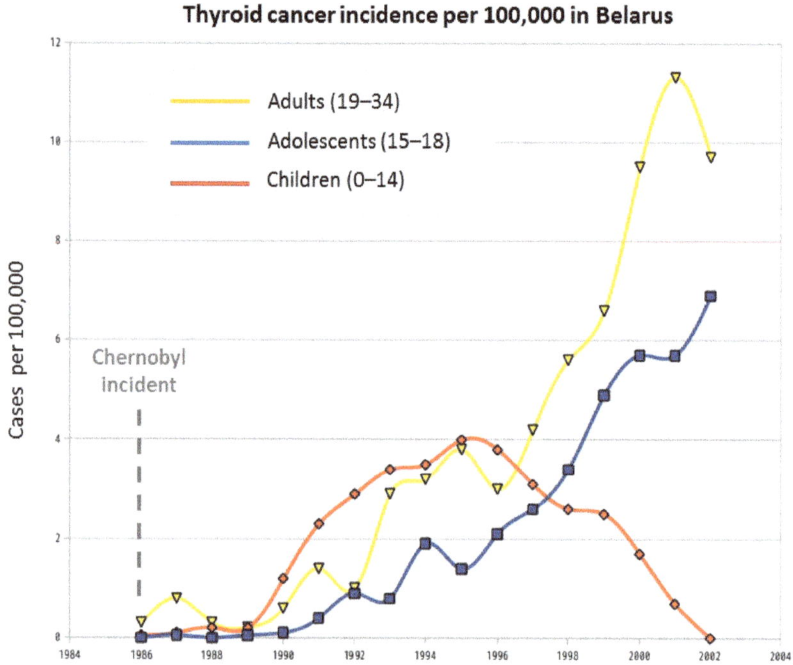

Fig. 2. Thyroid cancer incidence in Belarus after the Chernobyl accident (United Nations Scientific Committee on the Effects of Atomic Radiation, 2000).

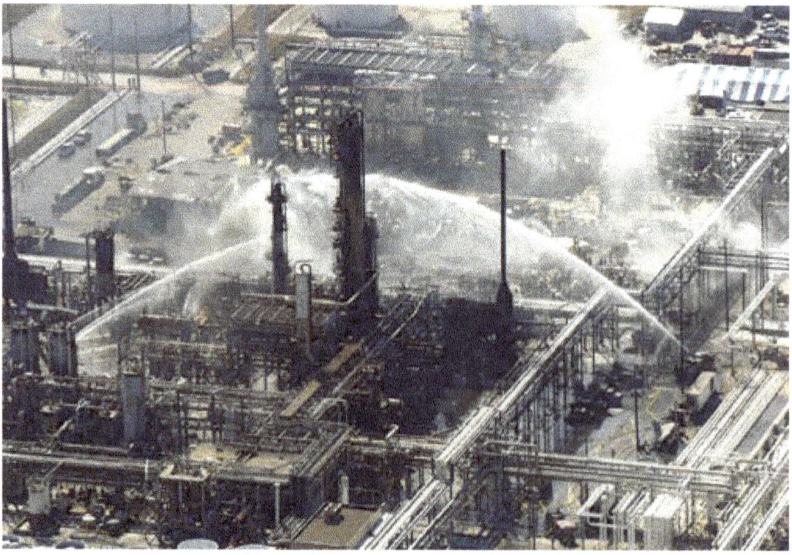

Fig. 3. Aerial view of the Texas City refinery soon after the explosion.

tion (OSHA) imposed an US$87 million fine on BP for failing to correct safety hazards revealed from investigations following the explosion. The fine was the largest in OSHA's history.

Case Study 4: Deepwater Horizon Drilling Platform Explosion and Oil Spill, 2010

20 April 2010: An explosion on the Deepwater Horizon Macondo oil well drilling platform killed 11 workers and injured 16 others. Ninety-four crew members were evacuated by lifeboat or helicopter in the ensuing rescue. The explosion also resulted in the largest accidental oil spill in history. Over the next 84 days, approximately 4.9 million barrels leaked, forming a slick over an estimated 75,000 sq. km of ocean and 1,770 km of shoreline. To help disperse the oil, 1.8 million gallons of chemical dispersants was used. Around 48,000 workers were employed in the clean-up operations, many of whom were exposed to the crude oil and the chemical dispersants (Fig. 4). By June 2010, 143 spill-exposure cases had been reported; 108 of those involved workers in the clean-up efforts, while 35 were reported by residents. The health effects from the exposure to the oil and chemical dispersant is still being studied.

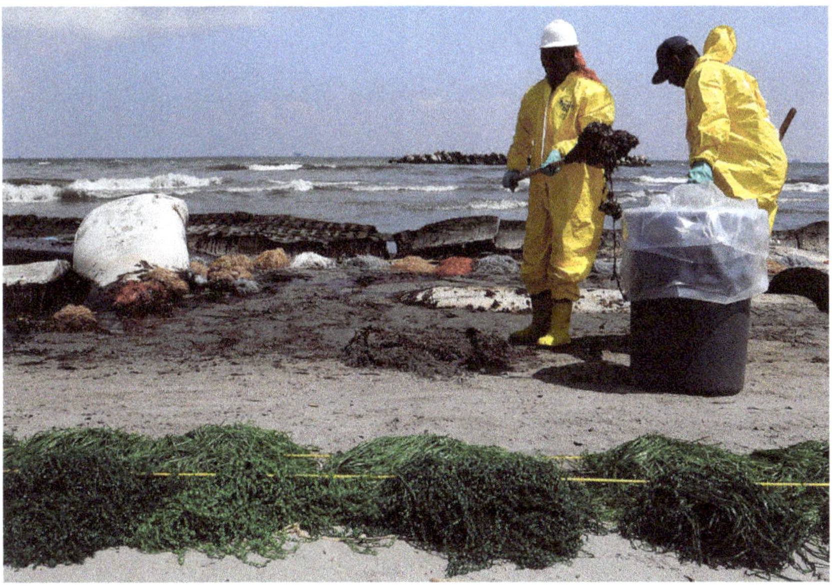

Fig. 4. Workers cleaning up oil spill from the Deepwater Horizon.

Case Study 5: Fukushima Daiichi Nuclear Plant Disaster, 2011

11 March 2011: A 9-magnitude earthquake occurred off the east coast of Japan, generating massive tsunamis that hit the Fukushima Daiichi nuclear power plant (Fig. 5). Although itself a natural disaster, the tsunami led to the loss of the plant's cooling capacity, causing severe damage to the nuclear cores, two explosions and radioactive release. Six hospitals designated as primary radiation emergency medical facilities provided initial treatment and decontamination. Whilst 16 workers were injured from the blast, there were no direct fatalities. However, during the urgent evacuation of more than 800 patients from hospitals and nursing care facilities on 14 March, no medical personnel were in attendance and no medical care was provided to the evacuees (Hasegawa et al., 2016). At least 50 elderly patients died during the evacuation. Hypothermia, deterioration of underlying medical problems and dehydration were cited as the potential causes of death (Tanigawa et al., 2012). In contrast, the evacuation done between 18 and 22 March were supported by the disaster medical assistance team. During this period, 509 patients were

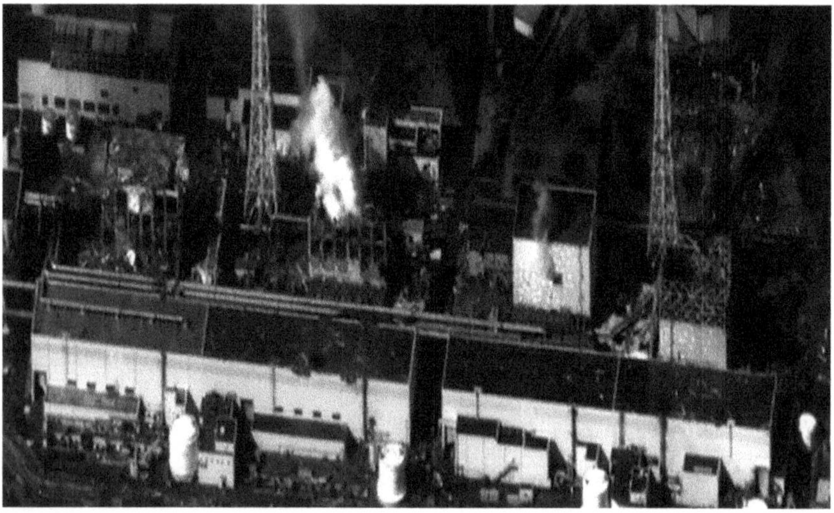

Fig. 5. The Fukushima I Nuclear Power Plant after the 2011 Tōhoku earthquake and tsunami.

safely evacuated with no loss of life. A recent study indicated that the severe health risk associated with the rapid evacuation of elderly residents from nursing care facilities after the Fukushima accident was 30 times higher than the radiation risk posed by the disaster itself (Murakami et al., 2015).

Challenges

In addition to overwhelming existing day-to-day medical emergency resources, major industrial accidents pose many unique challenges to the occupational physician. They include the following:

- Effective medical response requires a very high level of coordination between different agencies, including the police, fire department, ambulance services and local health facilities.
- Medical workers and emergency response personnel will themselves be at risk through contact with residual contaminants and contaminated casualties.
- The capabilities of the health facilities in the vicinity of high-risk industries are often limited. Mishandling of early cases may spread contamination and put these facilities out of action.
- Hospitals and roads leading to the hospitals may lie in the path of a chemical plume or discharge.
- Chemical (or radioactive) release may necessitate the immediate evacuation of neighbouring communities (e.g. Case Study 1 and Case Study 5).
- Communities may be affected by the contamination of water supplies or the food chain (e.g. Case Study 2).
- Weather and wind conditions may impact the MER.
- For many proprietary chemicals, there may be little or no information available regarding their effects on human health. The source chemicals in the accident may also be altered by fire, air, water, and reaction with each other.
- Certain chemical substances may give rise to delayed harmful effects following initial exposure (e.g. pesticides), even after rapid decontamination has taken place.

- Rapid evacuation may pose significant risk in addition to the risks of the disaster itself (Case Study 5).
- Major industrial accidents cause fear and anxiety which may dramatically increase the number of walk-in cases and referrals to treatment facilities. In addition, telephone helplines may be overwhelmed.
- The need to provide the public with useful, health-related information must be balanced against causing unwarranted fears (and litigation).

These challenges should be taken into account when developing the MER plans.

Medical Emergency Response Planning

MERPs help ensure that any injuries from major industrial accidents are managed as effectively as is practicable. This is achieved through the establishment of a set system of procedures and protocols, and by ensuring that it is followed during drills and actual emergencies.

MERP cannot be done in isolation. In order for the MER to be effective, it needs to be part of, and integrated with, the site's overall emergency response plan (ERP).

The MERP and its overarching ERP are vital for all workplaces where major accidents are reasonably foreseeable. These include sites where dangerous substances are present in significant quantities (e.g. toxic gases, flammable hydrocarbons, radioactive materials), and sites where the loss of control of work processes may generate dangerous substances, fire or explosions (e.g. oil platforms, nuclear plants, chemical manufacturing plants, oil terminals).

The aims of these ERP are to:

1. minimise harm to people, environment, and infrastructure;
2. facilitate recovery and business continuity; and
3. minimise legal liability and damage to reputation.

The ERP is typically divided into two parts: an on-site ERP (prepared by the site management) to specify response expected of those who work on site; and off-site ERP (prepared by the local authority) to specify the response of agencies to an emergency on the site. The importance of a combined, coordinated, multi-agency response cannot be overstated, and as such these two plans should detail how they integrate together.

The various stakeholders include the fire rescue service, ambulance service, the health authority, private health facilities, police, civil defense, coastguard, as well as the workers on site. Sometimes, competent authorities (e.g. Department of Occupational Safety and Health, Department of Environment, and poison centers) and the general public may also need to be consulted about these ERPs. A large part of the emergency plan preparation is about the exchange of information and ideas between people in these stakeholder organisations.

The plan should contain all the information that those involved can reasonably expect. The procedures should be simple and straightforward, should not be contradictory, and should enable maximum flexibility of response. In designing the MER plan, key components that must be included are covered in the next few sections.

Risk Assessment

Each site is unique. The types of foreseeable major accidents, the probabilities, and the extent of the consequences, will differ between sites. As such, MER plans must be developed in a way that matches the site's risk profile. The risk assessment should take into consideration:

- **Identification of significant sources and types of potential major accidents:** Specific questions that need to be considered include: What events could give rise to a release of dangerous substances? What dangerous substances are stored on-site? What are the quantities, and their locations? In addition to human errors, could natural disasters or malicious acts also initiate a major accident on this site (Case Study 5)?
- **An assessment of the likelihood of such an event:** In assessing the likelihood of a major accident, it is useful to ask: How often has such an event happened in the industry? Has there been any near misses within the site, or (in the case of a multinational corporation), in the Company's operations in other countries?

- **An assessment of the severity of the consequences of such an event:** In assessing how potentially serious are these events, the following questions must be considered: What could be the different impacts of such an event (e.g. on workers, neighbouring communities, environment and infrastructure)? What are the reactions of chemicals released and their behaviour in fires? Over what distances can these health hazards create harmful effects? What is the worst-case scenario? Could the impact extend beyond national and regional boundaries? How would such a scenario affect the local medical facilities? What could be the long-term health consequences?
- **An assessment of the adequacy of current controls and resources:** What is the site's current medical capability in providing first aid, stabilisation, advanced life support, and medical evacuation? What additional resources would be needed? How would these resources be obtained? What is the current level of collaboration between the site's medical department and the local agencies (e.g. the local hospitals, ambulance service, and emergency service providers)?

Initiation

The MERP should clearly define when and how to initiate the response, who the key players are (e.g. the incident commander, the emergency response team, the triage team, the ambulance team), how can they be contacted during the event, their rendezvous point (e.g. incident command post, emergency coordination centre, pre-designated medical treatment area), and how they will communicate with each other.

Structure and Organisation

The MERP must also clearly identify who will take charge, who will report to whom, each key players' roles, where will they be located (e.g. triage area, staging area, crisis centre), and how they can be identified during the chaos (e.g. coloured vests, badges).

Table 1. An Example of a Time Based, Tiered Response Model in Defining the MER Standard, Commonly Used in Remote Oil and Gas Operations

Tier	Description	Response Time (Practicable Response Times will Vary, Depending on the Nature of Operations, and the Site Location)
Tier 1: First Aid	First aid treatment, including defibrillation, by a designated first aider	4 min
Tier 2: Medical Stabilisation	Assessment and stabilisation by a health professional	1 h
Tier 3: Hospital Care	Admission to, and care at the nearest hospital	4 h

Standard of Care

In order to design an effective MER plan, it is important to first determine the expected standard of care during these major industrial accidents. Although there are various ways to do this, the authors believe the **time-based tiered response** model (Table 1) facilitates planning and implementation best. It is flexible enough to suit different operations and locations, as well as being proven in the field.

Resources

The medical resources required to provide effective mitigation during a major industrial accident include competent MER team members (e.g. first aiders, doctors, nurses and paramedics), effective means of communications, transportation, and local health facilities with adequate medical structures, equipment and supplies (Table 2).

It is unlikely for the worksite to possess all the medical resources necessary for major accidents. Additional resources will most likely be sourced through collaboration with the local hospitals, and local

Table 2. An Example of Medical Resource Requirements Based on a Tiered Response

Tier	Tier 1: First Aid	Tier 2: Medical Stabilisation	Tier 3: Hospital Care
Personnel Involved	Designated First Aider (DFA)	Nurse/Doctor	Emergency Physician
Location	Immediate on-site	Triage area (or Site Clinic)	Hospital
Equipment/ Transport Requirement	• First Aid Box • Automated External Defibrillator	• Trauma Bag • Ambulance Equipment • Site Clinic Equipment and Supplies	Ambulance
Training requirements	• Basic Life Support • First Aid	• Advanced Trauma Life Support (ATLS) or equivalent • Mass Casualty Incident (MCI)	ATLS and MCI refresher training (e.g. every 3 years)
Skills maintenance	Emergency Physician	Hospital	Ambulance

emergency agencies. This highlights the importance of integrating the on-site and off-site ERPs through multi-agency collaboration and drills.

The detailed list of medical equipment and supplies for a major industrial accident is not within the scope of this chapter. However, they are generally grouped into tiers 1 (first aid box) and 2 (trauma bag, site clinic equipment, and ambulance equipment). The chosen equipment, supplies, and their quantities must match the expected scenarios defined by the risk assessment.

First aid and medical stabilisation in the field is very different from a hospital setting. It has its own set of challenges. Consider the following when planning the equipment for major industrial accidents:

- **Portability:** Medical responders will need to rapidly mobilise to the worksite. The selected equipment (e.g. vital signs monitors, defibrillators, oxygen sets, ventilators) must be portable enough to be carried in a trauma bag by a single person. Consider the robustness of the equipment — as it may be exposed to difficult conditions (e.g. dust, ash, water, shock) over extended periods. Electrical supply for these medical equipment may also be either intermittent or absent.

- **User-friendliness:** During the early phases, the responders will often be overwhelmed by the number of casualties. Some emergency equipment is easier to use than others in these circumstances. They include the laryngeal airway, blind intubation devices, hemostatic dressings, disposable intra-osseous infusion systems, etc. They may save precious time, especially when support is limited or absent.
- **Containers/packs:** Where possible, pack medical equipment and supplies in durable, "ready-to-go" containers, bags or boxes. Weatherproof and impact-resistant cases (e.g. Pelican® cases) are ideal. These are best stored at a designated location off-site.
- **Quantity:** The quantity of items should be based on the number of casualties expected, the types of injuries, the duration of operations, and the likely duration before resupply. This will vary widely from site to site and must be defined by the risk assessment.

In many developing countries, local hospitals may not have the necessary expertise and capacity to deal with the types of injuries from major accidents caused by the industry (e.g. severe burns, chemical inhalation injuries, and radiation illness). A number of large industry players have chosen to work together with the local health authorities and upgrade the local hospitals' capability through the companies' social investment programmes. In addition to improving their ER plans, such demonstrations of corporate social responsibility (CSR) have been shown to help enhance the companies' reputation in their communities and host countries.

In some countries, different companies working in the same area formed mutual aid arrangements, with the aim of lending each other assistance during a disaster. Mutual aid may be ad hoc, requested only when such an emergency occurs. It may also be a formal standing agreement for cooperative emergency management on a continuing basis.

Escalation

The MER plan must indicate how the key players will recognise situations where the procedures and resources are not appropriate or sufficient, and define what needs to be done instead. Different countries have different systems of activating additional medical reinforcements. They include the Home Agencies (e.g. Civil Defense, Police, Fire Services, National Guard, Ministry of Health) and the Military.

Training

In order to plan effectively, the planners may need training in emergency planning and crisis management. These are now available in many countries.

Medical responders may also need specific training to ensure competent provision of care during major industrial accidents. These include Mass Casualty Incident (MCI) Training (Jenkins *et al.*, 2008), as well as Advanced Trauma Life Support (ATLS), Pre-Hospital Trauma Life Support (PHTLS), and their equivalents.

It is important to note that not all first aid or ATLS training covers the management of multiple casualties. As such, those likely to be involved in managing mass casualty incidents should preferably receive MCI training.

In addition, some sites may also have chemicals that require specific first aid measures (e.g. hydrogen sulphide gas). These skills may not be sufficiently covered in the first aiders' course, especially if the first aid course is "generic" or is very short. Where such competency gaps are identified, additional targeted training may help.

To prevent skill decay, it is recommended that first aid and advanced life support training are repeated every 3 years. Alternatively, the first aiders and medical professionals may complete a series of shorter, more frequent, modular skills maintenance training, which has been found to be more effective and practicable when compared to infrequent longer duration training. Such training may, for example, be implemented as practical, in-house, hands-on sessions organised regularly on-site (e.g. two hours every quarter) by the participants themselves. This training model has the advantage of being more practicable for busy employees, whose operational commitments may not allow them to be away from work for several days in a row.

Drills

Lessons from past major industrial accidents suggest that disorganisation and chaos are often the result of key personnel not fully understanding the ER plan, or their role within it. To address this, a regular programme of drills is essential. It verifies the effectiveness of the response, and exposes gaps and weaknesses in the MER. The scenarios chosen for these drills should reflect likely events as identified by the risk assessment.

Whilst the types of drills chosen will vary to suit the nature of operations, the drills commonly done shown in Table 3.

The procedures outlined in the MER plan should be followed and tested during these drills. It is helpful to include checklists in the plan to assist in decision-making, and to function as a series of reminders for the individuals involved.

Drill frequencies will vary, depending on the nature of operations, and the site location. It is also important to repeat drills whenever

Table 3. An Example of Various Types MER Drills and their Frequencies

Drill	Description	Frequency
Communications Test	Test all communication systems in the ERP, including external organisations (e.g. hospitals), and backup systems	Every quarter
Desktop Exercise	Key personnel discussing simulated scenarios and responses, without the actions being actually performed by the responders	Annually
Local Drill	Casualties are managed and treated by the site's responders, to the point when the casualties are ready for transport (e.g. ambulance ready to depart to the local hospital)	Annually
Full Scale Drill	Multi agency drill with simulated casualties delivered to the hospital	Every 3 years

there is a significant change in the site activities (e.g. construction of a new process area). Where possible, try and integrate medical scenarios whenever larger ER exercises are being planned for.

Consider assigning medically trained personnel to monitor, and evaluate the response (e.g. response time, adequacy of the provision of advanced life support, etc.) and to debrief the participants. Share the lessons learnt from these drills with the site stakeholders, and to use them to improve the MER Plan.

Review

The ER Plan is a "live" document. Changes in site activities, changes in work processes, employee turnover, and skill decay all contribute to reducing its effectiveness over time. It is thus important to conduct regular reviews of the site's existing ER plan, in order to continuously maintain and improve it. A periodic review cycles every 1–2 years is common. Additional reviews should also be done immediately after significant process or organisational changes (e.g. restructuring).

Emergency Response

Although the detailed circumstances may vary, the principles of medical management in a disaster, consisting of rescue, triage, stabilisation and casualty evacuation can be applied to all major industrial accident situations.

Scene Management

The incident site must be immediately isolated by controlling access to and from the area. Control the movement of contaminated victims and provide safe working methods for first responders. Immediate priorities for the first responders are as follows:

- Approach scene with caution (and where chemical release is suspected, approach upwind).
- Carry out scene assessment.

- Establish incident command.
- Estimate the number of casualties/victims.
- Estimate resource requirements.
- Carry out primary triage, decontamination, secondary triage, medical care, and transport.

Casualty Management Zones

The incident area is usually divided into three main areas or zones.

- The first is the danger area (sometimes called the *hot zone*). It may be contaminated by chemicals or are at risk of secondary explosions and fires.
- The safe area (sometimes referred to as the *cold zone*) is where the medical treatment area can be located. Where chemical contamination is a possibility, locate this zone at a safe distance upwind. Ideally, the treatment area may be on a vacant lot, an existing medical clinic, or any area that has good access to ambulance vehicles. The area should be large enough for triage (i.e. sorting of patients according to clinical condition), treatment areas and areas for evacuation assets (e.g. parking and circuit).
- A decontamination area, if needed, can be located in an area between the hot and cold zones (the *warm zone*). In such a scenario, all responders must leave the hot zone via specially designated pathways into the warm zone where they will be decontaminated.

Personal Protective Equipment

Depending on the nature of the major accident, it may be necessary to protect the first responders' airway, skin, and eyes prior to their entry the hot and warm zones (e.g. Case Study 4). Whilst necessary, the PPE may also restrict their physical activity, cause dehydration and heat-related illness. This highlights the importance of drills, where the proper choice and use of PPE is evaluated, and their impact on the response is appreciated.

Triage

As mentioned, major industrial accidents may produce an extremely large number of injuries, many of which will be life-threatening. In most instances, the number of patients will far exceed the capacity of available medical personnel. Until additional resources become available, some patients will receive treatment and others will not. For this reason, medical emergency responders must make difficult decisions based on resource-allocation. This is done through field triage — a systematic initial assessment and categorisation of victims based on the severity of their injuries. The objective is to do the greatest good for the greatest number of casualties within the confines of limited medical personnel, equipment and supplies.

The details of how to perform triage will not be covered in this chapter, as there are already many excellent publications on this subject.

In addition, there are significant differences in the way triage is done in various countries and organisations. Regardless of these differences, it is important to highlight that all medical responders involved in the site's emergency response must be familiar with triage and must use the same method of triage. Past incidents have repeatedly demonstrated that the use of a common medical language is vital for a coordinated MER. Different ways and terminology used to communicate a patients' condition results in confusion and poor clinical outcomes.

Recovery

Major industrial accidents are traumatic events that may result in a wide range of mental and physical health to the victims. The body of research over the past three decades suggests that the burden of psychiatric disorders among persons exposed to disasters is substantial (Neria *et al.*, 2008). For example, the prevalence of post-traumatic stress disorder (PTSD) was 73 percent among survivors of the Piper Alpha oil rig disaster in the UK North Sea in 1988 where a gas leak induced an explosion and fire took the lives of 167 men (Hull *et al.*, 2002). In addition to the victims, first responders and family members may also be vulnerable. Early intervention by mental health professionals may help reduce the psychological impact of disasters. This may include screening and identifying those who may be at risk of psychiatric disorders (e.g. acute stress disorder, depression and PTSD) and providing treatment as necessary. In addition to professional psychological support, the emotional support of family members, friends and social workers should also be encouraged.

Whilst early intervention is needed, the value of psychological debriefing (a type of early psychological intervention utilising some form of emotional processing/catharsis or ventilation by encouraging recollection/ventilation/reworking of the traumatic event) remains controversial.

On the other hand, a "business" debrief session should be conducted with all key personnel involved in the rescue operation soon after the event. The aim is to review the actions taken during the disaster with a view to identifying procedural lapses and recommending improvements to the ERP.

The occupational physician plays an important role in identifying the human factors and occupational safety lapses contributing to the disaster. Investigations of the Texas City refinery explosion (Case Study 3), for example, revealed that operator fatigue was a likely contributing factor.

Media

Whilst the occupational physician is not likely interface with the media directly, he/she must understand that the media can both facilitate or undermine the response and recovery efforts. As an ally, the media's role in mitigating the health impact of the disaster should not be underestimated. They can help to:

- Educate the public about the possible health impacts, as well as the preventive and preparedness measures.
- Warn the public about an impending hazard (e.g. gaseous release).
- Provide information regarding evacuation and sheltering.
- Relay what the responders are doing and how they are dealing with the disaster.

- List what organisations are providing relief and how assistance can be given or obtained.
- Generate support for medical emergency management (e.g. personnel, equipment).

However, depending on the segment of society they represent, the media may also have different goals (e.g. assigning blame, perpetuating popular myths). Other challenges include inaccurate reporting, misrepresentations of facts, interference with emergency response efforts, and even putting themselves in danger. In order to use the media effectively, the following strategies may be useful:

- **Communicate through the assigned public relations (PRs) professional:** A good ER plan will include a PRs focal point (or team), who will coordinate the information flow to the public. Assist him/her with accurate and timely situational reports. Highlight the importance of certain information — especially those that may help reassure the public or require them to take immediate action. As much as possible, avoid giving ad-lib comments to the media directly — unless you have been designated to do so by the company.
- **Educate the media:** Explain to the media about the hazards, the health risks, and how the current efforts are keeping the risks as low as reasonably practicable. Also tell the media (and your PR professional) that any adjustments to carefully worded medical statements can change the meaning dramatically and cause problems to the recovery efforts. Where possible, establish a relationship with media in advance.

The Potential Impact of a Pandemic on Major Accident Hazard

The recent COVID-19 pandemic has necessitated the conduct of hazardous operations under minimal staffing (e.g. in the energy sector). In addition, disruptions in travel and supply chain have negatively impacted maintenance, and thus plant reliability. Whilst this increases risk, to date there has been no reported major industrial accidents attributed (either directly or indirectly) to the pandemic. This may be due to advances in technical safety and their adoption as industry standard, as well as careful risk evaluations prior to de-manning the workforce.

Whilst the immediate risk of the pandemic to industrial disasters may have been mitigated, the long-term risks have yet to be defined. Anecdotal reports from the industry suggest that changes in work processes during the pandemic may have contributed to minor incidents and near misses. These include incidents due to fatigue (due to extended shifts of essential staff), bypassing of safety controls (due to task overload), and minor equipment failures (due to delayed maintenance). Over time, a prolonged pandemic may result in a build-up of the unsafe conditions, erode multiple safety barriers, and increase the likelihood of a major accident.

In order to mitigate these risks, it is important to perform risk assessments prior to a significant change in the work activity is envisaged (e.g. de-manning an industrial plant). Such risk assessments should include evaluations on process safety and asset integrity, as well as the necessary mitigations (e.g. emergency response) based on a defined risk tolerance.

Mitigating the overall impact of the pandemic (including that of a major accident hazard) can be done through the development of a Pandemic Preparedness Plan, communications with staff, and the identification of vulnerabilities through risk assessments (Staples, 2006). Where appropriate, such a plan may include policies and procedures for prompt identification and isolation of those affected, basic infection control measures, and workplace controls (e.g. engineering, administrative, safe work practices, personal protective equipment) in line with the workers' exposure risk classification (OSHA, 2020). This is especially important when resuming activities during recovery (Centers for Disease Control and Prevention, 2020a; Centers for Disease Control and Prevention, 2020b).

Conclusion

Although major industrial accidents are by their very nature unpredictable, it is nevertheless crucial to plan for them. Although they are by definition characterised by chaos and confusion, the greater the degree emergency response planning and organisation, the higher will be the chances of bringing order to an otherwise uncontrollable situation. The aim is always, to plan in such a way that when an emergency arises, a swift and effective response can be mounted to contain or minimise the effects of the incident, and to restore normality as soon as possible.

The occupational physician must exercise leadership and collaboration in planning. He/She must also be able to execute the MER plan under the most trying of circumstances and adapt when appropriate. He/She can best do this if he is sufficiently prepared.

References

Centers for Disease Control and Prevention. (2020a) *Resuming Business Toolkit, Coronavirus Disease 2019 (COVID-19)*. [Online] Available from: https://www.cdc.gov/coronavirus/. [Accessed on 28 March 2021].

Centers for Disease Control and Prevention. (2020b) *Guidance for Businesses and Employers Responding to Coronavirus Disease 2019 (COVID-19)*. [Online] Available from: https://www.cdc.gov/coronavirus/2019-ncov/community/guidance-business-response.html.

Centre for Research on the Epidemiology of Disasters. (2020) *Emergency Events Database (EM-DAT)*. [Online] Available from: https://www.emdat.be/. [Accessed on 28 March 2021].

Hasegawa A, Ohira T, Maeda M, Yasumura S, Tanigawa K. (2016) Emergency responses and health consequences after the Fukushima accident; evacuation and relocation. *Clin Oncol* **28**(4): 1–8. Available from: doi: 10.1016/j.clon.2016.01.002.

Hull AM, Alexander DA, Klein S. (2002) Survivors of the Piper Alpha oil platform disaster: Long-term follow-up study. *Br J Psychiatry* **181**: 433–438.

Jenkins JL, McCarthy ML, Saucer LM, Green GB, Stuart S, Thomas TL, Hsu EB. (2008) Mass-casualty triage: Time for an evidence-based approach. *Prehosp Disaster Med* **23**(1): 3–8.

McEntire DA. (2015) *Disaster Response and Recovery: Strategies and Tactics for Resilience* (2nd Ed). Hoboken, New Jersey, United States, Wiley.

Murakami M, Ono K, Tsubokura M, Nomura S, Oikawa T, Oka T. (2015) Was the risk from nursing-home evacuation after the Fukushima accident higher than the radiation risk? *PLoS One* **10**(9). Available from: doi: 10.1371/journal.pone.0137906.

Neria Y, Nandi A, Galea S. (2008) Post-traumatic stress disorder following disasters: A systematic review. *Psychol Med* **38**(4): 467–480.

OSHA. (2020) Guidance on Preparing Workplaces for COVID-19. *U.S. Department of Labor*, OSHA 3990-03 2020.

Ramesh AC, Kumar S. (2010) Triage, monitoring, and treatment of mass casualty events involving chemical, biological, radiological, or nuclear agents. *J Pharm Bioallied Sci* **2**(3): 239–247.

Reiners C. (2009). Radioactivity and thyroid cancer. *Hormones* **8**(3): 185–191.

Staples J. (2006) *Preparing for a Pandemic*. [Online] Available from: https://hbr.org/2006/05/preparing-for-a-pandemic. [Accessed on 28 March 2021].

Tanigawa K, Hosoi Y, Hirohashi N, Iwasaki Y, Kamiya K. (2012) Loss of life after evacuation: Lessons learned from the Fukushima accident. *Lancet* **379**(9819): 889–891.

United Nations Scientific Committee on the Effects of Atomic Radiation. (2000) *Sources and Effects of Ionizing Radiation*. New York, United Nations.

Chapter 22

Health Screening and Surveillance

Wee Hoe Gan and David Koh†*

Introduction

An important concept in occupational medicine is the interrelationship between work and health. While the primary strategy is the prevention of work-related ill health through eliminating or reducing hazardous work exposures, the ability to systematically monitor the health of a worker through his life cycle of employment (and even beyond) is a complementary strategy that has a place in occupational health practice. Occupational health surveillance enables the early detection and management of work-related disorders that could otherwise severely impact the work ability and quality of life of the individual.

The terms "health surveillance" and "health screening" are often used interchangeably. However, there are subtle technical differences. The United States (US) Occupational Safety and Health Administration (OSHA) defines health screening as "a method for detecting

*Department of Occupational and Environmental Medicine, Singapore General Hospital; Changi Aviation Medicine Centre, Changi General Hospital; and Duke-NUS Medical School, National University of Singapore, Singapore.
†PAPRSB Institute of Health Sciences, Universiti Brunei Darussalam, Brunei Darussalam *and* Saw Swee Hock School of Public Health and Yong Loo Lin School of Medicine, National University of Singapore, Singapore.
Corresponding author: Wee Hoe Gan (gan.wee.hoe@singhealth.com.sg).

disease or body dysfunction before an individual would normally seek medical care" (OSHA, 2021). On the other hand, health surveillance in the context of work connotes a more targeted reach only for workers who require such repeated health checks. It also has a feedback loop to the employer and workplace. Depending on the findings of occupational health surveillance, follow-on recommendations may be made on the interventions to be taken for worker health protection, as well as the reinforcement of workers' training and education (Health and Safety Executive, 2021a).

Whether health screening or health surveillance, the scope usually refers to some combination of the use of health questionnaires, limited clinical examination, and/or physiological or laboratory analytical investigations on biological samples. This is performed at different stages of employment, from pre-employment, pre-placement and job transfer, to pre-retirement and re-employment (for schemes that re-employ retired workers). Medical examinations may also be carried out prior to return to work following a period of sickness absence, and as part of occupational legislative requirements for workers with specified hazardous work exposures.

The terms "health screening," "health surveillance," and "periodic medical examinations" will be used in this chapter to refer to any form of regular assessment of health status, especially those performed by occupational health departments.

Definition and Rationale of Health Screening

The United Kingdom National Screening Committee (UK NSC) defined health screening as the process of identifying apparently healthy people who may have an increased chance of a disease or condition (UK NSC, 2021). It described screening as "a public health service in which members of a defined population, who do not necessarily perceive they are at risk of, or are already affected by a disease or its complications, are asked a question or offered a test to identify those individuals who are more likely to be helped than harmed by further tests or treatment to reduce the risk of disease or its complications" (UK NSC, 2000). In this respect, screening is different from tests that are applied to patients seeking consultation for an existing health problem with a doctor in the traditional doctor–patient therapeutic relationship.

In occupational health practice, the targets for health screening are individuals who are seeking to enter the workforce or those who are in employment. Health screening and periodic medical examinations are often advocated on the basis that undetected ill-health may pose a danger to the person, the public, or to third parties. There may also be a risk of damage to premises or property with accompanying costs to the employer, as well as adverse publicity. However, those who seek employment or remain in work are often individuals who are well, as those who have overt or severe disease will not seek employment nor are they likely to be at work.

The purpose of health screening in occupational health therefore seeks to achieve the following:

1. To detect occupational or work-related illnesses, so that any further need for preventive measures at the workplace can be considered and implemented before returning the individual to his regular job. This also has the benefit of improving the occupational health and safety of the workplace for other workers.
2. To detect diseases that are common in the general population, especially conditions that do not present early with symptoms, and diseases that have prospects for effective treatment. These disorders are not necessarily caused by occupational exposures, but may affect the safe, effective and efficient performance of work tasks. These disorders may also increase the likelihood of chronic clinical sequelae which could contribute to sickness absence and may incur costs to the worker, his family, and the organisation.

Risks and Benefits of Health Screening

Central to the definition of health screening is the concept of risks and benefits. Health screening and surveillance expend resources that could have been channelled to other aspects of occupational health and safety. If used judiciously and wisely, it allows the early detection of disease at an early stage which is amenable to effective treatment. The finding of a cluster of an occupational disease at a workplace suggests that there could be gaps or non-compliance with existing control measures. Even the detection of a single case may serve as sentinel event to prompt a proactive review of the workplace's safety and health system, as well as a heightened vigilance for yet-undiagnosed occupational disease in other workers.

With no perfect screening test for any condition, health screening can sometimes introduce physical and/or psychological harm to the individual. False positive results, overdiagnosis and overtreatment are possible outcomes of health screening (Gilbert, 2020). On the other hand, if a test is not sufficiently sensitive, it may not detect all persons with the disease, resulting in delayed diagnosis and a false sense of security.

Therefore, an understanding of the performance measurements of tests is important in occupational health practice. This enables the practitioner to develop screening and surveillance programmes that are fit-for-purpose, appropriate and cost-effective.

Principles, Criteria, and Indices for Screening

In 1968, Wilson and Jungner wrote a seminal paper on the principles and practice of screening for disease for the World Health Organization (WHO), which continue to guide the formulation, implementation and evaluation of screening programmes today (Wilson and Jungner, 1968). In the publication, they established the principles and criteria on which screening should be based. They advocated consideration of the following before beginning screening for a disease or risk factor/s:

1. Is the condition important?
2. Is the condition treatable?
3. Does the condition have a recognisable latent or asymptomatic stage?
4. Is the condition prevalent?
5. Is the screening test acceptable, safe, sensitive, specific, easily performed and affordable?

Persons who undergo a screening test for a particular disease may or may not have the disease. The screening test outcome can be positive (i.e. classifying the person as having the disease) or negative (i.e. classifying the person as not having the disease). The test results for each subject may or may not match the subject's actual health status. This will result in tests which are as follows:

1. **True positive:** Where diseased people are correctly identified as diseased;
2. **False positive:** Where healthy people are incorrectly identified as diseased;
3. **True negative:** Where healthy people are correctly identified as healthy;
4. **False negative:** Where diseased people are incorrectly identified as healthy.

The value of a screening test is governed by several indices.

The **sensitivity** of a test is its ability to detect "true positives," i.e. those who definitely have the disease being tested for. The higher the sensitivity, the better the test in picking up genuine cases. In practice, a negative result in a test with high sensitivity is useful for ruling out disease, since it rarely misdiagnoses those who have the disease. A test with 100% sensitivity will recognise all patients with the disease by testing positive. A negative test result would definitively *rule out* presence of the disease in a patient.

The **specificity** of a test is its ability to detect "true negatives," i.e. correctly showing that the screening test result is negative for those who definitely do not have the disease. The higher the specificity, the better the ability of the test to detect those without disease. In practice, a positive result in a test with high specificity is useful for ruling in disease, as the test rarely gives positive results in healthy patients.

A perfect screening test would be 100% sensitive (i.e. all diseased persons are identified correctly as diseased) and 100% specific (i.e. no healthy person is identified as diseased).

In practice, there are no perfect screening tests. For example, a screening test may have high sensitivity but low specificity. In this situation, most persons with the disease are likely to test positive during screening, as the test is highly sensitive. However, because of the low specificity, a large number of healthy persons could be incorrectly identified as diseased and test positive (i.e. a false positive test).

Conversely, there are screening tests that have low sensitivity and high specificity. With a low sensitivity, such a screening test will not be able to pick up all the cases of disease, and may incorrectly label many diseased people as "healthy." The high specificity of the test means that very few people who are healthy will have positive tests from the screening.

The **likelihood ratio** is the likelihood that a given test result is expected in an individual with the disease compared with the likelihood of the same result in an individual without the disease. It therefore provides an indication of the usefulness of the test. The likelihood ratio is defined by the formula Sensitivity/(1 – Specificity). For example, a likelihood ratio of 2 for a particular screening test means that a positive result would be twice as likely to be detected in an individual with the disease compared to another without the disease.

Case Study 1: Sensitivity and Specificity of Screening Tests for Asthma

Occupational asthma is one of the most common work-related pulmonary disorders in many industrialised countries. It can be a result of exposure to sensitisers such as antibiotics, animal and plant proteins (i.e. allergic occupational asthma), or it may be caused by exposure to irritant or noxious substances at the workplace, such as ammonia, chlorine and other chemical fumes (i.e. irritant-induced occupational asthma).

Workers in the motor vehicle repair (MVR) industry are exposed to a variety of substances that may potentially result in the development of occupational asthma (Mackie, 2008). These include solvents and diisocyanates in spray paint. An occupational health company is engaged to provide a health surveillance programme for MVR workers to detect occupational asthma at an early stage.

There are several modalities for screening and diagnosing asthma. A good clinical and occupational history will provide good sensitivity (>85%) but is generally of low specificity (Vandenplas et al., 2017). Spirometry, on the other hand, has high specificity (up to 90%) but poor sensitivity (Meneghini et al., 2017). An integrative approach combining history, spirometry and other modalities such as peak flow measurements will improve the overall diagnostic sensitivity and specificity

(Thorat et al., 2017) of a health surveillance programme for occupational asthma.

Addressing only sensitivity, specificity and likelihood ratio are insufficient to evaluate the usefulness of a screening test. **Pre-test probability** is an estimate of an individual's likelihood of a disease even before the test is performed. It takes into account the factors that may be related to disease causation (e.g. age, work hazard exposure), and use Bayes' theorem to calculate the probability of a positive result when these are considered prior to testing. Broadly, pre-test probability is equivalent to the prevalence of a disease in a population and is important for the interpretation of the results of the test in that population. If the pre-test probability of a disease is low, the implementation of a screening test may cause more harm than good by giving rise to more-than-acceptable number of false positive results, thereby subjecting the affected individuals to anxiety and more tests.

The probability of disease with a positive test result is called the **post-test probability** and is measured with predictive values. The **positive predictive value** of a screening test is the proportion of all those testing positive who are true cases of disease, and the **negative predictive value** is the proportion of all those who do not have the disease, out of all those who on screening are labelled "negative." Predictive values are affected by the prevalence of the disease or condition in the population screened (pre-test probability). For rare conditions, most of the individuals with a positive screening test result will eventually be found not to have the disease on further diagnostic or confirmatory tests, even if the screening test is of high sensitivity and specificity (hence, a low positive predictive value).

Case Study 2: Is There a Role for Occupational Surveillance for Carpal Tunnel Syndrome?

Carpal tunnel syndrome (CTS) is deemed as a costly disease in working adults as a result of the downtime from work and the cost incurred for treatment and rehabilitation. This has led to the implementation of surveillance programmes for the early detection of work-related CTS.

Such surveillance programmes commonly utilise questionnaires and physical examination tests (such as Phalen's and Tinel's tests), but these were found to be poor predictors of CTS in a general working population with a low prevalence of the condition. Dale et al. (2011) concluded that physical examination measures, employed either singly or in combination, are not useful or effective in screening worker populations for CTS prior to or during employment in view of their low sensitivities and positive predictive values. The addition of a nerve conduction study in post-offer, pre-placement screening for CTS also demonstrated no association between abnormal results and incident CTS, i.e. poor positive predictive value (Dale et al., 2016).

In addition to being a poor use of health and safety resources, ineffective surveillance tests may lead to inappropriate job placement or reassignment. The availability of suitable work-enabling devices and access to ergonomic programmes are recognised as more effective strategies to prevent CTS in workers.

Table 1 summarises the performance indicators of screening tests.

The **number needed to screen** (NNS) is defined as the number of people that need to be screened for a given duration to prevent one death or adverse event (Rembold, 1998). This index gives an indication of the extent of the task of screening. This can be used for planning and determining priorities for screening, and for assessing costs and benefits. This index can be directly calculated from clinical

Table 1. Sensitivity, Specificity, and Predictive Value

Test Result	Disease or Condition: Present	Disease or Condition: Absent	
Positive	a	b	Positive predictive value [a/(a + b)] × 100%
Negative	c	d	Negative predictive value [d/(c + d)] × 100%
	Sensitivity [a/(a + c)] × 100%	Specificity [d/(b + d)] × 100%	

Notes:
a = True positive: Sick people correctly identified as sick.
b = False positive: Healthy people incorrectly identified as sick.
c = False negative: Sick people incorrectly identified as healthy.
d = True negative: Healthy people correctly identified as healthy.

trials of disease screening, or it can also be estimated from clinical trials of treatment and the prevalence of yet unrecognised or untreated disease. To allow for comparisons, it is necessary for the index to be normalised to a duration standard.

As examples, Rembold (1998) determined that mammography significantly reduced deaths from breast cancer with a NNS of 2,451 over five years for women aged 50–59 years. For hypertension, the estimated NNS to prevent all-cause death ranged from 274 to 1,307 over five years, if detection was followed by treatment with a thiazide diuretic. The US Preventive Services Task Force recently reported that low-dose computed tomography scans afford a NNS of 130 over ten years of follow-up compared with no screening for high-risk current and former smokers aged 50–74 years (Jonas *et al.*, 2021).

Limitations of Health Screening

While the intent of screening and surveillance programmes is a good one, it is not without potential harm to the population on which screening is performed. As illustrated earlier in the different performance measurements of tests, misclassification of outcomes is possible. Other issues such as a short latent period, lead time, overdiagnosis, and lack of acceptability of the screening tests are also obstacles that could tilt the balance between the benefits and harm of subjecting a group of individuals to screening (Salmi *et al.*, 2016).

Lead Time Bias

The apparent long survival of a patient whose cancer has been detected by screening, followed by early intervention may be partly due to lead time bias. The screening brings forward the time of diagnosis. The time interval between diagnosis and death can appear longer compared to individuals with the same disease who are not screened, and may therefore be diagnosed at a later stage. This may be perceived as the screening conferring an improved prognosis even if there is no comparative advantage of treatment at an earlier than a later stage. Despite the apparently longer survival duration after diagnosis, the survival from the time of disease onset may not be significantly different between the two groups.

Length Bias

There could be a tendency for screening to favour the detection of less aggressive and less serious conditions. More rapidly advancing illnesses, by their very nature, will only be present asymptomatically for a short time, and are more likely to present as cases for diagnosis. Since it is more likely that screening detects slowly progressing illnesses much more than aggressive conditions, this could give an erroneous impression that detecting these conditions early confers improved survival.

Overdiagnosis

Screening may also detect the pre-clinical forms of a disease with a good prognosis. This is the phenomenon of overdiagnosis. An often cited example is the use of prostate-specific antigen (PSA) for prostate cancer screening. This remains controversial as prostate cancer has been detected in up to 50% of autopsy cases of men who died of unrelated causes, bringing into question the usefulness of screening and early diagnosis (Gilligan, 2020). A systematic review and meta-analysis showed that screening using PSA does not affect the overall mortality from prostate cancer. Instead, it may cause more harm by resulting in complications from biopsy and treatment, such as sepsis, urinary incontinence and erectile dysfunction (Ilic *et al.*, 2018).

Employers also need to be aware not all screening and surveillance programmes are appropriate nor cost-effective. There are rarely large financial returns from instituting screening. Indeed, it is very possible for healthcare and business costs to increase as a direct result of screening programmes, in part due to clinical abnormalities being detected that lead to further investigations and interventions. In spite of this, large-scale screening may have to be instituted at times not so much for the benefit of the individual, but to protect co-workers and even the wider community. An example is SARS-CoV-2 PCR testing at the workplace during the Coronavirus Disease 2019 (COVID-19) pandemic. While recognising that there could still be false positive and false negative results, it is generally accepted that the public health benefits of the early detection of COVID-19 cases outweigh the harm in order to reduce the occupational risk of transmission within a workplace (Health and Safety Executive, 2021b).

Components of an Occupational Health Screening

The procedures of an occupational health screening that are commonly performed by occupational health departments include:

1. Medical history, often using a standardised questionnaire. This includes a review of current and previous states of health, and the occupational history;
2. Limited clinical examination, the extent of which would depend on the history obtained. This usually includes baseline physiological parameters such as resting blood pressure and body mass index, as well as more detailed examination of specific organ systems, depending on the work hazard exposure;
3. Analysis of biological samples, which may include blood and/or urine;
4. Physiological tests such spirometry, audiometry and vision testing. Other tests, such as electrocardiograms and imaging studies (e.g. chest X-ray) are less common and useful as a routine procedure. The choice and range of procedures would depend on the hazards and risks at the workplace, and also on whether the aim is to encompass the screening of common chronic diseases such as obesity, diabetes mellitus and hypertension where early detection and control may improve general health status for the workforce.

The completion of an occupational medical examination results in a recommendation to the management as to whether the individual is:

1. Fit for the job;
2. Fit, but with specified temporary or permanent job task restrictions or job scope modifications; or
3. Not fit for the proposed job.

To make sound recommendations, the examining clinician needs to be familiar with the job requirements. This can be done through obtaining a job description, ideally specifying the main job tasks, with or without workplace visits to observe and to be familiar with the work activity and work environment. Decisions on fitness for work should not be made solely on the basis of diagnostic labels. Individuals with the same clinical condition may vary considerably in their inclination for or ability to do the same job. When there is uncertainty about ability or fitness for a job, one approach would be for a "trade test" to be conducted (refer to Section on "Pre-Placement Screening"). The ability of an individual to perform the work tasks in a particular job is best demonstrated by showing an assessor that the job duties can be done effectively, efficiently and safely despite the presence of an impairment, disability, or disease.

Fitness for work is multifactorial, and attempts to detect the presence of a clinical condition and use it as the sole or main factor in making a recommendation on work ability is inappropriate. There are at least several other relevant and important factors to consider:

1. The nature of the condition detected — its severity, stage, prognosis and the individual's response to treatment (including any side effects experienced), as well as the compliance with treatment, and any resulting impairment or disability because of the disease;
2. The nature of the job and the work tasks — whether it is mainly manual physical effort or office-based jobs; and the extent of exposure to and degree of control of exposure to hazards in the job;
3. The location of the job — whether it is in a remote area with extreme environmental conditions (as in desert surroundings, in the Arctic or Antarctica, or deep in tropical rain forests), the ease of access to healthcare, and the ability to transport the individual for emergency care if needed; and

4. The motivation of the individual for the job — whether there are aspects of previous training, experience, or physical and mental health that might indicate a poor fit between an individual worker and the job.

Types of Health Screening in Occupational Medicine Practice

Pre-Employment Health Screening

Medical examination of individuals for their fitness to commence work has long been advocated and practiced in many industries and countries. The justification has been that it would be inappropriate to put a person into work if he/she has a medical condition that may:

1. Be made worse by the proposed work demands or environment;
2. Affect the safe, effective and efficient performance of work tasks;
3. Affect the health and safety of co-workers and third parties in the workplace; or
4. Result in increased costs to the employer (e.g. where the costs of medical care or health insurance is provided by the organisation; or where the employer would have to meet the costs of emergency evacuation if a worker is placed in a remote location, and has a medical condition that could result in a need to be evacuated as an emergency from the work location for medical attention).

However, there is little good evidence that support the decisions made at pre-employment examinations regarding suitability or fitness of individuals for work (Pachman, 2009). A more recent Cochrane review also showed that general pre-employment medical examinations may not reduce the risk for employee sick leave, or the risk of musculoskeletal injuries when compared to no pre-employment examination (Schaafsma *et al.*, 2016).

There is now legislation in many countries that prohibit discrimination on the basis of health status. Pre-employment screening could result in treating individuals with a clinical condition (deemed "unfit") differently from those who do not have any abnormality detected (deemed "fit"). Examples of these laws include the Americans with Disabilities Act (ADA, 1990) and the UK Equality Act 2010 (United Kingdom, 2010). Both these laws require provision of equal access to employment and reasonable adjustments to be made at workplaces to accommodate any person with a medical condition that could be considered a disability.

Depending on the complexity of what is required, pre-employment health screening can be an expensive exercise. The cost effectiveness would depend on the pick-up rate of abnormalities, and whether the conditions are severe enough to affect the health and safety especially of the individuals and their co-workers.

In an audit of 9,139 pre-employment examinations in the UK National Health Service (NHS; one of the biggest employers worldwide with over a million employees), Whitaker and Aw (1995) showed that 98% of such examinations on new healthcare workers were considered fit for employment, without any restrictions. 1.3% were considered "temporarily unfit" with advice given for a temporary restriction of full work duties, and 0.7% were rejected from employment. The main reasons for rejection were an abnormal body mass index, skin problems, and mental health disorders. Hence, less than 1% of healthcare service applicants then were rejected for "health" reasons. A later audit carried out on pre-placement assessments in an NHS Trust had similar findings of 98.5% of employees passed fit without comment, 1.5% passed "fit with comments" (i.e. with some form of work restriction), and no employee found unfit for work (Lucey, 2008). This begs the question of an economic case for the practice of pre-employment medical screening.

Apart from the medical considerations, pre-employment medical examinations are sometimes advocated by employers to protect their economic interests (Lee and Koh, 2008). They may view candidates with risk factors for disease and having chronic illnesses, regardless of their ability to do the job, as being less preferable for employment because of perceived costs that may be incurred by their organisations. These business (and sometimes political) decisions should be distinguished clearly from medical decisions for screening based on sound evidence. Occupational physicians may face an ethical dilemma in performing health screening procedures that may have very limited value (e.g. checking for hernias or varicose veins as a matter of routine for every new employee) or may possibly be harmful (e.g. frequent x-rays of the chest or spine with no clear clinical justification). These are far from being theoretical dilemmas; they are commonly encountered by company medical officers engaged to conduct pre-employment health assessments.

There are industry guidelines and official guidance that recommend fitness standards for specific jobs such as firefighters, pilots, drivers, divers, sea-farers, and workers assigned to other safety-critical tasks (National Fire Protection Association, 2018; International Civil Aviation Organization, 2018; Driver and Vehicle Licensing Agency, 2021; International Maritime Organization, 2013). This is because any resulting safety incidents affect not just the worker, but have wider and direct implications on the safety of his co-workers and the public. Selection and periodic review of the health status of these vocationalists is therefore a continuing and stringent process.

Pre-Placement Screening

Pre-employment screening has been replaced by pre-placement screening in some countries. The main difference is that the individual is first offered employment on the basis of experience and ability to do the job, and then the pre-placement assessment is conducted to see if any adjustments are necessary to place the person in the assigned workplace.

Case Study 3: Pre-Placement Evaluation Prior to Disaster Response

Medical pre-placement evaluation was provided for workers engaged in the incident response to the Deepwater Horizon oil spill, one of the largest marine oil spill in history. The oil leak extended to more than 149,000 square kilometres of the Gulf of Mexico. Massive response and clean-up activities were carried out by over 47,000 workers, who were at risk of inhalational and skin exposure to crude oil, weathered oil, dispersants, solvents used to clean boats, and other chemicals (Michaels and Howard, 2012). Pre-placement assessment for the workers included obtaining medical and job activities information, a targeted physical examination, and additional procedures such as specific occupational health advice to workers of the risk posed by their medical conditions, and recommendations for specific training (e.g. use of respirator) prior to deployment (National Institute for Occupational Safety and Health, 2018).

Apart from targeted medical examinations and tests, some occupations also employ a "trade test", which is function-based testing as part of pre-placement screening. Harbin and Olson (2005) showed that the application of physical capacity testing for new hires, which is comparable with the lifting requirements in a food production plant, correlates with decreased work injury incidence. Visual demands analyses and testing have also been designed to complement standard visual evaluation for pre-placement screening of workers involved in quality inspection (Gowan, 2014).

Another example is the pre-placement vaccination screening of healthcare workers (HCWs) for infectious diseases common in the healthcare setting, such as measles, mumps, rubella, varicella and Hepatitis B. This allows unprotected HCWs to be vaccinated early and reduces their risk of occupationally acquired infections. In cases where HCWs refuse inoculation, such as against seasonal influenza, some institutions may implement a "vaccinate-or-mask" policy (Buynder *et al.*, 2015). A more contemporaneous topic is whether COVID-19 vaccination can be made mandatory for HCWs as a condition for employment, given their direct contact with populations at higher risk of SARS-CoV-2 infection. Most guidance issued advocate a process of informing and consenting (Faculty of Occupational Medicine (UK), 2021), though others have suggested that disincentives (such as placing unvaccinated HCWs on no-pay leave if they acquire COVID-19 infection, or even making vaccination a condition for employment for high risk occupations) may be employed as an indirect means to strongly encourage vaccination (WHO, 2021; Ministry of Manpower, 2021).

Periodic Medical Examinations

Medical examinations at periodic intervals may be prescribed by legislation, codes of practice, or offered as part of a company's policy or occupational health programme.

Statutory medical examination is prescribed by many countries' legislation for workers who are exposed to stipulated hazards at the workplace. These occupational hazards are highlighted for the closer monitoring of workers exposed to them because of their potential health impact. Statutory medical examinations are typically required for noise, asbestos, silica, lead, vinyl chloride monomer and other occupational hazards where the exposure limit for the worker exceeds the respective threshold limit values (or equivalent).

As an example, the United Kingdom has a provision under their Control of Asbestos Regulations (Health and Safety Executive, 2012) for medical surveillance for those involved in all work on asbestos-containing materials. They include a respiratory symptom questionnaire covering occupational information, respiratory symptoms, and a detailed smoking history; a clinical examination mainly of the respiratory system; and assessment of lung function at intervals of no more than two years as long as the worker is exposed to the work hazard. The US OSHA, in its medical surveillance guidelines for asbestos (OSHA, 1994), requires an annual review of workers' medical and work history; completion of a respiratory questionnaire; physical examination including a chest x-ray and lung function test; and any other investigations thought to be necessary by the examining physician. A medical review for the worker is also required at the point of employment separation. In addition to the frequency of medical screening, a major difference between the UK and US guidance is in the need for a chest x-ray. If the purpose of the x-ray is to detect early lung effects from asbestos, then routine x-rays may not show any relevant abnormality till many years after initial exposure to asbestos.

Companies may sometimes implement regular **screening to detect common chronic diseases** for their employees. Such screening can be included as part of a comprehensive occupational health programme and contribute to "total worker health," alongside measures to reduce risks from hazards at the workplace. Total worker health has been advocated by the National Institute for Occupational Safety and Health (2020) to improve worker health and well-being through a comprehensive programme of policies and practices that integrate workplace safety, protection from health hazards, and health promotion and prevention. Periodic health screening is an integral part of such programmes. By targeting the prevention, early detection and optimal control of chronic diseases in workers, this reinforces the important concept that a worker's health has a direct impact on work safety, and not only on work performance. A total and integrated approach that directly addresses the interdependency between health and safety has demonstrated benefits in positive health behaviours, and reducing employee medical leave consumption and medical claims (Chia *et al.*, 2014; Cooklin *et al.*, 2017).

Case Study 4: Statutory Medical Examination for Manganese

Workers from a ferroalloy smelting plant undergo a statutory medical examination every year. Their work involves maintaining and operating the smelting process, often requiring many of them to be within close proximity (less than 5 metres) of the smelting ovens. A reusable respirator is provided to every worker at the start of employment but these are not changed nor maintained regularly.

The urine manganese level of one of the workers was found to be 58 mcg/L (Biological Threshold Limit Value, or BTLV is 50 mcg/L). The affected worker did not report any symptoms. How should the worker be managed and what advice should be given to the plant's management?

Industries where workers may be exposed to manganese include production of steel and iron, welding operations with manganese-coated rods, manufacture of dry-cell batteries and chemicals such as potassium permanganate, among others. Inhalation of manganese fumes or dusts can lead to acute irritation of eyes and mucous members of the respiratory tract. Excessive chronic exposure may result in manganism, a central nervous system damage with clinical manifestations mimicking Parkinson's disease.

Statutory medical examination for manganese should be performed at pre-placement, as well as every 12 months with a focus on clinical examination of the central nervous system. Biological monitoring is performed with a urine specimen collected post-shift and at the end of the work week for urinary manganese estimation.

With urine manganese exceeding the BTLV, the worker should be suspended from his work involving further exposure to smelting fumes and clinically evaluated for signs and symptoms of poisoning. The urine manganese test should be repeated and if still elevated, a referral to a toxicologist may be considered. Serial monitoring of urine manganese should be performed every 3 months until it falls below the BTLV level. In the meantime, the worker should remain suspended from work on the production floor.

A workplace risk assessment should be carried out, which may involve measuring ambient air levels of manganese, and for the adequacy of control measures. Mandatory notification of the authority for workplace safety and health is required in most countries.

Return to Work Examinations

A period of prolonged illness with long periods of absence may have implications on fitness to work. Modern medicine has facilitated successful rehabilitation. In some cases, illness results in permanent impairment or disability. A review of current health, on-going treatment, and prognosis may be indicated. An example would be the case of a fireman recovering from a coronary event. Most fire departments would require a full medical assessment before allowing normal firefighting duties to be resumed.

In its position statement, the American College of Occupational and Environmental Medicine (ACOEM) advocated for the physician's role in facilitating an early return to work for the injured worker. This is through identifying barriers to work; providing recommendations on temporary restrictions on work activities, work function adjustment or workplace modifications; and care coordination with the employer and other stakeholders (ACOEM, 2017). Functional capacity evaluations (FCEs) are often used to assess the functional ability of the worker with a disorder, on his or her ability to undertake the physical requirements of the job. These are systematic approaches which translate work processes into physical constructs that can often be measured for the worker (e.g. static strength, physical endurance or stamina), which are then correlated back to what work tasks the worker can undertake upon return to work (Hoo, 2019). FCEs are often undertaken by the physician in conjunction with an occupational or physical therapist who is trained in assessing and interpreting the results of such evaluations. FCEs that are carefully selected or designed to be representative of the work requirements provide useful information to complement the assessment of the medical status of the worker by the physician.

Case Study 5: Return to Work Examination for a Worker with Stroke

A 54-year-old plumber presented with acute onset dizziness and left sided weakness while at work. He was quickly transferred to the Emergency Department of a nearby hospital, where he was diagnosed clinically with a cerebrovascular accident (stroke) even though the initial CT scan of the brain did not reveal any acute changes. Intravenous tissue plasminogen activator was administered in view of his early presentation. During inpatient monitoring over the next few days, his symptoms of left sided weakness improved but did not recover to the state which enabled him to ambulate independently. An MRI scan of the brain subsequently confirmed the diagnosis of a right middle cerebral artery stroke. He underwent physical rehabilitation for the next four months. He is now consulting his doctor for return to work assessment.

The severity of stroke is one of the most consistent predictors of return to work for stroke survivors (Ashley et al., 2019). The ability to walk and preserved cognitive ability are also indicators of a favourable prognosis of the ability to return to work (Vestling et al., 2003). Therefore, timely intervention with tissue plasminogen activator or thrombectomy if the patient presents early, are useful therapeutic options. Physical rehabilitation is effective for the recovery of function and mobility after stroke (Pollock et al., 2014). Secondary prevention with anti-platelet or anti-coagulant agent, good control of chronic diseases such as hypertension, dyslipidaemia and diabetes mellitus, as well as smoking cessation are important to reduce the risk of a future recurrence. This is also part of the longer term goal to improve the work ability of the worker.

In the return to work assessment, the physician should perform a physical assessment of the worker's neurological status, paying attention to any deficits in cognition, balance, gait, stiffness, strength and speech. Functional evaluation forms an important part of a holistic assessment and includes psychomotor abilities (e.g. control movement abilities), endurance and sensory abilities (e.g. visual, auditory and speech perception). If available, the services of a care coordinator can be engaged to coordinate return to work arrangements with the employer, in consultation with the worker, his physician and physical therapist, and identify job tasks that allow a graded return to work. Workplace interventions with components such as work ability assessments and workplace visits have been shown to be effective in facilitating return to work for stroke survivors (Ntsiea et al., 2015).

Genetic Screening at the Workplace

The success of the human genome sequencing has given further insights into the genetic influence of the human's biological effects to toxic hazards at the workplace. Genetic screening has been suggested as a basis for identifying workers with a predisposition for developing work-related diseases, and excluding them for specific jobs on the basis of "worker protection." Some genetic markers for disease are well established, but most are still at an early research phase, with uncertainty about the true level of risk especially following occupational exposures.

For example, individuals with sickle-cell anaemia have a genetically-determined haemoglobinopathy. Homozygotes with sickle-cell disease may develop haemolysis following exposure to low oxygen tension atmospheres as may be encountered in diving and flying. However, the risk for those with sickle-cell trait (heterozygotes) is much lower and adverse effects from occupational activity may be rarely encountered in practice. Screening for the presence of the abnormal haemoglobin (HbS) to detect affected individuals has led to difficulties in decisions regarding their exclusion from jobs as divers and pilots.

Another example is the increased susceptibility of individuals with the HLA-DPB1 gene to chronic beryllium disease if they are exposed to beryllium, a metal encountered in the telecommunications, automotive electronics and aerospace industries. Worker groups with specific high-risk genotypes have been found to have a prevalence of chronic beryllium disease from 42% to 72%, suggesting that genetic screening may be beneficial to identify vulnerable workers from cumulative over-exposure (Kreiss *et al.*, 2016).

The American College of Occupational and Environmental Medicine considers genetic testing conceptually as similar to other types of medical testing or screening, subject to the adherence to the relevant laws and codes of practice (Brandt-Rauf *et al.*, 2015). However, the organisation also recognises the ethical concerns such a form of testing may have on workers, such as the potential impact on the conditions of employment, work insurance coverage, and other considerations once such information is made discoverable. It therefore proposed that genetic screening related to work should be voluntary, and that the results should not be used to define the terms and conditions of employment.

The US National Institute for Occupational Safety and Health opined that "genetic monitoring may have some application in occupational health practice" insofar as how the understanding of the genetic influence on occupational exposures can improve prevention and control measures, and the identification of therapeutic targets for the development of better treatment modalities (National Institute for Occupational Safety and Health, 2014). However, it cautioned that genetic screening should not invidiously lead to the exclusion of the worker, when the focus remains to maintain a robust system for control of occupational hazards at the workplace.

Screening for Substance Abuse

Some organisations have programmes for periodic screening for alcohol and substance misuse amongst their workforce. The ethical, legal, and practical issues are considerable. If there is a need to introduce such screening, it should be conducted in accordance with an agreed policy that should apply to all employees regardless of rank. The practical issues include ensuring that there is a proper chain of custody for the biological sample collected, that those responsible for such testing, whether at in-house occupational health departments, or internal or external laboratory or clinical facilities, are trained for all stages from sample collection to dealing with the results of such testing.

The Civil Aviation Authority of Singapore introduced an Airport Alcohol Testing Programme to prevent and deter pilots from operating aircraft while under the influence of alcohol. The approach is calibrated to be risk-based random testing, taking into consideration factors such as whether a pilot displays signs of intoxication when reporting to work, or when reporting for work at overseas stations assessed to have a higher risk of alcohol misuse (Civil Aviation Authority of Singapore, 2019). If implemented, such a screening programme should be coupled with education on the health and occupational implications of the misuse of alcohol, and a support and rehabilitation programme to help pilots in need.

Conclusion

Different types of health screening in the occupational context carry specific objectives. Some are mandated by legislation or recommended as a standard under codes of practice, whereas others form part of a company's occupational health policy or programme. Notwithstanding, the occupational physician should also consider the preferences of the worker in decision making, especially if the health screening is for the purpose of determining work disposition. In formulating a recommendation, the physician should avoid being too prescriptive about inclusion or exclusion, and avoid prejudice and bias based on some imagined risk. Modern medicine has improved the therapeutic effectiveness and the prognosis in the work ability of workers across a spectrum of different disorders. Modern technology has also enabled those with an impairment to avoid it becoming a disability that prevents them from engaging in meaningful work. Health screening is therefore a tool that should be deployed judiciously to serve the purpose it is intended for, nothing more and nothing less.

References

ACOEM. (2017) *ACOEM Position Statement: The Personal Physician's Role in Helping Patients with Medical Conditions Stay at Work or Return to Work.* [Online] Available from: https://acoem.org/Guidance-and-Position-Statements/Guidance-and-Position-Statements/The-Personal-Physician-s-Role-in-Helping-Patients-with-Medical-Conditions-Stay-at-Work-or-Return-to. [Accessed on 7 July 2021].

ADA (Americans with Disabilities Act). (1990) *Information and Technical Assistance on the Americans with Disabilities Act.* [Online] Available from: https://www.ada.gov. [Accessed on 4 July 2021].

Ashley KD, Lee LT, Heaton K. (2019) Return to work among stroke survivors. *Workplace Health Saf* **67**(2): 87–94.

Brandt-Rauf P, Borak J, Deubner D. C, ACOEM Task Force on Genetic Screening. (2015) Genetic screening in the workplace. *J Occup Environ Med* **57**(3): e17–18.

Buynder PGV, Konrad S, Kersteins F, Preston E, Brown PD, Keen D, Murray NJ. (2015) Healthcare worker influenza immunization vaccinate or mask policy: Strategies for cost effective implementation and subsequent reductions in staff absenteeism due to illness. *Vaccine* **33**(13): 1625–1628.

Civil Aviation Authority of Singapore. (2019) *AC 99-3-1: Guidance on Airline Alcohol Management Programme (AAMP).* [Online] Available from: https://www.caas.gov.sg/docs/default-source/pdf/ac99-3-1-(rev-0)-guidance-on-aamp.pdf. [Accessed on 7 July 2021].

Chia SE, Chia A, Sng J. (2014) A total workplace safety and health service — what are the implications for the employees and employers? *Ann Acad Med Singap* **43**(9): 475–476.

Cooklin A, Joss N, Husser E, Oldenburg B. (2017) Integrated approaches to occupational health and safety: A systematic review. *Am J Health Promot* **31**(5): 410–412.

Dale AM, Descatha A, Coomes J, Franzblau A, Evanoff B. (2011) Physical examination has a low yield in screening for carpal tunnel syndrome. *Am J Ind Med* **54**(1): 1–9.

Dale AM, Gardner BT, Buckner-Petty S, Strickland JR, Evanoff B. (2016) Postoffer pre-placement screening for carpal tunnel syndrome in newly hired manufacturing workers. *J Occup Environ Med* **58**(12): 1212–1216.

Driver and Vehicle Licensing Agency. (2021) *Assessing Fitness to Drive: A Guide for Medical Professionals.* [Online] Available from: https://www.gov.uk/government/publications/assessing-fitness-to-drive-a-guide-for-medical-professionals. [Accessed on 4 July 2021].

Faculty of Occupational Medicine (UK). (2021) *COVID-19 Guidance on Vaccination and Testing.* London, FOM.

Gilbert N. (2020) The pros and cons of screening. *Nature* **579**(7800): S2–S4.

Gilligan T. (2020) Prostate cancer: To screen or not to screen? The question is complicated. *Cleve Clin J Med* **88**(1): 17–18.

Gowan NJ. (2014) Setting visual pre-placement testing in a technology manufacturing environment. *Work* **47**(3): 371–379.

Harbin G, Olson J. (2005) Post-offer, pre-placement testing in industry. *Am J Ind Med* **47**(4): 296–307.

Health and Safety Executive. (2012) *Guidance for Appointed Doctors on Medical Surveillance of Workers Doing Licensed Work With Asbestos.* [Online] Available from: https://www.hse.gov.uk/pubns/ms31.pdf. [Accessed on 5 July 2021].

Health and Safety Executive. (2021a) *Health Surveillance.* [Online] Available from: https://www.hse.gov.uk/health-surveillance/overview.htm. [Accessed on 29 June 2021].

Health and Safety Executive. (2021b) *HSE Workplace Health Expert Committee Report on SARS-CoV-2: Testing and the Workplace: Rapid Review to 16th February 2021.* [Online] Available from: https://www.hse.gov.uk/coronavirus/assets/docs/testing-and-the-workplace.pdf. [Accessed on 4 July 2021].

Hoo ERS. (2019) Evaluating return-to-work ability using functional capacity evaluation. *Phys Med Rehabil Clin N Am* **30**(3): 541–559.

Ilic D, Djulbegovic M, Jung JH, Hwang EC, Zhou Q, Cleves A, Agoritsas T, Dahm P. (2018) Prostate cancer screening with prostate-specific antigen (PSA) test: A systematic review and meta-analysis. *BMJ* **362**: k3519.

International Maritime Organization. (2013) *Guidelines on the Medical Examinations of Seafarers.* Geneva, IMO.

International Civil Aviation Organization. (2018) *Annex 1 to the Convention on International Civil Aviation — Personnel Licensing* (12th Ed), Geneva, ICAO.

Jonas DE, Reuland DS, Reddy SM, Nagle M, Clark SD, Weber RP, Enyioha C, Malo TL, Brenner AT, Armstrong C, Coker-Schwimmer M, Middleton JC, Voisin C, Harris RP. (2021) Screening for lung cancer with low-dose computed tomography: Updated evidence report and systematic review for the US Preventive Services Task Force. *JAMA* **325**(10): 971–987.

Kreiss K, Fechter-Leggett ED, McCanlies EC, Schuler CR, Weston A. (2016) Research to practice implications of high-risk genotypes for beryllium sensitization and disease. *J Occup Environ Med* **58**(9): 855–860.

Lee SM, Koh D. (2008) Fitness to work: Legal pitfalls. *Ann Acad Med Singap* **37**(3): 236–240.

Lucey S. (2008) Audit of pre-placement assessments undertaken in an NHS Trust. *Occup Med (Lond)* **58**(7): 512–514.

Mackie J. (2008) Effective health surveillance for occupational asthma in motor vehicle repair. *Occup Med (Lond)* **58**(8): 551–555.

Meneghini AC, Paulino ACB, Pereira LP, Vianna EO. (2017) Accuracy of spirometry for detection of asthma: A cross-sectional study. *Sao Paulo Med J* **135**(5): 428–433.

Michaels D, Howard J. (2012) Review of the OSHA-NIOSH response to the Deepwater Horizon oil spill: Protecting the health and safety of cleanup workers. *PLoS Curr* **4**: e4a83b7576b6e.

Ministry of Manpower. (2021) *Advisory on COVID-19 Vaccination in Employment Settings.* [Online] Available from: https://www.mom.gov.sg/covid-19/advisory-on-covid-19-vaccination-in-employment-settings. [Accessed on 4 July 2021].

National Fire Protection Association. (2018) NFPA 1583. *Standard on Comprehensive Occupational Medical Program for fire Departments.* Quincy, NFPA.

National Institute for Occupational Safety and Health. (2014) *Genetics in the Workplace.* [Online] Available from: https://www.cdc.gov/niosh/topics/genetics/default.html. [Accessed on 7 July 2021].

National Institute for Occupational Safety and Health. (2018) *Medical Pre-placement Evaluation for Workers Engaged in the Deepwater Horizon Response.* [Online] Available from: https://www.cdc.gov/niosh/topics/oilspillresponse/preplacement.html. [Accessed on 5 July 2021].

National Institute for Occupational Safety and Health. (2020) *NISOH Total Worker Health® Program.* [Online] Available from: https://www.cdc.gov/niosh/twh/default.html. [Accessed on 5 July 2021].

Ntsiea MV, Aswegen HV, Lord S, Olorunju SS. (2015) The effect of a workplace intervention programme on return to work after stroke: A randomised controlled trial. *Clin Rehabil* **29**(7): 663–673.

OSHA. (1994) *Occupational Safety and Health Standards No. 1910. Medical Surveillance Guidelines for Asbestos.* [Online] Available from: https://www.osha.gov/laws-regs/regulations/standardnumber/1910/1910.1001AppH. [Accessed on 5 July 2021].

OSHA. (2021) *Medical Screening and Surveillance.* [Online] Available from: https://www.osha.gov/medical-surveillance/screening. [Accessed on 29 June 2021].

Pachman J. (2009) Evidence base for pre-employment medical screening. *Bull World Health Organ* **87**(7): 529–534.

Pollock A, Baer G, Campbell P, Choo PL, Forster A, Morris J, Pomeroy VM, Langhorne P. (2014) Physical rehabilitation approaches for the recovery of function and mobility following stroke. *Cochrane Database Syst Rev* **2014**(4): CD001920.

Rembold CM. (1998) Number needed to screen: Development of a statistic for disease screening. *BMJ* **317**(7154): 307–312.

Salmi LR, Coureau G, Bailhache M, Mathoulin-Pelissier S. (2016) To screen or not to screen: Reconciling individual and population perspectives on screening. *Mayo Clin Proc* **91**(11): 1594–1605.

Schaafsma FG, Mahmud N, Reneman MF, Fassier J-B, Jungbauer FH W. (2016) Pre-employment medical examinations for preventing injury, disease and sick leave in workers. *Cochrane Database Syst Rev* **2016**(1): CD008881.

Thorat YT, Salvi SS, Kodgule RR. (2017) Peak flow meter with a questionnaire and mini-spirometry to help detect asthma and COPD in real-life clinical practice: A cross-sectional study. *NPJ Prim Care Respir Med* **27**(1): 32.

UK NSC. (2000) *Second Report of the UK National Screening Committee.* UK Department of Health.

UK NSC. (2021) *Guidance: The Pros and Cons of Screening.* [Online] Available from: https://www.gov.uk/guidance/the-pros-and-cons-of-screening. [Accessed on 29 June 2021].

United Kingdom. (2010) *Equality Act 2010.* [Online] Available from: https://www.legislation.gov.uk/ukpga/2010/15/contents. [Accessed on 4 July 2021].

Vandenplas O, Suojalehto H, Cullinan P. (2017) Diagnosing occupational asthma. *Clin Exp Allergy* **47**(1): 6–18.

Vestling M, Tufvesson B, Iwarsson S. (2003) Indicators for return to work after stroke and the importance of work for subjective well-being and life satisfaction. *J Rehabil Med* **35**(3): 127–131.

Whitaker S, Aw TC. (1995) Audit of pre-employment assessments by occupational health departments in the National Health Service. *Occup Med (Lond)* **45**(2): 75–80.

Wilson JMG, Jungner G. (1968) *Principles and Practice of Screening for Disease*. World Health Organization. Public Health Papers No: 34.

WHO. (2021) *COVID-19 and Mandatory Vaccination: Ethical Considerations and Caveats*. Geneva, WHO.

Chapter 23

Rehabilitation and Return to Work

*Nerys Williams**

Introduction

The links between health and work have long been recognised by many including physicians. However, it is only relatively recently that healthcare practitioners, employers and the general public have become aware of the benefits of employment and the disadvantages of unemployment for people with chronic long term health conditions.

Rehabilitation: Why Rehabilitate?

Rehabilitation and return to work is essential for both financial and health reasons, and for the individual and their family, their employer and society as a whole. In 2018 in the UK, sickness absence due to sickness or injury amounted to 141.4 million days, the equivalent of 4.4 days per worker. Groups with the highest sickness absence rates were women, part time workers, older workers with long term health conditions and workers in larger organisations of more than 500 employees.

*Consultant Occupational Physician, Birmingham, England, United Kingdom
Corresponding author: Nerys Williams (neryswilliams1443@gmail.com).

Trends suggest that sickness absence rates are reducing for some groups, at least in the UK. The largest reductions over the last 10 years are in workers with long term health conditions, those aged 50–64 and those in the public sector (Office for National Statistics, 2018). This excessive and sometimes prolonged sickness absence results in all round losses, for the employer, the employee and for society.

An independent review of evidence (Waddell and Burton, 2006; Office for National Statistics, 2018) found that "good" work was generally beneficial for both physical and mental health for people who develop long term illnesses. This was also true for disabled people and people with common health conditions (e.g. mental health disorders such as stress, anxiety and depression, which are the commonest cause of absence in developed countries such as the UK, parts of Europe and the Americas).

The physical and mental health effects of unemployment and being out of work have been well documented. The health effects of being out of work include a 20% excess mortality, 2–3 times the risk of poor general health and 2–3 times the risk of poor mental health (Young and Bhaumik, 2011).

At a social level, not having a job is also associated with poverty and social exclusion. As well as preventing the negative impact of unemployment, work can be an important part of recovery from illness although it is often not viewed as such by clinicians. A return or the gaining of employment can be used as an indicator of the success of medical treatment but unfortunately relatively few clinical studies consider employment as an outcome measure. This is changing in the field of mental health with documented outcome indicators such as employment status now routinely recorded by NHS mental health hospitals and community treatment in the UK.

The evidence of the health benefits of work means that the rehabilitation of sick and injured workers is crucial at an individual level but it is also important at a societal level for two reasons.

Firstly, because unemployed people have more ill health they also use more healthcare resources and are less successful at attempts to adopt healthy behaviours (Table 1). Secondly, due to the ageing populations across the UK, Europe and wider afield it is becoming more and more important that the workforce is capable of working and

Table 1. Specific Risks of Being Out of Work

Specific Risks of Being Out of Work
Out of Work Individuals are:
More likely to smoke (Wilson and Walter, 1993)
Drink alcohol (Janlert and Hammarstrom, 1992)
Indulge in sexual risk behaviours (Hammarstrom and Janlert, 1997)
Out of Work Individuals have a Higher Frequency of:
Use of healthcare services (Studnicka, 1991)
Admission to a psychiatric hospital (Agerbo *et al.*, 1998)
Out of Work Individuals are Likely to be:
Less physically active than employed people (Underlid, 1996)
Obese (Morris *et al.*, 1992)
Less successful at stopping smoking (Burgess *et al.*, 2009)

working longer in order to support both older and younger generations. This means workers need to stay fit and remain working for as long as possible and one way of achieving this is to ensure that countries have proactive approaches to promoting workers' health and active rehabilitation policies and programmes.

The evidence review (Waddell and Burton, 2006) on the benefits of work and the harm of a lack of work has had significant policy impact in the UK and has led to a change in the way sickness is certified, with the subsequent introduction of the "Fit Note" in 2010.

Why Rehabilitation is of Wider Importance

Being in work provides more than just money. Status, discipline and social contact are just some of the benefits. For people who are unemployed, being rehabilitated back into work can raise self-esteem and reduce psychological distress and minor psychiatric disorders as well as improving quality of life for the individual and their family.

Case Study 1: Importance of Proactive Rehabilitation

Jan is a 45-year old nurse working on a busy medical ward. She developed breast cancer and was off work for 6 months while she underwent surgery and chemotherapy. When she was well, in between courses of treatment, she would sit at home and watch daytime TV. Her husband, family and friends were all at work and her two children were at school, so she spent most of the day on her own. She became bored and started to worry about minor issues at home. When she returned to work, on part-time hours, she was initially tired at the end of her shift but found that the busy pace of the ward helped her to forget her domestic worries. Her psychological well-being improved within a few days and when the tiredness wore off, she felt much better and more like her old self.

Jan illustrates some of the basic points underpinning a proactive rehabilitation approach, namely:

1. Returning to work is generally good for both physical and mental health.
2. Employees do not need to be 100% fit to return to work.
3. Work can act as a therapeutic agent and facilitate recovery.
4. Flexibility about changes to the job/hours/tasks can aid return and reintegration.

Vocational Rehabilitation

There are many definitions of "vocational rehabilitation" but one which has become widely recognised is "whatever helps someone with a health problem stay at, return to and remain in work" (Waddell *et al.*, 2008). This definition recognises that it is more than just medical treatment which is needed for a person to return to work and that social and workplace factors are also important. Sometimes it is not the medical condition or its treatment at all which keeps someone away from work — it may be their attitude and beliefs towards their condition and the social milieu around them. Sometimes it is their relationship with their line manager or work colleagues.

Waddell *et al.* (2008) concluded that there was a strong evidence base for many aspects of vocational rehabilitation and more evidence on cost benefit than in many areas of health and social care policy. They suggested that common health problems be given priority for a vocational rehabilitation approach because these account for two-thirds of sickness absence and long term disability claims.

In terms of what was needed, the evidence suggests that in the first 6 weeks or so of absence, people can be helped to return to work with a few basic principles of healthcare and workplace management. This can be cost neutral. For only around 5–10% of the workforce, additional help may be needed at around 6 weeks of sickness absence.

The key messages from this review were:

1. Successful vocational rehabilitation requires work-focused healthcare and flexible workplaces. On their own, neither is sufficient; it must be a combined approach.
2. A stepped care approach is needed — i.e. providing what is needed at the right time. Do not waste resources on people who will get better anyway. Use resources for the people who need help at around 6 weeks or more.
3. Early intervention is key.
4. Co-ordinated communication between the individual, the employer and the general practitioner (GP), and other members of the healthcare team is very important to ensure a common shared understanding of who needs to do what, by when, to return someone to work.

It is this evidence which formed the basis of the British Fit for Work service (FFWS).

The Fit for Work Service

The FFWS was a British state funded health and work assessment and primarily telephone-based advisory service which operated from 2015 to 2018. The service was run in England and Wales by Health Management Limited (HML) and in Scotland by the Scottish Government via NHS Scotland on behalf of the Department for Work and Pensions (DWP). It aimed to provide impartial work related advice to GPs, employers and employees and can support an individual to both stay in and return to work. A key element of the service was "myth busting" and challenging attitudes and beliefs which kept people off work.

The service offered the following:

Advice

A free of charge advice line available for everyone, be they employed, self-employed, trade union or worker representatives, or members of the public. It was delivered by a website chat and separate telephone line.

Assessment

The assessment service was available for referrals from GPs for employees who had reached, or were expected to reach, 4 weeks of sickness absence and for employers when their employees reached 4 weeks of absence and had not been referred by the GP. The "4-week" referral point was important because evidence suggested that 4–6 weeks was the critical point for not returning to work. Referral was entirely voluntary and consent had to be obtained from the employee before the service contacted the individual or carried out an assessment.

The aim of the assessment was to identify all obstacles preventing a return to work and to recommend interventions that would aid return. This included advice on external organisations that could provide support. The output of the assessment was a return to work plan which, with the employee's consent, was shared with the GP and /or employer and any nominated third party, e.g. occupational health (OH) advisor. Assessment was primarily delivered by telephone but face to face assessments were undertaken for complex issues and for those which could not be dealt with on the telephone.

One of the key concerns of existing OH providers was how the new service would relate to them. In order to address this, the design of the service included always asking those individuals being assessed, if there was an OH service at their place of work and encouraging them to consent to OH getting a copy of the return to work plan.

The setting up of the service meant that small and medium sized businesses and even micro businesses (those with less than 10 employees) had access to work focused advice to help their employees return to work earlier than they may have done if just managed clinically by their family doctor or GP.

The FFWs was designed to operate according to several underlying evidence-based principles, namely:

1. that employees did not need to be 100% fit to return to work;
2. that treatment and return to work could occur together at the same time and should not occur one after the other;
3. that a shared understanding of who needs to do what by when is essential for the employee to return to work and finally;
4. that a return to work is facilitated by work focused healthcare and flexible workplaces.

The service was not primarily about providing more medical advice. The FFWs made the presumption that the GP and NHS were providing the healthcare that was needed but if there were delays, e.g. in accessing "talking therapies" such as cognitive behaviour therapy or physical treatments such as physiotherapy that may help a return, then the Government also introduced a financial incentive (a tax exemption for up to a specified limit, currently 500 GBP on medical treatments recommended by the assessment.)

Unfortunately uptake and referrals for the service from both GPs and employers were of low volume and so in 2019 the UK Government suspended the telephone and face to face elements of the service leaving the remaining aspects (website and chat function) to continue. The service demonstrated that even an evidence based approach which was clear and practical, could not succeed without better marketing and advertising of the service.

How Myths Impact Returning to Work

One of the key elements of the consultation with the healthcare professional within the FFWs was the exploding of myths about symptoms and workability. An example of how the service supported workers is shown in Case Study 2.

Case Study 2: Myths about Return-to-Work

Hans is an 18-year old office worker. He injured his back one day when reaching out to put some filing on a top shelf of a filing cabinet. His lower back was very painful for 3 weeks before it began to recover. The pain has gradually subsided and Hans is able to go to the gym and run on a treadmill for 30 minutes without any additional pain. He is off work and is reluctant to return until he is totally pain free as he thinks an early return before he is fully recovered will make the pain worse. He is afraid his back might be injured and damaged again.

In this case study, Hans is expressing some very common myths about back pain. He has a sedentary job yet he feels he must be 100% recovered and pain free to return to the office. He believes that returning to work will make his back pain worse and that will mean more damage to his spine. This again is a myth, pain does not equal damage. Despite the fact that Hans has recovered significantly (as evidenced by his gym schedule) he remains off work not because of the level of back pain or degree of disability but because of his beliefs about the pain. The intervention of a healthcare professional familiar with the biopsychosocial model of disability, using an evidence based approach, can address this myths and misconceptions and facilitate a return to work for Hans.

Models of Disability

The Medical Model

Doctors, nurses and healthcare professionals are trained in the "medical model" of disability, i.e. that it is the medical condition which prevents an individual from working. Their approach believes that if the condition is properly treated (and "cured") then the person will return to work. But the case study above and several studies show this is not the case. Research across many conditions rheumatoid arthritis (Bjork *et al.*, 2009), spinal cord injury (Young *et al.*, 2009), low back pain (Anema *et al.*, 2009) and common health conditions (Waddell *et al.*, 2008) shows that recovery from a health condition, reduction of symptoms and improvement in function does not directly lead to return to work. This clearly suggests that other, non-medical factors, are keeping a person from work, so what is needed is more than just additional or different treatment.

In the Medical model, the person has the disability — the problem — and what is needed is the doctor, nurse or therapist (the expert who has the power) to treat them. This is a single dimension approach which does not recognise the psychological and social factors impacting on return to work.

The Social Model

In the social model of disability it is the environment not the condition which is disabling the person and it is the environmental barriers to participation which need to be removed. The person is viewed as disabled because society has been designed to exclude them.

The Biopsychosocial Model

The biopsychosocial model contains elements of the medical and social models. This model considers not only the health condition (physical and mental) and its treatment but also the person's attitudes and beliefs about their health and work, the social and workplace environments and influencing factors such as finances and relationships with work colleagues and managers.

Case Study 3: Application of the Different Models of Disability to a Case

Tony is a 19-year old university student who is a wheelchair user due to spina bifida. He is unable to attend some of his lectures because they are held in a lecture theatre on the second floor of an old historic building that does not have a lift or wheelchair access.

Applying the medical model Tony is disabled by his spine bifida. If his spina bifida could be "cured" he could fully participate and attend his lectures. The solution appears to be to provide more treatment.

Applying social and biopsychosocial models Tony would be considered to be disabled by society and by his university which has selected a non accessible venue for the lectures. He does not need more treatment but instead the university needs to remove the barriers and allow him to participate and attend the lectures. Tony does not have a disability although he is being disabled by his surroundings and the man-made design of the space he occupies.

Case Study 4: Application of the Different Models of Disability to a Case

Pritti is a 35 year old secretary who was involved in a road traffic accident, injured her neck (a "whiplash injury") and became anxious about returning to drive her car but felt confident she could manage. But on returning to driving she noted that her anxiety symptoms were made much worse in busy rush hour traffic at the time when she usually travelled to work. Her neck pain gradually improved over 6 weeks and she was keen to return to work but when she got in her car on her first day she became very anxious and could not finish the journey. She panicked and returned home and phoned in to talk to her line manager to tell her what had happened. The line manager told Pritti that she really needed to come to work the following day as work was building up and she no longer had a valid "fit note." This made Pritti even more anxious.

The Medical model would suggest that Pritti has had an exacerbation of her anxiety and that is the problem preventing her from going to work. So what she needs is treatment for the heightened anxiety — medication such as anxiolytics for example, and/or counselling or cognitive behaviour therapy.

The social model would suggest that what Pritti needs flexibility from her environment is e.g. travelling before or after, but not during the rush hour. The social model would argue that Pritti is really being disabled, not by the anxiety, but by the fact her employer expects her to drive to and from work to start and finish at set times. If she did not have to travel in rush hour, then she would not have such disabling symptoms and may be able to participate in the workplace.

The biopsychosocial model encompasses both approaches — therapy may help in the long term to allow Pritti to travel in busy traffic in the future but for now, an adjustment of her start and finish time (thus keeping her hours worked the same) is one answer to remove the obstacle to Pritti returning to her job now. Another option may be to allow her to work from home while she undergoes treatment. Both adjustments achieve the same outcome — the lessening of the anxiety stopping her working, through the avoidance of rush hour traffic. But each option offers a different solution for the employer — one they could tailor to their specific business needs and how they arrange the work. Different employers may find one option more acceptable than the other or may achieve the same outcome with a different adjustment.

This is an example of work focused healthcare and a flexible workplace which the evidence suggests is the correct approach to take in vocational rehabilitation and the one most likely to yield return to work results.

Case Management

In the case study above what was needed was someone to facilitate the return to work and make suggestions as to how both parties could satisfactorily achieve their goals. Increasingly in OH practice, case managers are used to coordinate and facilitate a return to work in people on long-term sick leave. There are many definitions of case management. The Case Management Society of America (CSMA) describes case management services as "provided by healthcare professionals working with people to identify issues and barriers that may prevent them from getting better and uncovering mutually agreed upon solutions to achieve their healthcare goals." They describe case managers as working "with individuals and families to understand their illness or injury, what the individual/family needs to do to participate with the clinical team, follow the treatment plan and the path to reaching the best possible outcomes" (CSMA, 2015).

In contrast, the UK Case Management Society (CMS) describes case management as "a collaborative process which assesses, plans, implements, co-ordinates, monitors and evaluates the options and services required to meet an individual's health, care, educational and employment needs, using communication and available resources to promote quality cost-effective outcomes" (Case Management Society United Kingdom, 2020). This definition and approach has been most widely adopted in occupational medicine and OH practice.

In OH, the case manager is pivotal to the success of a vocational rehabilitation plan, and in the planning of an early return to work for the right type of employee at the right stage of their absence. Too early and it is a waste of case management resource as the person is likely to return anyway. Too late and any interventions become less likely to succeed.

The optimum time, according to Waddell, Burton and Kendall (Waddell *et al.*, 2008) is to intervene around the 6 week of sickness absence mark. Before this time, provided the employer does not put barriers in the way of return, the employee is likely to return to work anyway without intervention. In terms of contact with the employee this usually means managers requesting referrals at around 4 weeks of absence to allow for waiting times, holidays and leave, and so on, so that the person is seen around 6 weeks of absence when intervention is at its most effective.

Flags

When seen by the Case Manager, a history of the condition preventing work and its treatment is usually taken, and using a biopsychosocial approach, the person's attitudes and beliefs and those of relatives are sought. It is very important that the case manager explores relationships at work, with immediate managers and colleagues as well as these are often involved in the causation and prolongation of the absence.

The assessment also needs to include issues such as debt and financial trouble and relationship stressors outside of work as this is a holistic (whole person) approach rather than a focused workplace enquiry.

If the case manager identifies an issue which is an obstacle to return to work, they can use a system known as the "flags." These are a set of colored flags which denote health, psychological (attitudes and beliefs), workplace and societal factors which may influence a return to work. The flags act as a tool for the case manager.

Each flag denotes an obstacle that needs to be overcome and the case manager can use a variety of methods to achieve resolution including referral to external organisations for issues such as debt counselling, caring support and education.

Clinicians will be familiar with clinical red flags suggesting significant conditions such as cauda equina or cancers.

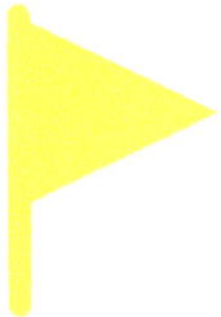

Yellow flags represent psychological factors (such as unhelpful beliefs about not recovering, catastrophising (believing that something is worse than it actually is) and adopting passive coping strategies).

Blue flags represent thoughts and views on work and health including the workplace. Can include fear of re-injury, lack of flexibility regarding work time and tasks, and problems with the line manager.

Black flags represent context and societal issues. This includes negative beliefs of family or employer, financial or legal issues with the employer (e.g. personal injury claim), and other family responsibilities.

The following case studies illustrate the flags at work and how the case manager can identify them and relevant in-place solutions to resolve the obstacles.

Case Study 5: Identifying Flags and Implementing Solutions

Jim is a 55-year old foundry worker who cares for his mother at home. She has early dementia and recently her cognition has deteriorated so that she becomes confused. Jim is reluctant to return to work after his recent hernia repair as he has been avoiding all lifting and bending and is concerned his job may cause injury and damage his surgical repair. He has also seen the benefit of his 24 hour a day attendance at home. It is his concern about re-injury and for his mother which prevents him returning. The case manager identifies this and discusses the operation and how his body is now stronger than before. She also signposts Jim to the local social work department and to the "Admiral nurses" (healthcare professionals specifically trained to help support people with dementia and their careers). They and the social worker can help Jim access social security benefits and career support such as a day center to help him feel happier about leaving his mother and returning to work.

Case Study 6: Identifying Flags and Implementing Solutions

Joachim is a 58-year old car salesman who has been away from work with 'stress' for the last 6 weeks. His case manager discusses the origins of his stress with him. He says that he has worked for the business for 30 years. He enjoyed his job until a new manager arrived 12 months ago and since then his life has "been hell". He feels that his manager asks for more sales and a higher standard of work than he does from the other salesmen. The manager gives the better jobs and cars which are easier to sell to newer, younger salesmen leaving Joachim to sell older less attractive cars which are more difficult to sell and so reduce his chance of his bonus. He has come to rely on the bonus to pay his mortgage and he is now in debt. The manager has been even more demanding than usual in the last 3 months and Joachim was reprimanded in front of the junior salesmen. He then felt that he could 'take no more' and so went off sick with stress.

He cannot see a solution– he must work to pay off his debt but cannot stand the manager and feels bullied by him. He is torn between resigning (but that would cause problems with debt) or returning (but that means he will face more stress from the manager).

The case manager identifies a blue flag indicating the workplace relationship as an obstacle. He signposts Joachim to a debt counselling agency and provides a contact number for a Government service which advises employees on their employment rights. Together they access a bullying helpline provided by trade unions. Joachim develops a clear plan to raise the issue with a Director of the company. The case manager offers support via a telephone call before and after the meeting. The Director listens to Joachim's concerns and follows the company procedure by asking another Senior Manager to investigate Joachim's claims. The manager apologises to Joachim as he says he was unaware of the problem.

The Fit Note, Adaptations and Adjustments

The findings of the evidence review by Waddell and Burton (Waddell and Burton, 2006) have profoundly affected the approach of the UK Government to sickness certification. For decades UK doctors (usually GPs/family practitioners) could certify workers only as fit or unfit. The worker would then take the "sick note" as it was called, to their employer and present it as evidence of their inability to work. The evidence review identified that workers did not need to be 100% fit to return to work and instead of being a "two-option only" decision as to their fitness or unfitness, there was a need for a middle ground.

After wide consultation and discussion, the "Sick note" was replaced by a new "Fit note" in 2010. The "fit note" allowed the examining doctor to suggest one or more types of adjustment to help the person return to work.

These include one or more of the following: A phased return to work, Altered duties, Altered hours, and Workplace adaptations.

Adjustments may be recommended by healthcare professionals, but in the UK it is the employer who has the decision to make as to whether the adjustment (whatever may be recommended) is to be implemented and is sustainable. The employer is best placed to know the demands of the work and what needs to be done to fulfil the requirements of the job, as well as how often and what other adjustment have been tried and are successful or have been stopped.

Phased Returns

A phased return need not always mean reduced hours. It is possible to phase a return to the specific component of the job that presents the challenge. Phased returns are the commonest applied adjustment to allow rehabilitation, but they are often overly long, unfocused on the issue that is the obstacle and sometimes open ended. The basic principles of phased returns are:

1. They should be aimed at returning the person to their usual job and are not a means of designing the dream job;
2. They should have a clear end date when the business reappraises whether it can continue to support any adjustments to the work schedule and times;
3. They should address the obstacle and not just gradually increase exposure/work;

4. They rarely need to exceed 3–4 weeks for most people except in conditions such as depression and chronic fatigue syndrome when it may take much longer.

Case Study 7: A Phased Return Following Injury

Anil is a 25-year old fabricator. His job is physical and involves considerable upper limb strength to assemble car seats by stretching fabric over a carcass and then stapling the fabric in place. He damaged his shoulder playing squash and required surgery to repair a torn rotator cuff muscle on his dominant side. Following a period of sickness absence, he was reviewed by Occupational Health who recommended a phased return to the job. Anil returned to work full time after an absence of 4 weeks and worked initially in the warehouse on dispatch duties using a computer for the first 3 days. He then returned to the job as a fabricator initially for 2 hours a day, then increasing the work hours so that he returned to his usual job as a full time fabricator in 4 weeks. At the end of each week his progress was reviewed with his supervisor who checked he was able to cope with the required work tasks. In some cases symptoms of fatigue may require a more gradual increase in work hours.

Case Study 8: A Phased Return for Chronic Fatigue Syndrome

Bella is a 49-year-old full-time university lecturer who has chronic fatigue syndrome (CFS). After a prolonged period of absence of 9 months she returns to work initially for 3 half days. During the first few weeks she updates herself on changes to the curriculum and staff, completes her mandatory training and works out lesson plans for her subjects. She is reintroduced to lecturing with a reduced commitment and no pastoral roles. Over the next 8 weeks she increases the amount of her usual job and increases her working day by an extra hour every 2 weeks. She had one setback when she was off for 4 days due to tiredness but on her return her duties and hours were modified slightly and she was able to continue. She returns to a ¾ time job in 8 weeks and decides that full time would be too much at this stage of her illness. Her employer agrees for her contract to be changed from full time to ¾ time.

Case Study 9: A Phased Return for a Cancer Patient

Marni is 40-year old dental receptionist who is undergoing treatment for breast cancer. She has been off work for 2 months during which time she has been fully investigated and has had a lumpectomy then a mastectomy. It is not expected that she will need chemotherapy or radiotherapy but her wound has broken down and she needs dressings three times per week at her local hospital. She reports tiredness but no other clinical symptoms. Her phased return to work begins midway into the 5th week initially working half days. She goes for dressings on her way home from the dental practice. The following week she works half days on the days she has dressings and full days on the other two days. The third week is the same and on the 4th week, as her dressings reduce in frequency, she works 4 days then the full 5 days. During this time, she undertakes her usual job of greeting patients, billing and typing referral letters. Her return to work plan also includes the availability of a rest room for her to rest, if needed, during her breaks (a workplace adaptation).

Case Study 10: Altered Duties

Pierre is a 20-year old retail assistant in a supermarket. He twists his back playing football and finds that stretching, bending and twisting is painful. He usually works stacking shelves, and on the checking out of purchased goods, both of which involve twisting of the back. The shelf stacking involves heavy lifting, stretching and bending. For a period of 3 weeks his employer moves him to a 'small items Kiosk' where he sits on a tall stool or stands and serves customers cigarettes, newspapers and lottery tickets, thus avoiding any bending, twisting and stretching.

His employer could have put him on the automatic scan section where customers scan their own groceries and the assistant verifies the customer's age to ensure eligibility to purchase alcoholic drinks, and deals with any problems with operating the machines–again avoiding bending, twisting and heavy lifting.

Case Study 11: Altered Hours

Jake is 18 years old and works as a kitchen assistant in a small restaurant in a rural area. He twists his ankle playing rugby and wears a supportive cast. He can do the job of the kitchen assistant as he can sit on a high stool to peel vegetables etc. and do washing up but he cannot drive and so cannot get to work. There is no suitable public transport. Jake normally works 9-1.30 pm returning again 4.30-6.30 pm for the lunch and supper sittings. His employer allows Jake to come in at 10 am and stay until 5.30 pm when he can get a lift home from his sister Pam who works in a neighboring shop. Jake undertakes the additional task of ordering and stock control.

Workplace Adaptations

Case Study 12: Change of Location

Myra, aged 52 years, has multiple sclerosis. She works as a data manager for a clothing company in an office which is located in a very old historic building which has a single lift and winding staircase. Myra is one of 3 data managers who work together at the single location on the first floor. Following her latest exacerbation of multiple sclerosis, she has to use a wheelchair as her mobility is greatly reduced. Her employer is concerned about how she will get out of the building in the event of a fire. Her employer conducts a risk assessment and concludes that Myra's current location carries too much of a risk so she relocates the whole team to the ground floor.

Conclusion

A review of the evidence has shown that the right type of work is beneficial for the majority of workers with disabilities and long term health conditions. But the workplace needs to be flexible to allow individuals who are less than 100% fit to return to work. A combination of flexible workplaces and work focused healthcare is needed to facilitate the return to work.

Good communication between clinicians providing treatment, the employee and employer is also crucial for success. Everyone needs a shared understanding of who needs to do what, by when, to overcome obstacles which can be identified by applying the "flags" approach. Intervention around 4–6 weeks of absence is likely to be the most cost effective in managing sickness absence.

Involving the employee themselves in finding workable solutions to obstacles can be beneficial and sometimes educational for the clinician but agreement by line managers as to what is feasible and the duration of proposed accommodation is important.

The decision as to whether any adjustment or adaptation is suitable and workable is a management decision, not an OH one, as only the manager knows the demands of the work and the capabilities of other work colleagues. Active management of absence using the evidence base, the biopsychosocial model and the system of "flags" can reduce sick leave and the risk of job loss due to prolonged absence thus benefiting the individual, their family, the employer and society.

References

Agerbo E, Eriksson T, Mortensen PB, Westergaard-Nielsen N. (1998) *Unemployment and Mental Disorders — an Empirical Analysis.* Centre for Labor Market and Social Research Working Paper No. 98-002.

Anema JR, Schellart AJ, Cassidy JD, Loisel P, Veerman TJ, Van der Beek AJ. (2009) Can cross country differences in return-to-work after chronic occupational back pain be explained? An exploratory analysis on disability policies in a six country cohort study. *J Occup Rehabil* **19**(4): 419–426.

Bjork M, Thyberg I, Balogh I, Gerdle B. (2009) Sick leave before and after diagnosis of rheumatoid arthritis-a report from the Swedish TIRA project. *J Rheumatol* **36**(6): 1170–0079.

Burgess DJ, Noorbaloochi S, Clothier B, Ricards J, Widome R, Van Ryn M. (2009) Employment, gender, and smoking cessation outcomes in low-income smokers using nicotine replacement therapy. *Nicotine Tob Res* **11**(12): 1439–1447.

Case Management Society of America. (2015) *What is Case Management?* [Online] Available from: http://solutions.cmsa.org/acton/fs/blocks/showLandingPage/a/10442/p/p-0003/t/page/fm/1. [Accessed on 2 Nov 2020].

Case Management Society United Kingdom. (2020) *What is Case Management?* [Online] Available from: https://www.cmsuk.org/case-management/what-is-case-management. [Accessed on 2 Nov 2020].

Hammarstrom A, Janlert U. (1997) Unemployment and sexual risk-taking among adolescents. *Scand J Public Health* **25**(4): 266–270.

Janlert U, Hammarstrom A. (1992) Alcohol consumption among unemployed youths: Results from a prospective study. *Br J Addict* **87**(5): 703–714.

Morris JK, Cook DG, Shaper AG. (1992) Non-employment and changes in smoking, drinking, and body weight. *Br Med J* **304**(6826): 536–541.

Office for National Statistics. (2018) *Sickness Absence in the UK Labour Market: 2018.* [Online] Available from: https://www.ons.gov.uk/employmentandlabourmarket/peopleinwork/labourproductivity/articles/sicknessabsenceinthelabourmarket/2018. [Accessed on 2 Nov 2020].

Studnicka M. (1991) Psychological health, self-reported physical health and health service use. *Soc Psychiatry Psychiatr Epidemiol* **25**(2): 86–91.

Underlid K. (1996) Activity during unemployment and mental health. *Scand J Psychol* **37**(3): 269–281.

Waddell G, Burton KA, Kendall NAS. (2008) *Vocational Rehabilitation — What Works, for Whom, and When?* Report for the Vocational Rehabilitation Task Group. London, The Stationery Office.

Wilson SH, Walter GM. (1993) Unemployment and health: A review. *Public Health* **107**(3): 153–162.

Young E, Murphy A, Gregory C. (2009) Employment status after spinal cord injury (1992–2005): A review with implications for interpretation, evaluation, further research, and clinical practice. *Int J Rehabil Res* **32**(1): 1–11.

Young V, Bhaumik C. (2011) *Health and Wellbeing at Work: A survey of Employees.* London, The Stationery Office.

Chapter 24

Workers' Compensation Schemes

Paul Cullinan and David Koh*[†]

Introduction

Rationale and Development of Workers' Compensation; Workplace Accidents

In most cultures, work is considered a "communal good," undertaken not only for the benefit of the individual but also that of their wider community. It follows, generally, that disease or an accident that arises from work — and would not otherwise have occurred — deserves recognition from the community; financial recompense, accompanied by provision of care to ameliorate the effects of the disease or accident, form the ethical basis of workers' compensation schemes. To the moral philosopher, workers' compensation is a matter of social justice owed to the harmed worker by a society that is dependent on its workforce to deliver its obligations to its members; to an economist, it is a

*Occupational and Environmental Respiratory Disease, National Heart and Lung Institute, Imperial College and Royal Brompton Hospital, London, England, United Kingdom.
[†] PAPRSB Institute of Health Sciences, Universiti Brunei Darussalam, Brunei Darussalam *and* Saw Swee Hock School of Public Health and Yong Loo Lin School of Medicine, National University of Singapore, Singapore.
Corresponding author: Paul Cullinan (p.cullinan@imperial.ac.uk).

correction to the failure of the market to provide employment that is free from the risk of adverse health outcomes.

The history of workers' compensation schemes stretches back further than many appreciate. Guyton (1999) describes Mesopotamian statutes, written on clay tablets around 4,000 years ago, which set out the sums to be paid for particular injuries to workers incurred during their employ, the fore-runners of modern injury schedules whereby specific injuries attract specified compensation. In medieval Europe, compensation was arbitrary and dependent on the *noblesse oblige* of more or less compassionate aristocrats but over several centuries a more formal system evolved through common law, a process accelerated by the mechanisation of industry and consequent increased risks of much employment.

The system became progressively hostile to claimants who found themselves increasingly restricted so that by the nineteenth century they were faced with what had become known as the "unholy trinity of defenses." "Contributory negligence" and the "common employment" or "fellow servant" defenses held that employers could not be found responsible for an employee's workplace accident if the worker — or a fellow employee — was in any way responsible for his injury. The consequence of these was that employees could mount a successful claim only if the employer had personally been negligent, an increasingly rare occurrence in large workforces such as those on the new railways or in mines. Another doctrine, that of the "assumption of risk", was especially restrictive as it held that an employee would know of the hazards of their job and that by agreeing to undertake it — generally at the start of employment — had assumed any risk it entailed, the so-called "right to die" contract.

The first shift away from this stance was probably a set of clauses in the Prussian Railroad Law of 1838 — at the time there were unmanageable numbers of railway accidents — which reversed the burden of proof and began the move towards "absolute" employer liability. In 1871, Chancellor Bismarck extended coverage to workers in mines, quarries and some factories through the Employers' Liability Law; and later (in 1884) championed Workers' Accident Insurance creating the world's first modern workers' compensation scheme. The government of Poland passed similar legislation in the same year and those of Austria and Czechoslovakia in 1887.

The principles were rapidly adopted in the United Kingdom (UK) where in the 1890s Joseph Chamberlain, president of the Board of Trade but originally a self-made businessman who owned a screw manufacturing company in Birmingham, argued for automatic compensation by employers for injuries occurring at work. Under the Workmen's Compensation Act of 1897, a fixed statutory scale defined somewhat limited payments for all injuries, regardless of whose negligence — if any — caused the accident. Workers were thus assured of at least modest compensation for all injuries they sustained at work, while employers could readily insure against a statutory maximum liability. As in Prussia, the Act removed the common law defenses described above, broadening the liability of employers who now had the same responsibility to their employees as they did to the public.

The Act was not passed without opposition. Member of Parliament Alexander Macdonald, originally a collier and a miners' leader, argued that "a system of insurance would be simply a system of license to destroy life." He — as did others at the time, and have since — suggested that a system of compulsory insurance with limited employers' liability freed them from both the legal and financial consequences of workplace accidents to their employees. As a consequence, incentives to improve worker safety and reduce the incidence of accidents at work were "sacrificed for minimum, albeit for the most part, assured payments for injuries." Sydney and Beatrice Webb (1897) described employers' contributions as "a flea-bite compared with the cost and trouble of adopting elaborate precautions that might totally prevent [the occurrence of workplace accidents]" and more recently, Mallino (1989) suggested that "employers for all practical purposes are paying little or nothing for occupational disease and, in fact, are being subsidised by the public welfare system and workers themselves." Markham Lester (2001), revisiting the matter in 2001, is uncompromising: "the economic compromise forged with the Workmen's Compensation Act of 1897 represented not a triumph of employer/employee co-operation, but rather the acceptance of the principle that workers' injuries were "nothing more than a cost of production." Whether workers' compensation schemes have an impact — positive or negative — on the rate of industrial accidents remains debated today.

At any rate, the principles espoused and enacted in Prussia and the UK were soon taken up elsewhere in Europe and in North America. By 1900, 11 countries had workers' compensation schemes; in 2012 this had risen to 136 (Williams, 2012), all except those in Australia, Canada and the United States of America (USA) based on a single national programme. In the USA, there was unusually fierce opposition, from both lawyers and doctors dealing with workers' claims, to the "blight brought to America from England and Germany" which was considered a "species of socialism" (Haller, 1988). In 1920, in comments which resonate still, WF Grinstead, the President of the Illinois State Medical Society complained about the "starvation rate" fees paid to doctors by insurance companies and about the plethora of forms they were required to complete.

Extension to Occupational Diseases

Compensation schemes aim to recompense workers for adverse occurrences that arise from their employment and would not otherwise have arisen. These criteria are, in general, readily obvious in the case of accidents in the workplace although there is some blurring around the edges, for example with accidents that occur during travel to or from work. Thus it is little surprise that workers' compensation schemes have — from antiquity — had their foundations laid in workplace injuries.

In the UK, the Workmen's Compensation Act of 1906 listed six *diseases* for which compensation was payable: poisoning by lead, arsenic, mercury or phosphorous, anthrax and anklyostomiasis (hookworm, at the time an occupational risk in bare-footed coal and tin miners). As with accidents, it was argued at the time that these were conditions whose occupational aetiology could readily be assumed in workers employed in relevant industries. Three of these (anthrax, lead and mercury poisoning) comprised, in 1925, the first List of Occupational Diseases of the International Labor Office (ILO). Kim and Kang (2013) provide an interesting history of subsequent iterations

Box 1. Recent Developments in Workers' Compensation — USA.

In the 1970s and 1980s, many states in USA passed legislation to expand the number of workers covered by Workers' compensation, and provide broader and more adequate benefits. Subsequently, from 1984 to 1990, employers' average costs per $100 of payroll rose by almost 50% from $1.49 to $2.18. In addition, the workers' compensation insurance industry was unprofitable every year from 1984 to 1992. The increased employer costs and reduced insurance profitability led to a pushback, with employers and insurers lobbying for legislation to reduce employer costs. The rationale was often framed as a means to improve one state's attractiveness to employers compared to other states. Unfortunately, this resulted in a "race to the bottom" for workers' compensation.

Boden (2020) has argued that since then, legislative efforts to reduce costs largely did not focus on improving safety or the efficiency of benefit delivery, but instead concentrated on reducing both medical costs and cash benefits to injured workers. Many of the laws passed since 1990 reduced costs by making it harder for people with occupational injuries and illnesses to receive compensation.

Over the last two decades, studies have demonstrated that many injured workers entitled to workers' compensation do not receive them. Benefits provided to those who receive them do not come close to replacing two thirds of lost earnings, the standard set by the National Commission on State Workmen's Compensation Laws. The failure of workers' compensation results in the costs of occupational injuries and diseases being transferred from this system of social insurance to families, communities, and other social programmes.

of this List with its heavy focus on industrial poisonings and classic disorders such as the pneumoconiosis and occupational skin cancer (first described in 1775).

The ILO list is the precursor of many others, such as those prepared by the member states of the European Union (2007) or in operation in Hong Kong (Hong Kong Labor Department, 2006), South Africa (Republic of South Africa Department of Labour, 2004), Germany (HVBG, 2002), Ontario (1994) and the Philippines; indeed most national jurisdictions have such a listing. It may surprise some that there are considerable variations in the diseases included in these lists and Kim and Kang record diseases which are considered occupational in some countries (such as snow blindness in India, or cerebral haemorrhage from psychological stress in Japan and Korea) that are *not* listed elsewhere. It follows that listing is not an entirely consistent practice.

Designation of an Occupational Disease

Case Study 1: Burnout and Covid-19: Are They Occupational Diseases?

Burnout - A survey of experts from 28 European Union countries revealed that burnout syndrome may be acknowledged as an occupational disease in nine countries (Denmark, Estonia, France, Hungary, Latvia, Netherlands, Portugal, Slovakia and Sweden). In Latvia burnout syndrome is explicitly included on the List of Occupational Diseases. Compensation for burnout syndrome has been awarded in Denmark, France, Latvia, Portugal and Sweden, with most of the compensated cases happening only recently. With growing recognition of psychosocial hazards at work, new systems to collect data on suspected cases have been developed. Furthermore, all the countries studied had an action plan to prevent workplace stress (Lastovkova et al., 2018).

Coronavirus Disease 2019 (COVID-19) — A direct attribution of COVID-19 to workplace exposure is often challenging, given that the virus can be contracted from other people in non-occupational settings. This area of law is evolving rapidly. At least four states in the USA (Alaska, Minnesota, Utah and Wisconsin) have legislated presumption of causation by work exposure for selected occupations, while several others (Arkansas, California, Florida, Kentucky, North Dakota, New Hampshire, New Mexico and Washington) have executive or administrative actions to institute such presumptions. Those covered differ by states, and have included healthcare workers, first responders, correctional officers, grocers, postal workers and the military. The worker's prior comorbidities or apportionment have not yet been directly incorporated into these new legislative and executive actions, although some states may have apportionment separately addressed in non-COVID regulations (Hyman et al., 2020).

In general, a disease is designated as "occupational":

1. If it appears to be specific to a particular occupation(s) in as much as it is not (or is only very rarely, in bizarre circumstances) observed elsewhere. Such diseases include, for example, coal workers' and other forms of pneumoconiosis, many types of poisoning and forms of musculo-skeletal disorders and, for the most part, pleural mesothelioma.
2. Others have an occupational aetiology that can be demonstrated at an individual level and in an individual claimant; these include occupational asthma or rhinitis, and many types of occupational dermatitis.
3. Others — probably many others — are not specific to an occupation, being seen in other circumstances also, but they occur more commonly in an occupational group than would otherwise be expected. Most occupational cancers fall into this category as do some types of osteoarthritis (such as of the hip, an affliction in farmers) and chronic obstructive airways disease (for example, in coal miners).

This third category gives rise to the greatest inconsistencies between national schedules. Driscoll and his colleagues considered the matter in some detail when reviewing the listing used in New Zealand (Driscoll *et al.*, 2011) and drew the distinction between lists designed formally to recognise that a disease *may* be related to work (and so be potentially compensable), and lists that formally identify disorders that are *likely* to be related to work and so can be attributed to work if sufficient relevant exposure can be confirmed.

These latter are commonly referred to as disease "schedules" and are used widely in workers' compensation schemes. Ideally, an occupational schedule would be confined to diseases for which there is strong, consistent scientific evidence of an association between its incidence and a work-related exposure. This is necessary to circumvent the need for an individual claimant to establish a connection between their work-related exposure and a resulting disease. Further, it is important that the work-related condition comprises a significant proportion of all cases of the disease in a population or in a readily identified subset of the population (such as an occupational group); more formally, the occupational population attributable fraction should be high. If applied carefully, this criterion allows the probable attribution of a workplace exposure (for example high cumulative exposure to asbestos) to a non-specific disease (such as lung cancer) in the case of an individual claimant. A third, pragmatic criterion is that scheduled diseases should be those in which a diagnosis is straightforward and — largely — unequivocal. While this is the case for many occupational disorders, others such as "anxiety" or some musculoskeletal conditions can prove problematic.

Internationally, the use of disease schedules in workers' compensation schemes is very variable; few European countries, for example, adhere strictly to the list prepared on their behalf by the European Union. In part this variation arises from strong cultural (and sometimes political) beliefs about what constitutes a work-related disorder. Coggon and colleagues, for example, in a survey covering 18 countries and six continents describe a ten-fold difference in the prevalence of "adverse" health beliefs about back and upper limb pain, and in awareness of terms such as "repetitive strain injury" (Coggon *et al.*, 2012). More significant determinants are probably historical, legal and administrative. Some countries, notably the UK, apply a strict schedule of "prescribed" diseases, with associated, qualifying exposures while the French list 112 scheduled diseases but have also a "systeme complementaire" which allows claims for unlisted conditions; in Finland, the schedule is "indicative" only. In contrast, the Swedish list includes only occupational infectious diseases and claims for all other diseases that could possibly have arisen from a workplace exposure are considered on an individual basis, an example of a so-called "open" system. The USA and Canada have no lists of compensable diseases and claims for any condition can be filed and are individually assessed by physicians and lawyers with adjudication by workers' compensation arbitrators.

Proponents of "closed" systems, with strict scheduling point to their administrative efficiency, their equity and their transparency. Under this approach, claimants do not have to prove that their disease was occupational in origin so long as the "prescribed" diagnosis is clear and they have met the statutory exposure criteria. In theory all claimants are treated consistently, and there are considerable savings on technical assessments of individual claims so that a greater proportion of what are usually limited funds can be directed to compensation.

The strict application of disease schedules, however, has several drawbacks. First, as above, the schedules themselves are internationally inconsistent. This is particularly so for diseases that are not specific to occupation; a good example is breast cancer. There is reasonably strong epidemiological evidence of a modest increase (a risk ratio of around 1.4) in the risk of breast cancer among women who have been shift-workers. In 2008, the International Agency for Research on Cancer (Straif *et al.*, 2007) classified shift working as "probably carcinogenic to humans," a decision that led the Danish National Board for Industrial Injuries to compensate women who developed breast cancer following a history of night working. In the UK, in contrast, the decision was made not to "prescribe" the condition on the grounds that the risk in shift-working women was not doubled (the attributable fraction is <50%) and thus it could not be ascertained with greater than 50% probability that an individual's breast cancer was attributable to their shift-work (Industrial Injuries Advisory Council, 2013). This inconsistency, between two countries that have most other practices in common, is driven not so much by science but by expediency, with a clearly inequitable result. In Denmark, some women whose breast cancer was not caused by their night work will be compensated; conversely, in the UK, individuals with cancer that was attributable, at least in part, to their night shifts will not receive compensation.

A second drawback of schedules is their failure to reflect modern working hazards. Again this applies chiefly to diseases that also have non-occupational causes for which there is often a lengthy lag in acquiring sufficient, robust scientific evidence to assess the occupational contributions to their aetiology. As a result, occupational disease schedules tend to be rich in the classic diseases of industry with a heavy gender bias towards working men; and in economically developed nations at least are likely to attract fewer and fewer claims. Walters (2007) remarks that all compensation schemes fail to deal with the predominant current conditions of work-related ill-health and there is no doubt that they reflect poorly the true burden of occupational disease. In this context it is notable that most European schemes and some in Asian countries (but not that in the UK) cover accidents incurred while travelling to or from work.

Eligible Benefits

Occupational injury and disease insurance systems are, in essence, designed to compensate workers for their loss of earnings arising from their inability to (continue) work consequent on the harm they have undergone. More advanced schemes aim also to help injured or disabled workers return to work and, in some cases, to improve the safety of work environments to reduce the incidence of future harm. This end may be achieved (or not) using several different means with, again, considerable variation between schemes.

Benefits for "incapacity" or "disability" are those paid to workers who have an inability, total or partial, temporary or permanent, to

Box 2. Terminology and Definitions (Knoblauch and Cassaro, 2020).

- Maximum medical improvement or maximum medical recovery: the employee has recovered from the injury at a level at which the provider states no further treatment will significantly change the outcome of the medical condition.
- Temporary total disability (TTD): the employee is unable to return to any continuous gainful employment due to an occupational illness or injury.
- Temporary partial disability (TPD): the employee is still under medical treatment for the work injury or illness but can return to work which has restrictions, or he/she is working at a lower-paying position than the pre-injury position.
- Permanent total disability (PTD): this is paid when the employee has a condition in which is permanent and completely incapacitates the employee, so the employee is not able to ever perform gainful employment.
- Permanent partial disability (PPD): this condition results in the loss of body part or lasting impairment that is estimated to be unlikely to improve, and there is a potential decrease in wage-earning ability.

perform one or more bodily or mental processes that are within the capacity of a normal person of the same age and sex; "disablement" generally refers to the sum total of all relevant disabilities. "Impairment" is a term generally used to denote the loss of anatomy or function of a body part or system. A permanent incapacity is one that remains after all medical, surgical or other forms of treatment have been completed, and is considered unlikely to improve spontaneously.

Determining and assigning the degree of incapacity is generally made by a specialist physician, guided by statutory schedules. This is a skilled task but one that is inevitably subjective, particularly so when assessing the incapacity arising from an occupational disease. Accidental injuries, especially those that have resulted in amputation, are more readily assessed through explicit schedules but most diseases require assessment and integration of several different dimensions. Guides to evaluation are available; perhaps the best known is that produced by the American Medical Association (2009) although this has been strongly criticised on several fronts, not least for its failing consistently to distinguish impairment from disability (Spieler *et al.*, 2000). The process is further complicated when assessing physicians are required to take into account the effects of pre-existing disease, or even predisposing factors. Unsurprisingly, most schemes incorporate a system of appeal for claimants who feel that their assessment has been inaccurate.

In some countries, such as the UK, benefits paid for incapacity are determined solely by the degree of disablement assessed as above and are independent of, for example, a worker's previous salary or future earnings prospects. In many other jurisdictions payments for both temporary and permanent incapacity are linked to a worker's reference salary. In some European countries (Austria, Belgium, Denmark, and Germany among them) the initial period of temporary incapacity is covered by the employer; after a defined period, payments are taken over by the state, usually — but not universally — at a reduced rate. The approaches to compensating workers for a permanent incapacity are very variable but generally follow one of two models. In the first, an indicative scale is used with more or less (or no) allowance for a worker's lost earning capacity. For accidents these scales are often derived from military compensation schemes; scaling for disability arising from occupational diseases is obviously more complex. The second model accounts not only for the physiological effects of a disability but also for the loss of any future earning power that is likely to arise from it. In some countries (such as Denmark) benefits are also tied to damage that affects life outside work. Payments may also be made for medical and associated expenses, generally in jurisdictions where these are not normally covered by the state.

Self-employed workers are seldom covered by state compensation schemes and must rely on individual pension arrangements. With the increasing use of zero-hour and other uncertain "contracts" of employment the distinction between true employment and self-employment is becoming blurred and a subject of concern for those who oversee and administer workers' compensation schemes.

In most schemes there is a threshold of disability below which benefits are not paid. As with most other aspects of workers' compensation these thresholds vary from, for example, very low levels in France and Portugal to much higher levels in Germany, Austria and Spain. In the UK, the minimum threshold for injuries and most diseases is 14%, equivalent to the loss of an index finger; workers may, however, "aggregate" percentage disabilities from separate conditions to reach a total of >14% even if each condition falls below the threshold. Most benefits are paid in regular instalments but some are covered by "lump sums" or by a combination of the two; there are good arguments for the use of both approaches, perhaps dependent on the nature of the injury or disease and the circumstances of the affected worker. A young man who has developed occupational asthma and as a result has to seek a new career may find a single "one-off" payment more useful in his re-training than a smaller payment made regularly throughout the period of his recovery.

When a worker has died from his injury or disease then payments are sometimes made to the surviving spouse or ex-spouse. The size of the benefit is generally linked to the age of the deceased (in relation to their loss of future earnings) and may further be determined by the existence of children. Some schemes provide payments for third-party assistance such as a personal career.

Barriers to Recovery and Rehabilitation

There may be barriers to recovery and rehabilitation among patients who are in the process of applying for workers' compensation (Knoblauch and Cassaro, 2020). Among these are:

- Prolonged treatment.
- Development of complex injury conditions after initial injury.
- Longer-than-expected recovery exceeding disability guidelines.
- Prolonged disability from a minor type injury.
- Multiple treating physicians, therapists, other practitioners.
- Co-morbidities.
- Lack of incentive (usually financial or psychosocial) to comply with medical treatment and return to work.

Claims in Civil Law and Other Available Payments

The common alternative to compensation through a social insurance system available to an injured employee, or one who has contracted an occupational disease, is to seek recompense through the courts by taking a claim "in common law" against an employer (or several employers) for personal injury. In general, this requires not only the establishment that the accident or disease arose during a defined period of employment but also that the employer was negligent in not preventing the harm. This process is inevitably adversarial and tends to be lengthy, expensive and distressing to claimants; in all but the most obvious instances (usually an accidental injury) its outcome is also uncertain and may be inequitable. Indeed, the no-fault, rapid settlement, explicit nature of most state compensation schemes was designed largely to combat the deficiencies and evident failings of the tort system; and in most countries, compensation is dominated by social insurance rather than civil litigation.

In some countries — for example, Canada and some parts of Australia — workers in receipt of state compensation forego the right to sue their employer who, by participating in an injury compensation scheme, is granted tort exemption. In the USA, while employees are free to sue third parties, any proceeds from such suits must first go to reimburse their employer's compensation insurance carrier. Similar arrangements operate in other countries such as the UK where workers are free to take both routes but the settlement reached in court may be adjusted to account for any benefits paid through the statutory system, the costs of which are also recovered.

Other Payments

Failures in common law — particularly common in diseases of long latency and highlighted by the legacy of asbestos — have in some jurisdictions been addressed by additional legislation. In the UK, for example, the Pneumoconiosis Act of 1979, and the Mesothelioma Act of 2014 provide, from the state, lump sums to workers who have developed pneumoconiosis/byssinosis/lung cancer or diffuse pleural thickening from asbestos exposure, or mesothelioma, respectively, who are unable to recover civil compensation because the relevant employer — and their insurer — are no longer in business or cannot be traced. The sums are higher in those whose diagnoses are made at a younger age, reflecting their greater loss in lifetime earnings. Similar schemes operate elsewhere; in Singapore, for instance, the Workers' Fund Regulations (2008) provide assistance to employees who have failed to obtain compensation because their employer has ceased trading or because their claim falls foul of the statute of limitations. In Sweden, a state-funded system known as AFA Insurance provides extra payments to those whose incomes were higher than the maximum provided by the general compensation scheme.

Organisation and Funding of Workers' Compensation

Workers' compensation is usually funded through a levy on employers with or without an additional contribution from the state. The details vary widely but on the whole, state contributions are used where employer levies fail; examples include the provision of payments to self-employed farmers in Finland and Germany, or the coverage of asbestos-workers in France. In the USA all workers' compensation schemes are employer-funded in full but handled by legislated state-compensation boards. Schemes for occupational accidents often have different funding arrangements — and in some countries, such as Denmark, are covered by private insurers — from those for occupational diseases. Moreover, there may be different arrangements for workers in different industries. Germany, for example, has a system of sectoral-based compensation provided through individual, largely self-governing schemes ("*Berufsgenossenschafts*"). In his account of the history of workers' compensation in South Africa, Erlich (2012) describes the evolution of separate systems for miners and non-miners in that country stemming, probably, from the urgent need to compensate gold and other miners in the wake of endemic "phthisis" (silicosis and silico-tuberculosis) in the early years of the 20th century. In a context of chronic underfunding, the separation appears to have poorly served miners, who are regionally dispersed (often in neighbouring countries) and often have limited access to the scheme.

Setting Premiums

Where they are used to finance a compensation scheme, employers' premiums, are generally set according to one of two models. In the first, a single rate is applied to all businesses based on their total payroll, irrespective of their risks and claims experience; this approach is used in several European countries such as Sweden, Belgium, Portugal and Austria. A difficulty with this approach is that as workforces in many countries are reduced through mechanisation and other means, the resources available to compensation schemes tend to fall.

The second model sets premiums based not only on the number of employees but also on the risk profile — and sometimes the extent of previous claims, known as "experience rating" — of a particular business or sector; this approach is used in Germany, Italy, Spain, Denmark and other European countries and also in the USA and Canada. In France a reduced rate may be applied to enterprises that can demonstrate effective health and safety systems designed to reduce the risk of workplace accidents and disease. Setting risk-based premiums is administratively costly and often a single, "pooled" premium is applied to all businesses in a sector irrespective of their individual risk profile. This may be counter-productive since there is some evidence that at least in some settings experience rating can be an effective lever to reduce the incidence of workplace accidents (Hyatt and Kralj, 1995; Lengagne, 2016). Others however have pointed out the dangers inherent in the approach; Harcourt and colleagues, for example, describe how the approach may lead to a harrowing list of discriminatory practices by employers (Harcourt *et al.*, 2007).

As with most aspects of worker's compensation, international variations in funding arrangements have arisen through an often conflicting complex of local historical, political, economic and expedient incentives. Such tensions have not disappeared and most countries continue to grapple with schemes that are imperfect. Arguably, the difficulties are most evident in compensating occupational diseases (rather than injuries) and in particular those of long latency that are the legacy of past industrial activity and a shrinking base of employer contributions.

Are Workers' Compensation Schemes Effective?

Effectiveness in this context has several dimensions. First, is that of the extent to which workers' compensation adequately and appropriately recompenses employees who have been injured or acquired disease through their occupation. Broadly, compensation schemes are more effective in their recognition of workplace accidents while it is widely accepted (as above) that they are inadequate in reflecting the true burden of occupational disease. Compensation schemes generally include, not unreasonably, a requirement that a compensable disease be one that arises out of and in the course of employment and is "peculiar to the workplace." This creates the "artificial barrier" of a "prescribed list" of compensable diseases with rigid exposure schedules that struggle to accommodate the contemporary recognition that most occupational diseases are multicausal in nature, with aetiological factors present both in and out of the workplace. As a result, many workers whose disease has at least a partial explanation in their occupation are disadvantaged. Watterson and O'Neill (2015), for example, point out that of the estimated 13,600 incident cases of occupational cancer that occur in the UK each year, just 2,600 are compensated by that country's scheme. Defendants of the scheme point out the difficulty in attributing cause in individual cases where the occupational contribution is relatively small. In riposte, some have argued that the burden of proof is too high and that a lower threshold should be applied; Mallino (1989) for example argued for a "30% rule" whereby if the incidence of a particular disease in an exposed population of workers is 30% higher than in a comparable non-exposed population, then that disease should be deemed to be work-related. While this approach would certainly come closer to accommodating the true burden of occupational disease in a community it would inevitably lead to the compensation of a high proportion of individuals whose disease did not arise from their work.

Case Study 2: Compensation for Occupational Tuberculosis (TB)

To investigate the experience of the workers' compensation system among health workers who suffered from TB while working in public service facilities in South Africa, 51 interviews were conducted among 300 health workers with claims for occupational TB (Van der Water et al., 2020). In nearly half of the cases, there was no record of claim status on the state Compensation Fund website. Of the 51 interviewees, only one had received all the compensation benefits for their particular claim circumstances. Health workers' experience of claiming for compensation was largely negative, with a perception of poor communication and administration. This added to the burden of being ill with TB.

Contemporary attitudes towards disability are focused on dignified, full integration, a fundamental shift from the outlook pertaining through the development and evolution of many compensation schemes. Schemes that protect workers' jobs and/or provide them with support to return successfully to work are probably more effective in integration than those that simple provide financial recompense. Lippel (2012), however, describes the several ways in which even the former may be adversarial, stigmatising and undignified; and contrasts the general model with that of New Zealand where in 1974 workers' compensation legislation and tort-based recourse were replaced by a no-fault compensation scheme for all types of accidents whether they occurred in the workplace or not. The scheme was deliberately organised to promote physical and vocational recovery and has probably resulted in a process that is less adversarial than most. Similarly, since 1967, disability insurance in the Netherlands has been provided regardless of its cause although in that country the right to a claim in civil law is unaffected (but rarely pursued).

Insurers — and their lawyers — often take a different perspective and are fond of discussing the potential "moral hazard" in workers' compensation, distinguishing *ex-ante* and *ex-post* hazards that arise from interactions between a system of compensation and the risk and claims behaviours of employees and their employers (Fortin and Lanoie, 1998). This is a highly complex field on which the players often take entrenched positions. One issue is the question of whether compensation arrangements influence the frequency and nature of employee claims through a variety of incentive effects; and to what extent an individual claims process is detrimental to recovery from an injury or disease.

Case Study 3: Are Patient Outcomes The Same For Those With And Without Workers' Compensation Claims?

Postoperative outcomes [Visual Analog Scale (VAS), American Shoulder and Elbow Surgeons (ASES), Veterans RAND 12 Item Health Survey (VR-12) mental and physical, Simple Shoulder Test (SST), and Single Assessment Numeric Evaluation (SANE) scores] of 925 patients after isolated biceps tenodesis for the treatment of a diagnosis of biceps tendinitis were studied.

139 patients had Workers' Compensation claims, while 786 patients did not. Both groups had similar demographic characteristics and comorbidities.

Compared to patients with WC claims, patients without WC claims had significantly improved VAS, VR-12, ASES, SANE, and SST scores at three months and one year after surgery. Furthermore, patients with WC claims had worse preoperative-to-postoperative improvements in most outcomes (Wagner et al., 2020).

On the other hand, the organisation of a workers' compensation scheme may offer no incentives for employers to identify and eliminate the causes of occupational diseases and injuries, a criticism levelled at compensation schemes from their inception. They may even be highly detrimental to employee rights. Guyton (1999) provides an egregious example from Oklahoma in the early 20th century where in an industrial accident a one-eyed man lost his remaining eye, a "second injury". Given the worker's consequent blindness, his employer was required to pay compensation for total, irreversible disability; very soon afterwards almost all one-eyed and one-limbed workers in the state were deemed by their employers to pose an undesirable risk and lost their jobs.

The broader question of how a compensation scheme might be designed so as to have the best chance of reducing, directly or indirectly, the incidence of occupational accidents and diseases remains largely unanswered (Tompa *et al.*, 2007). This is hardly surprising since the issue is not one that can be tested through experimental methods and the general approach using before-after designs fails to account for the multitude of competing influences.

Conclusion

Contemporary workers' compensation schemes evolved in response to two market failures; that of industry failing adequately to protect its workforce; and that of the tort system failing to provide speedy, equitable recompense to injured or diseased workers. Early systems had their origins in Europe and North America in an era of heavy industry with high rates of workplace accidents; newer schemes, in economically developing parts of the world, have borrowed heavily from the earlier approaches. Shifts in attitudes to disability and increasing pressure on public finances have forced those responsible for the design and administration of compensation schemes to consider whether they remain fit for purpose — considerations which have yet to result in any major new initiatives. While the approach to and management of claims for industrial accidents and the classic diseases of industry are fairly straightforward, schemes struggle to accommodate many of the risks of modern work and in particular those of diseases that are not unique to work and those that afflict persons in precarious employment.

References

American Medical Association. (2009) *AMA guides to the evaluation of permanent impairment* (6th Ed). United States, American Medical Association.

Boden LI. (2020) The Occupational Safety and Health Administration at 50-the Failure to Improve Workers' Compensation. *Am J Public Health* **110**(5): 638–639. Available from: doi: 10.2105/AJPH.2019.305549.

Coggon D, Ntani G, Palmer KT, Felli VE, Harari R, Barrero LH, Felknor SA, Gimeno D, Cattrell A, Serra C, Bonzini M, Solidaki E, Merisalu E, Habib RR, Sadeghian F, Kadir M, Warnakulasuriya SS, Matsudaira K, Nyantumbu B, Sim MR, Harcombe H, Cox K, Marziale MH, Sarquis LM, Harari F, Freire R, Harari N, Monroy MV, Quintana LA, Rojas M, Salazar Vega EJ, Harris EC, Vargas-Prada S, Martinez JM, Delclos G, Benavides FG, Carugno M, Ferrario MM, Pesatori AC, Chatzi L, Bitsios P, Kogevinas M, Oha K, Sirk T, Sadeghian A, Peiris-John RJ, Sathiakumar N, Wickremasinghe AR, Yoshimura N, Kielkowski D, Kelsall HL, Hoe VC, Urquhart DM, Derrett S, McBride D, Gray A. (2012) The CUPID (Cultural and Psychosocial Influences on Disability) study: Methods of data collection and characteristics of study sample. *PLoS One* 7(7). Available from: doi: 10.1371/journal.pone.0039820.

Driscoll T, Wagstaffe M, Pearce N. (2011) Developing a list of compensable occupational diseases: Principles and issues. *Open Occup Health Saf J* **3**: 65–72.

Ehrlich R. (2012) A century of miners' compensation in South Africa. *Am J Ind Med* **55**(6): 560– 569.

European Union. (2007) *Schedule of occupational diseases.* [Online] Available from: http://europa.eu/legislation_summaries/employment_and_social_policy/health_hygiene_safety_at_work/c11112_en.htm.

Fortin B, Lanoie P. (1998) *Effects of workers' compensation: A survey.* [Online] Available from: https://cirano.qc.ca/pdf/publication/98s-04.pdf. [Accessed on 22 March 2021].

Guyton GP. (1999) A brief history of workers' compensation. *Iowa Orthop J* **19**: 106–10

Haller JS. Jr. (1988) Industrial accidents--worker compensation laws and the medical response. *West J Med* **148**(3): 341–348.
Harcourt M, Lam H, Harcourt S. (2007) The impact of workers' compensation experience-rating on discriminatory hiring practices. *J Econ* **41**(3): 681–699.
Hong Kong Labor Department. (2006) *Guidance notes on the diagnosis of notifiable occupational diseases.* [Online] Available from: https://www.labour.gov.hk/eng/public/oh/Diagnosis.pdf.
HVBG. (2002) Hauptverband der gewerblichen Berufsgenossenschaften (German Federation of institutions for statutory accident insurance and prevention), List of occupational diseases. Bonn.
Hyatt DE, Kralj B. (1995) The impact of workers' compensation experience rating on employer appeals activity. *Ind Relat* **34**(1): 95–106.
Hyman MH, Talmage JB, Hegmann KT. (2020) Evaluating COVID-19 injury claims with a focus on workers' compensation. *J Occup Environ Med* **62**(9): 692–699. Available from: doi: 10.1097/JOM.0000000000001950.
Industrial Injuries Advisory Council. (2013) *Position paper 30; The association between shift working and breast cancer — an updated report.* [Online] Available from: https://www.gov.uk/government/uploads/system/uploads/attachment_data/file/328502/shift-work-breast-cancer-iiac-pp-30.pdf. [Accessed on 22 March 2021].
Kim EA, Kang SK. (2013) Historical review of the list of occupational diseases recommended by the International Labour organization (ILO). *Ann Occup Environ Med* **25**(1): 14.
Knoblauch DK, Cassaro S. (2020) *Workers compensation.* [Online] Treasure Island, Florida, StatPearls Publishing. Available from: https://www.ncbi.nlm.nih.gov/books/NBK448106/.
Lastovkova A, Carder M, Rasmussen HM, Sjoberg L, Groene GJ, Sauni R, Vevoda J, Vevodova S, Lasfargues G, Svartengren M, Varga M, Colosio C, Pelclova D. (2018) Burnout syndrome as an occupational disease in the European Union: An exploratory study. *Ind Health* **56**(2): 160–165. Available from: doi: 10.2486/indhealth.2017-0132.
Lengagne P. (2016) Experience rating and work-related health and safety. *J Labor Res* **37**(1): 69–97.
Lippel K. (2012) Preserving workers' dignity in workers' compensation systems: An international perspective. *Am J Ind Med* **55**(6): 519–536.

Mallino DL. (1989) Workers' compensation and the prevention of occupational disease. *Ann NY Acad Sci* 572, 271–277. Available from: 10.1111/j.1749-6632.1989.tb13613.x.

Markham Lester V. (2001) The employers' liability/workmen's compensation debate of the 1890s revisited. *Hist J* **44**(2): 471–495.

Ontario. (1994) Report to the workers' compensation board on IDSP revisions to Schedule 3: Phase one. Industrial Disease Standards Panel (ed.). Toronto: Workers' Compensation Board.

Republic of South Africa Department of Labour. (2004) Department of Labour. Compensation for Occupational Injuries and Diseases Act, 1993 (No. 130 of 1993). Amendment of Schedule 3-2004.

Spieler EA, Barth PS, Burton JF, Himmelstein Jr J, Rudolph L. (2000) Recommendations to guide revision of the guides to the evaluation of permanent impairment. *JAMA* **283**(4): 519–523.

Straif K, Baan R, Grosse Y, Secretan B, Ghissassi FEl, Bouvard V, Altieri A, Benbrahim-Tallaa L, Cogliano V. (2007) Carcinogenicity of shift-work, painting, and fire-fighting. *Lancet Oncol* **8**(12): 1065–1066.

Tompa E, Trevithick S, McLeod C. (2007) Systematic review of the prevention incentives of insurance and regulatory mechanisms for occupational health and safety. *Scand J Work Environ Health* **33**(2): 85–95.

Van der Water N, Yassi A, Ehrlich R. (2020) Workers' compensation claims for occupational tuberculosis in South African health workers: Outcomes and workers' experiences. *S Afr Med J* **110**(5): 389–395. Available from: doi: 10.7196/SAMJ.2020.v110i5.14247.

Wagner ER, Woodmass JM, Chang MJ, Welp KM, Higgins LD, Warner JJP. (2020) The impact of workers' compensation on recovery after biceps tenodesis. *J Shoulder Elbow Surg* **29**(9): 1783–1788. Available from: doi: 10.1016/j.jse.2020.01.095.

Walters D. (2007) *An international comparison of occupational disease and injury compensation schemes.* [Online] Available from: https://www.gov.uk/government/uploads/system/uploads/attachment_data/file/330347/InternationalComparisonsReport.pdf. [Accessed on 22 March 2021].

Watterson A, O'Neill R. (2015) *Mean test.* [Online] Available from: http://www.hazards.org/compensation/meantest.htm. [Accessed on 22 March 2021].

Webb S, Webb B. (1897) *Industrial democracy.* London, Longmans.

Williams CA. (2012) *An International Comparison of Workers' Compensation.* Dordrecht, Netherlands, Springer Netherlands.

Section 3 —

Multidisciplinary Occupational Health Practice

Chapter 25

The Multidisciplinary Nature of Occupational Health Practice

Ro-Ting Lin, Hathaichon Boonhat† and David Koh*

Introduction

Occupational health practice is multidisciplinary in nature. Case Study 1 demonstrates the complementary roles of the various disciplines required in occupational health practice. This example encompasses an investigation of an occupational disease outbreak, which required diverse areas of expertise — including clinical and epidemiological competencies, toxicology and occupational hygiene knowledge and expertise, and effective communication and follow-up.

Case Study 1: Investigation of a Cluster of Skin Rashes among Workers

Eighteen workers in a warehouse complained of rashes on their limbs, neck, and trunk within two weeks after their workplace was treated for termites. One day after the chemical treatment, the central air-conditioning unit, which cooled about two-thirds of the warehouse, ceased

*Department of Occupational Safety and Health, College of Public Health, China Medical University, Taiwan.
†Graduate Institute of Public Health, College of Public Health, China Medical University, Taiwan.

functioning. The workers believed that chemical exposure following the termite treatment and the poor ventilation were responsible for the outbreak of skin rashes.

A list of chemicals used for the termite treatment was obtained. The major chemicals in the termite treatment powder which was used were borax, arsenic trioxide, and iron oxide. The contractor who performed the treatment had not encountered similar problems in his previous operations.

A workplace investigation showed that the majority of workers with rashes worked in areas with non-functional air-conditioning. The majority of the rashes (9 cases; 50% of these workers) had the clinical appearance of miliaria rubra (Figs. 1 and 2), while the others had facial eczema, contact dermatitis, acne, urticaria, hyperhidrosis, tinea versicolor, pitted keratolysis, and dermographism. A walk-through survey of the warehouse revealed poor ventilation in the non-air-conditioned areas. The prevalence of heat rashes among employees working primarily in non-air-conditioned areas was 21%, while among those working

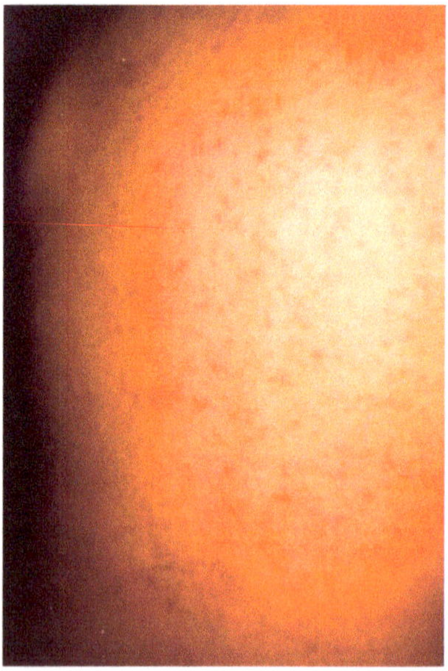

Fig. 1. Miliaria rubra of the upper back in a warehouse employee.

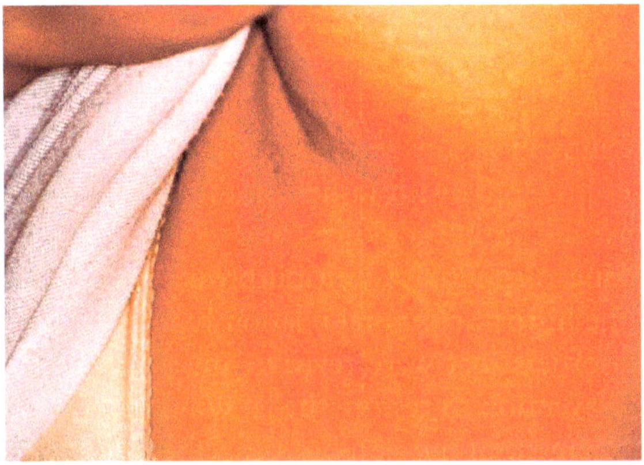

Fig. 2. Miliaria rubra of the axillary region in another worker in the warehouse.

mainly in air-conditioned areas, the prevalence of heat rashes was 11% (Koh, 1995).

The provisional diagnosis was an outbreak of heat rashes, and a recommendation (after the walk-through survey) was made for air-conditioning to be restored urgently. Heat stress was measured at various sites the following day. All the wet bulb globe temperature (WBGT) readings were within the threshold limit values (TLVs) recommended by the American Conference of Governmental Industrial Hygienists (ACGIH). To allay the workers' concern about arsenic exposure, environmental samples were collected and analysed for arsenic, but no arsenic was detected. The problem was resolved within two weeks after repairing the air-conditioner.

Interpretation of Results and Management: Lessons from Case Study 1

The interpretation of occupational health results requires a multidisciplinary approach encompassing clinical medicine, toxicology, epidemiology, and occupational hygiene. Besides, effective communication with management and workers is necessary to help understand and respond to their concerns.

In Case Study 1, the index case (a lady with endogenous facial eczema) presented with an itchy rash on the face within days of chemical treatment for termites. One week later, the air-conditioning ceased functioning in various sections of the workplace. Subsequently, 13 more cases presented with rashes on the head, neck, upper arms, upper back, axillae, flexures of knees, and elbows.

The working diagnosis was an outbreak of heat rashes, primarily based on the history, temporal relationships, and clinical diagnosis of the skin disorders that were reviewed by the occupational physician. Swift intervention to restore the air conditioning, followed by a marked improvement in the skin health of the workers, validated the preliminary diagnosis of heat rashes. However, toxicological, occupational hygiene, and epidemiological inputs were also important in characterising and managing the outbreak.

In terms of toxicology, important questions to be answered were:

1. What were the components of the chemicals used for the termite treatment, and could any of these components cause skin rashes? While information on the specific termite treatment chemical may be proprietary, some general information can be found in the safety data sheets (SDSs) and is available on the websites of the International Agency for Research on Cancer (IARC, 2021), Toxicological Profiles (Tox Profiles) (Agency for Toxic Substances and Disease Registry, 2021), and National Toxicology Program (US Department of Health and Human Services, 2021).
2. What types of skin disorders can occur because of exposure to the above chemicals, what is/are the mechanism(s) of action (e.g. irritant or allergic pathways involved), how long will it take the skin disorders to develop, and what levels of exposure are needed for such adverse effects to be seen? Sufficient knowledge of toxicology and clinical medicine is required to answer these questions.
3. Could there be other causes of skin disorders in this work environment besides the termite treatment powder? The familiarity of a particular workplace, a walk-through survey to assess for possible cutaneous hazards, and a literature search for similar past occurrences would help answer this question.

4. Are there any specific agents that the workers are concerned about, and how can they be addressed? It was ascertained that the workers were particularly concerned about arsenic, as it was labeled as a skin carcinogen and could cause dramatic skin changes. Consequently, measurements of arsenic in the work environment were performed to respond to the workers' concerns.

Regarding occupational hygiene inputs, one should consider the hazards to be measured, how the measurements can be performed, suitable sampling locations and strategies to be adopted, and interpretation of the results. In Case Study 1, WBGT measurements were recorded at six sites (Fig. 3) and measurement of arsenic levels at two sites. The environmental monitoring results are shown in Table 1.

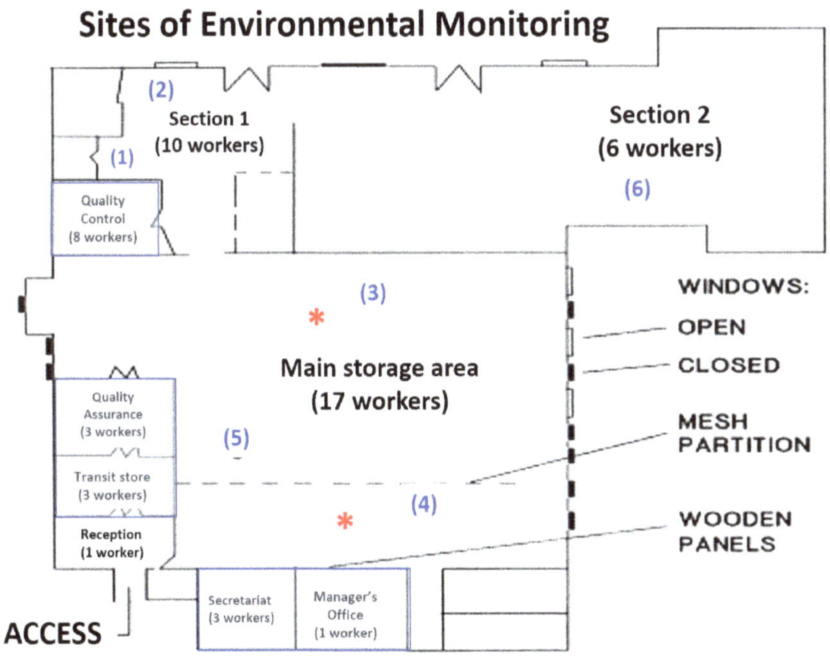

Fig. 3. Plan of warehouse, showing distribution of sites of environmental monitoring. Numerals (in brackets) indicate locations for WBGT measurements. Asterisks (in red) indicate air sampling locations for arsenic. The areas with functioning air-conditioning were the quality control and quality assurance rooms, transit store, and secretariat and manager's office (shaded in light blue).

Table 1. Environmental Monitoring Results

Location	Mean Dry Bulb (°C)	WBGT (°C)
Section 1 (2 locations)	31.0	26.4
Section 2 (1 location)	31.4	26.6
Main store area (3 locations)	31.0	26.1
Location	**Measurement of Arsenic Level**	
Environmental air samples (300 L) at 2 locations	Non-detectable for arsenic	

Table 2. Permissible Heat Exposure TLVs (ACGIH, 2020). Values are in °C, WBGT

Work/Rest Regimen	Light	Moderate	Heavy	Very Heavy
75% to 100%	31.0	28.0	—	—
50% to 75%	31.0	29.0	27.5	—
25% to 50%	32.0	30.0	29.0	28.0
0% to 25%	32.5	31.5	30.5	30.0

To interpret the results meaningfully, the measurement methodology and assumptions should be understood. For interpretation of the WBGT, for indoor and outdoor conditions with no solar load, the WBGT is calculated as:

$$\text{WBGT} = 0.7 \text{ Natural Wet Bulb Temperature} + 0.3 \text{ Globe Temperature}$$

The results obtained can be compared with established standards, such as the permissible heat exposure TLVs of the ACGIH shown in Table 2.

Notably, the work-rest regime of the worker must be considered in interpreting the TLVs. Furthermore, it is assumed that the WBGT of the resting place is the same or close to that of the workplace. Considering these factors, nearly all acclimatised, fully clothed workers (in light summer clothing) with adequate water and salt intake should be able to function effectively under the given working conditions without exceeding a core body temperature of 38°C.

Assuming that the workers in Case Study 1 were involved in continuous light work, all the WBGT measurements taken at the workplace were within permissible levels. Although this may initially appear not to support the diagnosis of heat rashes, it should be noted that the primary health outcome used to derive the ACGIH TLVs was not heat rashes but rather the core body temperature. Furthermore, the measurements were taken after the beginning of the outbreak, during a cool cloudy day — which may not accurately reflect the conditions of the preceding weeks, which were sunny and warmer.

The measured arsenic levels can be compared to a TLV of 0.01 mg/m^3 for arsenic and inorganic compounds, as As. Arsenic has an A2 notation, indicating that it is a suspected human carcinogen; i.e. the agent has been determined as carcinogenic in experimental animals at dose(s), by route(s) of exposure, at site(s), of histologic types, or by mechanism(s) considered relevant to worker exposure (Occupational Safety and Health Administration (OSHA), 2020). When a report states that no arsenic is detected, the detection limit of arsenic and the measurement instruments should be specified, in this case, a detection limit of arsenic using the measurement methodology was 0.0004 mg/m^3.

Following epidemiological investigations, the prevalence rate ratio of heat rashes among workers in non-air-conditioned sections to those working in air-conditioned sections was 21/11. This represents an almost two-fold increase in disease prevalence in the heat-exposed population compared to the non-heat-exposed population. While the finding was not statistically significant (p-value of 0.33 using Fisher's exact test), the result was judged practically and clinically significant. The lack of statistical significance is likely due to the small sample size (power studies can be performed to test whether a small sample size can be the explanation for this observation) and mobility of the employees (as they do not constantly remain in one location all day). The movement of workers in the course of their work will impact the actual exposure status of the workers and thus their subsequent disease status.

Additionally, risk communication is essential for the management of the outbreak. The findings had to be communicated to the management for quick repair of the air-conditioning systems to be initiated. Once management was convinced, this priority intervention by management resulted in a rapid resolution of the outbreak. Information was also provided to all workers, who were encouraged to ask questions and raise concerns. The workers were reassured by the concerns for their safety, and that action was being taken to alleviate their discomfort. The fact that the investigations were conducted by an independent, credible, non-partisan expert in occupational health was also important.

Interpretation of the results and arrival at a conclusion requires a synthesis of all sources of information, sufficient knowledge of the underlying principles of the various disciplines concerned, and astute judgment. Effective management of occupational hazards involves not only engineering controls but also communication with management and workers. Follow-up monitoring and evaluation can validate the diagnosis and effectiveness of the intervention.

Occupational Health Practice Requires Integration of Skills

Occupational health practice requires integration of skills from multiple disciplines, and a working knowledge and familiarity with other disciplines such as toxicology, epidemiology and occupational hygiene are necessary. Besides these skill sets, good occupational health practice involves effective communication, ethical behaviour, knowledge of and compliance with the law, good documentation practices, audits, and continuous improvement processes (these aspects are covered in other chapters in the textbook).

Toxicology

Toxicology is the study of the adverse effects of toxic agents (hereinafter referred to as toxicants) in chemical (e.g. arsenic), physical (e.g. radiation), or biological (e.g. snake venom) forms on living organisms and the ecosystem. In addition, it deals with the prevention and amelioration of such adverse effects (ToxTutor, 2018).

Each toxicant has an intrinsic toxicity characterised by its chemical and physical properties, such as molecular structure, stability, and reactivity. However, these properties do not determine the severity of adverse effects. The amount of toxicant exposure determines the potential effect. For example, the general population is exposed to various toxicants through air, water, food, living goods, and contaminants in their daily lives. The concentration and volume of these toxicants are often at low levels in the general environment. Hence, there are more concerns on their chronic health effect than on the acute effect in environmental settings.

In contrast, the concentration and volume of toxicants in workplaces are usually higher than those in the daily environment. Workers often directly handle high-volume toxicants used in manufacturing processes and production lines and consequently, they may be exposed to higher levels of toxicants and by-products. Acute and chronic health effects caused by exposure to toxicants are more frequent in occupational settings.

For a toxicant to be able to cause adverse health effects, it should be absorbed by the body. Each toxicant has specific route(s) through which it enters the human body and gets absorbed. The four main routes via which a toxicant can be absorbed into the human body are inhalation, dermal contact, ingestion, and injection. Once toxicants enter the body, they are distributed, metabolised, and/or excreted. Thus, the concentration to which a worker is exposed does not represent the concentration of the toxicant at the target organ inside the body or even the concentration that produces a biological response and adverse effect. The first concentration is usually called the administered dose, whereas the final concentration is the effective dose. All the above factors determine the ability of occupational toxicants to cause adverse effects in humans.

To protect the health of workers from exposure to toxicants, the best way is to prevent the use of toxicants. However, toxicants are difficult to eliminate from real settings if work processes remain unchanged or the raw materials are not substituted. Occupational toxicants mostly come from raw materials used in the work processes, as well as the accompanying by-products and wastes. Therefore, regulatory and recommended limits for the concentration of toxicants in workplaces have been established to regulate or control the concentration of toxicants in workplaces (Kacew and Lee, 2012).

Regulatory limits are set by regulatory authorities, including permissible exposure limit (PEL) by the United States (US) OSHA (OSHA, 2015) and occupational exposure limit (OEL) by the European Union and its nations (European Chemicals Agency, 2021). The recommended limits are usually established by research institutes of governments, such as recommended exposure limit (REL) by the US National Institute for Occupational Safety and Health (NIOSH, 2020), and professional associations, such TLV by ACGIH (as mentioned in Case Study 1). When assessing whether exposure exceeds the limits, the duration and frequency of exposure in workplaces should be considered because workers may be exposed to certain toxicants during the whole working day or only for a very short period. These limits are often categorised into time-weighted average (TWA), short-term exposure limit (STEL), and ceiling:

1. TWA refers to a concentration based on the average concentration for an 8-h workday and a 40-h workweek.
2. STEL refers to the average concentration within 15 min.
3. Ceiling refers to a concentration that should not be exceeded during any part of the working exposure.

Understanding the basic toxicology, chemical and physical properties of toxicants, work processes, and exposure assessment can help occupational health practitioners identify workers who are at a higher risk of developing occupational diseases.

The provision of integrated information, including chemical properties, hazards, and control measures, from manufacturers, suppliers, transporters, and employers to employees is required by several countries and in supply chain management as well. All hazardous substances and mixtures should be classified and labelled based on the United Nations (UN) Globally Harmonised System of Classification and Labelling of Chemicals (GHS) (UN, 2019).

The GHS classified hazards into physical hazards (covering 17 hazard classes, such as explosives and flammable gases), health hazards (covering 10 hazard classes, such as acute toxicity and carcinogen) and environmental hazards (covering two hazard classes, including hazardous to the aquatic environment and hazards to the ozone layer). Within each hazard class, hazard categories and sub-categories were used to indicate the hazard severity within a hazard class. Taking one hazard class under health hazard as an example, "carcinogenicity" can be categorised as 1, 1A, 1B, and 2 according to GHS.

Category 1 represents known or presumed human carcinogens based on epidemiological and/or animal data. If the judgment was based on evidence derived from human studies, the substance was categorised as 1A (known human carcinogen); alternatively, evidence derived from animal studies should be categorised as 1B (presumed human carcinogen). Category 2 represents suspected human carcinogens. To help workers, especially illiterate or foreign labourers, be aware of the potential hazards, GHS provides nine easily understandable symbols for each hazard (Fig. 4).

The aforementioned summary information (e.g. properties, limits, and toxicity) of hazardous substances and mixtures can usually be obtained from SDS. The information in the SDS should cover

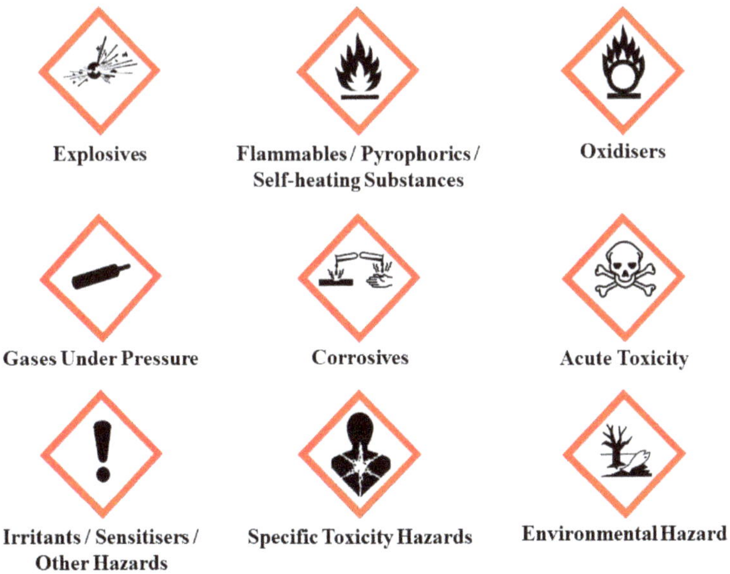

Fig. 4. Symbols for the globally harmonised system of classification and labelling of chemicals.

16 parts: (1) identification, (2) hazard(s) identification, (3) composition/information on ingredients, (4) first-aid measures, (5) fire-fighting measures, (6) accidental release measures, (7) handling and storage, (8) exposure controls/personal protection, (9) physical and chemical properties and safety characteristics, (10) stability and reactivity, (11) toxicological information, (12) ecological information, (13) disposal considerations, (14) transport information, (15) regulatory information, and (16) other information (UN, 2019). Occupational health practitioners should have knowledge to interpret the information obtained from SDS. Online resources such as the US Registry of Toxic Effects of Chemical Substances (NIOSH, 2011) and NIOSH Pocket Guide to Chemical Hazards (NIOSH, 2020) also provide compiled and updated data on toxicological information and chemical hazards.

Many people may regard regulatory limits as a safe level of exposure. However, these limits only specify the amount of chemicals in the workplace where workers are allowed to work, and some of these limits are outdated. Therefore, these limits should be based on updated scientific evidence. As noted by the US OSHA (OSHA, 2019), most PELs were issued shortly after the launch of the Occupational Safety and Health Act in 1970, and many PELs are outdated and inadequate to ensure the protection of workers' health. To solve this problem, the OSHA's Hazard Communication standard requires that SDS list both OSHA PEL and other alternative exposure limits, such as ACGIH TLV and NIOSH REL. OSHA also published a new menu on their website, PEL — annotated tables, to provide a side-by-side comparison of OSHA PEL with other limits. Table 3 shows the OSHA annotated table for acetone.

The establishment PELs and OELs should be based on the most recent scientific data available and also consider the availability of measurement techniques. The assumption underlying these limits (if not outdated) is that if healthy adult workers are exposed to hazardous chemicals in the workplace below these limits, workers should have been protected from occupational diseases or other adverse effects. However, this assumption hinders the settings of regulatory limits for some non-threshold carcinogens and may impact the efforts to

Table 3. OSHA Annotated Table for Acetone (OSHA, 2019)

Substance	CAS No.	OSHA PEL		Cal/OSHA PEL (as of 2/10/2019)	NIOSH REL (as of 18/10/2019)	ACGIH® 2020 TLV
		ppm	mg/m^3	8-h TWA (ST) STEL (C) Ceiling	Up to 10-h TWA (ST) STEL (C) Ceiling	8-h TWA (ST) STEL (C) Ceiling
Acetone	67-64-1	1,000	2,400	500 ppm (ST) 750 ppm (C) 3,000 ppm	250 ppm	250 ppm (ST) 500 ppm

Abbreviations: C = ceiling limit; CAS No. = Chemical Abstract Service number; mg/m^3 = milligrams/meter cubed; ppm = parts per million; ST = short term exposure limit; TWA = time-weighted average.

eliminate occupational cancer. In addition, regulatory limits consider workers' health but not socioeconomic and technological aspects, e.g. feasibility to regulate the hazard. Therefore, the European Union introduced binding occupational exposure limit values (BOELVs) for these non-threshold carcinogens, such asbestos, silica, polyaromatic hydrocarbons, and hexavalent chromium (Cr VI) (European Union, 1998; European Union, 2017). By taking other aspects into account, BOELVs may guide workplace protection moving towards a process of continuous improvement rather than answering passing/failing complying a standard (Cherrie, 2019). However, the use of BOE-LVs is arguable because parameters and scenarios used to estimate workers' lifetime excess death risk for exposure to certain substance remain incompatible with fundamental workers' rights of safe and healthy working conditions (Albin and Gustavsson, 2020; Johanson and Tinnerberg, 2019). Applying and interpreting these limits should be more stringent for occupational cancer prevention.

Epidemiology

Epidemiology is the study of the causes and distribution of disease in different populations (Coggon *et al.*, 2003). Besides examining study design, data analysis, and the interpretation of data, it emphasises the importance of precise case definitions and reporting of rates, in addition to the reporting of frequencies/counts. The comparison of rates of disease among exposed populations (relative to non-exposed populations) using measures such as rate ratios, rate difference, and risk ratios is another essential feature. Epidemiology also considers the effects of bias and interactions, and allows for the adjustment of confounding variables. In occupational health, special issues in epidemiology, such as the healthy worker effect, proportional morbidity/morbidity rates, and standardised mortality rates should be considered. A good understanding of the choice of correct statistical tests (when needed) is also important, as well as appropriate reporting of statistical data, for example, the use of confidence intervals. Case Study 2 illustrates how epidemiology and statistics can be integrated with clinical medicine and other disciplines to investigate a possible excess risk of tuberculosis among taxi drivers.

Case Study 2: Are Taxi Drivers More Prone to Contracting Tuberculosis?

A press release, quoting the annual report of a National Anti-Tuberculosis Association, "emphasised the belief that taxi drivers are more prone to developing tuberculosis." In the preceding year, chest X-rays (CXRs) of 69 persons applying for insurance with the tuberculosis and heart insurance scheme of the National Anti-Tuberculosis Association were found to have active tuberculosis when they had their pre-insurance CXRs. The Association's Deputy Medical Director noted that "It is interesting to note that of these 69, 10 (or 14.5%) were taxi drivers." Taxi drivers comprised only 5% of the total membership of the insurance scheme (which was 139,491 at the end of the surveyed year), but contributed to 14.5% of the active cases detected. The official also noted that the number of tuberculosis cases among taxi drivers was small, and stated that no firm conclusion should be drawn based on these figures (Koh and Phoon, 1986).

This report raised alarm among the public, as it was perceived that if taxi drivers were more prone to developing tuberculosis, passengers taking taxi rides (rather than other forms of public transport) and sitting in a confined space with infected drivers could also increase their risk of developing this communicable disease.

When contacted by the press to respond to this report, the management of the taxi driver co-operative requested its medical advisor to assist with preparing a response.

Integrated clinical, epidemiological, statistical, and management skills were needed by the medical advisor to address the question above. Mastery of these skills is required in the training of occupational physicians. Pertinent questions to consider when approaching the issue are as follows.

What are the possible mechanisms for an increased risk of tuberculosis among taxi drivers?

Taxi drivers work in a confined air-conditioned environment. They transport many passengers a day, and sick patients (if they can afford it) may prefer this mode of transport to other forms of public transport such as buses when they travel for medical consultations and treatment. These factors can potentially increase the risk of exposure to infectious diseases among taxi drivers. There have been anecdotal reports of taxi drivers contracting severe acute respiratory syndrome (SARS) and coronavirus disease (COVID-19) from patients traveling in their vehicles.

If there is an increased risk, is this for all types or specific types of tuberculosis?

Tuberculosis manifests in various forms, of which respiratory or pulmonary tuberculosis is the most common. In this case, the press report refers specifically to pulmonary tuberculosis (PTB) and does not mention other forms, such as, tuberculosis meningitis, osteomyelitis, or renal tuberculosis, which are much less common.

Does the data support an increased risk of PTB among taxi drivers, and if yes, what is the magnitude of the increased risk?

The initial report stated that, while taxi drivers form 5% of the population screened, they accounted for 14.5% of active PTB cases detected.

This information can be used to derive a proportional morbidity ratio (14.5%: 5% or 2.9), which is almost three times higher than expected, based on the % of taxi drivers in the screened population.

When interpreting the report, the case definition must be specified. The National Anti-Tuberculosis Association confirmed that the case definitions were as follows: New cases are persons with no past history of tuberculosis and no scars seen on previous CXRs, while relapse cases are persons who either have a past history of PTB or CXR lesions suggestive of past PTB; and either CXR changes suggestive of active disease or are sputum positive (by smear or culture) for tuberculosis.

On review of the individual clinical case notes of the infected taxi drivers by the occupational physician, it was ascertained that 11 of the reported cases were new cases, and four were relapse cases. All these cases occurred in male drivers. Informed consent was first obtained to review the individual medical records.

If there is an increased risk, what factors can explain the increased risk?

Besides occupational exposure, what are the other risk factors for PTB? The epidemiological characteristics of PTB show that males appear to be at higher risk than females, and that the risk of tuberculosis increases with increasing age. However, age and gender were not mentioned in the press report, and presumably, and their impact on the rates of PTB among the taxi-driver population was not considered.

The taxi drivers screened were predominantly male and were generally older than the other groups (of mixed gender and younger age) who participated in the National Anti-Tuberculosis Association insurance scheme. As information on the specific age distribution of the other occupational groups in the insurance scheme was not readily available, the taxi-driver data for PTB was compared to that of the general population.

The age distribution and observed and expected (based on the national notification rates of new cases of PTB in the general population) number of cases among male taxi drivers are shown in Table 4.

Table 4. Age Distribution of Male Taxi Drivers and Occurrence of Cases

Age in Years	Number of Drivers	New Cases in Last Year	Expected Number of Cases, Based on New Case Rate Notified to the National Authorities
20–29	24	0	0.016
30–39	1,817	1	1.199
40–49	2,641	5	3.513
50–59	1,634	3	4.314
>59	109	2	0.584
Total	6,225	11	9.626

This table shows the gender-specific rate for male taxi drivers, which are age-standardised to the general population rates by indirect standardisation. This results in an age-standardised morbidity ratio (SMR) of 11/9.6 or 1.14 (95% confidence interval 0.57–2.04), when the rate of new cases among taxi drivers is compared to the male general population rates.

This SMR suggests a 14% excess risk for the taxi-driver population compared to the general population, while the confidence interval indicates that the finding is not statistically significant and could therefore be due to chance.

Is the choice of a comparison population an appropriate one?

The choice of the general population as a comparison group is often driven by data availability. However, the general population may not be the best or the most appropriate comparison group. In this case, the comparison may be inappropriate or even invalid, as the general population rates rely on case notification of the national population — a population that is mostly unscreened for PTB. In comparison, the taxi drivers had a mandatory annual screening, and thus, the detection rates of new cases are likely to be higher. However, how much higher would this be, and can this figure be adjusted reasonably?

Information on previous community screening for PTB was available. A previous report indicated that 83% of the active cases were undiscovered before a community CXR survey in the unscreened general population. Thus, if the entire general population had been screened using CXRs, such as taxi drivers, the number of new cases notified from the general population would be about five times higher. If such a screened general population were the comparison population group, then the SMR would be considerably less than 1.27. An SMR of less than one among working populations can be expected due to what is termed "the healthy worker effect" (Li and Sung, 1999).

How can the findings be communicated to the drivers and public to assure them that appropriate measures are taken to protect the health of drivers as well as passengers?

The use of appropriate epidemiological and statistical tools indicated that the risk of tuberculosis among taxi drivers was less than that of the general population (if the general population were to be similarly screened), and that this is likely to be due to the "healthy worker effect." These findings were communicated to the taxi drivers as well as the general public, using non-technical terminology and avoiding jargon.

While the risk of tuberculosis among taxi drivers is not high, it does not mean that no further measures are needed. In view of the 11 new PTB cases among the taxi drivers found in the screening, guidelines on fitness to work and return to work were developed and implemented to safeguard both drivers and passengers. Guidelines on the frequency of periodic CXR screening were also developed, based on the need to increase the frequency of screening among older drivers, rather than having a standard screening protocol for all drivers, irrespective of age.

The successful outcome of this consultation was key in establishing an improved rapport between the medical advisor, occupational health management, and taxi drivers. This paved the way for subsequent consultations on other occupational health issues affecting taxi drivers, such as low back pain due to prolonged sitting while driving (which required ergonomic capability and input), risk of road traffic accidents (which required road safety knowledge), and management of unhealthy lifestyles due to spending long hours in a sedentary job (which required expertise and advice from health promotion and healthy lifestyle behaviour experts).

Occupational Hygiene

One example of an essential skill in occupational health practice is the ability to anticipate and recognise chemical, physical, biological, ergonomic, and psychological hazards in the workplace. The magnitude of these hazards should be evaluated through exposure assessment, followed by control. The ultimate goal is to protect workers from hazard exposure and safeguard their health. Occupational hygiene, defined as "the science of anticipation, recognition, evaluation, and control of environmental hazards in the working environment that may result in injury, illness, impairment, or affect the well-being of workers and members of the community (International Occupational Hygiene Association, 2021)" is important for occupational health practice.

Anticipation of Hazards

Anticipation refers to the expectation of potential health hazards before factories or operation processes are established in the workplace. Hazard anticipation ensures efficient use of resources by minimising costly retrofits and renovations as the problems discovered after establishing the factory or operating the process may be overly expensive to fix (Anna, 2011). To anticipate potential health hazards, the occupational health practitioner needs current knowledge of scientific developments and the awareness of other activities or processes in the workplace that may impact workers' health.

Recognition of Hazards

Recognition is the identification of workplace hazards and risk factors that may potentially harm the workers. Recognition of hazards requires the gathering of information about work processes and activities, sources of hazards, types of hazards, potential releases of hazards, and potential health effects associated with the hazards (including toxicological data) (Anna, 2011).

Walk-through surveys, onsite observations, and interviews with workers can provide information regarding potential health hazards. During a walk-through survey and onsite observation, occupational health professionals should carefully observe how workers perform their jobs and identify all potential exposure pathways, such as inhalation, ingestion, and dermal absorption. Interviews with workers also help collect information about their tasks, how they spend their time in each task, any exposure of concern, and any health signs and symptoms, particularly if they have contact with various chemical products or processes (Plog *et al.*, 2012).

Understanding the potential health effects associated with these hazards requires extensive knowledge and careful study of work processes and operations, the raw materials and chemicals used or generated, final products and by-products, and possibilities for the accidental formation of chemicals, decomposition of materials, and combustion of fuels.

Evaluation of Hazards

After identifying and listing potential health hazards, occupational health professionals should ensure that workers' exposure is well characterised. Exposure assessment seeks to determine the extent to which workers may be exposed to different types of hazards (i.e. chemical, physical, biological, ergonomic, and psychological hazards) in the workplace using quantitative, semi-quantitative, and qualitative methods (Anna, 2011). Occupational hygienists can collect quantitative data (e.g. air monitoring), perform semi-quantitative estimation (e.g. mathematical modeling), or perform qualitative assessments (e.g. interviews) to determine the magnitude of health hazards in the workplace. The exposure assessment seeks to answer the following questions (US Environmental Protection Agency, 2019):

1. What are the characteristics of exposure (e.g. magnitude, frequency, duration, and route of entry)?
2. How can exposure be reduced?
3. Has exposure changed over time?

In many situations, exposure scenarios vary over time because of process modifications, aging facilities, and task rotation. Assessing exposure over time is crucial to determine its association with adverse health effects. Exposure assessments may be conducted prospectively and/or retrospectively.

The following steps 1 to 5 can be applied to the prospective exposure assessment while steps 1 to 3 can be applied for retrospective exposure assessment.

Step 1: Establish the exposure assessment strategy

Occupational health professionals should first identify stakeholders (e.g. employees, labor unions, and communities) and other professionals (e.g. engineers, toxicologists, hygienists, physicians, nurses, and epidemiologists) and involve them in establishing an exposure assessment strategy (Bullock and Ignacia, 2006). There are two general types of exposure assessment strategies:

1. A compliance strategy assesses whether exposure to certain hazards complies with established regulatory standards (e.g. PELs and OELs). This approach can be employed in the case of a limited number of samples, in worst-case monitoring, based on a representative number of samples used.
2. A comprehensive strategy assesses the exposure to all potential hazards. Findings from this approach can help understand day-to-day distributions of exposure, address current health risks, and construct exposure profiles.

Step 2: Basic characterisation

This step encompasses the collection of data about the workplace (process/operation description and chemical, physical, and biological agent inventory), workforce (job title description, task analysis, and number of workers), agents (health effects data, PELs, OELs), characterisation of existing controls, past assessments/results, historical exposure data, environmental emission data, and biomonitoring (or biological monitoring) data. Information summarised from this step can help identify potential health hazards and workers at risk of exposure.

Step 3: Exposure assessment

This step assesses the intensity of exposure to listed workplace hazards and how it varies over time for a similar exposure group. In most situations, it involves measuring the exposure level of a few representatives from a similar exposure group rather than measuring all workers' exposure. A similar exposure group can be defined based on the frequency of the task(s) they perform, the similarity of the materials and work processes, and the similarity of the way they perform the task. With exposure profiles and information on the toxicity of certain hazards, occupational hygienists can judge whether each exposure is unacceptable, uncertain, or acceptable:

1. Unacceptable exposure is defined as high exposure to high-toxicity agents in the workplace. This is a priority for implementing health hazard controls.
2. Uncertain exposure is defined as exposure profiles in the workplace that may not be well understood. Additional information should be collected to make a conclusion about the exposure. Information that might be needed for uncertain exposure judgment includes exposure monitoring (e.g. noise monitoring, air monitoring, and dermal exposure monitoring), exposure modeling (used to estimate the potential exposures associated with new processes and products by mathematical modeling techniques to predict exposures based on workplace and worker parameters), biomonitoring (used to assess the exposure profile if there are concerns about exposure through skin absorption or ingestion), toxicological data (in case toxicity of the materials used in the workplace is unclear, the toxicologist or other experts may need to gather more health effects data on that environmental agent), and epidemiological data (used to identify the relationships between hazard exposure and disease to help determine whether the exposure is acceptable or unacceptable).
3. Acceptable exposure is defined as the level of exposure in the workplace that is appropriate and not harmful to human health. For this judgment, no further action is required. However, the collec-

tion of additional information such as air monitoring, toxicity, or epidemiological data may be needed to validate the judgment of acceptable exposure.

The above findings can help prioritise control of hazards based on the severity of health effects and the uncertainty associated with the exposure profile and adverse health effects. Unacceptable exposure requires the implementation of control strategies. However, acceptable exposure requires routine monitoring and reassessment to verify that acceptable exposures remain acceptable and update the exposure assessment findings.

Retrospective exposure assessment

Retrospective exposure assessment encompasses the estimation of past exposures to a particular hazard, type of task, or type of job title for an individual worker or groups of workers (Sahmel *et al.*, 2010). In investigating occupational diseases, especially chronic diseases and cancers, one essential criterion for confirming the causality is the exhibition of temporal relationships. In this case, a temporal relationship means that exposure must precede the outcome. This information is critical for workers who claim compensation for occupational diseases. The measurement of long-term exposure requires exposure data for individual workers during the entire working period.

Case Study 3: Evaluation of Hazardous Chemical Exposure Control System At A Semiconductor Manufacturing Company In South Korea

Epidemiological studies have shown increased cancer risk or mortality among workers employed in the semiconductor manufacturing industry. In South Korea, several workers from a semiconductor company were diagnosed with cancer or rare diseases and claimed for compensation (Park et al., 2019). To clarify the association between historical exposure and workers' diseases, the hazardous chemical exposure control system was reviewed in the semiconductor manufacturing company (Choi et al., 2018). The company operates chemical management programmes, including environmental safety and health quality review of newly purchased chemical products by an electronic system, SDSs, and a database of chemical products and their use.

The review found that these programmes and elements were fragmented, and some information was unavailable, for example, lack of information about the type and amount of chemicals used in the operation. Carcinogenic chemicals, such as arsenic, formaldehyde, nickel (insoluble inorganic compounds and metal), hydrogen peroxide, naphthalene, sulfuric acid, titanium dioxide, tetrahydrofuran, and welding fumes, were detected in the air. This semiconductor plant lacked a surveillance system to efficiently examine chemical exposure among workers according to the type of operation and job. Poor records system hindered estimation of past exposure to workplace hazards; hence, associations between the hazards and health effects such as cancers could not be accurately determined.

For Case Study 3, the company should conduct a retrospective exposure assessment (Borghi *et al.*, 2020). The measurement of past chemical exposure focuses on the duration of exposure and concentration of the chemical agent. Retrospective exposure assessment also considers different working scenarios (e.g. type of industry, job title, task performed, and materials involved) to classify the level of exposure in qualitative (yes/no) or exposure categories.

Table 5 summarises the necessary parameters that should be considered when performing a retrospective exposure assessment (Borghi *et al.*, 2020). Since some occupational data may be unavailable or incomplete in the company records, questionnaires specific to the occupation can be used to obtain more detailed information.

Occasionally, the time period between the first exposure and disease diagnosis is of decades. It becomes infeasible to reconstructive exposure timeline because factories may close. Case Study 4 demonstrates the implementation of a nationwide medical examination for former asbestos-exposed workers in Poland (Świątkowska *et al.*, 2016).

Table 5. Parameters for Assessing Retrospective Exposure Assessment in Semiconductor Manufacturing Industry (Borghi *et al.*, 2020)

Aspects	Parameters
Occupation data	• Type of industry • Job tittle • Length of the employment • Task performed, and materials used for each task • Information from plant personnel and documentations obtained from the industry historical databases • The use of collective protective measures and personal protective equipment • Possible sources of non-occupational exposure • Safety data sheets • Summary of process changes and process specification • Lab-tests for possible process intermediate • Accident and injury reports • Changes of the department during the employment • Movement of the employee among the process and the plant
Exposure data	• Duration • Frequency and distribution of the exposure related task (daily, weekly, and monthly)
Environment data	• Weather characteristics • Proximity to a major road and land use, working place characteristics (e.g. local exhaust ventilation, industrial mechanical dilution, location of the working area, proximity to the sources, process temperature and confinement of the space)
Individual data	• Health habits such as smoking

Case Study 4: Proactive Follow-Up Of Asbestos-Exposed Workers in Poland: A Nationwide Medical Monitoring Programme

Asbestos is a natural mineral that is widely used in cement, roofing, fire-proofing, textiles, and paint. After inhalation of asbestos fibers, asbestos may cause disorders of the lung and pleura (e.g., asbestosis, mesothelioma, and lung cancer). The health effects associated with asbestos exposure may manifest many years after the occupational exposure. The reported latency period for mesothelioma and lung cancer is approximately

30–40 years and the range for asbestosis wider, depending on the level of exposure. These delayed adverse health effects in former asbestos factory workers and asbestos-exposed workers continue to be an issue in health research and policy discussions.

Owing to the carcinogenic and pneumoconiosis characteristics of asbestos, approximately one-third of the member countries of the UN have banned the use of asbestos (Kazan-Allen, 2019). Poland banned the use, import, and production of asbestos and asbestos-containing products in 1997. The Polish procedures to certify occupational diseases involve three phases: "reporting of the suspected cases," "assigning a diagnosis to the case," and "certifying the cases as an occupational disease" (Świątkowska et al., 2016). Depending on the location of the workplace, employers, occupational physicians, or labour inspectors may be required to report the occupational case to the local authority for further documentation in the central registration system. Systematic data collection can be used to inform policies for occupational disease prevention and compensation. However, insufficient knowledge about asbestos-related diseases, lack of information about asbestos exposure history, and lack of specialised knowledge among physicians may contribute to the underreporting of asbestos-related diseases.

After banning asbestos, the Polish Ministry of Health introduced a nationwide medical examination for former asbestos-exposed workers in 2000, called the Amiantus programme. A typical recognition procedure usually starts when a patient is suggested of having an occupational disease on examination in the clinic. Unlike the traditional method, the Amiantus programme offers former workers of 28 Polish asbestos-processing factories periodic medical examinations and free access to medications for the treatment of asbestos-related illnesses. The criterion for a former employee to enter the Amiantus programme is that his/her factory uses raw asbestos material in the process. The long latency period of asbestos-related diseases necessitates long-term follow-up of occupationally exposed workers in asbestos factories. Compared with the average number of total registered asbestos-related diseases 10 years before the Amiantus programme (1991–2000), the average number 10 years after the programme (2001–2010) doubled.

Commentary

Asbestos-related diseases have long been underestimated in most countries because of their long latency period and difficulties in linking the disease to past workplace exposure. The Polish Amiantus programme demonstrates that the proactive follow-up of all asbestos-exposed workers, even after they stopped working or closure of the asbestos factory, can help address this gap. This proactive monitoring programme lengthens the period of medical observation, improves the level of awareness about asbestos hazards, raises physicians' competency in diagnosing asbestos-related diseases, and allows the government to generate a reliable estimate of the number of asbestos-related occupational diseases, all of which contribute to early diagnosis, prevention, and treatment of asbestos-related diseases.

Retrospective exposure assessment is useful for investigating the association between exposure and occupational diseases, but it requires several key parameters to better estimate historical exposures. Case Study 4 demonstrates that the government might still have to decide on a policy to adopt based on imperfect or missing historical or currently available data. The government policy stems from international trends of banning asbestos and the scientific evidence of the long latency period of asbestos-related diseases. The collaboration with multidisciplinary experts in occupational medicine, occupational hygiene, epidemiology, and public policy can prevent potential occupational disease victims from being neglected by the lack of comprehensive exposure records.

Step 4: Communication and documentation

Exposure assessment findings must be communicated appropriately to all workers and those involved in protecting workers' health. Workers have the "right-to-know" the chemical hazards present in the workplace and how they can be protected from exposure (OSHA, 2017). Employees can be informed through warning signs, color-coding, signals, and emails. Information used for exposure assessment, such as lists of similar exposure groups, exposure profiles, judgment on their acceptability, and recommendations, should be stored for future continuous improvement, re-evaluation, and occupational disease recognition.

Step 5: Adopting compliance and comprehensive strategies

In adopting a compliance strategy, occupational hazard data are compared with the existing regulations. Compliance requires the exposure to be below the standard at an acceptable level, whereas non-compliance occurs when the measured levels exceed the statutory level. The standard comparison requires the collection of workers' 8-h time-weight averages (8-h TWAs) exposure for direct comparison with PELs or OELs.

When a comprehensive strategy is adopted, the results are presented in the daily exposure distributions. The common measures for interpreting the comprehensive strategy results include:

1. TWA exposures: The values should be reported as 8-h TWAs.
2. Short-term exposures: This method is not accurate for estimating an 8-h TWA, although the full 8-h shift is monitored. It is appropriate for measuring peak concentrations for comparison within short-term exposures or ceiling limits. The short-term exposure report includes a 15-min average exposure. The ceiling limits are the instant values at that time.
3. Results comparison: This measure compares the results with previous results collected for the same exposure groups or operations. As mentioned above, occupational hygienists can examine whether exposure has increased or decreased over time. Controls may be needed for operations if the exposure has increased, even if the chemical exposure is below the regulatory and recommended limits.

Control of Hazards

Once exposure to a specific hazard is determined as unacceptable or one that should be reduced, occupational health professionals should recommend the most feasible and effective control plans. Hazard control is defined as the adjustment or regulation of an operation to meet a standard or guideline, the reduction or prevention of contaminant release, and the ability to contain a stressor. The control plans are prioritised as follows: elimination or substitution of hazards, engineering controls, administrative controls, education of workers, and the use of personal protective equipment. Case Study 5 demonstrates a potential measure to reduce workers' exposure to hazardous chemicals. Further details on control of hazards are provided in the chapter on Prevention.

Case Study 5: Reducing Workers' Hazard Exposure in Oil and Gas Extraction

Global demand for oil and natural gas has continued to increase over recent decades. During oil drilling and gas extraction, toxic chemicals, such as benzene and butadiene, can be released into the environment (Rosenfeld and Feng, 2011). Exposure to these chemicals is associated with cancer development, such as leukaemia. The US NIOSH reported that the average working hours for workers in the oil drilling and gas extraction industry were 41–43.9 hours per week, about 6–9.5 hours higher than the average of general workers (34.5 hours per week) in the US (NIOSH, 2019).

Increased working hours may prolong exposure to hazardous chemicals and the risk of developing occupational diseases. If elimination, substitution, and engineering control are not the most feasible or cost-effective plans, administrative controls such as rotating tasks and reducing the total duration of exposure to a specific hazardous working environment should be considered.

Biomonitoring

The four principles of occupational hygiene (anticipation, recognition, evaluation, and control) are generally practiced in large-scale companies with full-time occupational hygienists. Small-scale companies often have insufficient occupational hygienists and scarce exposure data and comprehensive occupational health surveillance. The use of biomonitoring may serve as a simple and practical tool for assessing the health risks of workers in small companies.

Case Study 6 demonstrates the use of biomonitoring to estimate occupational exposure to chromium (Cr), manganese (Mn), and nickel (Ni) and of workers performing gas-metal arc welding in small- and medium-sized enterprises (Persoons *et al.*, 2014).

Case Study 6: Using Biomonitoring to Determine Occupational Exposure: A Study of Urinary Metal Concentrations in Welders

Metal-arc welding is a process that uses electricity to heat and melt metals and connects metals as they cool. This process produces welding fumes containing gases and metal oxides in the form of ultrafine particles. Common metal oxides emitted from welding fumes include Cr, Mn, and Ni. Welding fumes were classified by the IARC as Group 2B carcinogens (possibly carcinogenic to humans) in 1989 and upgraded to Group 1 carcinogens (carcinogenic to humans) in 2017 (Guha et al., 2017; IARC Working Group on the Evaluation of Carcinogenic Risks to Humans, 2017).

To characterise welders' exposure, large-scale companies usually focus on metal concentrations in atmospheric particulates in the workplace. Workplace monitoring data can help identify determinants of health risk, such as the type of welding process, lack of ventilation, and the composition of consumables. However, very few small-scale companies have resources to perform such comprehensive workplace environmental monitoring, leading to a scarcity of exposure data and unknown risks. Biomonitoring is a practical tool for estimating occupational exposure to metals in welders.

A hundred and ten welders from small- and medium-sized enterprises were recruited, and their urine samples were collected (Persoons et al., 2014). Urinary Cr, Mn, and Ni concentrations were measured and compared with the biological limit values (BLV) and those of reference groups (non-welders and the general population). However, the determinants of exposure, such as welding experience, composition of base metal (stainless/mild/galvanised steel), weekly welding duration, welding in confined spaces, presence of mechanical ventilation, and hygiene practices (e.g. type of respiratory protective equipment), varied among welders.

Collaboration with occupational hygienists and welders to complete the basic characterisation step can help address this knowledge gap.

After urine samples were analysed, urinary levels of Cr, Mn, and Ni among welders were compared with those in the BLV and reference groups. In this case, urinary concentrations of these metals were lower than the guidance values but higher than those measured in the general population, suggesting a low but measurable occupational exposure. Statistical analysis can help interpret the data. Models such as multiple linear regression can be used to identify predictors of workplace metal exposure from the above-mentioned exposure determinants. In this case, significant predictors associated with higher urinary Cr levels included older age, welding in confined spaces, and longer welding hours. In contrast, lower urinary Cr levels were observed in welders who handled mild steel-based metals and worked in places with mechanical ventilation.

Biomonitoring has become an important tool for evaluating the internal dose of occupational toxicants. Case Study 6 shows that biomonitoring is useful in occupational settings for assessing chemical exposures when workplace environmental monitoring is not feasible or cannot reflect the total picture of multiple exposures. The selection of biomonitoring indicators and interpretation of biomonitoring data require toxicological knowledge and rely on the guidance values (Cocker, 2014). Examples of biomonitoring guidance values are biological exposure indices (BEIs) (ACGIH, 2021), biological monitoring guidance values (BMGV) (Health and Safety Executive, 2020), and human biomonitoring (HBM) values (Human Biomonitoring Commission, 2015). Occasionally, biomonitoring results are compared with reference or background values, which are basically data derived from the non-occupational exposure population. Guidance values are usually higher than the reference or background values. Thus, biomonitoring results can be interpreted using the "traffic light" approach: "green" for biomonitoring results below the reference/background value, "yellow" for those above the reference/background value but below the guidance value, and "red" for those above the guidance value (Cocker, 2014).

The integration of occupational medicine with knowledge of toxicology, occupational hygiene, epidemiology, and statistics can help identify workers at high risk and plan for hazard control. While biomonitoring is a useful tool in occupational settings, its use requires careful consideration of ethical issues (Manno *et al.*, 2014). Biomonitoring involves collecting bodily fluids, tissues, or other accessible samples and, therefore, requires informed consent from each individual. Confidentiality of the data is another important consideration.

Conclusion

Practicing occupational health requires multidisciplinary knowledge and expertise, e.g. clinical medicine, toxicology, epidemiological, occupational hygiene, and biomonitoring. Evaluation of hazards in the workplace by exposure assessment and the management of identified hazards are essential occupational health practices that require inputs from these various disciplines. Evaluation of hazard exposure in the workplace encompasses planning, data collection, analysing and interpreting the data, summarising and preparing a conclusion, and recommending appropriate remedies. After hazard control, reassessment is necessary to validate the exposures in the workplace. A team approach involving physicians, nurses, toxicologists, epidemiologists, occupational hygienists, ergonomists, and safety professionals is required for holistic assessment and control of the hazards as well as effective health communication.

References

ACGIH. (2020) *Threshold Limit Values for chemical substances and physical agents and Biological Exposure Indices.* Cincinnati, American Conference of Governmental Industrial Hygienists.

ACGIH. (2021) *TLV/BEI guidelines.* [Online] Available from: https://www.acgih.org/science/tlv-bei-guidelines/. [Accessed on 22 February 2021].

Albin M, Gustavsson P. (2020) A silent epidemic: Occupational exposure limits are insufficiently protecting individual worker health. *Scand J Work Environ Health* 46(1): 110–112. Available from: https://doi.org/10.5271/sjweh.3864.

Anna DH. (2011) *The occupational environment: Its evaluation, control, and management* (3rd Ed). United States, American Industrial Hygiene Association.

Agency for Toxic Substances and Disease Registry. (2021) *Toxicological profiles.* [Online] Available from: https://www.atsdr.cdc.gov/toxprofiledocs/index.html. [Accessed on 21 February 2021].

Borghi F, Mazzucchelli LA, Campagnolo D, Rovelli S, Fanti G, Keller M, Cattaneo A, Spinazze A, Cavallo DM. (2020) Retrospective exposure assessment methods used in occupational human health risk assessment: A systematic review. *Int J Environ Res Public Health* 17(17): 6190. Available from: https://doi.org/10.3390/ijerph17176190.

Bullock WH, Ignacia JS. (2006) *A strategy for assessing and managing occupational exposures* (3rd Ed). Fairfax, VA, United States, American Industrial Hygiene Association.

Cherrie JW. (2019) Binding occupational exposure limits for carcinogens in the EU — necessary but not sufficient to reduce risk. *Scand J Work Environ Health* 45(4): 423–424. Available from: https://doi.org/10.5271/sjweh.3836.

Choi S, Yoon C, Kim S, Kim W, Ha K, Jeong J, Kim J, Shin J, Park D. (2018) Comprehensive evaluation of hazardous chemical exposure control system at a semiconductor manufacturing company in South Korea. *Int J Environ Res Public Health* 15(6). Available from: https://doi.org/10.3390/ijerph15061162.

Cocker J. (2014) A perspective on biological monitoring guidance values. *Toxicol Lett* 231(2): 122–125. Available from: https://doi.org/10.1016/j.toxlet.2014.09.010.

Coggon D, Rose G, Barker D. (2003) *Epidemiology for the uninitiated* (5th Ed). London, United Kingdom, BMJ.

European Chemicals Agency. (2021) *Occupational exposure limits.* [Online] Available from: https://echa.europa.eu/oel. [Accessed on 24 February 2021].

European Union. (1998) *Council Directive 98/24/EC of 7 April 1998 on the protection of the health and safety of workers from the risks related to chemical agents at work (fourteenth individual Directive within the meaning of Article 16(1) of Directive 89/391/EEC).* [Online] Available from: https://eur-lex.europa.eu/legal-content/EN/TXT/?uri=celex%3A31998L0024. [Accessed on 28 February 2021].

European Union. (2017) *Directive (EU) 2017/2398 of the European Parliament and of the Council of 12 December 2017 amending Directive 2004/37/EC on the protection of workers from the risks related to exposure to carcinogens or mutagens at work.* [Online] Available from: https://eur-lex.europa.eu/legal-content/EN/TXT/?uri=CELEX%3A32017L2398#ntr3-L_2017345EN.01008701-E0003. [Accessed on 28 February 2021].

Guha N, Loomis D, Guyton KZ, Grosse Y, El Ghissassi F, Bouvard V, Benbrahim-Tallaa L, Vilahur N, Muller K, Straif K. (2017) Carcinogenicity of welding, molybdenum trioxide, and indium tin oxide. *Lancet Oncol* 18(5): 581–582. Available from: https://doi.org/10.1016/s1470-2045(17)30255-3.

Human Biomonitoring Commission. (2015) *Reference and HBM values.* [Online] Available from: https://www.umweltbundesamt.de/en/topics/health/commissions-working-groups/human-biomonitoring-commission/reference-hbm-values. [Accessed on 21 February 2021].

Health and Safety Executive. (2020) *Biological monitoring guidance values.* [Online] Available from: https://www.hsl.gov.uk/online-ordering/analytical-services-and-assays/biological-monitoring/bm-guidance-values. [Accessed on 22 February 2021].

IARC. (2021) *IARC publications.* [Online] Available from: https://publications.iarc.fr/. [Accessed on 27 February 2021].

IARC Working Group on the Evaluation of Carcinogenic Risks to Humans. (2017) *Welding, molybdenum trioxide, and indium tin oxide.* Lyon, France, International Agency for Research on Cancer.

International Occupational Hygiene Association. (2021) *Hazards.* [Online] Available from: https://www.ioha.net/resources/hazards/. [Accessed on 22 February 2021].

Johanson G, Tinnerberg H. (2019) Binding occupational exposure limits for carcinogens in the EU—good or bad? *Scand J Work Environ Health* 45(3): 213–214. Available from: https://doi.org/10.5271/sjweh.3825.

Kacew S, Lee BM. (2012) Occupational toxicology. In: *Lu's basic toxicology: Fundamentals, target organs, and risk assessment* (6th Ed). Boca Raton, FL, United States, CRC Press.

Kazan-Allen L. (2019) *Current asbesetos ban.* [Online] Available from: http://www.ibasecretariat.org/alpha_ban_list.php. [Accessed on 21 February 2021].

Koh D. (1995) An outbreak of occupational dermatosis in an electronics store. *Contact Dermatitis* 32(6): 327–330. Available from: https://doi.org/10.1111/j.1600-0536.1995.tb00620.x.

Koh D, Phoon WO. (1986) Pulmonary tuberculosis among NTUC comfort taxi drivers. *Bull Int Union Tuberc* 61(1–2): 40–42.

Li CY, Sung FC. (1999) A review of the healthy worker effect in occupational epidemiology. *Occup Med* 49(4): 225–229. Available from: https://doi.org/10.1093/occmed/49.4.225.

Manno M, Sito F, Licciardi L. (2014) Ethics in biomonitoring for occupational health. *Toxicol Lett* 231(2): 111–121. Available from: https://doi.org/10.1016/j.toxlet.2014.10.004.

NIOSH. (2011) *What is RTECS?* [Online] Available from: https://www.cdc.gov/niosh/rtecs/default.html. [Accessed on 25 February 2021].

NIOSH. (2019) *U.S. oil and gas extraction workers: Fatigue, sleep, and working hours (extended version).* [Online] Available from: https://www.cdc.gov/niosh/topics/workschedules/2019abstracts/oilgas2.html. [Accessed on 2 February 2021].

NIOSH. (2020) *NIOSH pocket guide to chemical hazards.* [Online] Available from: https://www.cdc.gov/niosh/npg/. [Accessed on 25 February 2021].

OSHA. (2015) *Preventing occupational illnesses through safer chemical management.* [Online] Available from: https://www.osha.gov/chemical-management [Accessed on 24 February 2021].

OSHA. (2017) *Workers' rights.* [Online] Available from: https://www.osha.gov/sites/default/files/publications/osha3021.pdf. [Accessed on 16 February 2021].

OSHA. (2019) *Permissible exposure limits — annotated tables.* [Online] Available from: https://www.osha.gov/annotated-pels. [Accessed on 25 February 2021].

OSHA. (2020) *Arsenic: Standards.* [Online] Available from: https://www.osha.gov/arsenic/standards. [Accessed on 22 February 2021].

Park DU, Choi S, Lee S, Koh DH, Kim HR, Lee KH, Park J. (2019) Occupational characteristics of semiconductor workers with cancer and rare diseases registered with a Workers' Compensation Program in Korea. *Saf Health Work* 10(3): 347–354. Available from: https://doi.org/https://doi.org/10.1016/j.shaw.2019.03.003.

Persoons R, Arnoux D, Monssu T, Culié O, Roche G, Duffaud B, Chalaye D, Maitre A. (2014) Determinants of occupational exposure to metals by gas metal arc welding and risk management measures: A biomonitoring study. *Toxicol Lett* 231(2): 135–141. Available from: https://doi.org/10.1016/j.toxlet.2014.09.008.

Plog BA, Quinlan PJ, Villarreal J. (2012) *Fundamentals of industrial hygiene* (6th Ed). Illinois, United States, National Safety Council.

Rosenfeld PE, Feng LGH. (2011) *The petroleum industry. In Risks of hazardous wastes.* Boston, MA, United States, William Andrew Publishing.

Sahmel J, Devlin K, Paustenbach D, Hollins D, Gaffney S. (2010) The role of exposure reconstruction in occupational human health risk assessment: Current methods and a recommended framework. *CritRev Toxicol* 40(9): 799–843. Available from: https://doi.org/10.3109/10408444.2010.501052.

Świątkowska B, Szeszenia-Dąbrowska N, Wilczyńska U. (2016) Medical monitoring of asbestos-exposed workers: Experience from Poland. *Bull World Health Organ* 94(8): 599–604. Available from: https://doi.org/10.2471/blt.15.159426.

ToxTutor. (2018) *Introduction to toxicology.* [Online] Available from https://toxtutor.nlm.nih.gov/index.html. [Accessed on 23 February 2021].

UN. (2019) *Globally harmonized system of classification and labelling of chemicals (GHS).* [Online] Available from: https://unece.org/ghs-rev8-2019. [Accessed on 21 March 2021].

US Environmental Protection Agency. (2019) *Guidelines for human exposure assessment.* [Online] Available from: https://www.epa.gov/sites/production/files/2020-01/documents/guidelines_for_human_exposure_assessment_final2019.pdf. [Accessed on 26 January 2021].

US Department of Health and Human Services. (2021) *Publications.* [Online] Available from: https://ntp.niehs.nih.gov/publications/index.html. [Accessed on 21 March 2021].

Chapter 26

Occupational Medicine Practice and the Law

See Muah Lee[*,†,‡] *and David Koh*[*,†]

Introduction

The State has an interest in the regulation of medical practice as it must, in all important spheres of public activity. The regulatory framework for this includes professional bodies, such as the national medical councils, which are vested with powers to investigate complaints and to sanction errant behaviour, the law of tort, through which claimants who are harmed because of negligence can seek redress, and legislation. The law of contract would also be operable for agreed occupational health work by providers performed for employers.

Occupational health stands out as one specialty that is very much legislatively influenced, because of its essential interphase between the worker and his work environment. The protection of the health and

[*] Ng Teng Fong General Hospital, National University Health System, Singapore.
[†] Saw Swee Hock School of Public Health, National University of Singapore, Singapore.
PAPRSB Institute of Health Sciences, Universiti Brunei Darussalam, Brunei Darussalam *and* Yong Loo Lin School of Medicine, National University of Singapore, Singapore.
[‡] Centre for Biomedical Ethics, National University of Singapore, Singapore.
Corresponding author: See Muah Lee (See_Muah_Lee@nuhs.edu.sg).

safety of workers has long been acknowledged as a social right in all modern states. Not surprisingly, in most countries, there would be legislation pertaining to health and safety at work. This would impact on the conduct of all parties, among them occupational physicians, responsible and accountable for the protection of the health of the worker.

Ethics and the Law

An important hallmark of the professions is self-regulation. This takes effect through national bodies like for example, the Singapore Medical Council in Singapore and the General Medical Council in the United Kingdom. The state grants such governing bodies the powers and with it, the responsibilities for regulation of professional conduct.

The governing medical bodies would normally comprise senior and experienced members of the profession. Furthermore, perhaps mindful of the popular belief that "all professions are a conspiracy against the laity (George Bernard Shaw)," most such bodies would include some lay representation as well.

This right to determination of standards for its members would not be complete without the power to impose censure and penalty when members fall short of such standards, regardless of whether a harmed victim can be identified or not. The traditional principles in biomedical ethics — autonomy, non-maleficence, beneficence and justice (Beauchamp and Childress, 2001) are applicable to all physicians, including occupational physicians. These principles, together with other ethical norms governing behaviour in the professional relationships of the physicians with other parties, besides patients, will inform the standards that such governing bodies expect its members to observe.

Many jurisdictions would allow for appeal against the decisions of the medical councils in a higher court of law. Reliance on medical ethics for the court decisions will also play an important role, as would be points of law. This has been extensively tested in the case of the traditional therapeutic relationship of doctor and patient and biomedical research. There is no reason to believe that such reliance would not happen in occupational health.

One distinctive feature of occupational health is the interests of many stakeholders, such as employers, workers, government officials (e.g. factory inspectors), worker representatives and other technical experts; set against the backdrop of the work environment, instead of the traditional hospital or clinic setting. Specialty specific guidance, such as those provided by the International Code of Ethics for Occupational Health Professionals (ICOH, 2014) from the International Commission of Occupational Health, and Ethics for Occupational Physicians by the Faculty of Occupational Medicine, United Kingdom (Faculty of Occupational Medicine, 2018) are helpful resources.

The status of workers, in any given situation, as patients construed in the traditional sense, has been perhaps a little over debated. How would biomedical guidelines apply? What is the status of a worker at screening but not seeking care, or a pre-employment candidate at a medical examination? Each will have to be determined on its own merit, including an understanding of the purpose of such a determination.

Laws will differ jurisdiction to jurisdiction, just as the rules of one country may not necessarily apply to another. One guiding principle ought to be that of a universal respect for the dignity of all individuals. This will not change, regardless of the individual being one among the group impacted by a management health decision, or being a patient with a clinical problem for consultation.

Where physicians are contracted with employers for occupational health work, it is also recommended that occupational physicians apprise the contracting parties of the fundamental ethical and legal obligations of doctors. This can help pre-empt problems in contract terms and its interpretation that might run contrary to these obligations.

Confidentiality of Information: Ethics and Law

Case Study 1: Sickness Absence

A company is trying to control its health care expenditure, which is increasing year by year. The Human Resource (HR) department has identified the twenty workers with the highest medical expenditure and another twenty workers with the highest sickness absence. The HR department now wishes to know about their health conditions so that they can understand the reasons and help the workers maintain better health and productivity.

Commentary

The doctor has a duty to maintain confidentiality of medical information that has been disclosed to the doctor. Breach of confidentiality, that is the disclosure of such information without consent, would be unethical and in certain countries, unlawful, for the purpose described. In Singapore and the United Kingdom, the Personal Data Protection Act 2012 and the Data Protection Act 1998 respectively gives legal protection to the confidentiality of medical information, restricting access by third parties. In the United Kingdom, the Data Protection Act 1998 also provides the statutory right of access by the patient/worker to his own health and medical information.

Businesses have a legitimate interest in controlling costs. This applies to employee benefits and welfare. The containment of health care costs is best achieved by the design of these benefits. The disclosure of medical information by doctors without informed consent from patients, nevertheless, would be a step too far in his assistance of this business objective.

Companies should have in place a management policy for dealing with sickness absences. Such absences may be long term or short term spells. The associated reasons are varied; from long term absences caused by serious illnesses to short term ones, sometimes, associated with stress and morale issues. Employers must act and be seen to be acting in a reasonable, fair and transparent manner.

If medical information is sought from the doctors, consent from the workers has to be obtained. When requesting for consent, the doctors should also explain to the workers the purpose for disclosure of such information, and who the recipient of such information would be. It is always good practice for occupational physicians, when preparing medical reports, to offer to show these reports to the workers or patients concerned before onward transmission to third parties, including employers.

Besides disclosure of information related to sickness absence, the control of sickness absence lends itself to ethical and legal controversies too when such absences are restricted, possibly as a result of management pressure. In 2013, the Ministry of Manpower, Singapore, has found it necessary to issue a circular to doctors addressing the issue of complaints alleging that medical practitioners have been issuing medical certification of absences to injured workers that are inadequate in relation to the nature and severity of their injuries (Ministry of Health Singapore, 2013). Restricting care, in this case, not giving the adequate amount of rest for injuries and illness to recover is unethical and risks liability to lawsuits.

The duty to maintain confidentiality of medical information is not absolute. The law may require disclosure, as in the notification of occupational illnesses, to the relevant authorities. In the event that the physician is the notifying person, then the delicate situation may also arise as to whether the employer should be informed as well. In most cases, it would also be good practice to seek the agreement of the worker in letting the employer know. This would allow the employer to investigate and manage the risks accordingly and cooperate fully with the authorities.

Public interest, such as the averting of real harm to others, has also been cited as grounds for justifiably breaching the duty to maintain confidentiality of information. Such was the reasoning in W v. Edgell (1990) and the United Kingdom Clinical Ethics Network (2010).

Fitness to Work; Medicolegal Challenges

Case Study 2: Physical Harm (Coffee, 1972)

Mr. Coffee applied for a position as a pilot with an aircraft manufacturer. He was required to undergo a physical examination at the corporation's clinic. It included, among other investigations, blood tests for haemoglobin count and erythrocyte sedimentation rate, which were found to be abnormal. The blood test results were filed and date and time stamped by the clinic secretary without review by the doctors. Mr. Coffee was hired and several months later, nearly collapsed and was discovered to have multiple myeloma.

Although the physicians, who were employees of the corporation, were exonerated, the corporation was nevertheless held was negligent in failing to exercise due care in handling blood test reports taken in a physical examination they required Mr Coffee to undergo.

Commentary

In *Coffee*, the claim involved physical harm. The court rightly expects a non-negligent medical assessment, one which requires the exercise of reasonable skill and care. There is no duty to explore and discover all manner of illnesses at such examinations. Whether the standard of care was breached has to be judged in "the light of all the circumstances" (Coffee, 1972). Thus, the failure to pay regard to the abnormal results of tests that were ordered, whatever the reasons may be, was judged to be inexcusable. Furthermore, the senior physician of the team had given evidence that had he been aware of the abnormalities, it would have prompted further inquiry and disqualification for the job. In this particular case, the employer did have a procedural system directed to their physicians, which was unfortunately flawed and resulted in the oversight. The employers were therefore found liable.

It is highly probable that the physicians would have been liable had they not been employees but independent contractors. The legal doctrine of "respondent superior," which briefly translated from its Latin origin means "let the superior answer," is widely applied in employer-employee relationships. Thus not only would employers be themselves liable for their own negligent actions, they would also be generally held liable for the negligent actions of their employees at work. *Coffee* should also serve as a deterrent to physicians against making careless and shoddy assessments.

We should also be mindful that work in occupational health may be conducted within a contractual framework between an occupational health service providing fitness to work assessments and the business organisation concerned. A legal duty thus exists to enforce competent performance of contractual obligations by the occupational health providers for these businesses, a breach of which can also potentially result in a claim by the business as well.

Case Study 3: Disability Discrimination (Kaltoft, 2014)

In November 2010, Mr Kaltoft, having worked for fifteen years as a childminder with the Municipality of Billund (Denmark) was terminated from employment. He alleged that his obesity was the motivation behind the termination. He then sought a declaration from the court for unlawful discrimination and compensation. The ruling from the European Court of Justice established that in general, the principle of non-discrimination is a fundamental right. However, in the area of employment European Union law does not lay down a general principle of non-discrimination on grounds of obesity as such.

Commentary

Statutory protection focuses on disability, with "substantial" effect on normal day-to-day activities regardless of cause. Following European Union case law, disability has come to be understood as a limitation arising from long term, physical, mental or psychological impairments which may hinder the full and effective participation of the person in professional life as compared to other workers. From a medical point of view, with all the known subjective as well as objective features of obesity affecting almost every organ system, proving disability from morbid or super obesity, a recognised medical condition should not be difficult.

In countries like the United Kingdom, statutory protection against disability discrimination under the Equality Act (United Kingdom, 2010) helps to clarify what constitutes discrimination and ensure the employment participation of people with disability and other statutorily defined "protected" characteristics. Many people with chronic diseases are however not disabled in the legal sense and therefore may not enjoy the protection of the Act.

Reliance on anti-discrimination statutes requires evidence of disability at the first instance. Where disability resulting from certain medical conditions is established, the occupational physician can assist in making a health risk assessment of the work requirements and its impact on the health and safety of the person concerned. Where appropriate, this can be translated into useful advice about how best to accommodate such workers. While occupational physicians can assist in dispelling myths and false beliefs about work-ability, it is a reality of the modern world, even in countries with anti-discrimination legislation that helps to improve the rights of people with disabilities, employers are generally free to choose who they wish to employ.

Some countries do not rely on hard legislations, instead turning to soft law in the form of codes to help workers who might feel they are unfairly treated, e.g. on grounds of their sickness, notwithstanding the fact that their work-ability is minimally affected if at all. In Singapore, the Tripartite Alliance for Fair and Progressive Employment Practices (TAFEP) is a government body with an advisory role and to a limited extent, an intercession role for people who might have "discrimination concerns," to which TAFEP would then respond by assisting the employers in the "adoption of fair employment practices." However, the decisions of such bodies may have limited binding force.

A Legal Duty to Non-Patients

Case Study 4: A Duty to Warn (Kaiser, 1965)

In Kaiser, the defendant physician prescribed a sedating antihistamine to his patient, whom the physician knew to be a bus driver. After taking the first dose of the medication the following morning, the driver went to work and was involved in an accident after falling asleep while driving the bus. The driver had apparently felt groggy before the accident but continued to drive nonetheless. A passenger on the bus was injured in the accident and sued the doctor and the bus company.

The Washington Supreme Court noted that the evidence suggested that the doctor may not have informed his bus driver-patient of "the dangerous side effects of drowsiness or lassitude" from the drug and that expert evidence suggested that it was negligent not to do so.

In remanding the case, the court held that: The jury should be directed that (a) in the event it finds no warning was given the bus driver as to the side effects of the drug, it shall bring in a verdict against the doctor; (b) in the event the jury finds the bus driver failed to exercise the highest degree of care, even though he was given no warning as to the side effects of the drug, the jury shall also bring in a verdict against the bus company and the driver; and (c) in the event the jury finds that a warning of the side effects of the drug was given to the bus driver, then the verdict shall be against the bus company and the driver only.

Thus, the basis of the doctor's duty to the non-patient bus passenger stemmed solely from the need to warn his patient, a bus driver, of the potential side effect of drowsiness.

Commentary

Kaiser is particularly instructive for the occupational physician. An occupational physician who has certified fitness in a worker who subsequently injures a third party because of a medical condition that has not been properly evaluated, or which the worker has not been cautioned about, may in turn be sued by the third party who has been injured by the worker. The necessity to warn and to advise cannot be overemphasised. An example would be the worker with diabetes on insulin treatment, who if considered stable and fit for employment, must be warned and be engaged in a discussion about hypogylcaemia. This is especially important if there are safety implications in the job (Lee *et al.*, 2009).

Whenever the standard of clinical care is in dispute, according to the judgment in Bolam v. Friern Hospital Management Committee (Bolam, 1957), "A doctor is not guilty of negligence if he has acted in accordance with a practice accepted as proper by a responsible body of medical men skilled in that particular art." Judicial scrutiny of the logic behind such expert opinion is allowed for, as decided in Bolitho v. Hackney HA (Bolitho, 1997). However, judges unwilling to accept the expert view as logical, especially for complex medical and technical issues would be rare.

When it comes to the duty to warn, a matter of which a nonmedical person can reasonably have an opinion of, the courts have shown they can be quite vigorous in defending patient interests.

The Bolam-Bolitho principle may have limited application in such cases where the duty centers on warning and cautioning patients about possible adverse effects and risks. Doctors are to ensure that patients are informed about material risks resulting from the treatment. "The test of materiality is whether, in the circumstances of the particular case, a reasonable person in the patient's position would be likely to attach significance to the risk, or the doctor is or should reasonably be aware that the particular patient would be likely to attach significance to it" (Rogers, 1995; Montgomery, 2015). Notably in Singapore, the area of consent is being codified into legislation. Reliance on peer professional opinion is retained, with the added caveat that the patient's individual factors must have been taken into account (Government of Singapore, 2020).

Occupational Health and Safety Legislation

The laws of most countries would mandate the duties of employers in the protection of workers at the workplace. In the developed countries, such legislations often have a long history. For example, in the United Kingdom, these date back to the Act for Better Regulations of Chimney Sweeps and their Apprentices of 1788. In 1802, the Health and Morals of Apprentices Act was enacted, and the Factory Act followed in 1819. The legislation has been continuously reviewed and updated, and subsequently led to the passing of the Health and Safety at Work etc. Act 1974.

These laws compel employers to think and reflect on their occupational health and safety responsibilities in the various areas of work. Duties, responsibilities, and competency issues will need to be addressed. The duties spelt out under the law in the United Kingdom are qualified by the principle of "so far as is reasonably practicable." Modern health and safety laws at work are generally based on risk assessment, risk management by competent persons, training and the setting up of emergency response procedures and the sharing of information with workers.

One continual challenge of occupational health law must be the necessity to respond to developments in work practices, such as the introduction of new substances, and new methods or new information about old substances and old methods used in the workplace.

The administration and enforcement of the legislation is usually provided for by establishment of national agencies with responsibilities for occupational safety and health, such as the US Occupational Safety and Health Agency (OSHA).

Case Study 5: Workplace Safety and Health Act

In 2004, three major industrial accidents happened in Singapore in quick succession. On 24 April, a subway tunnel being constructed under the Nicoll Highway collapsed, resulting in a cave-in across all six lanes of the road. Four people were killed and three injured (Committee of Inquiry Singapore, 2004). Five days later, on 29 April, steel latticeworks at a construction site for the country's latest high-tech business park at Fusionpolis gave way, killing two workers and injuring twenty-nine people (Ministry of Manpower Singapore, 2005). A month later, on 29 May, a flash fire occurred on board the tanker Almudaina while hot works were being carried out (Ministry of Manpower Singapore, 2004). Seven workers died. Upon investigation, all three incidents were found to have resulted from lapses in workplace health and safety processes. Multiple irregularities and warning signs at the Nicoll Highway worksite were disregarded, resulting in the catastrophic collapse of the tunnel. The design of the foundation of the steel latticeworks' design at Fusionpolis was fundamentally flawed, leading to its failure and collapse. Safety procedures on the Almudaina were not complied with. Sludge at the bottom of a tank was not cleaned out prior to the hot works. Sparks and molten metal from the hot works ignited the sludge and caused the flash fire.

Commentary

Following the accidents, the Singapore Parliament moved to tighten up the laws and regulations governing workplace health and safety. The Workplace Safety and Health Act (Cap. 354A) ("WSHA") came into effect in 2006. It brought Singapore in line with the regulatory practices of other developed countries.

The WSHA covers all workspaces, not just those at high risk of industrial accidents, like shipyards and construction sites. Both employers and occupiers of workplaces are liable. For instance, someone who owns a building who employs a contractor to carry out building works is liable if the contractor's workers (who are not directly employed by the owner of the building) suffers an injury during the works. Unpaid volunteers, loaned employees and illegal workers are also covered, and employers cannot disclaim liability due to the nature of an employee's legal status.

As in the United Kingdom, stakeholders are required to take "all reasonably practical measures" to ensure the safety and health of their workers and the public. This standard is similar to the standard of "reasonable care" in the common law.

If companies fail to comply with the standards of the WSHA, they would be subject to a remedial order to rectify the lapses. If the company does not comply then it may also be prosecuted and fined — even if no injury has resulted from the breach. Financial penalties were raised and all breaches of the WSHA criminalised, to better reflect the true cost of workplace accidents. If a company commits a criminal act, its directors and senior management are liable.

Fundamentally, the WSHA sought to create a "culture of safety." To usher in this cultural change, the government also set up a Workplace Health and Safety Council ("WHSC"). Its membership comprises leaders of industry, the unions, the government and professional organisations. WHSC is in charge of setting safety and health standards in the form of Codes of Practice across the different sectors, from metal working to healthcare.

Features of Occupational Health and Safety Legislation

Common features found in such legislation would cover areas such as requirements for:

Risk assessment

Employers should assess the risks to employees and others who may be affected by the work. Such assessments should include identification of significant hazards and the control measures. The questions to ask are: (a) what measures are necessary and sufficient to prevent a breach of law, and (b) are these measures reasonably practical? Practically, this means conducting comprehensive risk assessments and coming up with detailed plans to minimise or eliminate risks. This helps to create a mindset amongst employers and employees to take active steps in improving workplace safety and health. There should be arrangements in place for the effective planning, organisation, control, monitoring and review of the preventive and protective measures, including the provision of personal protective equipment.

First-aid and emergency measures

Adequate facilities must be provided. There should also be trained personnel, such as first-aiders and rescuers, who must be readily available to respond to emergency situations.

Appointment of trained and competent persons

This is to ensure that employers have trained competent persons appointed to monitor and effectively control health and health problems. Competence can be described as a combination of training, skills, experience and knowledge that a person has and their ability to perform a task safely.

Training in occupational health and safety and hazard communication

All employees should understand their role and responsibilities in preventing accidents and diseases and promoting health at work. They should be made aware of the preventive measures required and given specific training on safe work procedures. Persons exposed to hazardous substances or processes have a right to know of the risks and the preventive measures. Information provided can be in the form of Safety Data Sheets (SDS), warning signs and labeling.

Statutory medical examinations

Persons employed in certain occupations, or who are exposed to prescribed hazards at the workplace may require medical examinations to ensure that they are fit for such work, as well as to monitor their health and detect any early evidence of work-related ill-health.

There may be requirements for such examinations to be performed by medical practitioners who have training in occupational medicine.

Reporting of occupational accidents and diseases

It is important that accidents and diseases caused by work are reported as soon as possible so that investigations can be conducted and measures implemented promptly to prevent recurrence of such cases.

Health and safety committees

Health and safety committees should comprise management as well as worker representatives. This partnership would enable collective wisdom to be brought to bear on the interpretation and compliance to health and safety laws, bearing in mind the particular circumstances of the business. Their functions are to review safety and occupational health performance regularly, as well as to promote occupational health and safety. In some countries, the occupational health physician is a designated member of the Committee.

Case Study 6: Breach of Statutory Duty in Civil Claims (Cookson, 2007)

Mr. Cookson had worked for Novartis in the production of dye-stuffs from 1964. In 2001, he developed bladder cancer and alleged that this was caused by negligent exposure to beta-naphthylamine, among some other substances of varying carcinogenicity found in the dye manufacturing process. Throughout this period, the regulations regarding beta naphthylamine use have been updated in tandem with new knowledge about its properties and health effects.

The process of making dyestuff consisted of mixing and heating various chemicals in liquid form in reaction vessels. The work environment to which the claimant was exposed was extremely dusty and the claimant alleged a breach of the section 63(1) of the Factories Act in force at that time. Furthermore, it was alleged that the employer failed to warn the claimant of the risk of exposure and did not provide him with appropriate protective clothing. At one time, the claimant was given only a gauze mask and later a paper mask.

Having established that there was exposure and that the exposure was in breach of duty, the final issue of the claim turned on causation. An independent epidemiologist invited to submit his views on the issue on causation, concluded that the risk of harm from smoking was probably the greater compared to occupational exposure. However, Mr. Cookson's urologist did not agree and went on to prepare a full report refuting the findings of the epidemiologist. He referred also to the epidemiologist's own published work that the risks due to smoking decreased with the passage of time after cessation. Mr. Cookson has by that time, given up smoking many years. He also made references to the exposure levels to which Mr. Cookson was subjected.

The appeal by the employer, against the judgment of the lower court which found the employer liable, was subsequently dismissed.

Commentary

Claims can arise in tort for breach of health and safety duties created by statute. Employees who are injured because of the employers' breach of these duties would find the courts in general to be quite sympathetic in respect to such breaches being applied as a cause of action. Such claimants belong to the class for whose benefit the legislation was enacted.

Self-Regulation

State resources are often not available for intensive inspection and scrutiny of all workplaces. Moreover, legislation can never be completely comprehensive in addressing issues given the varied nature of workplaces and work processes. The statutes will need to be interpreted in the context of each workplace.

Therefore, regulatory agencies could adopt a strategy of cooperative compliance or industry self-regulation with a strong coercive foundation. Self-regulation does not mean that the State would observe with idle indifference serious breaches in health and safety performance of a business, even if these activities have been negotiated in agreement with the workers.

A responsible State would not condone risky and poorly managed activities voluntarily undertaken by workers, induced perhaps by the prospect of more pay. Thus, regulations are issued for specific activities deemed too hazardous or dangerous to be left to its discretionary management by the business. These regulations include those for chemical handling (Health and Safety Executive (HSE), 2002), work in confined spaces (HSE, 1997), noise exposure (HSE, 2005), and asbestos (HSE, 2006), among many others.

Standards and Codes of Practice

Occupational health and safety legislation is often supplemented by standards developed to provide more detailed guidelines and performance measurements for the purposes of compliance and/or adoption of best practices.

Two examples of these standards are exposure standards that set limits on exposures to harmful substances (such as noise, radiation, chemicals), and Occupational Health and Safety Management Systems (OHSMS). Key components of OHSMS include policy setting, hazard and risk analysis, implementation of measures to manage risk, training and hazard communication and measures for continuous review and improvement. Audits of these management systems must be conducted at regular intervals to ensure that they remain relevant and are effectively implemented.

Codes of practice provide practical examples of good practice. Adherence to codes of practice, analogous to clinical practice guidelines, would have evidentiary value in court proceedings. These codes of practice would usually have been approved by the relevant regulatory bodies. Examples include those for respirator use and ear defenders (CP74, 2006; CP76, 2006). The regulatory bodies can exercise their powers in enforcing compliance, providing advice and in the gravest of cases, prosecution.

The following two case studies demonstrate the importance of both external as well as internal guidelines and performance measurements for the purposes of compliance and/or adoption of best practices.

Case Study 7: Failure to Provide Adequate Occupational Health Services (Health and Safety Executive, 2017)

Ramsay Health Care (UK) Operations Ltd, a healthcare provider, was fined £550,000 plus £36,000 costs under ss.2 and 3 of HSWA for failing to ensure the health and safety of employees and non-employees.

An occupational nurse employed by the company raised concerns with the Health and Safety Executive (HSE) about the operations of the company's internal occupational health service in June 2014. On investigation, the HSE determined that the company had failed to appoint sufficient occupational health professionals to run its service, which compromised the health and safety of employees, patients and the public. Four improvement notices were served on the company. It was also deemed that the company has also failed to provide adequate health surveillance for its workers, resulting in a nurse developing occupational dermatitis.

Commentary

In 2013, Ramsay Health Care (RHC) brought its OH Service inhouse from an external provider. A well-being coordinator with a Master's degree in occupational health was appointed. However, this person had a background in physiotherapy and had never worked in an OH department. The rest of the team had broad healthcare qualifications, including health and safety, sports science and rehabilitation and speech therapy but limited OH experience. A single temporary agency OH nurse was employed by the department, to cater to approximately 4,500 employees. This agency nurse had no access to an occupational physician.

According to the HSE, staffing at RHC was "inadequate both in numbers, organisation and qualifications." The lack of an adequate OH service meant that RHC was not complying with relevant legislation such as the Health and Safety (Sharp Instruments in Healthcare) Regulations 2013 and the Control of Substances Hazardous to Health Regulations 2002.

In general, an employer is required to assess workplace risks to determine what is appropriate in terms of OH provision. This assessment has to take into account factors such as the size of the workforce, the risks present, the distribution of those risks throughout the workplace, and the relevant legislations that apply to the workplace. In this particular instance, the Association of National Health Occupational Physicians (ANHOP) guidelines for staffing an occupational health department in the NHS — Assessing the Occupational Health Manpower Levels for NHS Trusts, 1/7/1999 — might be an appropriate external guideline, and competent persons should be appointed to provide the OH service. It would be appropriate that the service in this context be either nurse-led or doctor-led, with qualifications in OH and experience working in OH (Webber, 2018).

Case Study 8: Occupational Health Standards vs Public Interest (R, 2012)

In September 2009, the volunteer fire department in the town of Meaford in Canada responded to an early morning fire in an apartment above a local restaurant. The fire department employed appropriate tactics in the response, including an interior search and seizure. However, during the rescue attempt, the self-contained breathing apparatus of a firefighter malfunctioned and, although extricated from the burning building, two firefighters suffered smoke inhalation.

Following this incident, the Ministry of Labour prosecuted the Town of Meaford Fire Department under the OSHA.

Commentary

Fire and Rescue Services and similar agencies throughout the world have to balance public expectations to perform heroic emergency services on one hand while maintaining high standards of occupational health and safety on the other. This dilemma was demonstrated in the above case, where the Ontario Court of Justice eventually acquitted the Town of Meaford Fire Department from charges under the OHSA, when it ruled that a standard of perfection regarding worker safety in this instance is both unfair and contrary to public interest. However, a fire department should have its own internal standard operating guidelines and should also refer to available provincial or national level guidelines for its standard practices. If the Fire department does not adhere to these guidelines, it may find itself liable to prosecution and be convicted (Norm, 2013).

Qualifying Disclosures

In many countries, there are laws to protect whistleblowers against reprisals by employers if they make disclosures which are in the "public interest". Such reprisals may range from detrimental treatment at work to outright dismissal. Disclosures about threats to health and safety are included as matters of public interest. They should logically be followed up with the employer or management.

However, if the worker is not comfortable with disclosures to the employers, she may do so to the authorities. In the United Kingdom, under the Public Disclosure Act 1998, these are prescribed bodies, which in the case of occupational health and safety issues would be the "Health and Safety Executive". To be protected by the law, the worker must make the disclosure in good faith and believe the disclosure to be substantially true.

Occupational Health Legislations and the Occupational Physician

The involvement of occupational health physicians as specialist service providers is often needed when health risk assessments are undertaken. This can be varied, from statutory medical examinations for workers, e.g. those exposed to prescribed hazards such as noise, to workplace assessment, e.g. noise level measurements. Reliance on such advice by employers which turn out to be inept or negligent could be potentially litigable (Lee *et al.*, 2009). The case of the occupational health providers being invited to court to defend such decisions, though seldom heard of, is a distinct possibility.

Notification of occupational illnesses is also another statutory duty in most countries. This would usually follow a prescribed list in the regulations, which in the United Kingdom is the Reporting of Injuries, Diseases and Dangerous Occurrences Regulations (RIDDOR).

Compensation for Injuries Suffered at Work and Occupational Diseases

Case Study 9: Workplace Injury and Compensation

In 2008, Mr. Hafizul, a foreign worker from Bangladesh working at a construction site in Singapore was injured (Vijayan, 2010). A 50kg bag of cement fell onto his back, fractured his spine and left him paralysed from waist down. He rejected the workmen compensation of SGD182,000 authorised by the Commissioner for Labour and decided to pursue the claim in the civil court. In June 2010, the High Court found in his favour and ordered the employers to compensate Mr. Hafizul SGD910,000.

Commentary

The Workplace Injury and Compensation Act (Cap. 354) ("WICA") is, in its essence, a no-fault compensation scheme. Similar schemes can be found in other countries. Currently in Singapore, an employer who suffers a workplace injury has up to one year to choose to pursue a claim under common law, or WICA, but not both at the same time. Mr Hafizul's High Court claim following assessment by the Commissioner of Labour would not be possible today.

Under WICA, as long as an injury or a disease was acquired in the course of employment, an employee can make a claim for compensation without having to prove that her employer was negligent. This includes psychiatric injury, as well as situations where a worker is injured in a traffic accident while travelling on company transport.

WICA covers any local or foreign employee (like Abdul) who is under a contract of service or contract of apprenticeship, regardless of salary, age or nationality. However, independent contractors, the self-employed, domestic workers, and those considered "uniformed personnel" are not covered.

WICA compensation comprises medical leave wages, medical expenses up to a maximum limit and lump-sum compensation for permanent incapacity or death. Claims must be made within one year from the accident.

In contrast, an action brought in tort law would entitle the claimant to damages in the form of current and future medical and hospital expenses, current and future loss of earnings, miscellaneous expenses (such as cost of caregivers and transport costs), and pain and suffering. If a worker succeeds in a civil suit against his employer, she is likely to obtain a higher quantum of damages than if she had filed for a claim under WICA. However, this is based on the assumption that she is able to prove that the employer was at fault, and was able to produce sufficient evidence in support of her claim. The cost of legal fees as well as the longer time it would take to see through the lawsuit may prove to be prohibitive to many injured workers.

Case Study 10: Pandemic Issues: COVID-19 and Legislation

The impact on work caused by the COVID-19 pandemic has been significant. Shops, offices, factories and construction sites were shut, save for those providing essential services and sectors critical to the global and local supply chain. Work from home was encouraged. Social distancing and use of masks were mandated. Cross boundary travels were prohibited, and this affected foreign workers. Quarantine measures were instituted.

Singapore with a population of 5.7 million, was heavily dependent on 1.42 million migrant workers for mostly low skilled jobs. Many of these workers were housed in "foreign worker dormitories." While dormitory conditions reportedly complied with standards that the World Bank imposed on their construction projects, they were nonetheless cramped, with workers often sleeping in bunk beds and sharing communal kitchens and toilets. This created conditions that allowed the virus to spread rapidly. The epidemic in Singapore was subsequently brought under control through a series of measures including testing, isolation, quarantine and vaccination when it was subsequently available.

The government's powers to impose sweeping, restrictive public health measures were derived from a number of statutes. Chief amongst those was the Infectious Diseases Act (Cap. 137), which provided the legal basis for monitoring and reporting the disease by practitioners, and for the declaration of isolation areas. From 2 April to 1 June 2020, the Infectious Diseases (Workplace Measures to Prevent Spread of COVID-19) Regulations 2020 was also implemented to mandate telecommuting and social distancing measures in the workplace. These devolved to become the Safe Management Measures issued by the Tripartite Partners, which would become relevant as companies resume business.

Conclusion

Many stakeholders are involved in occupational health. The agenda of these stakeholders may not be necessarily congruent. Profits and the bottom line would be a pressing concern for all commercial enterprises. Employment issues for workers would revolve round career progression, perks and pay. Safety, with its immediate consequences and impact may tend to overshadow occupational health concerns, some of which have long latency before harms are obvious. Adherence to sound occupational health practice requires commitment, training, greater awareness and the resources of a multidisciplinary team. The State has an important role in balancing the interests of all these stakeholders, through the application of laws and regulations and the use of the "carrot and stick" approach.

References

Beauchamp TL, Childress JF. (2001) *Principles of Biomedical Ethics*. Oxford, Oxford University Press.

Bolam v. Friern Hospital Management Committee. (1957) 2 ALL ER118.

Bolitho v. Hackney HA. (1997) 4 All ER 643.

Coffee v. McDonnell-Douglas Corporation. (1972) 503 P2d 1366 Cal 1972.

Committee of Inquiry, Singapore. (2004) *The Incident at the MRT Circle Line Worksite that Led to the Collapse of the Nicoll Highway On 20 April 2004: An interim report on the investigations, by The Committee of into the Collapse of Nicoll Highway on 20 April 2004.* [Online] Available from: https://www.nas.gov.sg/archivesonline/data/pdfdoc/2004091398-MOM.pdf. [Accessed on 14 June 2021].

CP74. (2006) Code of Practice 74 Code of Practice for selection, use and maintenance of respiratory protection devises, approved under Workplace Safety and Health Act Singapore.

CP76. (2006) Code of Practice 76 Code of Practice for selection, use and maintenance of hearing protectors, approved under Workplace Safety and Health Act Singapore.

European Court of Justice. (2014) *Kaltoft v Municipality of Billund.* Info-Curia Case-law, C-354/13.

Faculty of Occupational Medicine. (2018) *Ethics Guidance for Occupational Health Practice 2018.* London, Faculty of Occupational Medicine of the Royal College of Physicians.

Government of Singapore. (2020) *Civil Law (Amendment) Act 2020.* [Online] Available from: https://sso.agc.gov.sg/Bills-Supp/33-2020/Published/20200903?DocDate=20200903. [Accessed on 14 June 2021].

Health and Safety Executive v. Ramsay Health Care (UK) Operations Ltd. (2017) Southwark Crown Court, 30 October.

Health and Safety Executive. (1997) *Confined spaces regulations.* [Online] Available from: http://www.opsi.gov.uk/si/si1997/19971713.htm. [Accessed on 14 June 2021].

Health and Safety Executive. (2002) *Control of substances hazardous to health (COSHH).* [Online] Available from: http://www.hse.gov.uk/coshh/index.htm. [Accessed on 14 June 2021].

Health and Safety Executive. (2005) *Control of noise at work regulations.* [Online] Available from: http://www.hse.gov.uk/noise/regulations.htm. [Accessed on 14 June 2021].

Health and Safety Executive. (2006) *Control of asbestos regulations.* [Online] Available from: http://www.hse.gov.uk/asbestos/regulations.htm. [Accessed on 14 June 2021].

Health and Safety Executive. (2013) *Reporting Accidents and Incidents at Work: A Brief Guide to the Reporting of Injuries, Diseases and Dangerous Occurrences Regulations 2013 (RIDDOR).* [Online] Available from: https://www.hse.gov.uk/pubns/indg453.htm. [Accessed on 14 June 2021].

ICOH. (2014) *International Code of Ethics for Occupational Health Professionals.* [Online] Available from: http://www.icohweb.org/site/multimedia/code_of_ethics/code-of-ethics-en.pdf. [Accessed on 14 June 2021].

Kaiser v. (1965) *Suburban Transportation System.* 398 P.2d 14 (Wash. 1965).

Kaltoft v. Municipality of Billund. (2014) CJEU Case C-354/13.

Lee SM, Sng J, Koh D. (2009. The doctor in claims for work injuries and ill health. Legal Pitfalls. *Ann Acad Med Singap* **38**: 727–732.

Lee SM, Sum CF, Koh D. (2009) Legal issues in the management of patients with diabetes mellitus. *Singap Med J*, **50**(12): 1200–1206.

Ministry of Manpower Singapore. (2005) *Outcome of Investigations into the Cause of the Collapse of the Steel Latticework at the Fusionpolis Worksite Located at Ayer Rajah Avenue on 29 April 2004.* [Online] Available from: https://www.nas.gov.sg/archivesonline/data/pdfdoc/20050505994.pdf. [Accessed on 14 June 2021].

Ministry of Manpower Singapore. (2004) *Outcome of Investigations into the Cause of the Fire Onboard the Vessel "Almudaina" at Keppel Shipyard Limited at 15 Benoi Road on 29 May 2004.* [Online] Available from: https://www.nas.gov.sg/archivesonline/data/pdfdoc/20041215-MOM.pdf. [Accessed on 14 June 2021].

Ministry of Health Singapore. (2013) MOH Circular 17/2013 Issuance of Medical Certificates to Injured Workers.

Montgomery (Appellant) v. Lanarkshire Health Board. (2015) 2 WLR 7687.

Norm K. (2013) *5 Cases OHS Managers Need to Know.* [Online] Available from: https://www.thesafetymag.com/ca/news/opinion/5-cases-ohs-managers-need-to-know/187298. [Accessed on 14 June 2021].

Novartis Grimsby Ltd v. John Cookson. (2007) EWCA Civ 1261.

R. v. The Meaford and District Fire Department. (2012) ONCJ 573.

Rogers v. Whitaker. (1995) 175 CLR 479.

United Kingdom. (2010) *Equality Act 2010.* [Online] Available from: https://www.legislation.gov.uk/ukpga/2010/15/contents. [Accessed on 14 Jun 2021].

United Kingdom Clinical Ethics Network. (2010) *Ethical Issues — Confidentiality.* [Online] Available from: http://www.ukcen.net/ethical_issues/confidentiality/legal_consider. [Accessed on 14 June 2021].

Vijayan KC. (2010) *$1M Awarded to Paralyze Bangladeshi.* [Online] Available from: http://www.zappiling.com.sg/journal-ehs-others-judge-made-law.html. [Accessed on 14 June 2021].

W v. Edgell. (1990) 1 ALL ER 835.

Chapter 27

Ethics in Occupational Medicine

See Muah Lee[*,†,‡] *and David Koh*[*,†]

Introduction

The occupational physician functions at the interface between the employer (management) and the employee (non-management or trade-union). It is important to recognise that the physician's primary concern is to protect the worker from adverse health effects resulting from work. The ethical principles of the doctor in medicine — autonomy, non maleficence (do no harm), beneficence (do good) and justice, first championed by Childress and Beauchamp in 1965, are just as relevant in the doctor worker relationship in occupational health as the doctor in the traditional therapeutic relationship (Beauchamp and Childress, 2001).

In addition, there may be discipline specific considerations and issues. The complex and sometimes competing roles and responsibilities of occupational physicians towards workers, employers, the public, national public health and labour authorities and other bodies,

*Ng Teng Fong General Hospital, National University Health System, Singapore.
†Saw Swee Hock School of Public Health, National University of Singapore, Singapore.
PAPRSB Institute of Health Sciences, Universiti Brunei Darussalam, Brunei Darussalam *and* Yong Loo Lin School of Medicine, National University of Singapore, Singapore.
‡Centre for Biomedical Ethics, National University of Singapore, Singapore.
Corresponding author: See Muah Lee (See_Muah_Lee@nuhs.edu.sg).

e.g. unions, social security and the courts necessitate the reference to established and updated ethical guidelines.

Duties to Employees, Management, National Authorities and Himself

The occupational physician has a duty to educate workers about work hazards and prevention in an objective and prudent manner, and to disclose the purposes and procedures of health surveillance, while emphasising his or her professional independence.

There is also the duty to advise management on all factors in the work environment that may affect the health of employees, and its management. At the same time, while there is a duty to protect commercial secrets which may be learnt during the course of duties, the occupational physician cannot conceal information which is needed to protect the health of workers or the community.

There are often legal requirements for notifications of occupational or infectious diseases and workplace accidents and injuries, and to report results of statutory medical examinations. In such cases, reporting is mandatory, even if the management or workers do not give their consent. However, the occupational physician should explain the necessity of such notifications to both management and workers.

Finally, the occupational physician has a duty to maintain professional independence and impartiality, and to practise according to the highest standards of professional conduct and moral principles (Koh *et al.*, 1995).

Examples of Occupational Health Codes of Ethics

Codes of ethics or guidelines can be physician specific (Litchfied and Brecker, 2012), but increasingly cater to occupational health professionals in general, which reflects the multidisciplinary nature of occupational health practice.

United Kingdom

The latest ethics guidance produced by the Faculty of Occupational Medicine (FOM), UK (FOM UK, 2018), in its eighth edition, takes into account the multidisciplinary nature of good occupational health practice and would be relevant to all health care professionals in occupational health practice. The guidance covers topics such as governance, consent, confidentiality, access and disclosure of information, workplace ethical issues, research in occupational health and the legal-ethical interface of fitness for work, including attendance and performance management. The guidance also incorporates discussion on the implications of recent legislation in the UK, such as the General Data Protection Regulation which came into force in 2018.

United States of America

The American College of Occupational and Environmental Medicine (ACOEM) lists seven ethical principles of occupational and environmental medicine (ACOEM, 2010). It states that occupational and environmental health professionals have an obligation to:

1. Promote a safe and healthy workplace environment
2. Uphold ethical standards
3. Avoid discrimination
4. Maintain professional competence
5. Protect patient confidentiality
6. Advise and Report
7. Address conflict of interest

International

The third edition of the International Code of Ethics for Occupational Health professionals was produced by International Commission on Occupational Health (ICOH) in 2014 (ICOH, 2014). Among the issues covered in this publication are commercial secrets, danger to a third party, health surveillance and biological monitoring and investigations. The document also emphasises the importance of professional independence, competence, integrity and impartiality.

Confidentiality

The occupational physician, like his or her colleagues in other medical specialties have a duty to safeguard the confidentiality of medical information.

However, the occupational physician will often have to engage the works supervisors and the employers to understand the health and safety risks associated with work. The duty to maintain confidentiality in the doctor worker relationship is particularly exercised because, besides employers and management, other parties such as the state regulatory authorities, work representatives and insurers also have a vested interest to be informed and be given notice in the event of any suspected or confirmed work related illness. In some ways, it may not be possible to operate absolutely within the confidential domain of a doctor-patient relationship if the interests of the patient and also co-workers, are to be protected and promoted.

Being Impartial

The occupational physician must not take sides with either the management or the trade union, in the discharge of his duties. This may appear obvious but conflict of interest may arise, as the physician is often paid either by the management or the employee. His role as an impartial expert can be particularly sorely tested in an atmosphere of tense industrial relations. In this context it is always important to fully apprise both management and trade unions of the ethical responsibilities of a physician.

Case Study 1: Autonomy

A worker consulted his doctor several times for an eczematous rash. After several treatments, the doctor suspects that the rash could be due to some unidentified workplace allergen. The doctor sought the patient's consent for this clinical information to be released to his employer. The worker refused, fearing economic reprisals.

Commentary

What is the purpose of disclosure?

A causal relationship, if confirmed, will assist the doctor in the management of this patient. It could also be argued that the disclosure is to alert the management to the possible harmful nature of the products to enable remedial measures to be taken. This could be an especially compelling argument in the case where large numbers of employees are exposed, as opposed to a small workplace where there are few employees, and where affected individuals are likely to be more easily identified.

What is the extent of harm?

If it is a minor skin condition, the need to disclose may be less as opposed to another condition with potentially fatal consequences, such as occupational asthma. Disclosure under such serious circumstances, even where the worker has accepted the risk of self-endangerment and refused consent for disclosure, could qualify under the grounds of "public interest" and therefore be ethically justified. If it is a condition, which on analysis, poses a threat to the safety of others, again the "public interest" argument may prevail to override the consent of the worker. Examples include the poorly controlled epileptic patient operating in a safety sensitive environment.

Case Study 2: Health Risk Assessment

An environmental exposure measurement for a certain hazard mandated by legislation has been carried out. The majority of the measurements were within normal limits and the management has used these results, sanctioned by the occupational physician, to repel allegations of unsafe working conditions by the workers. In any case, the management has advised the occupational physician that the workers, admittedly working under hazardous conditions, have been compensated more favorably compared to workers in the other departments.

Commentary

How accurately do the environmental exposure readings represent a safe working condition?

Exposure measurements are part of the total information matrix in a health risk assessment. It cannot be considered in isolation to prove (management interest) or to disprove (worker interest) a safe work environment in a dispute, which in some cases, may have overtones of an industrial conflict. The evidence has to be objectively evaluated against other factors, such as the tasks of the workers, the duration of the exposures, and the environmental control measures. An exposure measurement, even if properly undertaken by accredited experts, does not replace the need for primary prevention efforts at the workplace to reduce exposure to as low as reasonably practicable.

Is it ethically acceptable to pay workers more to compensate for higher risk jobs?

Workers are free to choose and negotiate their terms of employment with their employers, including the voluntary assumption of work related risks. To some it may appear paternalistic and unacceptable to interfere with this, so long as the laws of the land are not violated.

However, the more ethically tenable view is that whilst payment may be increased for higher risk jobs, the financial incentive should not replace the need for measures to minimise such risks to as low as reasonably practicable. A globalised workforce with transient migrant labour across the world has made such issues all the more pressing.

Case Study 3: Commercial Secrecy

A factory manufacturing electronic components recently introduced a new cocktail mix of solvents in one of its processes. This improves the quality of the product and shortens the processing time. However, workers using this solvent cocktail reported minor skin itch. Some felt giddy after working with the new solvent mix. This occurred in spite of the use of respirators, gloves, and other protective clothing while handling the solvent mix.

The occupational physician requested for information on the chemical composition of the new solvent cocktail but the technical management was not keen to release the information, stating that it was a "commercial secret" which gave the company an edge over its rivals. Besides, the health complaints were felt to be relatively minor in nature, and the technical management stated that the workers were already provided with gloves and respirators to protect themselves adequately.

Commentary

What is the duty of the occupational physician with respect to such "trade" information?

The doctor who obtains information about the business during the course of his work has an ethical duty to maintain the confidentiality of such information.

Along a similar vein, should the doctor wish to publish the findings in medical journals, it would be best if the employers are given notice and a chance to discuss the findings. At its most extreme, if a pressing "public interest" need arises for disclosure of information that has been intentionally suppressed because of a grave endangerment to health, then legal advice has to be sought.

Is there a way to obtain the required information with minimal risk to the business interests of the employer?

This should be properly explored before a foreclosure of the possibilities of a medical investigation.

Other Ethical Dilemmas

The occupational physician who manages some categories of workers, e.g. the chronic sick and migrant workers may face unique ethical dilemmas.

The Chronic Sick

In free market economies, where labour relationships are freely bargained, the economic motive to employ the young and healthy may lead to the exclusion of the aged and people with chronic diseases from the workplace, even though work undertaken by this group of people may not affect their health. Such a perspective taken to its extreme reflects the ethically troubling view of reducing labour to a mere commodity where human dignity can be sacrificed (Henk, 2016).

Work undertaken by those willing and able, which keeps a person socially engaged with the community, would have a positive impact on well-being and health. That there is an economic cost in the employment of workers with chronic diseases, e.g. diabetes mellitus cannot be refuted (Dray-Spira *et al.*, 2013). This can be due to the direct financial costs of care, if it is subsidised by the employers as a "staff benefit." Indirect costs incurred by lowered productivity and absenteeism caused by sick days, medical appointments and hospitalisation would invariably be borne by employers. This was noted to be in excess of 5.9 days for males and 9.4 days for females among those with body mass index exceeding 40 kg/m^2 (Finkelstein *et al.*, 2010).

Minimising business cost is a legitimate objective. However, instead of a policy of exclusion, employers can be encouraged and assisted by state sponsored initiatives, including fiscal subvention, that promote care and inclusiveness at work. Occupational physicians can be advocates for this, especially in the organisation of occupational health programmes aimed at physical and mental well-being for all. Assisting the employers to design jobs to accommodate those whose work ability is compromised because of diseases would be an important role for the occupational physician.

Migrant Workers

In 2015, 244 million people (3.3% of the world's population) lived outside their country of origin (International Labour Organization, 2020). The vast majority are migrants in search of economic opportunities, working in sectors that locals shun, such as domestic work, commercial sex and other hazardous jobs such as construction. Access to health care can be challenging for this group of workers, due to language barriers, cultural differences and unfamiliarity with the healthcare system and relevant local laws and policies (Office of the High Commissioner for Human Rights, 2013). For documented migrant workers, employers may be de facto gatekeepers of their healthcare decisions, particularly in receiving countries where responsibility for their healthcare costs fall on the employers.

Case Study 4: Health Care for Migrant Workers

A migrant worker working in a developed country suffered from seizures. He was hospitalised and found to have a tumor in the brain. His seizure was stabilised. This is neither a workplace injury nor an occupational disease.

Once the acute condition was stabilised and the patient is rendered safe for repatriation, what information should be given to the employer?

In addition, while it may be in the best interest of the patient to remain in the developed country (where medical treatment is superior to that available in the worker's less developed home country) — who is responsible for the financial cost of treatment?

Commentary

In many countries, employers may have to bear the medical costs of care of the foreign worker, often through mandated insurance schemes, which often, may not cover the entire costs in complex cases. Sending the migrant worker back home to some villages often may mean death, not imminently but nevertheless in the near future.

While imminently life threatening conditions should be managed without question, the situation is different when the patient can be stabilised and rendered safe for repatriation to home countries, sometimes with medical escort to a home country medical facility with all the relevant information for continuity of care. Employers may be allowed by the authorities to exercise this option.

While the confidentiality of medical information is to be respected, the nature of the employment relationship, the fact that foreign workers are often without kinship support while in a foreign land, and the fact that the employer may be permitted rightfully to exercise the justification of repatriation of sick but stable workers makes the involvement of the employers unavoidable. This is especially so for migrant workers; whose welfare are predominantly dependent on the employer.

Host countries with advanced treatment options, including its follow-up care, are expensive and unsubsidised. This may be a preferred option in the best interest of the patient. However, the financial cost imposed on the employers poses a profound ethical dilemma, especially in countries where citizens themselves are not entitled automatically to full state funded care. Ensuring an equitable access to health care for migrant workers against such a backdrop is always challenging. A practical solution to this is to involve employers and the families for the best way forward and working within the boundaries set by the authorities (Voo *et al.*, 2020).

During infectious disease outbreaks, migrant workers face heightened risks of infection due to barriers to public health information, infection and prevention control, and social distancing both at work and their residences. As clearly shown by the COVID-19 pandemic, it is not only ethical, but a public health priority to address the health needs of migrant workers — as safeguarding their health also mitigates the risk of community spread, thus benefiting local residents and communities (Koh, 2020). Many of these health needs overlap with welfare provisions as well. Accommodations in the form of dormitories, e.g. must have proper hygiene standards and provisions to facilitate social distancing and avoid overcrowding.

Conclusion

Different decisions made in occupational medicine frequently involve consideration of the competing interests of different parties. These decisions must have ethically sound foundations, such as the duty to tell the truth, upholding the dignity of the individual, justice and transparency. Taking into account the autonomy of the worker, public interests and the interests of the employer is often a fine balancing act.

References

ACOEM. (2010) *The Seven Ethical Principles of Occupational and Environmental Medicine*. Illinois, United States of America, ACOEM. [Online] Available from: https://acoem.org/acoem/media/pdf-Library/About_ACOEM/Code-of-Ethics-Condensed-Version.pdf. [Accessed on 25 December 2020].

Beauchamp TL, Childress JF. (2001) *Principles of biomedical ethics* (5th Ed). Oxford, Oxford University Press.

Dray-Spira R, Herquelot E, Bonenfant S, Guéguen A, Melchior M. (2013) Impact of diabetes mellitus onset on sickness absence from work — a 15-year follow-up of the GAZEL Occupational Cohort Study. *Diabet Med* **30**(5): 549–556.

Finkelstein EA, DiBonaventura MD, Burgess SM, Hale BC. (2010) The costs of obesity in the workplace. *J Occup Environ Med* **52**(10): 971–976.

FOM, Royal College of Physicians. (2018) *Ethics guidance for occupational health practice* (8th Ed). London, Faculty of Occupational Medicine of the Royal College of Physicians.

Henk TH. (ed.) (2016) *Encyclopedia of Global Bioethics.* Switzerland, Springer International Publishing.

ICOH. (2014) *International Code of Ethics for Occupational Health Professionals* (3rd Ed). Rome, ICOH. [Online] Available from: http://www.icohweb.org/site/code-of-ethics.asp. [Accessed on 25 December 2020].

International Labour Organization. (2020) *International Labour Standards on Migrant Workers.* [Online] Available from: https://www.ilo.org/global/standards/subjects-covered-by-international-labour-standards/migrant-workers/lang--en/index.htm. [Accessed on 25 December 2020].

Koh D. (2020) Migrant workers and COVID-19. *Occup Environ Med* 77(9): 634–636.

Koh D, Lee SM, Jeyaratnam J. (1995) Health and safety ethics for management. *Asia-Pac J Public Health* **8**(2): 144–147.

Litchfield P, Brecker N. (ed.) (2012) *Ethics Guidance for Occupational Health Practice.* London, Faculty of Occupational Medicine.

Office of the High Commissioner for Human Rights. (2013) *Migrant Workers: Their Right to Health Care.* [Online] Available from: http://www.ohchr.org/EN/NewsEvents/Pages/Migrantworkerstheirrighttohealthcare.aspx. [Accessed on 25 December 2020].

Voo TC, Kaur S, Rajaraman N. (2020) Ethical medical repatriation of guest workers: Criteria and challenges. *Developing world bioethics.* [Online] Available from: doi:10.1111/dewb.12286.

Chapter 28

Audit and Evidence-Based Occupational Medicine Practice

*Yue-Liang Leon Guo**

Introduction

Clinical audit, initially named medical audit, was introduced to the National Health Service (NHS) of the United Kingdom (UK) by the 1989 White Paper "Working for Patients" (NHS, 1989). To ensure the delivery of the best health care, clinical audit involves reviewing of clinical diagnosis, care processes, and resultant patient outcomes (Health and Social Care Information Center, 2021). One definition of audit in medical care has been "a review and evaluation of health care procedures and documentation for the purpose of comparing the quality of care provided with accepted standards" (O'Toole, 2007).

Occupational medicine is the practice of clinical medicine concerning with keeping people physically and mentally well at work. The practice includes diagnosis of diseases, assessment of work-relatedness, health promotion, preventive care, intervention and treatments, fitness for work evaluation, prognosis and return-to-work for the injured or ill workers. Audit of occupational medicine practice thus should be

*Environmental and Occupational Medicine, College of Medicine, Graduate Institute of Occupational Medicine and Industrial Hygiene, College of Public Health, National Taiwan University (NTU) *and* NTU Hospital, Taipei, Taiwan.
Corresponding author: Yue-Liang Leon Guo (leonguo@ntu.edu.tw).

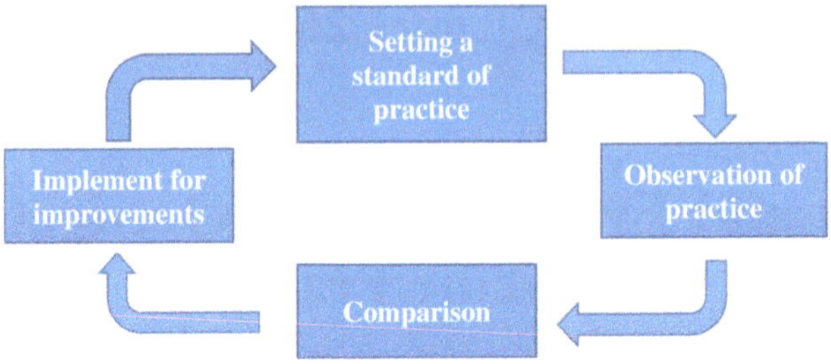

Fig. 1. Audit cycle.

"a review and evaluation of curative and preventive healthcare in the workplace and documentation for the purpose of comparing the quality of care and prevention provided with accepted standards".

An "audit cycle" involves repeating cycles of continuous improvements (Fig. 1), each cycle begins with setting a standard of practice, then observation of the practice. Comparison of observed practice with the set standard will lead to the needs of improvements to fulfill the standards. Changes will be made to implement these improvements. Thereafter, the second cycle will begin, again with setting a presumably higher standard, followed by the other steps. Therefore, with such repeating cycles, audit should result in progressive improvement and eventually sustained assurance of quality. These concepts can be applied to many disciplines, including medicine and occupational medicine.

Purpose of Audit in Occupational Medicine

The purposes of audit in occupational health and medicine have been reviewed (Agius, 2010). These are:

1. For workers: improving the standard of care and prevention, while keeping personal and clinical information confidential;
2. For employers: improving overall health of the workforce, working morale, work ability, effectiveness and efficiency;
3. For occupational health providers: understanding the state-of-the-art practice in occupational health; and improving the processes and quality of professional performance;

4. For all: to determine knowledge gaps in the current practice, enhancing further research, which will lead to improvement in quality of care.

Quality Assurance of Audit

Quality assurance is of utmost importance in medical care and related activities, including occupational health services and their audits. The quality of audit is highly dependent on the following:

1. Staff conducting audits on occupational medicine practice are competent to perform this task;
2. Staff conducting audits are independent from the activity being audited;
3. Audits identify both strengths and weaknesses in the occupational health service system;
4. Audits verify that the organisation is achieving its occupational health service performance targets;
5. Audit results are communicated to all relevant individuals and the managers/employers;
6. Results of audit are used as the basis for corrective action.

Topics of Audit in Occupational Health and Medicine

Selection of Topics to Audit

The selection of topics to be audited has to be based on the following factors.

Relevance

The topic is common to the workers in the target industry. For example, high prevalence rates of carpal tunnel syndrome in one similar exposure group in the industry of interest.

Influence on outcome or resources

The topic is of significant health risk, or of high cost to the workers or the employers. For example, high accident rates in workers, which required hospitalisation, or high sick absence rates.

Effective and efficient methods exist for such audit

Effectiveness indicates high probability of achieving the purposes when an intervention, regimen, or service is deployed in the workplace. Efficiency indicates a high result/effort ratio, where the effort includes money, time and other resources. Actually, from a higher organisational point of view, the effectiveness and efficiency of the occupational health service should be included as a topic of audit.

Examples of clinical audits can be seen in the website of The Health and Social Care Information System, UK (HSCIC, 2021). Cardiac rehabilitation, pulmonary hypertension, bowel cancer, diabetes care, pregnancy in diabetes, head and neck cancer, lung cancer, esophago-gastric cancer, etc. have been audited at a national level.

Types of Audit in Occupational Medicine

Several types of audits have been proposed, including:

1. Audit of Structure: the organisational framework and the quantity and quality of resources available;
2. Audit of Process: curative and preventive care to the workers carried out by way of problem identification, assessment, medical advice and other interventions;
3. Audit of Outcome: the results of the above-mentioned processes by the occupational physician or related health service, such as reduction in symptoms, morbidity or health risks; and
4. Audit of Communication: including oral and written, personal and mass. The results of communication should be the improved understanding and practice of preventive measures in the workplace as well as at the personal level.

Audit of structure

The following points can be included in the audit of structure in OM services:

1. Whether workers' health is integrated into business performance;
2. Whether published workers' health policy is available to all employees;
3. Whether appropriate resources are available to implement workers' health policy;
4. Degree of employee commitment to workers' health policy and active participation;
5. Whether personnel working for OM services have received appropriate training and are competent to carry out their duties and responsibilities;
6. Availability of health risk assessment programme, and the control measures;
7. Whether a top manager is allocated with full responsibility for workers' health;
8. Existence of confidentiality policy concerning individual health data;
9. Whether contingency plans for emergencies are available, including emergency evacuation, liaison with the emergency services, and urgent casualty referrals.

Existing policy and plans, competent personnel, medical facility and supplies, and participation of the employer and employees are the essence of the structure of occupational health services. Amongst these, competence in personnel is probably the most critical component. Delivery of occupational health services can be done by primary care physicians trained in occupational health, free-standing occupational medicine clinics, hospital-based occupational health services, group occupational health services, company-based occupational health services, etc. In any model, occupational health professionals who have received appropriate training are more likely to produce a higher quality process of "care" than inadequately trained professionals. Core personnel of occupational health services include physicians, physician assistants, nurses, nurse practitioners, industrial hygienists, and other clinical staff. Potential supplementary staff includes psychologists, physical and occupational therapists, health educators, counselors, safety engineers, ergonomists, toxicologists, emergency medical technicians, etc. However, the distinction between core staff and supplementary staff is somewhat artificial. The composition of the occupational health team depends upon many factors including the availability of personnel and equipment, the range of industries covered, and the nature of anticipated hazards.

Audit of processes

The processes of occupational health services include workers' health policy and its periodic review for the purpose of continual improvement, health status of employees and its periodic review, training and retraining of the occupational health personnel, consultations and related record-keeping, investigation of health and safety events, etc. These processes require regular audit to optimise their function.

The following can be included in the audit of process in OM services, e.g.:

1. Whether workers' health policy is understood and implemented;
2. Whether there is continual cost-effective improvement in workers' health;
3. Whether periodic review is carried out for the policy and management system on workers' health;
4. Whether there are periodic measurement and audit for workers' health performance, followed by necessary corrective and preventive actions;
5. Whether there are periodic training and retraining of personnel responsible for occupational medicine services;
6. Whether documents including records are kept up to date and relevant;
7. Whether the emergency response programme is periodically tested;

8. Whether workers health performance and the effectiveness of preventive measures are routinely assessed;
9. Whether health and safety incidents are reported and investigated, and necessary corrective measures taken;
10. Whether the workers' health management system is periodically reviewed;
11. Whether a proactive approach is taken towards improving the workers' health management system.

For each employee covered by occupational health services, a complete medical record and the results of preplacement and periodic health examination should be kept and stored appropriately. This will facilitate the efficiency in auditing activities.

Box 1. Auditing Individual Occupational Health Consultation.

Individual consultation is one of the most frequent activities in occupational health services. Many types of consultations can happen in the workplace, including follow-up of abnormal physical examination findings, respiratory conditions, musculoskeletal conditions, stress, sickness leave, etc. Auditing of individual consultation is thus important. The audit should include the following components

1. The nature of the consultation. This provides the basis for the comparison and for determining the relevance of items included in the records.
   - Is it an initial or a follow-up consultation?
   - Is it self-referral or referred by management?
   - The purpose of referral: e.g. pre-employment, periodical health surveillance, sickness absence, symptoms, etc.
2. Clinical information gathered
   - Demographics: age, gender, etc.
   - Chief complaints and history
   - Physical and laboratory examinations
3. Occupational information gathered
   - Job title and job description
   - Workplace

(*Continued*)

Box 1. (*Continued*)

- Shiftwork
- Number of hours worked per week

4. Decision making process
   - Evidence-based diagnosis
   - Evidence-based judgment of work-relatedness
5. Communication
   - Oral and/or written communication to the employee
   - Oral and/or written communication to the manager/employer
   - Oral and/or written communication to other specialists
6. Conclusions and the actions taken
   - Diagnosis
   - Assessment of work-relatedness
   - Occupational implications for the employee
   - Follow-up plan
   - Needs for workplace assessment or modifications
7. Effectiveness and efficiency issues
   - Adequacy and legibility of relevant information provided
   - Time interval between referral request and appointment
   - Legibility — identifiable signature, date, marked corrections
   - Implementation of the follow-up, referral, and workplace assessment or modifications

Case Study 1: Prospective Internal Audit of Peer Reviewed Occupational Health Reports

A prospective internal audit of all peer reviewed occupational health (OH) reports was performed (Lalloo et al., 2012). The audit utilised an abbreviated assessment form, based on Questions 4–12 of the Sheffield Assessment Instrument for Letters (SAIL). The results found that 27% of OH reports required modifications, including 18% related to minor reasons and 9% to more complex reasons. The latter included all the manager's questions were not being addressed, review arrangements were not clear, and the report was not clear and understandable to the intended readership. The authors concluded that audit using peer review approach can be a useful tool in improving the standard of OH reports.

Furthermore, the audit can be a valuable educational tool in terms of personal feedback, benchmarking, and exposure to different styles of report writing. This audit was repeated approximately one year later (Lalloo et al., 2015), OH reports requiring modifications were reduced from 27 to 14%, including 8% related to minor reasons and 6% to more complex reasons. Clinical complaints about OH reports from customers were also reduced from three in the preceding year to none 2 years later.

Audit of outcome

Health endpoints are obvious outcomes to be audited in any workplace. In the modern workplaces, frequently encountered health outcomes include:

- Musculoskeletal disorders;
- Psychological health and socio-organisational issues;
- Absence attributed to sickness;
- Respiratory disorders, e.g. occupational asthma and pneumoconiosis;
- Health issues related to specific occupational hazards such as: noise, skin problems in the workplace.

Box 2. Audit of Musculoskeletal Conditions at Individual Level.

Musculoskeletal conditions are important health problems facing workers and hence occupational health professionals. If an occupational medicine doctor receives a consultation due to musculoskeletal complaint from an employee, the following are some points to be considered;

1. History
    - Description of symptom
    - Time of onset of symptom
    - Time of onset of symptom
    - Time of symptom during a day and a week
    - Aggravating and relieving factors

(Continued)

Box 2. (*Continued*)

- Limitation in activity
- Relevant past history

2. Physical examination
   - Distribution of tenderness, numbness or difficulty in movements
   - Signs of inflammation or nerve compression
   - Neurological symptoms and signs
3. Other laboratory or imaging studies
4. Diagnosis and conclusions
5. Advice/action
   - Medical treatment or surgical consultation
   - Advice on fitness for work, or sickness leave
   - Physical and occupational therapy
   - Workplace assessment and modification

Box 3. Audit of Musculoskeletal Conditions at Group Level.

If similar musculoskeletal complaints come from more than one employee, a cluster of medical conditions should trigger the consideration of a potential sentinel event in occupational health. Therefore, a more in-depth investigation will be warranted. In addition to the above personal level evaluation, the following should be considered:

1. Survey of the coworkers for symptoms and signs with an instrument such as the Nordic Musculoskeletal Questionnaire (NMQ);
2. Workplace assessment with careful observation of the working procedures, and the relevance to the reported symptoms and signs;
3. Assistance from an ergonomist should also be considered if a disease cluster is highly suspected;
4. Such investigation will result in understanding whether certain deficiencies in ergonomics or human work physiology might have caused musculoskeletal conditions in similarly exposed workers. If such a deficiency is identified, further actions are required to improve working condition and to minimise the risk of musculoskeletal disorders in the workers. This kind of audit can lead to immediate effective remedial actions.

Box 4. Audit of Mental Health Conditions.

Psychiatric conditions have become one of the most important ailments causing a burden on health in the world. In the workplace, stress and depression are important conditions encountered by occupational health services. Existing assessment instruments are available, e.g. for job control and psychological demands, for workplace support, for effort and reward imbalance, for burnout, and for depressive mood. However, the interpretation of the scores of the instruments has to be cautious when applied at an individual level, since many factors may cause deviations of the scores. Sound epidemiologic knowledge has to be applied when these instruments are used in individual workers, as well as in a group of symptomatic workers.

If an occupational medicine doctor receives a consultation request from an employee regarding a psychological condition, the following are some points to be considered;

1. History
   - Symptom onset — Timing and description, and triggering event
   - Medicinal therapy
   - Relevant past history
   - Somatic complaints and symptoms
   - Possible substance misuse
   - Social support — especially non-occupational
2. Examination
   - Mental state examination — (affect)
   - Intellect/other higher functions
   - Behaviour
3. Job history
   - Job description — Title and tasks
   - Recent change in job content and work environment
   - Qualitative and quantitative workload
   - Social support — occupational
4. Diagnosis
   - Medical diagnosis (physical/psychological/psychiatric)
   - Occupational or organisational factors
   - Non-occupational factors and other risk factors

(*Continued*)

Box 4. (*Continued*)

5. Advice/action
   - Work assessment
   - Fitness for work and needs for work modification
   - Reduction of other risk factors
   - Counseling and rehabilitation

Less frequently, clustered psychological conditions may attract the attention of the occupational medical services. In such situations, assessment of affected individuals, and using epidemiological approaches that include comparisons with similarly exposed asymptomatic groups can be considered. When this is applied, the following factors are relevant in regards to audit:

1. Robustness of the instrument used in the specified situation encountered
2. Representativeness of the participants from the exposed group
3. Soundness of the statistical techniques used in analysing the data obtained
4. Caution in the interpretation of the data
5. Communication with involved employees, the direct managers, and the employer

Box 5. Audit of General Health Conditions (Cardiovascular and Cerebrovascular Risks).

With modernisation of lifestyle, risks for cardiovascular and cerebrovascular diseases have increased. Occupational health services have ready access to workers' periodic physical examination records, and can thus identify those with elevated risks for cardiovascular and cerebrovascular diseases. Public health and lifestyle preventive measures can be recommended to reduce workers' risk for cardiovascular and cerebrovascular diseases.

A risk estimation can be made based on the Framingham studies and other long-term follow-up investigations (Wilson *et al.*, 1998). Factors including age, blood pressure, total cholesterol, high density lipoprotein, low density lipoprotein, diabetes, and smoking are used for the risk estimation of cardiovascular and cerebrovascular diseases. The other useful indicator is the identification of workers with metabolic syndrome. Metabolic

Box 5. (*Continued*)

syndrome has been known to be an important predictor for cardiovascular and cerebrovascular diseases. It is generally agreed that obesity, insulin resistance, dyslipidaemia and hypertension are the most important components for metabolic syndrome. One of the definition for metabolic syndrome by International Diabetes Federation (IDF) is meeting three of the following five conditions:

1. **Waist circumference:** men ≧90 cm; women ≧80 cm.
2. **Triglyceride:** ≥150 mg/dL.
3. **HDL cholesterol:** <40 mg/dL (male) and <50 mg/dL (female).
4. **Blood pressure:** systolic BP ≥130 or diastolic BP ≥85 mm Hg, or treatment of previously diagnosed hypertension.
5. **Fasting plasma glucose:** ≥100 mg/dL, or previously diagnosed type 2 diabetes.

Measures should be taken to reduce any of the above criteria. In the audit process, the following should be considered:

- Availability of individual physical examination data to the occupational health service;
- Availability of computerised physical examination data to the occupational health service;
- Confidentiality of workers' health data management;
- Prevalence rates of workers with elevated risk for cardiovascular and cerebrovascular diseases;
- Measures taken to reduce individual risk of cardiovascular and cerebrovascular diseases and/or metabolic syndrome;
- Comparisons across years the prevalence rates of workers with elevated risks of cardiovascular and cerebrovascular diseases;
- Comparisons across years the prevalence rates of workers with metabolic syndrome.

Box 6. Audit of Fitness for Work

Fitness for work is an important responsibility of the occupational health services. The evaluation for fitness for work includes preplacement assessments, periodic health examination, and return-to-work after illnesses and

(*Continued*)

Box 6. (*Continued*)

injuries. In evaluating a person's fitness for work, an occupational physician has to take the following three important issues into consideration: (1) the person's functional capacity, (2) safety and health risk involved to the person in undertaking the work, and (3) potential risks to others. To address these issues, a detailed understanding of the person's functionality is important, as well as the knowledge of the requirements and the potential risks of the work. In general, occupational physicians are trained to be able to characterise the above three issues. However, in many cases, careful evaluation of the person with assistance of a physical therapist, an occupational therapist, or a psychologist, as well as evaluation of the workplace with assistance of an industrial hygienist, an ergonomist, etc., are required.

An audit of fitness for work thus should involve the following:

1. Whether the clinical diagnosis is adequately made;
2. Whether the work-relatedness of the clinical diagnosis is clearly assessed and understood;
3. Whether treatment and rehabilitation are optimised;
4. Whether the evaluation of functional capacity of the worker is adequately conducted, considering his/her medical condition. As an example, a worker with a cardiac condition or respiratory disease might have impaired exercise tolerance, thus having difficulty in performing regular strenuous work duties. On the other hand, a worker with a recent accident and a fractured fibula might have impaired lower extremity movements, thus limiting his/her work capacity for tasks including climbing ladders, but only temporarily. In evaluation of functional capacity, other relevant factors have to be taken into consideration, such as long-term prognosis, and exacerbation. For example, people having chronic obstructive pulmonary diseases or severe asthma can have exacerbation of the condition beyond his/her average limitation of capacity. While a less permanent condition is of question, there are references which can be useful guides to refer to (Reed, 2007). However, careful tailoring of the disability duration by clinical assessment of individual functionality is required, rather than taking the recommended duration wholly. In addition, job requirements can be categorised into sedentary, light, medium, heavy, and very heavy. In general, sedentary work involves exerting up to 10 pounds of force occasionally and/or a negligible amount of force frequently to lift, carry, push, pull, or otherwise move objects, including the human

Box 6. (*Continued*)

body. Whereas heavy work involves exerting 50–100 pounds of force occasionally, and/or 25–50 pounds of force frequently, and/or 10–20 pounds of force constantly to move objects. Duration of disability can vary greatly according to the job requirements, even in those with the same medical condition;

5. Whether potential adverse effects by workplace exposure on a worker's health is adequately evaluated. For example, a worker with carpal tunnel syndrome conservatively treated can have his/her condition aggravated by repetitive hand movements during work activity. A worker developing sensitisation to epoxy resin in the workplace can have recurrence of allergic contact dermatitis when working with the chemical again. He or she may have to be removed from the workplace with such exposure if contact cannot be avoided effectively;
6. Whether potential excessive risk to coworkers or the public is adequately assessed, considering the medical condition in the context of his/her work. An obvious example is recent onset epilepsy following brain trauma in a bus driver, that can prohibit him/her from performing work safely. Since many workers drive cars, public service vehicles, heavy goods vehicles, and use machinery during work or during commuting to work, some published guidance can be useful in such assessment (Driver and Vehicle Licensing Agency, 2018);
7. Whether the occupational physician who conducted fitness for work evaluation made adequate efforts to accommodate workers with various degrees of physical or mental abilities;
8. Whether specialists are adequately consulted when the medical condition requires such consultation.

Box 7. Audit of Sickness Absence

In day-by-day practice of occupational medicine, sickness absence and fitness for work are probably the most frequently encountered issues. Requests for advice regarding sickness absence may come from various sources, namely, the employee, his/her primary care doctor, or the employer.

To a certain extent, sickness absence overlaps with fitness for work. Therefore, the following are important components of auditing sickness absence, namely, evaluation of clinical diagnosis and work-relatedness,

(*Continued*)

Box 7. (*Continued*)

optimisation of treatment and rehabilitation, assessment of functional capacity, addressing potential adverse effects from workplace exposure, and estimating potential excessive risk to co-workers or the public. References to consult for the generally recognised shortest, optimal, and longest duration of sick leave after specific injury types for different work types from sedentary to very heavy are available (Reed, 2007). However, for the evaluation of injured workers for return-to-work, an occupational physician should not just focus on physical fitness, but also mental. Among injured workers, some can develop trauma and stress-related disorder (TSRD) and/or major depression, or other psychiatric conditions months or years after injury (Chin *et al.*, 2017). Those with psychological symptoms and psychiatric disorders as a result of the traumatic event are known to encounter difficulty returning to work (Chu *et al.*, 2019). Therefore, early psychological intervention or counseling has to be considered if an occupational physician detects such needs.

In auditing sickness of absence, in addition to the above-mentioned points, the following questions may have to be addressed:

- Whether there is compliance with the sickness policy of the industry;
- Whether rehabilitation is started in good time;
- Whether residual disability is adequately assessed;
- What is the basis of the estimated duration of absence?;
- Whether psychological assessment and counseling is applied at an early stage;
- Whether attendance and safety for any future work is considered;
- Whether adjustment for future work performance is considered;
- Whether the time of redeployment is chosen appropriately;
- Whether consideration is given to the need for workplace improvements or modification.

Box 8. Audit of Infection Prevention During Pandemic for the General Workplace (Excludes Healthcare Settings)

The COVID-19 pandemic had great impact to industries. Workplaces are considered potential locations of disease transmission because of frequent interpersonal contact, enclosed spaces, etc. Prevention programme are

Box 8. (*Continued*)

required to minimise the probability of disease transmission in the workplace. The following areas are important for the audit of infection prevention while an epidemic is active.

- Whether a committee is formed to overlook the situation of the epidemic, to update the current knowledge concerning the epidemic, to estimate the probability of infection among the employees, and to form preventive strategies according to the prevalence or incidence of the infectious disease?
- Whether international and domestic situation about the contagion is updated?
- Whether methods of identifying employees with sickness are installed, such as self-report forms or applications, analytical algorithms for the reports, and thermometers at entrances?
- Whether a requirement of adequate PPE is installed? Whether availability of PPE is ensured?
- Whether a strategy for continual surface cleaning has been implemented?
- Whether dual work teams in each department are formed to ensure the continuity of productivity if a certain percent of employees become infected?
- Whether guidelines for sick-leaves, including the consideration of their work-relatedness are written and reviewed by interested personnel and party, e.g. the union?
- Whether adequate arrangements for work-from-home is set up? These must include percent of workforce, punch-in and punch-out mechanisms, and online security.
- Whether written rules for employees or clients with needs for international travel are available, this will need to include testing, vaccination, and quarantine.
- During pandemic, the changes of disease occurrence and prevalence has been rather rapid, and the audit process may need be conducted frequently, such as once per week, to respond to the epidemic efficiently. Concerning the above, a good source of reference can be obtained from Center for Disease Control and Prevention (Centers for Disease Control and Prevention, 2021).

Audit of group health data

An important proportion of health promotion consists of annual or biannual health examination. The overall effect of health promotion activity can be evaluated by comparing group data through the years. This practice provides an overall understanding of general health conditions in the workforce. Conditions such as cardiovascular risks as estimation by Framingham scheme, metabolic syndrome and its components, job stress and satisfaction, etc. can be compared from year to year. It is important to adjust these outcomes for age, because the cardiovascular risks and metabolic syndrome are highly related to age. A successful health promotion programme can be considered if the across-year comparison shows lower risk in cardiovascular system, or reduced metabolic syndrome while adjusted for age.

Audit of communication

An essential part of occupational health services is communication to the employee and employer. This not only includes oral and written report as a result of clinic visit, but also risk communication for preventive measures, and communication with the employer for policy considerations. In addition to curative medicine, the nature of occupational medicine practice includes preventive measures. Therefore, communication for the purpose of enhancement of proactive and preventive measures is important.

In auditing communication, the following questions should be addressed:

- Whether effective and efficient communication is delivered to the employee when a clinical assessment or care is provided;
- Whether potential occupation-relatedness is included in the communication if clinically indicated;
- When occupation-relatedness is in question, whether effective communication with relevant personnel is done, such as industrial hygienists, occupational health nurses, ergonomists, and psychologists, etc.;

- When communicating with the employer, whether confidentiality issues are carefully addressed;
- Whether updated information on preventive medicine concerning general health is provided to the employers and employees on a regular basis.

In dealing with several of the above issues, evidence-based practice of occupational medicine is stressed. In principle, evidence-based medicine (EBM) has to be applied in every aspect of medical practice in all specialties. However, in occupational health services, lacking of exact scientific-based answers to specified circumstances occurs frequently. It is important to understand the general principle of EBM in occupational health services, as well as its limitations when occupational health services are to be delivered.

Completion of Audit Loop

For any selected topic in occupational health services, when auditing of structure, process and outcome is done, completion of the audit loop usually requires consensus among the auditors on,

1. The points of strength of the service.
2. The major deficiencies identified by the audit.
3. How these deficiencies are to be remedied:
    - By whom?
    - By what means?
    - In what time frame?
4. How will the remedial steps be evaluated?
    - By a repetition of the original audit?
    - By a different audit approach?
5. What is the next potential weak spot to be audited?
    - By whom?
    - By what means?
    - In what time frame?

Consensus on the above must be documented, reported to the appropriate persons, and used for further improvement of the audited services.

Evidence-Based Medicine in Occupational Health Services

EBM is commonly used in the clinical setting, and involves the integration of best research evidence with clinical expertise and patient values (Evidence-Based Medicine Working Group, 1992; Sackett *et al.*, 1996). EBM has been proven to enhance the quality of health care in several medical specialties (Straus, 1997). In general, occupational physicians are believed to be less aware of the high number of relevant questions that can be derived from their daily practice and of the opportunities to answer most questions when following EBM strategies. Before the year 2000, a relatively high percentage of occupational physicians relied on their own experience or on advice from colleagues and "experts," as compared to other medical specialties. However, it was shown that the advice occupational physicians received from colleagues may not reflect the best evidence from the literature. Around the early 2000s, attempts to promote EBM in the occupational medicine and public health care were started. In general, occupational medicine physicians have a demand for medical, para-medical, and non-medical information on a broad range of topics. A survey in the early 2000s showed that occupational physicians generally chose to contact colleagues when pursuing answers to unfamiliar clinical questions. However, their attitude towards EBM was fairly positive (Schaafsma *et al.*, 2004). In occupational medicine practice, types of medical information resources used to deal with a case include advice from colleagues, and use of internet resources/computer databases. Textbooks and guidelines can also be a source of information. Relevant information and reviews have been published concerning application of research information to improve the quality of occupational health practice (Verbeek and van Dikj, 2007).

The application of EBM in occupational health services include the following components covered in the next few sections.

To Formulate an Answerable Question

The clinical question can belong to any of the following categories:

- Diagnosis
- Causation, including work-relatedness
- Therapy or intervention
- Prognosis
- Legal or legislation
- Return to work
- Prevention
- Statistics

To Search and Acquire Relevant Literature

This step includes searching a wide-range of most up-to-date guidelines, databases, systematic review articles, and original research findings from medical journals

Evidence from occupational cohort studies, randomised controlled studies, and/or case-control studies can be used in this regard. In the meantime, evidence obtained from studies performed by a wide variety of medical specialties, psychology, industrial hygiene, ergonomics, and other disciplines can also be used. Pitfalls during the literature search may include typing mistakes, using medical subject headings that are not optimal, and unreliable search strategies. Continuing education and training of occupational physicians concerning literature search is warranted to minimise these problems. On line search has become more and more important, due to the apparent efficiency and the broadness of coverage. Usually, the primary sources from the literature should include systematic reviews and original investigations. Other sources are considered secondary, such as advisory reports, quality websites or apps, practice guidelines, Wikipedia, etc. For effectively obtaining evidence-based information, adequate use of search engines and databases is essential, e.g. PubMed/MEDLINE, Cochrane Library, Google Scholar (van Dikj and Caraballo-Arias, 2021).

To Appraise the Literature for Quality

Training for the appraisal of the presented data and results from the literature is important. The following points should be considered:

- Clinical importance (will the use of this information make an important difference in clinical decision);
- Validity (can I trust this information);
- Impact (size of the reported effect);
- Applicability (can I use the information in this particular situation).

Frequent application of these techniques, regular instruction and training are needed for most occupational physicians to increase their literature searching and critical appraisal skills. In addition, many busy occupational physicians obtain or just use the abstracts only. Although a reasonable proportion of clinical questions can be answered satisfactorily by just reading the abstract, details of concrete risk estimates and clear dose-response relationship between exposures and outcomes are often lacking in abstracts. The lack of availability of full text journals decreases the reliability of the critical appraisal and risk estimation. Therefore, the occupational health services' provision of full-text services and/or connection to membership of, e.g. a medical institution with access to full text journal articles, is important in promoting occupational physician's capability for practicing EBM.

In cases where a topic has been critically appraised, e.g. in a review article, meta-analysis, or editorial comment, the conclusion can be viewed as a useful summary. This significantly reduces the time and effort of the critical appraisal by the physicians. Since year 2000, more and more published work based on meta-analysis have been available, and are useful in summarising the current understanding of diseases and their work-relatedness. Where available, referring to these resources is an efficient way for occupational physicians to practice based on scientific evidence. Some available sources have already undergone rigorous critical appraisal, such as Cochrane Reviews (John Wiley and Sons, 2021) and American College of Occupational and Environmental Medicine (ACOEM) practice guidelines (ACOEM, 2021).

Despite the growing database of pre-appraised resources making a "search" mode more and more feasible for busy clinicians, occupational physicians encounter clinical problems not yet pre-appraised more frequently than in other medical specialties. In such occasions, searching for the primary research, with the recommendations from authorities in the relevant branch of medicine or opinions from communications with experts can efficiently help evidence-based practice.

A special field of knowledge in occupational physicians has been the relationship between environmental exposure at work and health outcomes. Such knowledge should also include dose–response relationship between the specific exposures and outcomes. Relevant information has been available at least for a proportion of the following exposure-outcome combinations:

- Dust exposure and respiratory cancer;
- Metal exposure and cancer of certain organs;
- Metal exposure and neurodegenerative disorders;
- Solvents and neurological disorders;
- Solvent exposure and cancers;
- Chlorinated aromatic hydrocarbons and skin eruptions;
- Cumulative trauma and musculoskeletal diseases;
- Heavy lifting and degenerative intervertebral disc disorders;
- Stress and mental disorders;
- Mental strain and hypertension, cardiovascular disease, etc.;
- Shiftwork and breast and prostate cancers;
- Sedentary job and certain cancers;
- Pesticide exposure and neurodegenerative disorders;
- Sensitiser exposure and allergic conditions;
- Cooking fumes and respiratory cancer.

To Apply the Findings

The application of the findings from the literature involves integrating the critical appraisal with the occupational physician's clinical expertise and with the patient's or employer's perspectives. The following points have to be considered:

- Clinical problem of the worker;
- Unique concerns;
- Values, organisational issues, and circumstances.

For the exposures mentioned in the appraisal of the literature for quality, although increased occurrence has been found associated with relevant exposure, the dose has to be taken into consideration. Taking degenerative intervertebral disc disorders as an example, there is sufficient evidence to support a causal relationship between heavy lifting exposure and the disease. However, the weight and shape of the objects lifted each time, the number and duration of objects, the posture adopted during lifting, and the total years of lifting with or without adequate rest breaks are some important dose considerations when applying the findings from the literature. Individualised assessment of exposure condition is therefore critical when making clinical judgments on work-relatedness.

To apply the findings, integration of medical evidence found against the patient's or the employer's unique perspective or question is made. From formulating of an answerable question to applying the findings, the process varies greatly and is dependent on the specific clinical conditions. For conditions that we encounter every day (e.g. assessment of metabolic syndrome, treatment of hypertension or control of blood glucose levels) we need to be particularly up-to-date and knowledgeable about our medical decisions. Accordingly, more time and effort are required to carry out both searching and critically appraising the literature. For the conditions we encounter less often in occupational health (e.g. determination of the causal relationship between dust exposure to pneumoconiosis, level of noise exposure to noise-induced hearing loss, pesticide exposure to neurodegenerative diseases), we can conserve our time by seeking out critical appraisals already performed by other experts.

To Make Recommendations

Recommendations based on clinical evidence will be made to the worker(s), other related personnel, and the employers.

The occupational physician should use information acquired from scientific evidence-based methodology to derive good practice guidelines, in balance with their experience, and with workers' and other stakeholders' preferences. Respiratory health surveillance in a workplace with potential exposure to respiratory sensitisers is an example. The scientific knowledge that prognosis of occupational asthma is highly dependent on early removal from workplace will guide the physician to relocate the workers diagnosed or suspected as having occupational asthma. In some workplaces, this may be done easily. On the other hand, if relocation of a worker requires considerable effort, unwillingness, and/or loss of resources for either the employee or the employer, a more definitive diagnosis of occupational asthma may be required. In which case, a clear demonstration of ventilatory defects when exposed to the potential sensitiser (for example, by demonstration of pre-shift and post-shift differences in lung function, or by specific Bronchial provocation test) may be required. However, these tests are not always easily available, and some, e.g. bronchial provocation, should be conducted in hospitals with adequate support facilities.

To Evaluate the Effectiveness and Efficiency and to Seek Ways to Improve

This step actually can be considered an equivalent to auditing as described in the first half of this chapter.

In summary, application of EBM in occupational health services can enhance the quality of patient care, as in most other medical specialties. Occupational physicians should apply the methodologies of

EBM in their daily practice, balancing the improved quality with the efforts and time required.

Conclusion

This chapter provides information how to carry out occupational health audit in the workplaces. Examples are provided for some of the more frequently encountered situations in industries, including musculoskeletal, mental, and general health conditions. Evaluation for fitness for work and sickness leave are common occupational health practices, and auditing of these practices are useful to ensure the quality of occupational health services. Despite the general valuation of experience in occupational health practices, the importance of evidence from scientific literature cannot be overly emphasised, especially considering the nature of preventive care in occupational health practices.

References

Agius RM. (2010). *Standards and Audit in Occupational Health.* [Online] Available from: http://www.agius.com/hew/audit/index.htm. [Accessed on 23 January 2021].

ACOEM. (2021) *Practice guidelines.* [Online] Available from: https://acoem.org/Practice-Resources/Practice-Guidelines-Center. [Accessed on 15 March 2021].

Centers for Disease Control and Prevention. (2021) *Guidance for Businesses and Employers Responding to Coronavirus Disease 2019 (COVID-19).* [Online] Available from: https://www.cdc.gov/coronavirus/2019-ncov/community/guidance-business-response.html. [Accessed on 28 January 2021].

Chin W, Shiao JS, Liao S, Kuo C, Chen C, Guo YL. (2017) Depressive, anxiety and post-traumatic stress disorders at six years after occupational injuries. *Eur Arch Psychiatry Clin Neurosci* [Online] **267**(6): 507–516. Available from: doi: 10.1007/s00406-016-0762-x.

Chu P, Chin W, Guo YL, Shiao JS. (2019) Long-term effects of psychological symptoms after occupational injury on return to work: A 6-year follow-up. *Int J Environ Res Public Health* [Online] **16**(2): 235. Available from: doi: 10.3390/ijerph16020235.

Driver and Vehicle Licensing Agency. (2018) *Assessing Fitness to Drive: A Guide for Medical Professionals.* [Online] Available from: https://www.gov.uk/guidance/assessing-fitness-to-drive-a-guide-for-medical-professionals. [Accessed on 21 January 2021].

Evidence-Based Medicine Working Group. (1992). Evidence-based medicine. A new approach to teaching the practice of medicine. *JAMA* [Online] **268**(17): 2420–2425. Available from doi: 10.1001/jama.1992.03490170092032.

Health and Social Care Information Center. (2021) *Workplace Health: Applying All Our Health.* [Online] Available from: https://www.gov.uk/government/publications/workplace-health-applying-all-our-health. [Accessed on 28 January 2021].

Health and Social Care Information System. (2020) *Clinical Audit.* [Online] Available from: https://www.gov.uk/guidance/clinical-audit-descriptive-studies. [Accessed on 3 April 2021].

Lalloo D, Ghafur I, Macdonald EB. (2012) Peer review audit of occupational health reports-process and outcomes. *Occup Med (Lond)* [Online] **62**(1): 54–56. Available from: doi: 10.1093/occmed/kqr152.

Lalloo D, Demou E, Macdonald EB. (2015) Impact of peer review audit on occupational health report quality. *Occup Med (Lond)* [Online] **65**(6): 440–443. Available from doi: 10.1093/occmed/kqv077.

National Health Service. (1989) Working for patients. NHS White Paper. New diagnosis — new prescription. *Health Service J* [Online] **99**(5136): 134–137.

O'Toole MT. (ed.) (2017) *Mosby's Pocket Dictionary of Medicine, Nursing & Health Professions* (8th Ed). St Louis, Missouri, Elsevier.

Reed P. (2007) *The Medical Disability Advisor: Workplace Guidelines for Disability Duration.* Westminister, Colorado, Reed Group.

Sackett DL, Rosenberg WMC, Gray JAM, Haynes RB, Richardson WS. (1996) Evidence based medicine: What it is and what it isn't. *BMJ* **312**: 71–72. [Online] Available from: https://doi.org/10.1136/bmj.312.7023.71.

Straus SE, Glasziou P, Richardson WS, Haynes RB. (1997) *Evidence Based Medicine: How to Practice and Teach Evidence Based Medicine* (5th Ed). Edinburgh, United Kingdon, Churchill Livingstone.

Schaafsma F, Hulshof C, van Dijk F, Verbeek J. (2004). Information demands of occupational health physicians and their attitude towards evidence-based medicine. *Scand J Work Environ Health* **30**(4): 327–330. Available from: doi: 10.5271/sjweh.802.

van Dijk F, Caraballo-Arias Y. (2021) Where to find evidence-based information on occupational safety and health? *Ann Glob Health* **87**(1): 6. Available from: doi: 10.5334/aogh.3131.

Verbeek J, van Dijk F. (2007). *A Practical Guide for the Use of Research Information to Improve the Quality of Occupational Health Practice: For Occupational & Public Health Professionals/Editors.* [Online] Available from: https://apps.who.int/iris/handle/10665/43463. [Accessed on 15 March 2021].

Wilson PW, D'Agostino RB, Levy D, Belanger AM, Silbershatz H, Kannel WB. (1998) Prediction of coronary heart disease using risk factor categories. *Circulation* [Online] **97**(18): 1837–1847. Available from: doi: 10.1161/01.cir.97.18.1837.

Chapter 29

Cultural Aspects of Occupational Medicine Practice

*Adul Bandhukul**

Introduction

Culture is commonly defined as shared beliefs and attitudes of a group. Undoubtedly, culture influences work behaviour, the perception of disease and options for and choice of treatment. Differences between cultures are helpful in understanding discrepancies when several nationalities are working together (European Agency for Safety and Health at Work *et al.*, 2013).

Successful occupational health and safety programmes for migrant workers will require a good understanding of the cultural background of the workforce. This is especially true as globalisation increases the movement of workers between countries; and constitutes a continuing challenge for occupational physicians and other occupational health practitioners, particularly among low skilled migrant workers in poorly paying jobs as well as higher skilled workers working as professionals or in multinational organisations abroad.

* Occupational Medicine Institute, Nopparat Rajathanee Hospital, Bangkok, Thailand.
Corresponding author: Adul Bandhukul (adulstorage@gmail.com).

Globalisation and Mobility of Workers

Currently, there is a trend towards increasing economic cooperation among countries around the world. The regional cooperative initiatives take advantage of the resources in each country and attempt to reduce taxes and other barriers to free trade. Examples include the Asia Cooperation Dialogue (ACD), Asian Development Bank (ADB), ASEAN Economic Community (AEC), Asia-Pacific Economic Cooperation (APEC), the European Union (EU), Forum for East Asia-Latin America Cooperation (FEALAC), the International Monetary Fund (IMF), the Organisation for Economic Co-operation and Development (OECD), United Nations Conference on Trade and Development (UNCTAD), the World Bank (WB) and the World Trade Organization (WTO).

The world population is growing older with the population aged 65 and over growing faster than all other age groups, resulting in a falling proportion of working-age population group. The potential support ratio, which compares the number of working-age population aged 25–64 to those over age 65, is falling around the world with Japan having the lowest potential support ratio of 1.8. By 2050 most countries in the world are expected to have potential support ratio lower than two (United Nations, 2019). There is a trend toward a decrease in working-age population and migration can be a potential solution to the predicted shortage of this group which will become a necessity for all nations and not an option (Abubakar, 2020).

There is a constant stream of movement of labour for "migrant workers" to be employed usually in multinational organisations in many countries away from their homes. Multinational corporations are enterprises operating in several countries but managed from one (home) country. They also refer to any company or group that derives a substantial part of their revenue from trading outside their home country. Migrant workers are an increasingly permanent feature of today's labour market (International Labour Organization (ILO), 2007). They are subject to important occupational health and safety issues because of differences in characteristics such as ethnicity, culture, religion, language and beliefs. Multinational corporations can experience problems dealing with migrant workers from many different countries and cultures. Occupational physicians employed by these corporations can face difficulties in communicating and implementing occupational health and safety initiatives, especially if the workers are not native to these countries, and have newly arrived in these locations for the first time. Behaviour and mannerisms that are acceptable in one culture may be considered rude and inappropriate in other cultures. Religious beliefs may also require certain accommodations to be made in the workplace. It is usual for human resource departments to organise introductory briefings for new foreign workers, so that they can familiarise themselves with socio-cultural aspects of their new job locations. Occupational health team members may contribute to these introductions either directly or indirectly.

Case Study 1: The Expatriate Worker

Many Asian multinational corporations send their own engineers and managers to work in various countries globally. Some of these expatriate workers do not adapt easily to the native culture in the countries they are sent to, and with other factors such as loneliness through being away from their family for prolonged periods and social isolation, they may resort to risky health behaviours, e.g. alcohol consumption, cigarette smoking, unsafe sex. Expatriate workers can be held in high regard in the foreign community, but not necessarily so when they return home. This can lead to depression, and a reduced feeling of sense of worth. The converse is also true, when expatriate professionals take on a job of lower status, despite possible higher salaries.

Migrant Workers

Migrant workers, as defined by the ILO, refer to "people who leave home to find work outside of their hometown or home country." Persons who move for work in their own country are "domestic" or "internal" migrant workers. Person who move for work in another country are commonly called "foreign" or "international" migrant workers (ILO, 2007). Often, the intention for moving to work outside their homeland is a result of economic factors, instead of any keenness to "migrate" and make a permanent home at their place of work. The ILO estimates that there are 244 million migrants around the world (ILO, 2020a).

Some migrant workers obtain work overseas through legal channels, and others ae illegal. The pay and terms and conditions of employment vary depending on the grade and expertise level of the person hired. Higher grade, skilled expatriate staff often get a large expense allowance which may include additional benefits such as housing, children's education costs, and medical care. At the other end of the spectrum, some illegal workers are victims of human trafficking, which is often accompanied by a higher risk of succumbing to injuries and illnesses.

Migrant workers should have the same degree of occupational health and safety protection as nationals of the country in which they work. Countries should take all appropriate measures to prevent any special health risks to which migrant workers may be exposed (ILO, 1975).

Characteristics of Migrant Workers

A review of published articles regarding migrant workers from various countries (Ahonen *et al.*, 2007) indicated that:

a) Work is conducive to good health. Swedish studies of unemployment and sickness found that 50% of migrant workers thought that they were not in good health, with unemployment contributing to poor physical and mental health (Akhavan *et al.*, 2004). Similarly in Germany, many unemployed foreign workers experienced chronic health problems (Elkeles and Seifert, 2004).
b) Mental ill-health is featured prominently in many groups of migrant workers. Migrant workers also recognise how work can affect their health. In Israel, a positive association was found between mental stress and exposure to pesticides in Thai workers (Griffin and Solskone, 2003). A study of migrant nurses in Australia found that as a result of changing residence, loneliness and stress were experienced (Jackson, 1996). This was also true in Sweden where a study

found that there was an association between inappropriate work environment and low "life satisfaction" among migrant workers (Rosmond *et al.*, 1998).

c) Health, safety, and security are often accorded a lower order of priority amongst migrant workers, who are concerned about their job security. This was found in a study of taxi drivers in Canada (Facey, 2003). In San Francisco, some migrant workers experienced job insecurity, especially where there appeared to be an over-supply of readily available labour (Walter *et al.*, 2002).
d) Fatal occupational injuries occurred at a higher rate. In the United States (US), it was found that fatal occupational injuries were high in migrant workers (Loh and Richardson, 2004), while in Australia there were no differences between natives and migrant workers. However, the rate of injuries was higher among migrant workers in some occupations, and in those who had just arrived from non-English speaking countries (Corvalan *et al.*, 1994).
e) Non-fatal occupational injuries also occurred at a higher rate. Data from Singapore showed that there was a slight increase in non-fatal injuries in migrant workers, with a longer duration away from work as a result (Carangan *et al.*, 2004). Latino migrant workers in the US also experienced higher injury rates, and more days away from work. The latter was attributed to a greater severity of injuries (Pransky *et al.*, 2002). Middle school students who had jobs as migrant farm workers in the US had twice the non-fatal injury rate compared with their native US colleagues doing similar work. The injury rate was four times higher when high school students were compared (Cooper *et al.*, 2005). Similar findings regarding extent of injuries, and duration of sickness absence, were noted in studies in the Netherlands, Germany, Switzerland, and France (Bollini and Siem, 1995).

Migrant Workers and the Coronavirus Disease 2019 (COVID-19) Pandemic

The COVID-19 pandemic represents a major public health challenge, which has serious economic and social impacts on origin, transit and destination countries, as well as migrant workers and their families and business and their operations. Most of the migrants worked in the most affected occupations such as hospitality, construction, in health-care and domestic work.

Additionally, migrant workers often belong to minority ethnic groups, who have been identified as a higher risk group for COVID-19 (Public Health England, 2020).

ILO estimates that full and partial lockdown measures affected almost 2.2 billion workers or 68% of the global workforce. As a result, migrant workers now have fewer options to access support services such as money, social protection or access to medical care. Those who illegally worked in countries will not seek help in any form because of their fear of deportation (ILO 2020b).

Unsatisfactory housing conditions for migrant workers is another concern. Millions of low-skilled migrant workers live in housing conditions where social distancing is difficult to practise, with poor hygiene. Unsatisfactory housing and social overcrowding in accommodation for low-skilled migrant workers need to be addressed before any pandemic occurs. If this is not done, epicentres of the disease can arise in these housing areas during a pandemic and these housing sites could be flash points for spread of infection among these workers which may spread to the general population. For example, from early April 2020, a marked escalation of new cases of COVID-19 was observed among low-skilled migrant workers living in dormitories in Singapore (Koh, 2020). By the end of 2020, these infected workers formed the vast majority of cases of COVID-19 confirmed in Singapore.

Case Study 2: Support for Migrant Workers During the COVID-19 Pandemic

These are samples of communication and financial support for migrants in some countries during the COVID-19 pandemic:

a) Italy's online "JsUMA" portal provides refugees and asylum-seekers with access to information in 15 different languages on COVID-19.
b) Canada provides information in multiple languages on financial assistance for migrants who face financial hardship.

c) Brazil has a monthly emergency basic income, to be paid for up to three months to the unemployed, self-employed and those working in informal economy including migrant workers with irregular status.
d) In Myanmar, the consortium of international donors under the Livelihoods and Food Security Fund is financing an emergency COVID-19 cash transfer targeted at vulnerable groups, including internal and returning international migrants.
e) The Overseas Worker Welfare Administration in the Philippines has created an emergency fund targeted at Filipino migrant workers. This fund provides a one-time payment to land-based and sea-based workers who have been displaced because of COVID-19.
f) Thailand sent aircraft to repatriate Thai workers and students who wish to return home from "locked-down" countries. Many migrant workers in Thailand went home during the early stages of the pandemic because there were more COVID-19 cases in Thailand than in their countries.

Migrant Workers and Hazardous Work

Migrant workers often face the risk of working in hazardous occupations or with dangerous processes in the workplace. In the US, the work includes agriculture, construction and the service and garment industry. In Italy and Germany, migrant workers are mainly "blue collar workers" and perform unskilled work tasks. Key factors contributing to occupational injury and ill-health include language barriers and poor communication in daily work. In Australia, the fatal injury rate of migrants only decreased to the same level as natives after they worked more than 5 years (Corvalan *et al.*, 1994); and in Taiwan most fatal injuries among migrant workers occurred in the first six months of work (Wu *et al.*, 1997). Misunderstandings arising from cultural differences play a role in about 70%–80% of all maritime accidents (Horck, 2006).

Ill-health in Migrant Workers

Studies of health problems in migrant workers have identified work place exposure to pesticides, lead, and a variety of chemicals and fumes. Musculoskeletal disorders were commonly reported among agricultural and garment workers. Other health effects reported are respiratory irritation, and non-specific symptoms such as headache and dizziness. These effects were often attributed to a lack of safety training among migrant workers, and especially training that was not conducted in a familiar language (Pransky *et al.*, 2002).

This association between ill-health and lack of safety training has however not been consistent. Migrant workers are often reluctant to report work-related health effects and minor injuries. This may be due to their uncertain migration status (legal or illegal), type of work, economic circumstances, access to health care, barriers to compensation, delays in administration, a lack of knowledge about the process for reporting, language barriers, and a fear of consequences of reporting.

Even in countries with a long history of labour representation, the struggle continues for better occupational safety and health provisions for migrant workers. Coordination through a network of countries with substantial numbers of migrant workers, in order to gather data, better understand their occupational safety and health problems, and share cost-effective measures for preventing occupational injury and ill-health, would be a welcome development.

Cross Cultural Issues and the Importance of Communication

In communicating occupational health and safety issues to a workforce with a large group of migrant workers, an ideal approach would be to use the workers' native language. This is not always practicable, since migrant workers in some countries such as in the Middle East and in Malaysia, Singapore, and Hong Kong, originate from many different countries such as India, Bangladesh, Thailand, Burma, Philippines, and Indonesia. Also, occupational health and safety professionals may not be conversant in the languages of these countries. Use of the workers' friends or relatives as interpreters can also be problematic, because of non-availability and confidentiality.

Misunderstandings may arise from the use of the spoken language or body language. Postures and gestures could have different connotations in different cultures. Occupational health and safety professionals need to have "cultural competency," which refers to possession of knowledge, awareness, and respect for other cultures. This is essential for a proper understanding of the attitude and behaviour of migrant workers regarding their health, home life and work.

Possible issues of communication should be considered when dealing with foreign workers. These include the following:

a) Use of the worker's formal name instead of a nickname. In some cultures, individuals prefer to be addressed by their formal name, especially when they deal with persons deemed to be in positions of authority, e.g. a doctor or a government official.
b) Avoiding unnecessary body contact. In many Asian and Middle-Eastern cultures, touching or shaking hands especially between members of the opposite sex is discouraged. Strong displays of affection in public are unacceptable, and wearing modest attire is often the rule. It can be considered impolite to touch someone on the head, or to insist that a person should be clean shaven when considering, for example, the choice of respiratory protective devices. These cultural norms need to be borne in mind for healthcare and occupational health and safety professionals working with a multinational workforce in foreign countries.
c) Body language during communication can enhance or confuse the interaction between healthcare professionals and their clients. In some cultures, patients or their relatives may attempt to agree with physicians by seemingly nodding in agreement or smiling approvingly, even when they do not understand what is said.

Family relationships and influence of family members is important in many cultures. In Asian countries, the extended household family structure with several siblings and their families living together with their parents is common. Knowledge and attitudes to occupational health and safety may be influenced by the views of other family members and close friends, and this could be a major factor determining the success or failure of preventive measures at the workplace.

Socio-Cultural and Religious Beliefs

Culture and religion can affect the perception of what causes diseases or injuries. Many Buddhist workers believe in "karma" affecting life events. "Karma" is a spiritual principle linking cause and effect, where the intent and actions of an individual (cause) influences his/her future (effect). Similarly, some cultures believe that good or bad life events are pre-ordained. Others believe in the role of spirits in causing illness or injury. In some religions, the use of helmets at work may be impractical, because of requirements to keep long hair; and the use of respirators may be ineffective among workers who keep beards and facial hair because of religious beliefs.

An understanding of the socio-cultural and religious beliefs of all workers can assist occupational physicians and clinicians in the effective management of the illnesses and concerns of the workforce.

Case Study 3: The Role of "Karma" in Occupational Accidents

An occupational health investigation into several cases of workers with traumatic amputation of the fingers at a factory in Thailand revealed that part of this occurred as a result of the workers' belief in the inevitability of life's incidents. The affected individuals placed more importance on the role of "karma" than on the relevance of safe working practices, and safety devices and tools.

Case Study 4: Shamans and Health

An occupational health investigation was initiated following an outbreak of severe pruritic rashes on the extremities and neck in many workers at a factory in a suburban area of Thailand (Fig. 1). The rashes occurred mainly in outdoor workers. The factory owners thought that this was because they had upset the land spirits, and invited a shaman

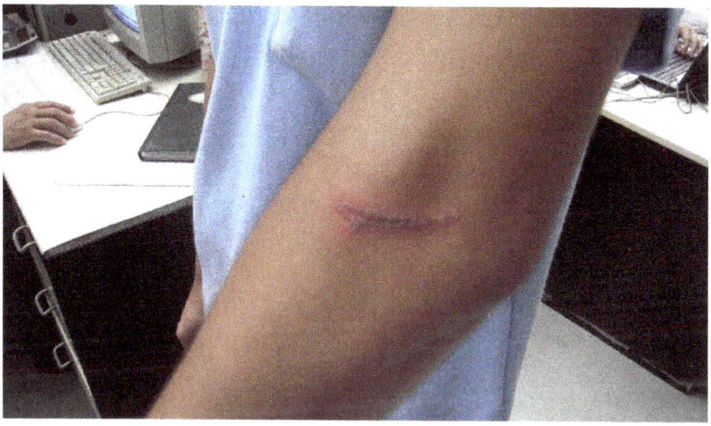

Fig. 1. Skin lesion in a worker with "paederus dermatitis."

to perform a ritual to appease the spirits. Meanwhile, the occupational physician who was invited by worker representatives to investigate the cause found that this rash also occurred in people who lived around the factory. Working with colleagues in dermatology, the cause was traced to skin contact with the haemolymph from a rove beetle (Paederus fuscipes). Extermination of the beetle, with screening of the open area of the workplace reduced the number of new cases of paederus dermatitis amongst the workers. The rituals of the shaman were believed by the factory owner and some of the workers to have played a major role in halting the outbreak.

This case study demonstrates that the effectiveness of the occupational health measures can be enhanced by taking into account employers and workers beliefs in the investigation and management of outbreaks of disease at workplaces, regardless of the personal knowledge and/or beliefs of the investigating physician.

Folk Medicine

Folk medicine is common in many countries. Resorting to the use of folk remedies and self-medication to promote and maintain health or to treat ailments is a practice by workers in many cultures. The ingredients in the medicines used for this practice have been known to cause harmful effects. Even when these medications exert only a placebo effect, there is no quality control scheme that ensures the quality, safety, and efficacy of many of these remedies. Occupational medicine practitioners working in countries with a multicultural workforce need to be aware of this approach by workers in dealing with their symptoms. Non-awareness by the doctors could well be detrimental to their efforts to prevent and manage ill-health at work.

Case Study 5: Folk Medicine

A worker from a chemical factory developed skin lesions around his trunk. He attributed this to the chemical used at work. The occupational physician investigated and found no evidence of exposure to the chemical. He asked about the possible use of any medicines by the worker. It transpired that the worker had been taking folk medicines for "strengthening his health" over a considerable period of time. Analysis of a sample of the medicine consumed by the worker showed the presence of arsenic. The skin lesions were consistent with arsenical keratosis. The worker was advised to discontinue using the specific preparation; and some subsequent improvement in his skin condition ensued.

Health Perception

Prejudices against migrant workers exist, often strongly held, through erroneous views about the economic and health burden imposed by migrant workers on the indigenous population. Migrant workers are sometimes viewed as a cause of the spread of communicable diseases. Hence, extensive and complicated health screening procedures are often required for migrant workers before they can commence employment in a foreign country. Protection of public health is often invoked as a reason for requiring initial and periodic chest X-rays and a battery of laboratory tests for all expatriate workers seeking employment. The requirements often do not take into account the specific jobs or work tasks that the workers are hired to do.

In the EU, there is evidence that the migrant population could have a significant effect on communicable and vaccine preventable diseases. A study of United Kingdom (UK) enhanced surveillance data for tuberculosis (TB), human immunodeficiency virus (HIV), malaria and enteric fever among the migrant (non-UK born) population (Wagner *et al.*, 2014) showed that South Asia was the most common region for TB and enteric fever cases (57% and 80% of migrant cases respectively). Subsaharan Africa was the predominant region of HIV in heterosexual and malaria cases (80% and 75% of migrant cases, respectively).

A study of perception of occupational risk in employee contact with migrant workers in the Hungarian border in EU found that significant gaps in health awareness of these employees (Istvan *et al.*, 2014). There was a lack of training about the risk in work that have effect on the migrant health and the infectious diseases in migrant workers and for health care workers who take care of migrant workers. Provision of training and improving knowledge and skills to healthcare workers, especially on aspects of migrant health, will likely improve public health and occupational health and safety.

Case Study 6: Annual Physical Examinations of Migrant Workers

In the annual physical examination of workers in a factory, 14 migrant workers were suspected to be infected with pulmonary TB. When investigated, the doctor found that each small room in the dormitory in the factory was allocated as living quarters for six or more workers. Hence, there was considerable overcrowding. The doctor made appointments for the infected workers to be examined, investigated clinically, and treated if warranted, but they absconded from the workplace because of a fear of deportation. The owner of the factory promptly hired other workers instead.

A study (Fellmeth *et al.*, 2015) of pregnant migrant and refugee women's perception of mental illness on the Thai–Myanmar border focused on five main themes: symptoms of mental illness, causes of mental illness, suicide, mental illness during pregnancy and the postpartum period, and managing mental illness. Symptoms included emotional disturbances, somatic symptoms and socially inappropriate behaviour. The main causes were described as current economic and family-related difficulties. Suicide was mainly attributed to shame on economic hardships, domestic and family issue. Mental illness was most common during and following pregnancy due to a lack of family support and worries about the future. The study suggested that more formal and systematic training including the development of assessment tools in the local languages would enable better ascertainment and treatment of mental illness in this population.

Conclusion

An appreciation of the socio-cultural factors relevant to the background of foreign workers will help in the effective provision of occupational medicine services. This is especially where workplaces have a high proportion of foreign workers. Similarly, in the investigation and management of occupational illnesses, the physician should appreciate the worker's social and cultural perception of illness and treatment.

References

Abubakar I. (2020) The future of migration, human populations, and global health in the Anthropocene. *Lancet* **396**(10258): 1133–1134.

Ahonen EQ, Benavides FG, Benach FG. (2007) Immigrant populations, work and health — a systematic literature review. *Scand J Work Environ Health* **33**(2): 96–104.

Akhavan S, Bildt CO, Franzén EC, Wamala S. (2004) Health in relation to unemployment and sick leave among immigrants in Sweden from a gender perspective. *J Immigr Minor Health* **6**(3): 103–118.

Bollini P, Siem H. (1995) No real progress towards equity: Health of migrants and ethnic minorities on the eve of the year 2000. *Soc Sci Med* **41**(6): 819–828.

Carangan M, Tham KY, Seow E. (2004) Work-related injury sustained by foreign workers in Singapore. *Ann Acad Med Singap* **33**(2): 209–213.

Cooper SP, Weller NF, Fox EE, Cooper SR. (2005) Comparative description of migrant farmworkers versus other students attending rural south Texas schools: Substance use, work, and injuries. *J Rural Health* **21**(4): 361–366.

Corvalan CF, Driscoll TR, Harrison JE. (1994) Role of migrant factors in work-related fatalities in Australia. *Scand J Work Environ Health* **20**(5): 364–370.

Elkeles T, Seifert W. (1996) Immigrants and health: Unemployment and health-risks of labour migrants in the Federal Republic of Germany, 1984–1992. *Soc Sci Med* **43**(7): 1035–1047.

European Agency for Safety and Health at Work, Starren A, Luijters K, Drupsteen L, Vilkevicius G, Eeckelaert L, Eeckelaert L. (2013) *Diverse Cultures at Work: Ensuring Safety and Health Through Leadership and Participation.* [Online] Available from: https://op.europa.eu/en/publication-detail/-/publication/e3b26a4a-ed09-415d-9f6e-85705f6dfb7e/language-en. [Accessed on 25 December 2020].

Facey ME. (2003) The health effects of taxi driving: The case of visible minority drivers in Toronto. *Can J Public Health* **93**(4): 254–257.

Fellmeth G, Plugge E, Paw MK, Charunwatthana P, Nosten F, McGready R. (2015) Pregnant migrant and refugee women's perceptions of mental illness on the Thai-Myanmar border: A qualitative study. *BMC Pregnancy Childb* **15**(1): 93.

Griffin J, Solskone V. (2003) Psychological distress among Thai migrant workers in Israel. *Soc Sci Med* **57**(5): 769–774.

Horck J. (2006) The gender perspective in maritime education and training. *WMU J Marit Aff* **9**(1): 93–119.

ILO. (1975) *Migrant Workers Recommendation.* [Online] Available from: https://www.ilo.org/dyn/normlex/en/f?p=normlexpub:12100:0::no:12100:P12100_instrument_id:312489:no. [Accessed on 25 Dec 2020].

ILO. (2007) *International Labour Standards on Migrant Workers' Rights: Guide for Policymakers and Practitioners in Asia and the Pacific.* [Online] Available from: https://www.ilo.org/wcmsp5/groups/public/---asia/---ro-bangkok/documents/publication/wcms_146244.pdf. [Accessed on 25 Dec 2020].

ILO. (2020a) *International Labour Standards on Migrant Workers.* [Online] Available from: https://www.ilo.org/global/standards/subjects-covered-by-international-labour-standards/migrant-workers/lang--en/index.htm. [Accessed on 25 Dec 2020].

ILO. (2020b) *COVID-19 and the World of Work* (3rd Ed). *Updated Estimates and Analysis.* [Online] Available from: https://www.ilo.org/wcmsp5/groups/public/---dgreports/---dcomm/documents/briefingnote/wcms_743146.pdf. [Accessed on 25 Dec 2020].

Jackson D. (1996) The multicultural workplace: Comfort, safety and migrant nurses. *Contemp Nurse* **5**(3): 120–126.

Koh D. (2020) Migrant workers and COVID-19. *Occup Environ Med* 77(9): 634–636.

Loh K, Richardson S. (2004) Foreign-born workers: Trends in fatal occupational injuries, 1996–2001. *Monthly Lab Rev* **127**(6): 42–53.

Istvan S, Katz Z, Berenyi K, Csepregi P, Huszar A, Barath A, Marek E. (2014) Perception of occupational risks and practices of self-protection from infectious diseases among workers in contact with international migrants at Hungary's border. *J Rural Med* **9**(2): 59–73.

Pransky G, Moshenberg D, Benjamin K, Portillo S, Lee JT, Hill-Fotouhi C. (2002) Occupational risks and injuries in non-agricultural immigrant Latino workers. *Am J Ind Med* **42**(2): 117–123.

Rosmond R, Lapidus L, Björntorp P. (1998) A cross-sectional study of self-reported work conditions and psychiatric health in native Swedes and immigrants. *Occup Med (Lond)* **48**(5): 309–314.

Public Health England. (2020) *Mitigation of Risks of COVID-19 in Occupational Settings with a Focus on Ethnic Minority Groups — Consensus Statement from PHE, HSE and FOM.* [Online] Available from: https://www.gov.uk/government/publications/covid-19-mitigation-of-risks-in-occupational-settings-with-a-focus-on-ethnic-minority-groups/mitigation-of-risks-of-covid-19-in-occupational-settings-with-a-focus-on-ethnic-minority-groups-consensus-statement-from-phe-hse-and-fom. [Accessed on 25 Dec 2020].

United Nations, Department of Economic and Social Affairs, Population Division. (2019) *World Population Prospects 2019: Highlights.* [Online] Available from: https://population.un.org/wpp/Publications/Files/WPP2019_Highlights.pdf. [Accessed on 25 Dec 2020].

Walter N, Bourgois P, Loinaz HM, Schillinger D. (2002) Social context of work injury among undocumented day labourers in San Francisco. *J Gen Intern Med* **17**(3): 221–229.

Wagner KS, Lawrence J, Anderson L, Yin Z, Delpech V, Chiodini PL, Redman C, Jones J. (2014) Migrant health and infectious diseases in the UK: Findings from the last 10 years of surveillance. *J Public Health* **36**(1): 28–55.

Wu TN, Liou SH, Hsu CC, Chao SL, Liou SF, Ko KN, Yeh WY, Chang PY. (1997) Epidemiologic study of occupational injuries among foreign and native workers in Taiwan. *Am J Ind Med* **31**(5): 623–630.

Chapter 30

Crisis Communication in the Pandemic Era for Occupational Medicine

*Max Lum**

Introduction

During epidemics and pandemics, and humanitarian crises and natural disasters, effective risk communication allows people most at risk to understand and adopt protective behaviours. It allows authorities and experts to listen to and address people's concerns and needs so that the advice they provide is relevant, trusted and acceptable (World Health Organization (WHO), 2017a).

On 11 March 2020, WHO formally declared coronavirus disease 2019 (COVID-19) a pandemic, highlighting the uncertainty that has impacted lives, and livelihoods into a worldwide health crisis. Outbreaks continued to grow and subside, and mortality rates created anxiety and severely impacted workers, workplaces and our economic future.

There is enough of crisis communication literature that exists on how to respond to high consequence of environmental events like fires, floods, hurricanes and earthquakes and what steps are needed to assure that appropriate communication strategies are available and implemented to protect populations at risk (Schoch-Spana *et al.*,

---

*National Institute for Occupational Safety and Health, Center for Disease Control and Prevention, Washington, D.C., United States of America.

2019). However, global catastrophic biological risks such as COVID-19 jeopardise humanity by posing a different type of risk communication challenge due to its debilitating effect on work and workplaces, the necessity of a speedy country response and the absolute necessity for occupational health and safety professionals to be involved in the early stages of pre-planning championing evidenced-based preventive actions targeted to both the workplace and the community at large.

The Global East and West have divergent perspectives on the communication strategies needed to respond to hazardous biological events. Historically past biological threats such as Severe Acute Respiratory Syndrome (2002–2004), Influenza A H1N1 (2009), Middle East respiratory syndrome–related coronavirus (2012), Zika (2013–2016), Ebola (2014–2015) and COVID-19 (2019–) all presaged the need for prior planning. Apparently only scientists and policy makers mainly in Asian countries thought about how they would respond to a serious biological event. Although the pandemic hit the Asian region first, its countries — including emerging Association of Southeast Asian Nations (ASEAN) — have to date recorded significantly lower transmission and fatality rates per capita than other regions (Statistica, 2020). Lack of best pre-planning practices in western countries poses a clear need for a more responsive and efficient way to raise awareness among policy makers and design effective preventive actions.

The argument that an epidemic or pandemic is a surprise event seems nonsensical, yet many western nations seem to believe the opposite. Escalating international travel, increased urbanisation and climate effects made the case more probable that hazardous biological events were ever more likely. In addition, global warming contributes to new disease carrying vectors that do not follow geographic boundaries. The increase association of humans and animals in wildlife markets and other venues create an ideal environment for increased biological exposure and spread. The COVID-19 response was further exacerbated due to the lack of health professionals rigorously trained to understand the interplay between culture, climate, politics and biology such that they can effectively communicate health messaging to exposed populations.

Definition and Phases of Crisis Communication

In every industry, in business of all sizes, crisis communication should be a common topic of discussion and training. Crisis communication in larger industries is often a sub-specialty of public relations that views its role as defending an individual, company or organisation facing some type of public challenge to its reputation. Increasingly the public relations "protect the reputation" approach is not effective in handling larger biological health risk communication requirements. Timothy Coombs, a leading communication scholar warns that a more expansive view is necessary where crisis communication is more appropriately defined as the "collection, processing and dissemination of evidence-based information to address a crisis that generates negative outcomes for stakeholders" such as workers, employers and the local community (Coombs, 2012). Occupational safety and health professionals have an important responsibility in steering workplace crisis communication pre-event planning and crisis response strategies away from public relations approaches toward more evidenced-base solutions heavily influenced by scientific practice. The main goal of every workplace crisis communication strategy must be to implement appropriate engineering and/or administrative controls and provide useful information to workers for protective decision making. Administrative control requirements used in crisis communication strategies must be designed to provide evidenced-based knowledge and the appropriate dissemination tools to assist the reach and application of preventive measures tailored for the emergency.

Three Phases of Crisis Communication

a) Crisis prevention, preparation and training to include pre-event risk communication strategies identifying practical preparedness solutions, risk scenarios and anticipated threat characteristics.
b) Crisis response and management including: crisis communication and guidance regarding protective actions to be taken, appropriate risk messaging with consideration for technological tools to expand reach and speed immediate action.

c) Post-crisis evaluation of the control strategies undertaken during the crisis response and management stage and the feedback of findings to improve future crisis event planning and control.

Disease prevention and control involves strategies, training and specific leadership actions required to reduce known risk. Both global health organisations such as the WHO, country institutes, universities, and leading communication professionals document that organisations are better able to handle crisis situations when they "(1) have a crisis management plan that is updated annually, (2) have a designated crisis management team, (3) conduct exercises to test the response plan, and (4) have pre-draft communication messages" (US Centers for Disease Control and Prevention (CDC), 2018).

Phase I Crisis Prevention, Preparation, and Training

Champion for science in crisis planning

Occupational health professionals must be strong proponents and stewards of the application of timely and evidenced-based data to design and implement emergency response pre-planning initiatives in a crisis. In western countries some political leadership expressed extraordinary skepticism about the SARS-CoV-2 virus and the steps needed to curb it. Some disease experts in the United States (US) felt that government culture demonstrated a fixed way of thinking creating delays in providing laboratories and public health agencies around the country with an effective strategic plan and local guidance. Early in the pandemic several European Union (EU) countries, particularly the UK and Belgium, faced similar bureaucratic hurdles resulting in the delay of important messaging for at risk citizens (Walsh, 2020; Stevis-Gridneff *et al.*, 2020).

Assure outside guidance and expert participation

Occupational health professionals' input in pre-crisis planning is essential to assure that evidenced-based planning forms the foundation of control initiatives. Like any other workplace strategy, crisis communication needs a comprehensive plan with clear goals and measurable objectives. Without the proper plan with appropriate public health input organisations may not be able to adapt to unanticipated consequences are handicapped to align employee actions with larger country control strategies. This is particularly true in a pandemic crisis where guidance from outside experts and government leadership is required to assure comprehensive planning and implementation.

To be effective, pre-crisis planning must seek evidence to identify and understand what control measures are accountable and in sync with country culture and government guidance. When that guidance is missing or delayed, businesses must consider the importance of assuming a pro-active leadership role in moving forward.

With the pandemic in full swing Mexican federal political leaders (as with the political leadership of other nations) minimised the pandemic, questioning the science behind wearing face masks, testing and limiting response planning.

Case Study 1: Enlightened Leadership is Essential

The mayor of Mexico City with the support of the strong pro-active support of the business community pushed aggressive testing, and a contact tracing campaign which included setting up testing kiosks where people could get tested for free. Larger organisations voiced their support of the mayor's face-covering policies. "The virus has thrived in the dense capital, home to nine million people, half of them poor. But while the toll has been horrific analysts say it could have been worse without the mayor's interventions" (Kitroeff, 2020).

Occupational health professionals must develop effective pro-active communication skills

To speak persuasively during an epidemic or pandemic crisis requires more than knowing one's audience, government requirements, and developing an appropriate style. It requires applying knowledge to develop discreet tailored messages specifically targeted to those populations most at risk. Occupational professionals should be part of the employer's pre-planning outreach team to assure the best evidenced-based strategies are selected in the planning process to support tailoring employee messages to those workers most at risk. The health and safety spokespersons must be trained and experienced in how to handle crisis communication, be able to provide employees with useful information for their decision making, assist in explaining the science supporting control measures and always be ready to answer employees' specific questions and concerns. Appropriate training and skills development are essential to help health professionals to achieve success. Good communication skills build trust with employees and assist working towards common goals.

Occupational health professionals must understand and address the potential leadership gap between "feeling ready" versus "being ready"

There is a real opportunity for occupational health professionals to champion and support quality planning outcomes. According to research on communication, 47% of employers say that they have the capabilities or processes they would need to meet a crisis with the best possible outcome but only 49% of corporate board members have engaged with management to understand what has been done to support crisis preparedness and only half say that they and management have special discussions devoted to crisis communication and prevention. Additional findings found that only 32% report their companies engage in crisis simulations or training. This indicates a significant gap exists between people "feeling ready" as opposed to "being ready" to cope with and handle "crisis situations" (Smarp, 2020; Deloitte, 2020). Businesses of all kinds must be prepared for a wide range of potential crisis, including environmental and biological incidents. Crisis communication pre-planning ensures that all relevant leadership personnel have developed and tested strategies and tools that provide quick and effective communication with each other as well as protecting workers and business assets ensuring continuity.

Phase II Crisis Response and Management

Crisis communication messaging must be evidenced-based

The WHO responding to crisis information being disseminated concerning the COVID-19 pandemic identified an "infodemic" defined as an "over-abundance of information-some accurate and some not rendering it difficult to find trustworthy sources of information and reliable guidance" (WHO, 2020).

Business organisations must address the infodemic and keep policies and messages delivered to employees up-to-date as expert knowledge evolves. Occupational safety and health personnel with their training in science and their intimate knowledge of the workplace are strategically placed to forewarn business leadership, managers and workers to impending expected health threats and in suggesting appropriate preventative strategies.

Case Study 2: Evidenced-Based Information is Essential

According to Belgium's Federal Health Minister: "It isn't a very aggressive virus. You would have to sneeze in someone's face to pass it on" (Stevis-Gridneff et al., 2020).

Limit public pushback on threat messaging

The message of uncertainty and unpredictability is not emphasised nearly often enough to respond and limit public criticism about expected morbidity and mortality data during a crisis. The assumptions behind mathematical modelling concerning changing infection and outcome data is rarely if ever explained in understandable language. Failure to incorporate clear messaging into emergency response modelling plans is a familiar weakness worldwide. Universities and business organisations especially those with an active staff of well-trained health professionals can assist message clarification by providing clarifying information, answering questions of why outbreak modelling and analysis is not an exact science and providing insight into evolving data changes.

An area that needs continuous and specific attention is vaccine safety and efficacy. Communications must be clear that vaccine availably is not immediate for all and how well it works is a question that can be answered only by science driven evidence.

Health organisations need to get it right

Studies have concluded that face masks have helped reduce contagion by reducing droplets being sprayed into the air. "It may be that they work in a small amount of cases and/or just wearing them helps to promote healthy behaviours with COVID-19, but facemasks are seen as beneficial for protection of both health-care workers and the public" (Holger *et al.*, 2020).

Case Study 3: Organisations Must Avoid Contradictory Messages

After initially recommending that all health professionals encountering coronavirus patients wear N95 respirators, the US CDC announced that less protective surgical masks were an "an acceptable alternative" except in some cases that were not explained. Further confusion was created when the US Surgeon General earlier stated that those without symptoms didn't need to wear a mask (Sandman, 2020).

Case Study 4: Recommendations Must Adapt to Actual Available Evidence

"The virus is not spreading in the general community... we don't routinely recommend the use of face masks by the public to prevent respiratory illness. And we certainly are not recommending that currently for this new virus" (CDC, 2020a).

Crisis communication messaging must be targeted

It is critical to design and deliver relevant safety messages to the most venerable workers especially to the elderly and those employed in health care. Occupational health professionals especially those working in a public health capacity have a critical role to assure that communication outreach during a crisis deliberately focuses upon the most vulnerable workers, including minority workers, health care professionals, nursing home workers, and the myriad of workers most directly servicing the public (Mckinsey and Company, 2020).

Worldwide public health officials excluded nursing home workers from pandemic preparedness plans and initially omitted community residents from mathematical threat modelling. "During the COVID-19 pandemic some European countries forced health care professionals to ration care to the elderly because of shortages of space and equipment. In some European cities' public health officials and hospitals sometimes flatly failed to communicate appropriate health and safety messages to the elderly and their health care givers" (Stevis-Gridneff *et al.*, 2020). It is important to note that even countries like Australia that developed and implemented a relatively effective emergency response plan sustained a high rate of nursing home fatalities.

Messaging must be targeted to minority populations

In the United States the targeting of health messaging and mitigation efforts which focused on prevention and early detection generally failed to reach working black Americans who were already disproportionately likely as their white peers to die from diabetes, hypertension, and asthma — all risk factors that exacerbate COVID-19 symptoms.

Case Study 5: Minority Populations Must be Targeted

A CDC analysis of 114,411 US COVID-19–associated deaths from May to August 2020, found that 24.2% were Hispanic or Latino (Hispanic), and 18.7% were non-Hispanic (Black). The percentage of Hispanic decedents increased from 16.3% in May to 26.4% in August (CDC, 2020b).

Risk messaging must account for disabled populations

There is a clear need to identify and provide targeted response and mitigation information to disabled persons to better anticipate and plan for their personal safety during a disaster event. Such efforts must be provided to disabled workers with specific regard for their working conditions and response ability.

Case Study 6: Messaging for Disabled Individuals

The American Red Cross with federal support has published a booklet that provides information and tips to disabled individuals to assess their personal disaster preparation and provides resources and suggestions for gathering and making their personal risk safer (American Red Cross and The Federal Emergency Management Agency, 2004).

Messaging to small and medium-sized enterprises (SMEs) and micro-SMEs creates a special outreach challenge

Occupational health professionals can alert business leadership to the need to be especially aware of service delivery barriers, administrative control challenges and the importance of designing and implementing effective crisis communication outreach efforts to their SME and micro-SME stakeholders. This is especially needed for corporations' dependent on SME supply-chain workers. Where appropriate businesses may want to consider supporting direct financial incentives toward communication capacity-building programmes.

Case Study 7: Messages Must be Targeted to SMEs and Micro-SMEs

Singapore offered the Industry 4.0 Human Capability Programme, which helped 300 SMEs implement digital communication use cases and redesign jobs to support them (Daly et al., 2020).

Avoid providing mixed messages

The public is often skeptical of those who manage risk and crisis situations. To create trust, it is important for health professionals to correctly respond and address information which is wrong but not deliberately misleading and disinformation which refers to organised falsehoods that are intended to deceive. "In a biological hazard crisis, inaccurate information doesn't only mislead but can be a matter of life and death if people start taking unproven drugs, ignoring public-health advice, or refusing a vaccine when one becomes available" (Heath, 2010; Palenchar, 2008).

Case Study 8: Message Myth Comparisons Need to be Avoided

"Last year 37,000 Americans died from the flu. Nothing was shut down, life and the economy go on," President Trump stated in March 2020 and then a few days later made a U-turn on that statement: "Nothing would be worse than declaring victory before victory is won." But changes were not forthcoming (Bump, 2020).

Modelling good messaging behaviour is essential

Wearing masks is perceived as normal and effective in many Asian counties but in western countries mask-wearing spiraled into confusion and outright misinformation concerning their efficacy. Political leaders delayed and were often unwilling to model good mask wearing behaviour. Mask wearing became a politically polarising issue and political leadership resisted the recommendations of public health officials to wear masks when in public. In the US top public health officials pushed former President Trump to advise everyone — even people who appear to be healthy — to wear a mask when in public places. But the former US President and other White House officials resisted.

Case Study 9: Political Leadership Must Model Scientifically Sound Protective Behaviours

The former US President had offered tepid endorsement for masks, saying: "The mask, perhaps, helps." He had also raised doubts about the science, noting that health experts who now advocate public mask-wearing were once opposed to it. "I guess I'm somewhere in the middle," Trump said recently and "I understand both sides of the argument" (Farley, 2020).

Business leadership have a role in clarifying government messaging

Conflicting and erroneous messages received from government sources and political leaders can have a seriously negative impact. Beyond modeling good behaviour, clear, authoritative, communication of evidence-based information by business leadership can clarify and reduce worker skepticism and misunderstanding of unclear or mixed messages from outside experts and government sources. For crisis communication, workers' ability to perceive the correctness of the information can hamper trust and useful decision making. Numerous studies have examined how people perceive policies toward risk messaging and regulation. Where public skepticism is high, and trust is low, message recipients are unlikely to accept recommendations and risk messages (Palenchar, 2008, 2010). Business organisations where there is substantial corporate employee loyalty can serve as a conduit to build trust by providing evidence-based information free of political concerns. Research has provided evidence for the "*critical trust*" concept — where a high degree of trust in a person or institution such as a business organisation or industry can co-exist with a relatively high degree of skepticism from government sources and misstatements (Sanders, 2019).

Case Study 10: Businesses Can Anticipate Employee Misinformation

Coats (a thread manufacturer) and Viessmann (heating and refrigeration systems) concerned about government censorship, unclear messages and highly invasive technology developed and deployed their own corporate designed messaging apps to be used for their Chinese employees "to limit political messaging, improve evidenced-based preventive measures and provide real-time health and safety updates" (Staffbase, 2020).

The changing world of work effects messaging

The COVID-19 pandemic has started a debate as to whether in-building office workplaces are still appropriate. Occupational health and safety officials and business teams have an increasing role to play in being alert to the changing remote workplace and in identifying the corresponding effective digital communication tools to assist their employees.

Case Study 11: The Changing World of Work Will Affect Communication Strategies

Les Stanley, CEO of Barclays Bank, believes that the notion of putting his 7,000 employees in a building may be a thing of the past. Whether this is true or not, employee friendly communication digital tools and strategies need to be developed to optimise workplace flow in addition to providing for the speedy delivery of health and safety requirements as people increasing work outside of the office setting (White, 2020).

The increasing trend for remote working arrangements will challenge business leadership and safety professionals to develop useful, speedy and efficient health and safety digital tools to confront this new reality.

Case Study 12: Deployment of Information for Non-Resident Employees

A global fashion house in northern Italy shared reliable and immediate emergency information to employees in their headquarters and worldwide creating a dedicated channel in their employee app. "The employee app through thoughtful pre-planning was already in-place and provided an immediate pathway for two-way digital communication to the workforce" (Max Mara, 2020).

Case Study 13: Corporate Deployment of Information Applications (Apps) Increases Reach

A major international automaker working with its suppliers found the employee app particularly useful during the coronavirus crisis. "Under normal circumstances, the company sees about 100 employees per week register as new app users. As the coronavirus epidemic intensified, health personnel reported getting about 100 new users per hour. Later the company reported more than 1,500 new registered users in just two days. The reason? Employees demand official communications that are clear, reliable, fast and trustworthy" (Staffbase, 2020).

Digital tools (Fig. 1) are becoming mainstream

An additional challenge that businesses face is how to keep employees safe, even when one of them tests positive for COVID-19. Occupational health professionals can provide evidenced-based guidance as employers consider the possible use of mobile friendly digital apps for contact tracing and information outreach in the workplace. Traditional contact tracing involves a team of workers who talk to people on the phone or often face-to-face in business settings. This time-con-

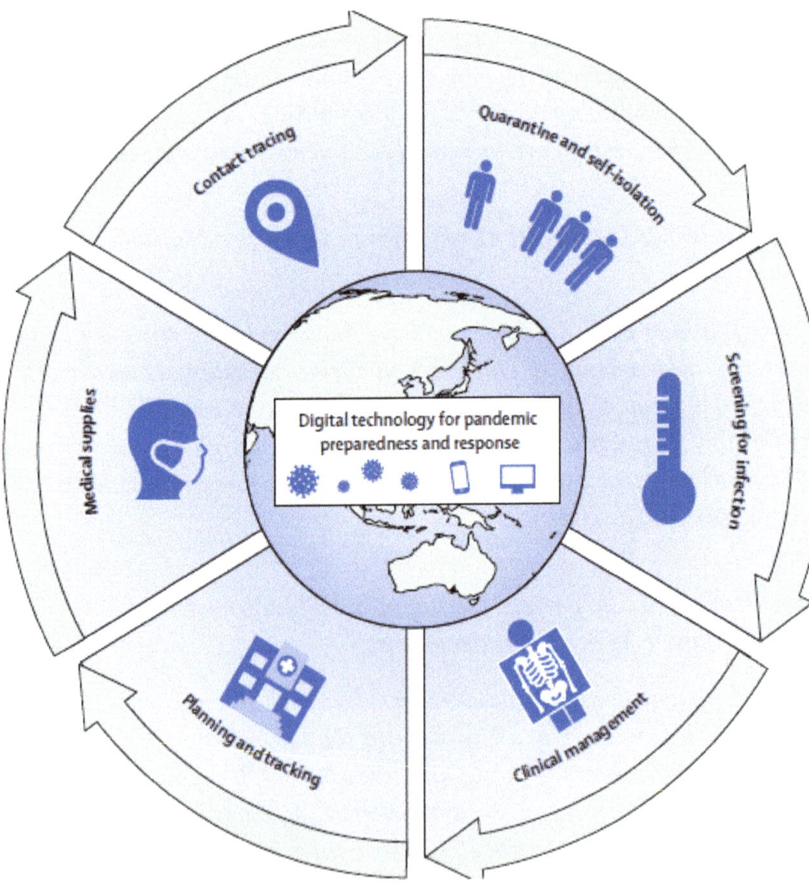

Fig. 1. Digital Technology as a Tool for Preparedness and Response (Whitelaw, 2020).

suming, methodical process for businesses in complex situations with multiple geographic locations can be onerous. Even in the best of situations the process can take days and weeks-too long to effectively respond to a biological hazard crisis. Mobile friendly apps offer the promise of exposure tracking and real-time information dissemination within a workplace setting utilising a geolocation feature that creates maps of impacted areas or otherwise only tracks contacts within a specified area. Other options are available. Occupational health professionals should be familiar with the range of health and safety apps. Because of their training and knowledge of the workplace and workers, occupational health professionals can suggest appropriate apps and recommend features such as a pro-active information alert system apps that employers may want to consider for their outreach initiatives to employees.

Case Study 14: Traditional Contact Tracing Methods are too Slow to be Effective

"Early in the pandemic, a British research group studying outbreaks in China and Singapore, and with a focus on prevention, compared the different routes of transmission, including from people with and without symptoms and concluded that traditional manual contact tracing was initially too slow to keep pace with the rapidly spreading COVID-19 *outbreaks" (Ferretti et al., 2020).*

Contact tracing apps show success

The success of contact tracing apps in Asian countries limiting virus exposure and workplace disruption provide evidence that employers where appropriate and with employee input should consider a range of digital applications. The key advantage is that the use of apps as part of a comprehensive two-way exposure notifications system is quicker and more efficient than traditional contact tracing manual investigations in identifying exposed individuals in the workplace.

Case Study 15: Contact Tracing is Impactful

"China and Singapore were consistently able to show a correlation between the roll-out of smart phone contact-tracing apps and the emergence of what appears to be an early sustained suppression of COVID-19 infection. Analyses showed that the same held true in Taiwan and South Korea where data collected using smart phone apps were used to recommend quarantine and provide essential safety information" (Collins, 2020).

Since country and business culture relates directly to citizen acceptance of risk communication outreach tools, information transfer must be transmitted in a form that makes individuals' acceptance compatible with core cultural beliefs. The understanding of the importance of country information culture is necessary to inform not only risk messaging but to gauge citizen acceptably of digital platforms necessary to deliver and receive risk messages. A governments overall commitment to the level of digital intrusion that its population can tolerate is key to understanding which digital platforms may be more acceptable in receiving and providing risk information.

Coming to terms with digital intrusion

If business leadership can come to terms with the use of digital communication techniques that mirror country public health tools as displayed in Table 1, a pathway for employee communication utilising apps may be possible (Table 2). A more voluntary approach while not technically ideal may be more realistic for western countries. A trade-off between personal privacy and economic disruption must be a driver of a sound digital communication approach.

Case Study 16: Reinforce Outreach Efforts with Additional Resources

Unlike in the UK, where early test and trace efforts were largely outsourced to private companies that proved unsuccessful, in Germany the effort relied on local public health services reinforced with redeployed civil servants, extra staff, additional resources and supported by state institutions (Joe, 2020).

Table 1. Applications of Digital Technology in Covid-19 Pandemic Planning and Response in Selected Countries (Howell *et al.*, 2020; Whitelaw *et al.*, 2020)

Location	Name	Voluntary	Limitation	Destroyed	Transparency
Australia	COVID SAFE	Yes	Yes	Yes	An issue
Notes	Privacy an issue. Adoption a concern.				
China	Health code	No	No	No	No
Notes	Little public information on the app. Highly invasive.				
Denmark	Smittestop	Yes	Yes	Yes	Yes
Notes	Useful but withdrawn- security issues.				
Germany	Corona-warn	Yes	Not known	Yes	Yes
Notes	Google/Apple app. Non-invasive but adoption level an issue of concern.				
Ireland	COVID tracker	Yes	Yes	Yes	Yes
Notes	Accuracy issues. Google/Apple app. Adoption level issues.				
Japan	COCOA	Yes	Not known	Yes	Yes
Notes	Many early problems. Withdrawn twice but later implemented.				
Malaysia	MyTrace	Yes	Not known	Not known	Not known
Notes	Android only. Data security concerns.				
Singapore	Trace Together	Yes	Yes	Yes	Yes
Notes	First Bluetooth tracing app. Appears successful.				
Vietnam	BlueZone	Yes	Not known	Not known	Yes
Notes	Access to photos, contacts other media. Invasive concerns.				
United Kingdom	NHS COVID-19	Yes	Yes	Yes	Yes
Notes	False start but a September launch. Google/Apple app.				
United States	No federal apps.	Not applicable	Not applicable	Not applicable	Not applicable
Notes	Some states (Virginia) have developed apps. Apple/Google app.				

Table 2. Key to Defining Terms (Howell *et al.*, 2020; Whitelaw *et al.*, 2020)

Terms	Definition
Limited	Are their limitations on how the data will be used?
Destroyed	Will data last forever or be destroyed at some point?
Minimised	Is data collected only for what is needed and for what the app is required to do?
Location Tracking	Some apps identify a person's contacts by tracking the phone's movements and looking for other phones that have spent time in the same area or near location and where appropriate linked to external third parties
Bluetooth	Some systems use tracking in which phones use proximate encrypted "chirps" with any other nearby phones. The approach is considered better for anonymity and privacy.
Google/ Apple	Google and Apple's apps will rely on this jointly developed free platform It allows iOS and Android phones to communicate with each other through a Bluetooth connection. Plans are being considered to build the system right into both phones' operating system.

Case Study 17: Digital and Traditional Outreach Tools must be Compatible

"As a part of a larger outreach control programme Ireland's national government developed an app which fits hand in glove with its manual tracing programme. The app widely supported by businesses safety personnel was credited according to government sources as equally if not more important in keeping the coronavirus at bay" (Joe, 2020).

Case Study 18: Involving the Business Community Enhances Quality and Support

The Republic of South Korea effectively involved the business community and their safety personnel early during the COVID-19 response planning stage. "Communications went out immediately to representatives of 20 major medically related companies who attended emergency planning meetings to assist government initiatives to develop an effective intervention strategy utilizing a contact tracing app" (Shaw and Kim, 2020).

The main problem with the use of contact tracing Apps

Using apps in a country as well as a business setting must be timely and achieve scale. In a corporate setting, if workers don't download the app to their mobile phones the systems are unable to gather enough data quickly enough to support effective digital tracing. Most researchers estimate that about 50–60 percent of new COVID-19 cases would need to be detected and traced to have a realistic chance of an effective response to the virus (Simmons-Duffin and Stein, 2020).

Tips for occupational health professionals on developing and implementing useful apps for trial in the workplace during biological health emergencies.

Surveillance and clinical management

Most of the more successful Asian countries and businesses relied on adopting digital technology and integrating the platforms into the countries emergency response policy. China, Taiwan, Japan, Singapore, South Korea, were able to quickly target the use of digital apps to develop essential administrative controls and provide and receive important population-based information. "In part their approach lies in applying best practices by health professionals from the outbreak of SARS experienced in their countries in 2002" (Kluth, 2020; Whitelaw, 2020).

Distancing and spacing

The use of apps that focused on safety and health distancing measures within the workplace were effective in providing tips for maintaining required distance between fellow employees and provided real-time feedback to assure a proper response. In addition, mobile apps allowed employers and employees to manage their shared office before returning to the office (Beekman, 2020).

Employer deployment of less invasive contact tracing apps

An Apple and Google joint venture has resulted in the development of a less invasive app which traces the contacts of those infected with COVID-19 but relies heavily on self-reporting. "Apple plans to maintain strong user privacy and will openly publish information about the app for others to analyze. Both Google and Apple also have said publicly that the technology will not track users' specific locations or reveal an infected users' identity" (Nicas and Wakabayashi, 2020). Google and Apple have teamed up to load software into billions of phones worldwide that will permit contact tracing on an opt-in basis (see Table 1 for examples of country adoption).

Assessing employee health status

Some apps are designed to help employers monitor and test the health status of their employees during the COVID-19 outbreak. While highly invasive this approach allows companies to monitor workforce health in real time and make necessary modification to accommodate workers and the enterprise (Zielinski, 2020).

Limiting direct contact with employees through telemedicine

Telemedicine and telehealth have emerged during the pandemic as a significant alternative for direct contact with clinicians, employees and patients thus limiting the potential exposure and spread of the virus. In addition, "the technology holds the promise to solve some of the most significant problems related to global healthcare systems, such as access to care, cost-effective delivery, and distribution of limited providers" (BIS Research, 2020).

Case Study 19: Telecommunication Provides an Increasingly Important Remote Communication Tool

"Sweden's KRY International, one of Europe's biggest telehealth providers reported that registrations were up more than 200 percent. France and Korea have both changed regulations to ease access to telemedicine" (Beekman, 2020)

Tips for occupational health professionals for improving the adoption of protective behaviours in the workplace

Fundamental to the adoption of safety and health measures is the need to understand human behaviours that deeply effect perceptions and the incentive to adopt helpful actions. Health professionals need to guide corporate leadership toward the use of health behaviour-based interventions. Increasingly, controlling a virus needs to address the behavioural science challenge. How can we get people to adopt unfamiliar behaviours to limit exposure and maintain their health and safety? The application of consistent and appropriate evidence-based messaging in the workplace is key to the success of any behavioural change strategy. Because of a deep understanding of the importance of science coupled with a rigorous understanding of workplace culture occupational safety and health professionals have an opportunity to encourage the design of messages that respond to their community's specific values and needs. A clearly proactive behavioural-based crisis messaging approach by its very nature illustrates a true concern for the wellbeing of employees (Brossard *et al.*, 2020).

Link existing business functions with health and safety

Case Study 20: Consider Linking Human Resources with Safety and Health Personnel

"A New York City based human resources company assisted by internal safety and health personnel developed app based digital communication templates for improving internal communication, sharing accurate safety and health information, and updating safety tips so that their employees remain safe and secure" (Staffbase, 2020).

Involve local public health authorities

Case Study 21: Linkage with Public Important External Health Networks

The Anthrax attack in 2011 in the United States (New Jersey) identified how pre-existing business and public health communication networks and political relationships increased trust of key business leaders and communicators during the crisis (Chess et al., 2007).

Provide real-time broad-based information tools that show immediate value

Case Study 22: An Employee App Already in Place Enhances Communication

A Brewery Group in Germany published regular health and safety postings on the homepage of its employee app. The focus was on preventive measures to protect workers and the production site, provide guidance on traveling safely, videos with hygiene tips and rules to follow concerning the employer information chain (Staffbase, 2020).

Mandate adoption

Some businesses following the culture of the country can effectively mandate adoption; others can strongly encourage it. Privacy protections may require alternate less invasive strategies. Forced measures will be difficult to implement in many countries where personal freedoms and privacy are paramount.

Case Study 23: Corporate Culture can Enhance Mandated Requirements

One of the largest banks in Italy, required all employees to use its corporate information and contact-tracing app focused on providing updated information to assist employees returning to their offices. "The app was automatically installed on company smartphones which initially covered over 40% of the employees and after evaluation was reported to be scaled up to the other 60%" (Staffbase, 2020).

Provide watchful oversight for evidenced-based health messages from government sources

Case Study 24: Assure Data and Data Systems are Properly Vetted

The premier public health agency in the US made early missteps in the rollout of its testing protocol. In addition, it encountered a major disconnect

between hospital record keeping systems and local health department reporting which resulted in message confusion delaying timely counts of COVID-19 infections and deaths. Public health agencies and those involved in data collection were quick to highlight needed changes to the policy and corrected the initial errors in messaging (Shear, 2020).

Provide an outreach tool for improving public engagement

It is critical to target specific essential workplaces for digital involvement. Identify those with high public contact such as airlines, restaurants, food stores, public transportation, and critical services and encourage or require employees and patrons to download the safety and distancing app before connecting with the business.

Case Study 25: High Public Contact Workers Need Special Tools

The BVG Berlin's major transport company with so many of its employees at risk interacting with the public updated its employee app with articles on hand washing techniques, how to avoid panic, advice on how to deal with public criticism, and authoritative information on health and safety from the German Institute responsible for disease control and prevention (Staffbase, 2020).

Start with small manageable initiatives

Health professionals should encourage businesses, organisations and communities to start with small initiatives. Launch strategy can benefit by thoughtful targeting rather than launching an app indiscriminately. Consider targeting a small part of the industry to test the app and review employee response to work out unexpected problems before expanding a larger corporate roll-out.

Case Study 26: Implementation of Ride-Share Apps can Serve as a Model

Small incremental roll-out approaches worked well for ride-sharing apps that began in a few selected cities as a trial and then expanded as success was achieved. This approach seems particularly relevant for large businesses that might consider testing in a defined geographic area or specific production facility.

Make the case for the "collective good" for fellow employees and colleagues

Key predictors of preventive behaviours often include worker confidence in business ability to provide protection and solace from worry and anxiety about one's close associates. Human behaviour points to the need, where appropriate, to invoke the "collective good" approach particularly for face mask protection and personal distancing.

Case Study 27: Be Proactive in Providing Regular Updates to Lower Worker Anxiety

"Workers who believe that their employer provides a safe and healthy workplace are more likely to report for work during a pandemic. Clear communication promotes confidence in the employer's ability to protect workers and reduces absenteeism" (Occupational Safety and Health Administration, 2020).

Be proactive and add a two-way communication function

Avoid the trap of one-way app communication strategy by adding a two-way information function so users can enter their concerns and where appropriate be guided on finding local medical help and testing facilities. Consider adding more information to the app on local contagion so users know their area risks. Perhaps add a PPE section with real-time purchasing information.

Case Study 28: Consider Tailored Digital Cross-County Boundary Tools

"One of the largest insurance groups in Europe operating in over 30 countries have been using the Employee Experience Intranet including an app news feed form for submitting questions, a directory of important contacts, hygiene tips, and a list of Frequently Asked Questions (FAQs)" (Staffbase, 2020).

Be innovative in the design and implementation of response strategies

While China created major impediments to information sharing among local, national and global authorities early on which severely limited an effective comprehensive response to COVID-19 it did move aggressively to build an innovative digital response for the country's administrative controls.

Case Study 29: Innovation Comes in Many Useful Forms

The Chinese government deployed robotic mail delivery in quarantined locations and built and required the downloading of an app to track daily temperatures, show overall health status using a QR code, deployed location tracking, and linked to an updated health portal with pandemic information. "The app had a unique invasive mapping feature that worked with WeChat messenger to display which communities and businesses have cases and their physical distance of employees and citizens from the exposure" (Shaw, 2020).

Make changing a behaviour rewarding and fun

For many cultures wearing a mask is not rewarding or fun. In the United States certain minority populations believe wearing a mask is out-right dangerous. When behaviours are rewarding and accepting, citizens are likely to repeat them often enough for a habit to form.

Case Study 30: Make Mask Wearing Interesting and Unique to the Audience

Decorating a mask with the logo of your favorite sports team or even your business (but not political slogans) may increase a positive commitment and habit.

Consider deployment of apps that can reward workers for positive behaviour

Consider rewarding people in the workplace for downloading an app by simply recognising their contribution. "In response to the pandemic, a mobility incentive platform has been released that enables companies and organisations to encourage and reward employees for sheltering in place and maintaining appropriate physical distancing including, encouraging employees to engage in safe and health habits that benefit themselves, their family, their team and community; ease the financial burden of being furloughed; provide telework and ensure that work from home team members are actually at home" (Stone, 2020).

Make sure messaging is easy to understand and contains understandable suggested actions and where appropriate an element of fun

Case Study 31: Health Behaviour Theory Can Inform Risk Messaging

Past research has supported the effectiveness of implementing a strategy for getting children at home and at school to wash their hands during flu season by distributing translucent bars of soap with a toy inside (Burns et al., 2018).

Tie a new behaviour to existing habits. Consider "habit stacking" as an appropriate strategy

Case Study 32: Consider A Way to Support Habit Stacking

"Habit stacking is a term to describe linking a new behaviour onto an existing habit, to take advantage of automaticity" (Ovenden, 2017). For example, keeping a protective mask in a convenient location perhaps in a sock drawer or near the car steering wheel can lead to automatic stacking of the behaviour in favor of adoption. "Start the car put on the mask."

Provide clear, specific descriptions of the behaviour to be adopted

Case Study 33: Language Structure and Words are Important

A sign saying, "wear a mask" when you are inside is a clearer direction than "if you're inside masks are required when you have extended

contact with people." Using a phrase like "personal distancing" has a clearer and more appropriate message then using the term "social distancing" (Gale, 2020). Generally, we don't want to encourage people to be distanced socially.

Use trusted messengers

Use the best messengers trusted most by employees to spread the word. Identifying trusted credible sources can spread health messages and prove to be especially effective. The effectiveness of such a strategy is well supported by research suggesting that the greatest effects of behaviour change comes not from direct effects on workers but from direct efforts on their social contacts who then copy the behaviour (Sanders, 2019).

Case Study 34: Search out Trusted Individuals for Messaging

During the West African Ebola crisis, for example, well respected and trusted religious leaders across faiths in Sierra Leone effectively advocated for such practices as regular hand washing and safe burials seen as a positive health and safety turning point in local communities (Manguvo and Mafuvadze, 2015).

Understanding digital media as a communication tool

Respected heath organisations use digital media

Globally WHO and other national health organisations took to social media early posting on YouTube, Spotify, Instagram, Facebook, Twitter and other social media platforms to spread the word about staying home, wearing-masks, personal distancing and hand washing. By its very nature social media platforms can be effective in communicating information in real time. As coronavirus infections surged globally, people turned to social media platforms to learn how to protect themselves from the emergent threat. Social media may be important during times of crisis, but the downside is evidenced in the extensive spread of COVID-19 misinformation through online social networks (Frenkel *et al.*, 2020).

The two conflicting faces of Twitter

On the positive side scientists and clinicians have used Twitter to disseminate scientific information to an academic audience and link with their professional networks. Health professionals should be aware that conflicts created by the Twitter algorithm has created two distinct Twitters in constant conflict with each other often cancelling out evidenced-based messaging. It is important to distinguish the non-academic context of Twitter in the COVID-19 era where the focus is often on public perception. Misleading information exacerbates health problems and increases the workload of health organisations who must exert resources to responding the false claims. Health professionals must be aware that there is significant variation of accuracy of information related to COVID-19 and exercise a high degree of caution in trusting posts from the non-academic networks.

Case Study 35: Non-Academic Supported Personal Tweets have Major Trust Issues

"A recent commentary published in the American Journal of Medicine reported that researchers analyzed 13,596 nonacademic tweets associated with COVID-19. They identified seven important misinformation categories of individuals attribution of COVID-19: (1) the influenza vaccine could lead to positive COVID-19 test results; (2)attributions of influenza deaths or cases to COVID-19; (3)prior influenza infections could cause positive COVID-19 tests; (4) influencers quoted the 'Flu shot leads to a positive COVID-19 test"; (5) 5G networks could be a link to COVID-19 cases or symptoms; (6) 5G is used to track individuals with a vaccine; and (7) specific activities or seasonal effects causing allergies may led to COVID-19 infection" (Krittanawong, 2020).

Case Study 36: Super-Spreaders of Misinformation Are Active

Researchers from the Queensland University of Technology found that celebrities are the major so-called "super-spreaders" of misinformation during the current COVID-19 crisis through use of their Twitter accounts (Shahi et al., 2020).

Case Study 37: Hold Your Breath Twitter Myth

This specious recommendation is how to take a simple coronavirus test: "Take a deep breath and hold your breath for 10 seconds…after you have held your breath for 10 seconds and you're not coughing, experiencing chest pains, tightness or any discomfort you probably are not infected with the coronavirus" (Landsverk, 2020).

Facebook can be useful but is overwhelmed with fact-checking

Facebook claims it is supporting the global public health community's work to keep people safe and informed during the coronavirus crisis and over 2 billion people have used the resources from health authorities through the COVID-19 Information Center and pop-ups on Facebook and Instagram (Avaaz, 2020). Nevertheless, health professionals must exercise a high degree of caution in using Facebook because its algorithm favours misinformation.

Case Study 38: Facebook is Losing the "Fact Check" Battle Against Misinformation

The COVID-19 Facebook Information Center has providing a gateway for millions of information seekers but conversely, a recent research report published by global activist group Avaaz in April 2020 (data collected up to May 27) states "that pages from the top 10 sites sharing misinformation and conspiracy theories about health received almost four times as many views on Facebook as the top 10 reputable sites for health information" (Avaaz, 2020). Examples of misinformation included harmful claims that you could stop the virus by using a hair dryer, taking a variety of drugs, eating specific foods and bogus theories like physical distancing being ineffective in preventing the disease from spreading.

Case Study 39: Over-Reporting Facebook Myth

A recent research analysis of Facebook posts noted that a single article that falsely claimed that the American Medical Association was encouraging doctors and hospitals to overestimate COVID-19 deaths, was seen over 160 million times (Avaaz, 2020).

Case Study 40: Quarantine Facebook Myth

"Two Emergency Medicine Doctors writing on Why Quarantine Just Doesn't Make Sense" contained multiple false claims to support the argument that quarantine harms public health. The post received 2.4 million views (Avaaz, 2020).

LinkedIn an overlooked digital resource with 30 million corporate members

When it comes to social media comparisons Instagram, YouTube, Facebook and Twitter get the attention. But LinkedIn is an ideal place for professionals to connect. LinkedIn is easily the most boring of the social networks. It's not fun filled entertainment or posts of snarky comments. "LinkedIn reports over 660 million users spread over 200 countries, (including China) as of late November 2019 representing 30 million companies" (Linkedin, 2020). Most importantly, a high majority of the LinkedIn profiles seem to be fully public and the platform hasn't experienced a great deal of turmoil. Having a LinkedIn profile may help disseminate information among its business membership and stimulate discussions about the best approaches to crisis management relatively free of harassment.

Case Study 41: Consider Linkedin as an Effective Outreach Social Media Tool

During COVID-19, with increased professional lives migrating online the LinkedIn platform has helped to drive increased professional engagement. According to recent data LinkedIn is seeing "record levels of engagement across the platform" and a 26% rise in sessions for the 3rd quarter of 2020 (Hutchinson, 2020).

Tips for handling social media misinformation and criticism (Reid, 2019)

Current standard advice is that it is critically important to reply to criticism given that social media criticism can spread around the globe instantly. The type of response given will have a significant impact on how the rest of the digital platform membership views and trusts the poster. We may appease the critic, relieve tension, or escalate things to become worse if we don't respond to criticism and misinformation appropriately.

Criticism comes in many forms, but online criticism tends to fall into just a few categories, such as disagreements and criticism; trolling; and bullying and threatening.

Suggested responses to social media posts

- Always be gracious. If a post provides a criticism make sure to thank them for the insights. Gracious response is a positive troll killer.
- Resist the urge to delete. Deleting a critical comment can damage you and your organisation. If a poster claims your data is incorrect or not supported, it is best to follow up with an explanation and possibly a link that provides the source of your information and acknowledges the concern.
- Admit, apologise, and make a simple useful suggestion if the criticisms leveled against you are accurate. People appreciate posters taking responsibility. Consider taking the conversation offline. It can be beneficial for others to see how you deal with criticism but drawing out the conversation in a public forum may give more visibility than necessary.
- Understand how to handle social media trolls. Interacting with trolls usually encourages them. If you are certain that a critical person is a troll best to provide an appropriate comment once, cite evidence and then disengage.

Understanding traditional media as a communication tool

Health professionals must exercise a high degree of caution with traditional news outlets. While television news is still one of the top outlets for both routine and crisis communication messaging the accuracy of information is the most important factor desired by the public. "Research has indicated that exposure to fake news on social media is rare compared to exposure to other types of media and news content, such as television news. In the United States to the extent that the public does consume news, it is overwhelmingly from television, which accounts for roughly five times as much as news consumption as online" (Allen *et al.*, 2020).

Case Study 42: Always Consider the Power of Traditional Media

When faced with the SARS outbreak in 2003 the Singapore Ministry of Health created a dedicated SARS television channel, which exclusively played updates and recordings of daily press conferences and received high praise for its efforts (Menon and Goh, 2005).

Case Study 43: Misconceptions Abound on Traditional Media

A recent American Academy of Science report suggests that the origins of public misinformation and polarisation are more likely to lie in the content of ordinary news or the avoidance of news altogether as they are in overt fakery (Allen, 2020). Correcting misconceptions about health through all forms of media involves timely expert advice, regular public health awareness, and alertness to the sources and their use of evidence-based information. Responding to criticism on social media requires special care.

Phase III Post-crisis Evaluation

Examine better ways to prepare for the next crisis and evaluate how well actions fulfilled commitments made during the crisis-response phase.

The findings of a post-crisis review of global COVID-19 response provides occupational health professionals an opportunity influence the development of the initial emergency response and mitigation plan of the enterprise and its communication outreach initiatives.

<u>What worked and what didn't?</u>
The post communication crisis evaluation phase for business organisations focuses on a detailed review of the level of success of the initial crisis communication goals and objectives with an aim to: (1) understand

what information strategies and initiatives accelerated or proved a barrier to the initial communication plan; and (2) what will be required to ensure the elimination of communication vulnerabilities that contributed to less effective communication outreach engagement. In this phase, communication evaluation approaches should engage a wide audience in a collaborative and interactive process toward understanding the expected outcomes of the communication plan and strategic initiatives (Seeger and Padgett, 2010).

Were health professionals actively involved?

A common request from occupational health professionals, is the desire for "a seat at the table." Occupational health training and practice provides a deeply science-based approach which can be extremely helpful in the post-evaluation phase assuring that ineffective crisis communication strategies during the pandemic are not repeated, and new lack-of-science vulnerabilities are not inadvertently created to generate a less resilient and robust response.

Key cross cutting challenges for post crisis evaluation that need to be addressed.

- Evaluating how well the pre-crisis crisis communication plan and initial goals were implemented and the effectiveness and extent of involvement of key external public health officials and stakeholders.
- Evaluating communication policies and strategies implemented during the crisis that hindered appropriate employer surveillance, administrative controls, worker behaviour, outreach techniques and the effectiveness of disease prevention and mitigation.
- Evaluating the balance between health communication messaging speed to the workforce, employer uncertainty and the necessary deliberations from internal or external sources.
- Evaluating how well planning and response strategies fostered employee engagement and used effective digital and/or traditional approaches to enhance the scope, speed and effectiveness of the outreach effort.

- What was the result of crisis communication objectives? Was risk communication training provided to managers, senior staff and business leadership? Was business leadership trained on how to manage remote workers to assure respect for workers privacy and work/life balance and to encourage the separation of employee work hours from home life?
- Were privacy and security guidelines developed with worker input to ensure clear understanding of the scope and limitation of digital technology strategies? Can benefit of technology against its risk be successfully demonstrated? What is the evidence?
- If contractors were employed in the workplace, were plans developed with their involvement? Were plans designed to communicate with contract employees directly about changes to work processes and requirements needed to protect their health and safety? Where appropriate, was communicating with the hard-to-reach SME workforce an integral and successful part of the communication plan?
- Did the enterprise manage the communication aspects or regular connections with important and/or required external partners and stakeholders?
- Did the health information have a strong evidence-base? Was it presented in clear and understandable language and did it provide a reasonable and culturally appropriate call to action? Did employers and employees acknowledge and agree to the use of the specific communication approaches provided? What is the evidence?
- Was the deployment of health and safety apps used? Was it successful? Was an appropriate level of scale reached quickly? Was data stored within encrypted platforms? Was data automatically deleted within a given time frame?

The application of digital applications and data collection needs specific attention

The use of invasive digital technology raises important policy questions about data control and how privacy is protected. The effective use of technology particularly apps requires a clear acceptance of the necessity of the adoption of technology by the workforce — whether required or strongly encouraged. How effective has been the planning for digital security? For western democracies agreement on a responsible trade-off between personal privacy and public safety is essential. To be optimistic concerning privacy in the digital age we need joint social, legal and technical aspects in place to manage and assure a better cyberspace (Ran, 2016).

Case Study 44: Global Collaboration for Developing an Effective App

WHO's Digital Health Technical Advisory Group is working with the United States Centers for Disease Control and Prevention, foundations, and various national governments to develop less invasive communication tools that have worked well in some countries. "CoEpi short for Community Epidemiology in Action, has focused on a 'privacy-first' system using an anonymous Bluetooth-based contact tracing smartphone app that provides anonymous and inaudible 'chirps' that will alert other users if they may have been exposed to someone with the virus" (CoEpi, 2020).

Conclusion

This chapter summarises the call for an expanded role for occupational health professionals in the development, implementation and evaluation of emergency response crisis communication plans and their implementation. The COVID-19 global response shows a clear need for the input of health professionals trained in evidenced-based science and an understanding of the limits and promise of the changing nature of the workplace.

References

Allen J, Howland B, Mobius M, Rothschild D, Watts DJ. (2020) Evaluating the fake news problem at the scale of the information ecosystem. *Sci Adv* [Online] 6(14). Available from: doi: 10.1126/sciadv.aay3539. [Accessed on 14 March 2020].

American Red Cross, Federal Emergency Management Agency. (2004) *Preparing for Disaster for People with Disability and Other Special Needs.*

[Online] Available from: https://www.redcross.org/content/dam/redcross/atg/PDF_s/Preparedness___Disaster_Recovery/General_Preparedness___Recovery/Home/A4497.pdf. [Accessed on 12 June 2020].

Avaaz. (2020) *Facebook's Algorithm: A Major Threat to Public Health.* [Online] Available from: https://secure.avaaz.org/campaign/en/facebook_threat_health. [Accessed on 14 March 2020].

Beekman J. (2020) *Telehealth Services are Gaining Attention During the COVID-19 Outbreak.* [Online] Available from: https://iotmktg.com/telehealth-services-are-gaining-attention-during-covid-19-outbreak. [Accessed on 14 March 2021].

BIS Research. (2020) *Spread of COVID 19 Has Pushed the Global Telemedicine Market to the Forefront.* [Online] Available from: https://blog.marketresearch.com/spread-of-covid-19-has-pushed-global-telemedicine-market-to-the-forefront. [Accessed on 4 August 2020].

Brossard D, Wood W, Cialdini R, Groves RM. (2020) Encouraging adoption of protective behaviours to mitigate the spread of COVID-19, strategies for behaviour change. *Nation Acad Sci Eng Med.* Available from https://doi.org/10.17226/25881.

Bump P. (2020) *210,000 Deaths Later, Trump Reverts to Comparing the Coronavirus to the Flu.* [Online] Available from: https://www.washingtonpost.com/politics/2020/10/06/210000-deaths-later-trump-reverts-comparing-coronavirus-flu/. [Accessed on 4 November 2020].

Burns J, Maughan-Brown B, Mouzinho A. (2018) Washing with hope: Evidence of improved handwashing among children in South Africa for a pilot study of a novel soap technology. *BMC Public Health* [Online] **18**(1). Available from: https://bmcpublichealth.biomedcentral.com/articles/10.1186/s12889-018-5573-8.

CDC. (2018) *Crisis and emergency risk communication (CERC).* [Online] Available from: https://www.emergency.cdc.gov/cerc. [Accessed on 14 March 2021].

CDC. (2020a) *United States National Center for Immunization and Respiratory Disease.* [Online] Available from: https://www.cdc.gov/ncird/index.html. [Accessed on 8 August 2020].

CDC. (2020b) *Morbidity and Mortality Weekly Report May–August 2020.* [Online] Available from: https://www.cdc.gov/mmwr/index.html. [Accessed on 8 August 2020].

Chess C, Clarke L. (2007) Facilitation of risk communication during the Anthrax attacks of 2001: The organizational backstory. *Am J Public Health* [Online] **97**(9): 1578–1583. Available from: 10.2105/AJPH.2006.099267.

CoEpi. (2020) *Community Epidemiology in Action.* [Online] Available from: https://www.coepi.org. [Accessed on 14 March 2021].

Collins F. (2020) *Can Smart Phone Apps Help Beat Pandemics.* [Online] Available from: https://directorsblog.nih.gov/2020/04/09/can-smart-phone-apps-help-beat-pandemics. [Accessed on 12 April 2020].

Coombs WT. (2012) *On Going Crisis Communication: Planning, Managing and Responding* (3rd Ed). Thousand Oaks, California, Sage.

Daly E, Das K, Yeah R. (2020) *Reimagining Emerging ASEAN in the Wake of COVID-19.* [Online] Available from: https://www.mckinsey.com/featured-insights/asia-pacific/reimagining-emerging-asean-in-the-wake-of-covid-19. [Accessed on 14 March 2021].

Deloitt. (2020) *Addressing the Impact of COVID-19. 'How Deloitte Can Support You.* [Online] Available from: https://www2.deloitte.com/an/en/footerlinks/pressreleasespage/ddc-pressrelease-COVID19-DeloitteSupport.html. [Accessed on 14 March 2021].

Gale R. (2020) *Is Social Distancing the Wrong Term? Expert Prefers "Physical Distancing" and the WHO Agrees.* [Online] Available from: https://www.washingtonpost.com/lifestyle/wellness/social-distancing-coronavirus-physical-distancing/2020/03/25/a4d4b8bc-6ecf-11ea-aa80-c2470c6b2034_story.html. [Accessed on 14 March 2020].

Heath R. (2015) Crisis Communication: Defining the beast and de-marginalizing key publics. In: Coombs, W, Holladay, S. (eds.), *The Handbook of Crisis Communication.* Malden, Massachusetts, Wiley Blackwell.

Farley R. (2020) *Trump has not been Clear in Support of Masks', Fact Check 25 September.* [Online] Available from: https://www.factcheck.org/2020/09/trump-has-not-been-clear-in-support-of-masks. [Accessed on 30 September 2020].

Ferretti L, Wymant C, Kendall M, Zhao L, Nurtay A, Abeler-Dörner L, Parker M, Bonsall D, Fraser C. (2020) Quantifying SARS-CoV-2 transmission suggests epidemic control with digital contact tracing. *Science* **368**(6491). Available from: doi: 10.1126/science.abb6936.

Frenkel S, Alba D, Zhong R. (2020) *Surge of Virus Misinformation Stumps Facebook and Twitter.* [Online] Available from: https://www.nytimes.

com/2020/03/08/technology/coronavirus-misinformation-social-media.html. [Accessed on 21 March 2021].

Holger J, Akl EA, Chou R, Chu DK, Loeb M, Lotfi T. (2020) Use of face-masks during the COVID-19 pandemic. *Lancet* **8**(10): 954–955. Available from: doi.org/10.1016/S2213-2600(20)30352-0. [Accessed on 14 March 2021].

Howell OP, Tate R, Johnson B. (2020) *A Flood of Coronavirus Apps are Tracking us. Now it's Time to Keep Track of Them.* [Online] Available from: https://www.technologyreview.com/2020/05/07/1000961/launching-mittr-covid-tracing-tracker. [Accessed on 7 August 2020].

Hutchnson A. (2020) *LinkedIn's up to 690 Million Members, Reports 26% Growth in User Sessions.* [Online] Available from: https://www.soialmediatoday.com. [Accessed on 24 April 2020].

Joe C. (2020) *Is a Successful Contact Tracing App Possible? These Countries Think so.* [Online] Available from: https://www.technologyreview.com. [Accessed on 13 August].

Kitroeff N. (2020) *Between the Pandemic and the President: Mexico City Mayor's Balancing Act.* [Online] Available from: https://www.nytimes.com/2020/09/05/world/americas/mexico-mayor-amlo-sheinbaum.html. [Accessed on 7 April 2020].

Kluth A. (2020) *If we Must Build a Surveillance State Let's do it Properly.* [Online] Available from: https://www.bloomberg.com/opinion/articles/2020-04-22/taiwan-offers-the-best-model-for-coronavirus-data-tracking. [Accessed on 30 April 2020].

Krittanawong C, Narasimhan B, Virk HUH, Hahn J, Wang Z, Tang WHW. (2020) Misinformation dissemination in Twitter in the COVID-19 era. *Am J Med* [Online] **133**(12): 1367–1369. Available from: https://doi.org/10.1016/j.amjmed.2020.07.012. [Accessed on 13 August 2020].

Landsverk G. (2020) *Holding Your Breath Can't Help You Self-diagnose the Coronavirus. Here's What You Should Do Instead.* [Online] Available from: https://www.businessinsider.com/holding-breath-10-seconds-drinking-water-wont-cure-diagnose-coronavirus-2020-3. [Accessed on 19 April 2020].

Linkedin. (2020) *50+ Users' Statistics for 2020.* [Online] Available from: https://www.foundationinc.co/lab/b2b-marketing-linkedin-stats/. [Accessed on 14 March 2021].

Manguvo A, Mafuvadze B. (2015) The impact of traditional and religious practices on the spread of Ebola in West Africa: Time for a strategic shift.

Pan Afr Med J [Online] **22**(Suppl 1)(9). Available from: doi: 10.11694/pamj.supp.2015.22.1.6190. [Accessed on 14 March 2021].
Max Mara. (2020) *Coronavirus News Update', Dedicated Coronavirus News Feed.* [Online] Available from: https://www.maxmarafashiongroup.com. [Accessed on 2 March 2020].
McKinsey & Company. (2020) *Safeguarding Lives and Livelihoods, Cultivating Resilience in Crisis.* [Online] Available from: https://www.mckinsey.com. [Accessed on 14 March 2021].
Menon KU, Goh KT. (2005) Transparency and trust: Risk communications and the Singapore experience in managing SARS. *J Commun Manag* [Online] **9**(4): 375–383. Available from: doi: 10.1108/13632540510621614.
Nicas J, Wakabayashi D. (2020) *Apple and Google Team Up to Contact Trace the Coronavirus.* [Online] Available from: https://www.nytimes.com/2020/04/10/technology/apple-google-coronavirus-contact-tracing.html. [Accessed on 21 April 2020].
Occupational Safety and Health Administration. (2020) *Fact Sheet. Protecting Workers During a Pandemic.* [Online] Available from: https://www.osha.gov. [Accessed on 14 March 2020].
Ovenden O. (2017) *Habit Stacking: How to Train Your Brain with Routine.* [Online] Available from: https://www.esquire.com/uk/life/fitness-wellbeing/a15489/habit-stacking-chaining/. [Accessed on 28 June 2020].
Palenchar M. (2008) Risk communication and community right to know: A public relations obligation to Inform. *Public Relat J* **2**(1): 1–26.
Palenchar M. (2010) Historical trends of risk communication. In: Heath, R, O'Hair, D. (eds.), *The handbook of crisis and risk communication.* Routledge, New York.
Ran J. (2016) *Striking the Balance Between Privacy and Governance in the Age of Technology.* [Online] Available from: https://repository.upenn.edu/cgi/viewcontent.cgi?article=1054&context=spice. [Accessed on 12 April 2020].
Reid C. (2019) *7 Tips for Handling Social Media Criticism.* [Online] Available from: https://www.jotform.com/blog/handling-social-media-criticism/. [Accessed on 14 March 2021]
Sanders R. (2019) *Everything is Connected. Nothing is Trusted the Critical Trust Gap.* [Online] Available from: https://www.keyfactor.com/critical-trust. [Accessed on 14 March 2021].
Sandman P. (2020) *Commentary: Public Health Share of the Blame: US COVID-19 Risk Communication Failures.* [Online] Available from: www.cidrap.umm.edu.8/24/2020. [Accessed on 14 March 2021].

Schoch-Spana M, Hurtado C, Meyer D, Moore-Sheeley K, Ravi S, Snyder M. (2019) *Risk communication strategies for the very worst cases.* John Hopkins School of Public Health, Center for Health Security. [Online] Available from: https://www.centerforhealthsecurity.org/our-work/pubs_archive/pubs-pdfs/2019/190304-Risk-Comm-Strategies.pdf. [Accessed on 14 March 2021].

Seeger MW, Padgett DRG. (2010) From image restoration to renewal: Approaches to understanding post crisis communication. *Rev Commun* **10**(2): 127–141. Available from doi.org/10.1080/15358590903545263.

Shahi GK, Dirkson A, Majchrzak TA. (2020) An exploratory study of COVID-19 misinformation on Twitter. *ArXiV.* [Online] Available from: https://arxiv.org/pdf/2005.05710.pdf. [Accessed on 6 June 2020].

Shaw R, Kim YK. (2020) Governance, technology and citizen behaviour in pandemic: Lessons from COVID-19 in East Asia. *Progress in Disaster Science.* [Online] Available from: 10.1016/j.pdisas.2020.100090. [Accessed on 6 April 2020].

Shear M. (2020) *They let us down: 5 takeaways on the CDC Coronavirus response.* [Online] Available from: https://www.nytimes.com/2020/06/03/us/cdc-virus-takeaways.html. [Accessed on 15 July 2020].

Simmons-Duffin S, Stein R. (2020) *CDC Director: 'Very Aggressive' Contact Tracing Needed for U.S. to Return to Normal.* [Online] Available from: https://www.wbur.org/npr/831200054/cdc-director-very-aggressive-contact-tracing-needed-for-u-s-to-return-to-normal. [Accessed on 14 March 2021].

Smarp. (2020) *Crisis Communication: Definition, Importance and Best Practices.* [Online] Available from: https://blog.smarp.com/crisis-communication-definition-importance-best-bractices. [Accessed on 3 March 2020]

Staffbase. (2020) *8 Examples of Effective Crisis Communication.* [Online] Available from: https://www.aamc.org/news-insights/address-covid-19-and-future-pandemics-we-must-answer-fundamental. [Accessed on 6 March 2020].

Statistica. (2020) *Number of Novel Coronavirus (COVID-19) Deaths of Selected Countries in the Asia Pacific Region as of October 27, 2020.* [Online] Available from: https://www.statista.com/statistics/1104268/apac-covid-19-deaths-by-country. [Accessed on 14 March 2021].

Stevis-Gridneff M, Apuzzo M, Proncuk M. (2020) *When COVID-19 hit, many elderly were left to die.* [Online] Available from: https://www.

nytimes.com/2020/08/08/world/europe/coronavirus-nursing-homes-elderly.html. [Accessed on 8 August 2020].

Stone T. (2020) *US Smart Mobility App Offers Cash Awards to Users Who Stay at Home During COVID-19 Pandemic.* [Online] Available from: https://www.traffictechnologytoday.com/news/multimodal-systems/us-smart-mobility-app-offers-cash-rewards-to-users-who-stay-at-home-during-covid-19-pandemic.html. [Accessed on 14 March 2021].

Walsh D. (2020) *Coronavirus: Belgium Death Toll Passes 10,000, UK Breaks New Daily Cases Record.* [Online] Available from: https://www.euronews.com/2020/09/30/coronavirus-belgium-death-toll-passes-10-000-uk-breaks-new-daily-cases-record. [Accessed on 14 March 2021].

White L. (2020) *The Changing Face of Work.* [Online] Available from https://www.reuters.com/news/picture/how-covid-is-changing-the-way-we-work-idUSRTX7XPL8. [Accessed on 14 March 2021].

Whitelaw S, Mamas AM, Topol E, Van Spall H. (2020) Applications of digital technology in COVID-19 pandemic planning and response. *Lancet Digital Health* **2**(8): 435–440. Available from: https://doi.org/10.1016/S2589-7500(20)30142-4.

WHO. (2017a) *Communicating Risk in Public Health Emergencies. A WHO Guideline for Emergency Risk Communication (ERC) Policy and Practice.* [Online] Available from: https://www.ncbi.nlm.nih.gov/books/NBK540729. [Accessed on 14 March 2021].

WHO. (2020) Joint statement by WHO, UN, UNICEF, UNDP, UNESCO, UNAIDS, ITU, UN Global Pulse, and IFRC. https://www.who.int/news/item/23-09-2020-managing-the-covid-19-infodemic-promoting-healthy-behaviours-and-mitigating-the-harm-from-misinformation-and-disinformation.

Zielinski D. (2020). *New Apps Address Employers' COVID-19 Challenges.* [Online] Available from: https://www.shrm.org/resourcesandtools/hr-topics/technology/pages/new-apps-address-employers-covid19-challenges.aspx. [Accessed on 14 March 2021].

Chapter 31

Prevention of Occupational Diseases

David Koh and Wee Hoe Gan†*

Introduction

The International Labour Organization (ILO) estimates that 2.34 million people die from work-related accidents and diseases annually. The vast majority, approximately 2.02 million, succumb to a wide range of work-related diseases, as opposed to accidents or injuries. In addition, the ILO further estimates that 160 million cases of non-fatal work-related diseases occur every year (International Labour Organization, 2013). Worldwide, it is estimated that workplace hazards account for at least 2.1% of all deaths and 2.7% of all DALYs (Wolf *et al.*, 2018). Prevention of these risks would reduce the global burden of disease, especially in the productive and economically active working population.

Occupational and work related diseases are caused or aggravated by excessive exposure to specific chemical, physical, biological or psy-

* PAPRSB Institute of Health Sciences, Universiti Brunei Darussalam, Brunei Darussalam *and* Saw Swee Hock School of Public Health and Yong Loo Lin School of Medicine, National University of Singapore, Singapore.
† Department of Occupational and Environmental Medicine, Singapore General Hospital; Changi Aviation Medicine Centre, Changi General Hospital; and Duke-NUS Medical School, National University of Singapore, Singapore.
Corresponding author: David Koh (david.koh@ubd.edu.bn and ephkohd@nus.edu.sg).

chosocial agents at the workplace. The causes of these diseases are known, and as such, they are eminently suited for prevention. The aim of preventive medicine is to stop the occurrence of disease in the individual or a specific population group. This is usually achieved by attempts to reduce the risk of contracting a disease. If this is not possible, then activities should be targeted at early detection of disease, in order to halt disease progression. This should ideally occur before the disease is irreversible.

Levels of Prevention

Primary prevention reduces the occurrence of disease by eliminating or reducing exposure to the causal agent. For example, the prevention of noise induced hearing loss could be through elimination of the source of noise, or the use of hearing protectors.

Secondary prevention detects early effects of harmful exposure, or subclinical disease. Examples are the monitoring of blood lead (BPb) levels among lead exposed workers; or conducting periodic audiograms among workers working in noisy environments. If early effects are detected, corrective action is introduced to the work environment, while the worker is temporarily removed from further exposure. In many instances, the early health effects are reversible, and the worker can then be returned to a safer work environment.

Tertiary prevention aims to minimise adverse consequences in persons who already have disease. This activity is largely a curative and rehabilitative process. Primary and secondary prevention will be the focus of this chapter.

Health Promotion

Occupational health services should provide total health care to the working population. In view of the two-way relationship between WORK and DISEASE, it is widely accepted that a more holistic approach to occupational health is appropriate. Such an approach allows for the use of the workplace as the focal point for general health promotion and disease prevention activities.

Health promotion activities for employees at their workplaces have the following advantages — convenient location, a readily available target group, peer pressure to conform to healthy lifestyle, workers accustomed to receiving and following health and safety advice from health workers, and facilities available for incorporation of healthy lifestyle practices, e.g. provision of healthy choices of food at the canteen. Besides an improvement in health, there may also be additional benefits of health promotion programmes at work. These include potential reduction in health care costs, decrease in sickness absenteeism, increase in job performance, decrease in work-related injuries and reduced employee turnover.

Total worker health (TWH) programmes aim to advance worker well-being by integrating injury and illness prevention efforts with reduction of work-related safety and health hazards. To date, evidence suggests that while integrated TWH interventions might improve health behaviours such as reducing tobacco use, encouraging exercise and physical activity, and improving diet, the effects of these interventions on injuries and overall quality of life are largely unknown (Feltner *et al.*, 2016).

Prevention of Work-Related Diseases

The World Health Organization has identified the following important diseases as being work-related — behavioural and psychosomatic illness, hypertension, ischaemic heart disease, chronic non-specific respiratory disease and musculoskeletal disorders.

Work-related diseases have multiple causes which may include several workplace factors and non-work factors. The work-relatedness of these diseases could be due to partial occupational aetiology or through exacerbation of ill-health by adverse workplace exposures.

Case Study 1: Death from Isocyanate Exposure

Mr. L was a 52-year-old furniture factory manager who died of an acute asthmatic attack after being exposed to diisocyanate vapour. He had a past history of asthma which was poorly controlled in the past few months, requiring several instances of emergency treatment at the family clinic. Many of his asthmatic attacks had been provoked by exposure to diisocyanate fumes from spray-painting work at his factory.

Case Study 2: Musculoskeletal Disorder Caused by Poor Work Posture

Mr. T, aged 30-years, worked as a technical officer in a semiconductor manufacturing company. He suffered from worsening neck and shoulder pain which was only temporarily relieved by analgesics. In his job, he had to clean the spin-coater several times a day (Fig. 1). The machine, which is used to deposit uniform thin films to flat substrates, was placed on a low bench, requiring him to work with his neck flexed for prolonged periods.

The workplace and non-occupational factors associated with the WHO list of important work-related diseases are shown in Table 1. In order to prevent work-related diseases, the associated workplace risk factors should be minimised to safe levels. In addition, it is not only necessary to reduce workplace factors contributing to disease but also to identify and control the known non-occupational risk factors for disease.

A rapidly expanding area of work-related activity is frequent travel and commuting. Road travel has associated risks of road traffic incidents and injury, some of which are related to the driving skills of other

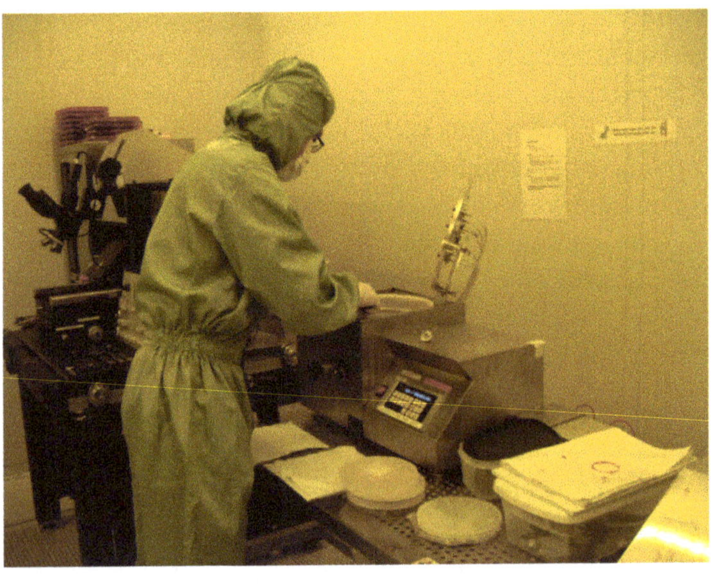

Fig. 1. Mr. T. operating the spin coater at his work bench.

Table 1. Selected Work-related Diseases, Workplace Factors, Non-occupational Risk Factors and their Control

Disease	Adverse Workplace Factors	Risk Factors and Control
Behavioural and psychosomatic illness	Stress caused by: • Work overload • Work underload • Shift work • Career development • Migration/travel • Role conflict • Role ambiguity	Type A behaviour, reduction of organisational stress
Hypertension	Stress	Stress relief; screening, diet and weight control
Ischaemic heart disease	Stress, workplace exposures, e.g. CS_2, CO	Stress relief; screening for risk factors and intervention
Chronic nonspecific respiratory disease	Dusts and irritants	Smoking cessation, control of dusts and irritants
Musculoskeletal disorders	Ergonomic factors; weight bearing, trauma, whole body vibration, poor work posture	Ergonomic design, healthy back programme

drivers and behaviour of other road users. For the business traveler or expatriate worker, travel-related illness such as infections and sleep disorders from jet lag are common and can contribute to poor performance and sickness absence. Thus, preventive activities would include immunisations, giving advice on how to avoid travel-related risks as well as general advice on management of jet lag and food hygiene.

For air crew who operate long haul flights, fatigue and performance may raise concerns of flight safety. Several measures can be taken to minimise fatigue and improve performance.

Case Study 3: Fatigue Among Air Crew Operating Long Haul Flights

Fatigue, sleepiness and impaired performance are safety issues for air crew operating long haul flights of 14 hours of more. Several ways to address these issues include regulations for flight time limits, having augmented crews, i.e. extra air crew members on flights, provision of purpose built sleeping berths on board the aircraft and scheduling of departure times to optimally coincide with circadian rhythms. Assessments of the flight sector should be conducted for the risk of delays in order to plan for extended flight times. In terms of rostering, advance notice of the flight should be given to allow air crew to prepare themselves with adequate sleep before the flight. An extended layover period may be considered, as well as adequate recovery time given after the return flight before the next long-haul flight. Such crew should also be monitored for possible long-term effects of these extended flights on sleep, performance and health.

Prevention of Occupational Diseases

The types of occupational diseases seen today have evolved. This is due to technological, economic and social changes — which may worsen existing health hazards and create new ones. Traditional occupational diseases, such as pneumoconiosis and noise induced hearing loss, remain widespread. On the other hand, relatively new occupational diseases, such as mental health and musculoskeletal disorders, are increasing in prevalence.

There is great scope for the prevention of occupational illnesses, as the causal agents are known and exposure can often be controlled and maintained at safe levels. The occurrence of occupational disease must be viewed as a failure of prevention.

Case Study 4: Fibreglass Dermatitis from Printed Circuit Boards

Two production lines in an electronics factory that assembled printed circuit boards (PrCB) were shut down because all the workers complained of itch of the hands and fingers. Workers noted that the problem started when a new "dusty" PrCB was used. Examination of the workers revealed only excoriation marks. Skin stripping with adhesive tape after the workers washed their hands showed fibreglass spicules in the epidermis (Fig. 2). Samples of the PrCBs from the production line and two

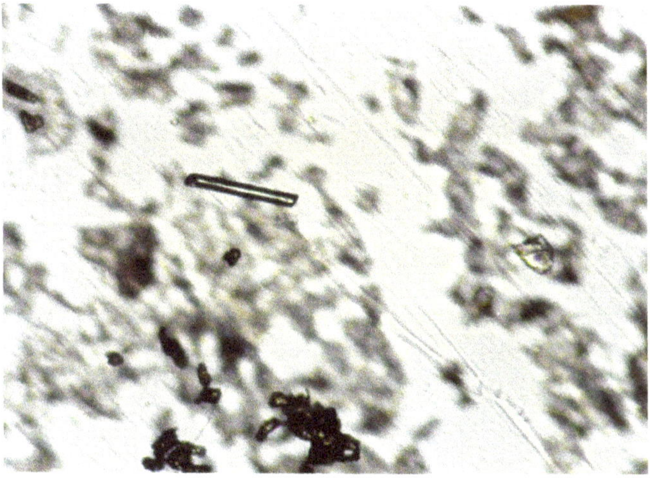

Fig. 2. Skin stripping of worker, showing fibreglass.

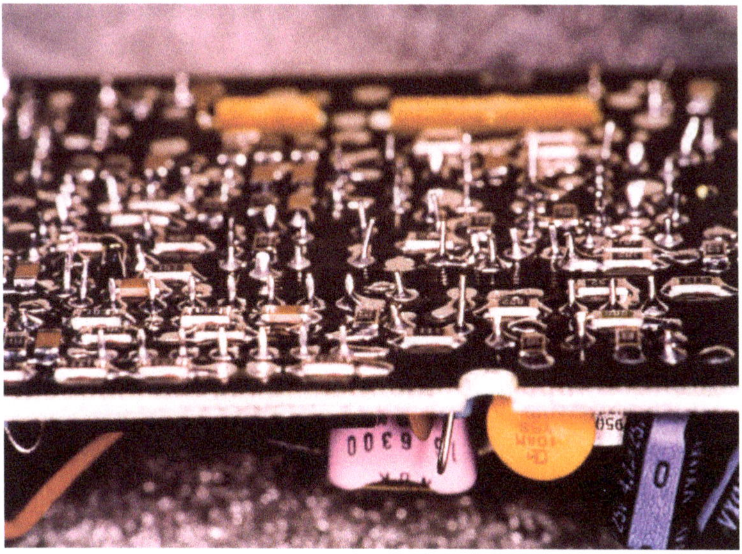

Fig. 3. Fibreglass can be found at the free edge of the printed circuit board.

other unaffected lines were examined. The samples from the problem line showed substantial amounts of free fibreglass from the edge of the PrCB (Fig. 3). The diagnosis was fibreglass itch from PrCBs. The problem was resolved by requesting workers to apply powder, wear cotton gloves, and to wash their hands during breaks. At the same time, other measures were taken. These included the use of sharper cutting tools to minimise free fibreglass at the edge of the PrCBs, and vacuuming of the free edges before the PrCBs were sent to the assembly lines. Plans were also made to inform the supplier to produce PrCBs with less freely dislodged fibreglass.

Case Study 5: Minimising Solvent Exposure

A group of display artists working in a retail store complained of tiredness, loss of concentration, exhaustion and difficulty in sleeping. They worked with solvent-based paints to prepare the sales displays in a fairly confined space.

The artists were young, fit and had no previous health problems. Clinical examination by the company doctor did not reveal any remarkable findings. Liver function tests were performed and liver transaminase enzymes were raised. Common causes of hepatic damage, e.g. viral hepatitis, alcohol ingestion, were excluded. Workers with more severe symptoms were sent for neurophysiological assessment, with inconclusive results. It was not possible to ascertain the exact chemical constituents of the solvent from the suppliers to determine hepatotoxicity.

In spite of the lack of a definitive diagnosis, the management was advised of the risk of solvent exposure, and work in the confined area was stopped. The potential hazard was communicated to the staff concerned through several dialogue sessions. Staff were also briefed on the control measures to be taken while working with the solvents. Subsequently, a management decision was taken to reduce solvent use in decorative work. All solvent spray work was relocated to another part of the workplace, which had proper ventilation and exhaust fans. Workers undertaking work using solvents were provided masks, gloves, and other personal protective equipment, and worked for shortened periods at these operations. Following these changes, all the workers recovered uneventfully.

Primary Prevention of Occupational Diseases

Primary prevention refers to efforts to reduce the occurrence of occupational disease by eliminating the cause or preventing harmful exposure to the agent.

Control of New Hazards

Animal toxicity studies of chemicals to be used in industry are a reasonable predictor of potential health hazards to humans. On the basis of such studies, the legislation in manufacturing nations would control the usage of such chemicals in industrial processes. One limitation is that the legislation for such controls in many countries apply only to new chemicals which are to be introduced into the market. For instance, it is estimated that only 10% of pesticides in current use have undergone such toxicological evaluation. In addition, animal toxicity studies often do not provide adequate information on long term human health effects, such as the potential for cancer causation.

Control of Known Hazards

Several countries have legislation to ban the use of substances known to be harmful to human health. Since 1991 the United Nations has compiled and regularly updated a "Consolidated List of Products — whose consumption and/or sale have been banned or severely restricted by governments". This publication is a tool which helps governments to keep up-to-date with regulatory decisions taken by other governments and assists them in considering the scope for eventual regulatory action.

In 1989, the United Nations Environment Program (UNEP) developed a mechanism for Prior Informed Consent (PIC) to inform governments of banned agents so that these governments can take appropriate action for their control. The Rotterdam Convention on the Prior Informed Consent Procedure for Certain Hazardous Chemicals in International Trade came into force on 24 February 2004. The objective of this Convention is to "promote shared responsibility and cooperative efforts among Parties in the international trade of certain hazardous chemicals in order to protect human health and the environment from potential harm and to contribute to their environmentally sound use, by facilitating information exchange about their characteristics, by providing for a national decision-making process on their import and export and by disseminating these decisions to Parties" (United Nations Environment Programme Rotterdam Convention, 2020).

As an example, in the European Union (EU), the PIC Regulation (PIC, Regulation (EU) 649/2012) apply to the import and export of certain hazardous chemicals and imposes obligations on companies that wish to export these chemicals to non-EU countries. The regulation applies to various banned or severely restricted chemicals such as industrial chemicals, pesticides and biocides, e.g. benzene, chloroform, atrazine and permethrin. Export of these chemicals is subject to export notification and explicit consent (European Chemicals Agency, 2020).

Monitoring of Workplace Exposures (Box 1)

Box 1. Monitoring of Workplace Exposures.

Ambient Environment ← Environmental Monitoring → Permissible Environmental Level (e.g. TLV)

Internal Monitoring ← Biological Exposure → Permissible Biological Dose (e.g. BEI)

Environmental Monitoring

Environmental or ambient air monitoring is undertaken to measure external exposure to harmful agents. This is to ensure that environmental levels are kept within permissible levels so as to prevent the agent from causing disease. The concept of permissible levels assumes that for each substance, there is a level of exposure at or below which the exposed worker is unlikely to suffer any health impairment.

There are limitations when permissible levels of exposure are applied. Such levels are based on current understanding of health effects which may not be complete (especially for long term effects such as carcinogenesis and reproductive system effects). Previously unsuspected health risks have arisen from substances assumed to be comparatively safe, e.g. glycol ethers in the electronics industry and abortions. As such, every effort must be made to keep exposure levels as low as possible.

The determination of permissible levels is based on several considerations, such as the physical and chemical properties of substance (including nature and amount of impurities), toxicological studies (using animal models), and available human data.

In some countries, permissible levels are derived after consultation with employers, workers, unions and other interested parties. In other countries, they are issued by governmental enforcement agencies as a directive following agreement through consensus or expert opinion, or in accordance with current evidence or levels set by international bodies. For example, threshold limit values (TLVs) are permissible levels for workplace exposure recommended by the American Conference of Governmental Industrial Hygienists (American Conference of Governmental Industrial Hygienests (ACIGH), 2020). There are three categories of TLVs:

1. Threshold Limit Value — Time Weighted Average (TLV-TWA), based on an average exposure over an 8-hour work period for a 40-hour workweek.
2. Threshold Limit Value — Short-Term Exposure Limit (TLV-STEL), based on an exposure over a 15-minute period. This short-term exposure standard allows a less stringent standard for short periods of exposure, e.g. for rescue operations.
3. Threshold Limit Value — Ceiling (TLV-C), an absolute limit that does not permit any excursions above this level.

Biological Monitoring

Biological monitoring is the analysis of a biological sample from a worker. It aims to detect the presence and amount of a toxic substance or its metabolite as an indicator of exposure. The measurement value obtained by biological monitoring is evaluated as a health risk by comparing it with the corresponding biological exposure index (BEI) or biological limit value (BLV). The BEI is based either on the relationship between intensity of exposure and the biological levels of the toxicant (or its metabolite), or on the relationship between

Table 2. BEIs for Some Chemical Toxicants (ACGIH, 2020)

Toxicant	Source	BEI	Sampling Time
Carbon monoxide	Blood	3.5% of haemoglobin	End of shift
Carboxyhaemoglobin carbon monoxide	End exhaled air	20 ppm	End of shift
Cadmium and	Urine	5 ug/g creatinine	Not critical
inorganic compounds	Blood	5 ug/L	Not critical
n-hexane 2,5-hexanedione	Urine	0.5 mg/L	End of shift at end of workweek
Lead	Blood	200 ug/L	Not critical
Mercury (Inorganic)	Urine	20 ug/g creatinine	Prior to shift
Phenol	Urine	250 mg/g creatinine	End of shift

biological level and health effects. In some countries, the biological monitoring standards are based on what can be achieved following best workplace practice in industries where various chemicals are encountered.

BEIs as used by ACGIH (2020) for some toxicants are shown in Table 2.

Identification of Susceptible Workers

Pre-placement/employment medical examination aims to achieve proper job placement according to the mental and physical capabilities of the worker. During such examinations and job placements, susceptible workers can be identified and their exposures can be limited to prevent adverse health effects. Such examinations are also undertaken for different purposes, e.g. to protect other workers and the general public; for insurance purposes; and to obtain baseline information on health and fitness.

There are genetic disorders that may make a worker more vulnerable to certain workplace exposures. One example is a deficiency in red cell glucose-6-phosphate dehydrogenase (G6PD), which increases susceptibility to haemolytic anaemia, especially following exposure to fava beans, naphthalenes and other chemicals. As such, G6PD deficient individuals should be protected from exposure to these agents.

Another example is alpha-1 antitrypsin (AAT) deficiency. Persons with AAT deficiency are at high risk of developing chronic obstructive pulmonary disease and should be advised against work involving substances that can hasten the onset of or worsen respiratory function. However, there is continuing debate regarding the ethics of genetic screening, and many genetic screening tests have not been developed to a stage where they can be advocated and accepted for workplace screening (See section on genetic testing).

Lifestyle factors such as smoking and alcohol consumption, and pre-existing diseases such as chronic bronchitis, liver or kidney disease may increase the susceptibility to certain agents encountered in the workplace.

Control of Exposure

Successful prevention of occupational disease can be achieved by limiting exposure to harmful agents to what are considered as safe levels, or by eliminating exposures where feasible. A well accepted preventive approach is via a hierarchy of prevention, which goes from the most to the least effective desirable intervention (National Institute for Occupational Safety and Health, 2016), viz.

1. Elimination of the hazard;
2. Substitution of the hazard;
3. Engineering controls, i.e. use of mechanical or technical measures such as enclosure, ventilation and workplace design to minimise exposure;
4. Administrative controls, i.e. changes to the way people work to minimise exposure; and
5. Personal protective equipment (PPE).

Engineering Controls

Engineering controls minimise or eliminate hazards at the source. This is a preferred means of prevention. Unlike other measures, such as the use of personal protective equipment, engineering controls do not rely on workers' compliance for their effectiveness.

Engineering controls can include the following:

1. Removal (or replacement with safer alternatives) of toxic hazards in the manufacturing process, e.g. using a cadmium free brazing filler in Case Study 6, or using a benzene-free organic solvent;
2. Automation, enclosure, or segregation of a work process to minimise worker exposure (although in such situations, exposure could still occur among maintenance and repair staff);
3. Modifications to reduce the emission of hazards from the work process, e.g. dampeners or mufflers to reduce vibration or noise, reducing the open surface area for the evaporation of volatile chemicals; and
4. Exhaust ventilation to remove hazardous fumes, vapours or dusts from the work process.

It is often more cost effective to incorporate the engineering controls at the initial setting up of the work process. Such controls should also be considered when new processes or machinery are introduced to existing manufacturing operations. It is important that the effectiveness of the engineering controls be monitored periodically, and regular maintenance be conducted.

Case Study 6: Cadmium Exposure from Brazing

Brazing is a process where a filler metal (of lower melting point than the two metals to be joined) is melted and allowed to flow by capillary action into a close fitting joint of two metals. A common type of brazing filler metal is a copper-zinc-silver-cadmium alloy. This is used to join brass, cast iron, nickel or stainless steel. Torch brazing was performed in a factory that manufactured compressors. A review of the safety data sheet of the filler revealed that it contained a significant amount of cadmium. Cadmium is a nephrotoxic agent that is used to reduce the melting point of the filler metal. While cadmium-free alloys are available, these cost more, as a higher silver content is needed to achieve an equivalent melting temperature.

Environmental monitoring showed that cadmium in air levels were above the recommended threshold limit values in that country. Biological monitoring of exposed workers showed that a large proportion of exposed workers had blood cadmium values higher than 10μg/L, the recommended biological exposure index in that country. Note: The BEI for Cadmium in blood recommended by the ACGIH is 5 μg/L (ACGIH, 2020). Some of the workers also had beta-2 microglobulins in their urine samples. This is a biological effect marker that results from cadmium exposure.

The health risk was deemed to be unacceptable, and as a result, the brazing alloy was replaced with a cadmium free substitute.

Redesign of the Workstation or Process

Workstation design can help reduce the risk of work-related symptoms. For example, redesign of a food processing station to reduce unnecessary and repetitive bending, and to prevent excessive stretching to the limit of the range of movement in the workers shown below can minimise an ergonomic risk (Fig. 4).

In the case of computer operators, the use of adjustable equipment, the positioning of the workstation to reduce glare, and appropriate work rest pauses can help prevent the development of eyestrain and musculoskeletal complaints.

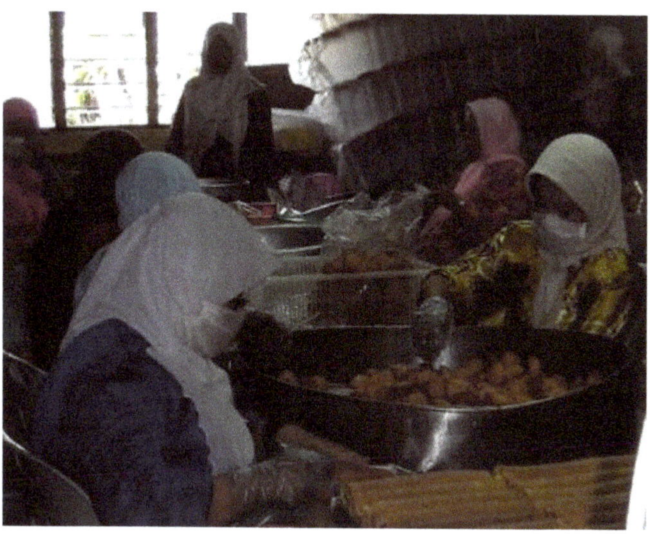

Fig. 4. Ergonomic improvements of this workplace can reduce the risk of musculoskeletal disorders among the workers.

Administrative Controls

Administrative controls may be a viable alternative or additional measure to reduce worker exposure to occupational hazards. These measures could take the form of job enlargement and job rotation, restriction of hours of work at a hazardous operation, or even temporary job re-assignment. Travel illness prevention for the frequent business traveler (such as immunisation, advice on food safety and hygiene) could be considered as a form of administrative control for occupational hazards.

Training of workers to recognise work hazards, how to work safely, and what to do in the event of an emergency or when occupational diseases occur, is another important aspect of prevention.

Personal Protective Equipment

The use of personal protective equipment is often widely practiced. It has its merits — a major one being its relative low cost, and it is especially useful for short term or occasional exposure to occupational hazards.

However, protective equipment has to be properly selected to be effective against specific hazards, e.g. the choice of an appropriate glove for use with a particular solvent. Workers have to be trained to use the equipment correctly and to ensure that they are working effectively, e.g. the use of respirators and respirator fit testing. Worker compliance in the use of the equipment must be high; otherwise the protective effects may be less than desired, e.g. hearing protectors. Finally, personal protective equipment has to be regularly maintained and replaced when necessary.

The Occupational Safety and Health Administration (1995) stipulates that personal protective equipment should NOT be used as a substitute for engineering, work practice, and/or administrative controls. Instead, personal protective equipment should be used in conjunction with these controls to provide for employee safety and health in the workplace.

Secondary Prevention of Occupational Disease

Secondary prevention is the detection of disease at an early stage before the worker would normally seek clinical care. For such an activity to be truly preventive, detection of the disease in the preclinical, asymptomatic or early symptomatic stage must have clear benefit for the workers. This means that the pathological process must be reversible on discontinuation of exposure and prognosis is better than if it were detected at later stages.

Screening for Disease

The discussion on screening for disease in this chapter is confined to early detection of disease. Biological monitoring may sometimes be wrongly classified as a screening procedure. This is not accurate as the purpose of biological monitoring is to detect the presence of a toxicant or metabolite so as to keep exposure levels within safe limits. Thus biological monitoring precedes screening as it is indicative of exposure and not health effect or disease (Fig. 5).

Advances in Monitoring and Screening

Technological advances in molecular biology over the last few decades have offered more sophisticated techniques that can be used to study the role of specific exogenous agents and host factors in causing ill-health.

These advances have resulted in the development of newer molecular biomarkers of exposure, response, and genetic susceptibility. These include measurements for structural gene damage, gene variation, and gene products in cells and body fluids, e.g. oncogenes and tumour suppressor genes, DNA adducts, gene products and genetic polymorphisms, and metabolic phenotypes in environmentally exposed populations.

An understanding of biochemistry and genetics at the molecular level, specific knowledge on metabolism and mechanisms of action,

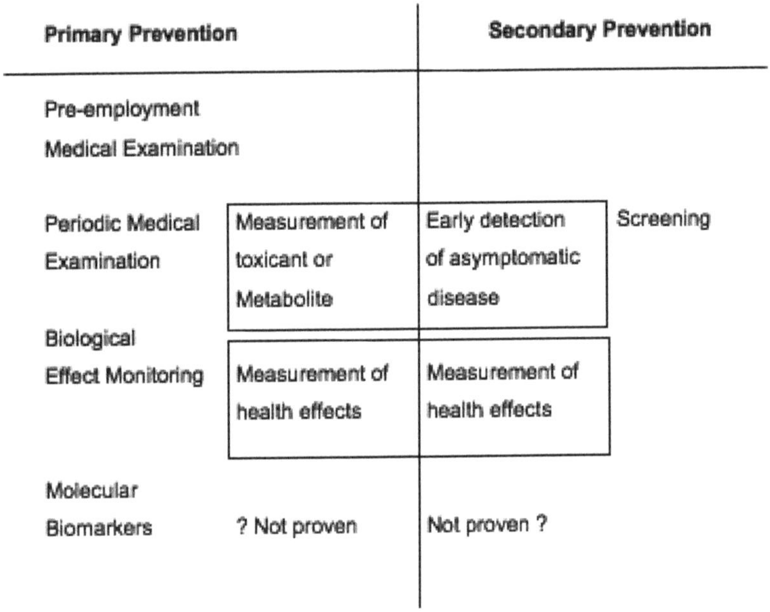

Fig. 5. Levels of prevention in occupational disease.

and epidemiology has become increasingly important. This is necessary in order to address the major question of validation and relevance of these molecular biomarkers.

For example, the availability of genetic tests to identify susceptible workers raises issues of ethics, individual privacy, right to work and the relevance of such tests. Several studies have presented data on the association of environmental measurements and various biomarkers for internal and biologically effective dose, genetic polymorphisms, and early response markers (Table 3).

There are limitations of individual molecular biomarkers in assessing health risk, and more importantly, environmental and occupational diseases are multifactorial in nature. It is likely that a combined approach which examines several of these biomarkers simultaneously will increase our understanding of the complex issue of disease mechanisms and further refine the process of risk assessment.

In the last few decades, new biomarker discovery tools have emerged that can potentially be applied to occupational and environmental health

Table 3. Examples of Molecular Biomarkers Measured in Occupational Health

Molecular Biomarkers	Application	Study Population
Exposure Marker		
8-hydroxy-2-deoxyguanosine (8-OHdG)	Oxidative stress and increased cancer risk from exposure to benzene, chromium, cobalt, fine particulate matter (PM2.5)	Petrol station attendants, electroplating workers, boilermakers
Urinary 1-hydroxypyrene (1-OHP)	Cooking oil fumes exposure	Restaurant workers
Urinary malondialdehyde (MDA)	Oxidative stress marker	
PAH-DNA adduct	Workplace and community exposures and exposure to cigarette smoke, and risk of lung cancer	Foundry workers, coke oven workers, general community in industrial areas
Early Effect Markers		
p53 tumor suppressor gene or its protein product	Specific fingerprint mutation in certain gene codon and risk of liver, breast, lung, and esophageal cancer	Radon exposed miners, vinyl chloride monomer workers, general population with environmental exposure to AFB1
H-*ras* and K-*ras* gene or its protein product	Increased risk of various cancers, e.g. lung, liver and bladder	Firefighters, hazardous waste workers, foundry workers, vinyl chloride monomer workers
Hypermutations/Mutational Signatures		
30-fold higher somatic mutations detected per Mb in the genome of workers' cholangiocarcinoma tissues	Occupationally related Cholangiocarcinoma	Printing workers with high exposure to organic solvents, mainly halo alkanes, e.g. 1,2-dichloropropan (1,2-DCP) and/or dichloromethane (DCM)

(*Continued*)

Table 3. (*Continued*)

Molecular Biomarkers	Application	Study Population
C:G-to-T:A transitions with substantial strand bias; unique trinucleotide mutational changes of GpCpY to GpTpY and NpCpY to NpTpY or NpApY		
Host Susceptibility Markers		
Functional polymorphisms in GST genes	Increased risk of lung cancer with exposure to indoor cooking fumes (wood smoke, cooking oil fumes)	Cooks, kitchen workers (especially Asian- style cooking)
CYP1A1 polymorphism	Increased risk of lung cancer with exposure to Benzo[a]pyrene	Foundry workers
NAT2 polymorphism	Increased risk of bladder cancer	Workers exposed to arylamine and hydrazine

practice. The five most developed technologies are genotyping, transcriptomics, epigenomics, proteomics and metabolomics. At present, their use has largely been limited to research studies. Examples of utilisation of these technologies have been in the investigation of human health effects from benzene and arsenic (Vlaanderen *et al.*, 2010).

Screening usually aims at the detection of disease at an early asymptomatic or sub-clinical stage. The following are criteria to be fulfilled prior to screening:

1. The screening test/procedure is validated as being able to detect the disease at an early (usually asymptomatic) stage;
2. Early intervention in the management of the disease is of benefit to the individual screened and facilities are locally available for its management; and
3. The physician undertaking the screening procedure should not be the one who will subsequently treat the disease. This is important as it eliminates the potential for observer bias and a possible con-

flict of interest, particularly in situations where there exists a financial benefit in over-diagnosing for treatment. Such a problem will not arise where the physician is a salaried employee — as opposed to a physician whose income is influenced by the number of interactions and consultations undertaken.

Periodic Medical Examinations

Periodic medical examinations are undertaken on occupational groups in order to effect primary, or failing that, secondary prevention of disease. In many countries, by convention most employees undergo pre-employment medical examinations. The main focus of such examinations is not necessarily as a pre-placement procedure but rather for assessing routine fitness for work as well as for medical insurance needs. In some countries, there are legal and administrative regulations mandating pre and periodic medical examination. And in other countries, discrimination on the basis of health or illness or disability is prohibited.

Statutory Medical Examinations

An example of statutory examinations can be found in Singapore, where since 1985, all workers exposed to a list of prescribed hazards have to undergo pre-employment and periodic medical examinations. The list includes hazards such as arsenic and its compounds, asbestos, benzene, cadmium and its compounds, raw cotton, lead and its compounds, manganese and its compounds, mercury and its compounds, excessive noise, organophosphates, perchloroethylene, silica, tar, pitch, bitumen, creosote, trichloroethylene, vinyl chloride monomer and any occupation or process carried out using compressed air. Such examinations are to be conducted by physicians trained in occupational health and registered with the Ministry of Manpower. In addition, periodic examinations are required for other categories of workers such as migrant workers, food handlers, professional drivers and radiographers.

Notification of Occupational Diseases

Most countries require the statutory notification of occupational diseases to the government. Notification should be done on the suspicion of occupational disease. The notified case is subsequently investigated and confirmed by the relevant government specialists. Either the employer or health practitioner who sees the worker can notify. In many countries, a list of notifiable occupational diseases is available.

Notification serves as an additional means of control of occupational diseases, undertaken by occupational health and safety professionals in the public sector. It initiates a chain of events, which often includes investigation and confirmation of the index case, and active case finding of other affected persons.

Recommendations for specific preventive measures at the workplace are then prescribed. The authorities would follow up by ensuring that the recommendations have been implemented. If necessary, further evaluation of the effectiveness of the preventive measures can be made. However, compliance with notification in many countries is often poor, and there are practical and logistical reasons for this. It includes non-familiarity with occupational diseases, and how they can be recognised. There are also legitimate concerns by employers, workers, and physicians about the consequences of notification.

Figure 6 summarises the continuum of various means of prevention in occupational health practice.

Tertiary Prevention

Tertiary prevention activities are largely curative and rehabilitative procedures. Workers should be removed from further exposure, and the appropriate medical treatment given if indicated. Examples of appropriate treatment include the rendering of first aid promptly after an injury, chelation for severe cases of symptomatic heavy metal poisoning, and hyperbaric treatment for cases of compressed air illness. Following treatment and attention to any resulting disability, affected workers should not be returned to their usual work until adequate preventive measures have been put in place.

Disaster Planning

Occupational health personnel can also assist in planning for dealing with disasters in the workplace and the community. Planning and

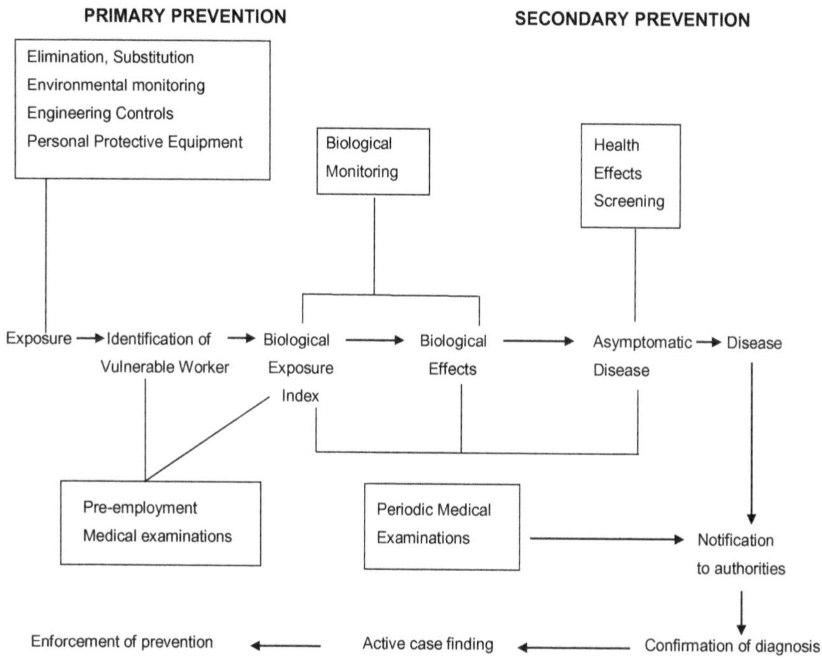

Fig. 6. Continuum of preventive actions in occupational health practice.

practice drills should be done jointly between occupational health and safety staff and services such as the fire and emergency response department and other relevant local community agencies. This topic is covered in an earlier chapter.

Post Illness or Injury Evaluation

An evaluation of the health status of the employee returning to work after a prolonged absence from work attributed to illness or injury is important. The aim is to ensure that the worker has sufficiently recovered from the illness or injury, and that he or she is fit to return to full performance of work tasks. Two issues to consider would be:

1. Can the worker perform his or her duty without adverse health and safety risks to himself/herself or fellow workers?
2. Should he or she return to full time unrestricted duty, or should some modified, restricted or alternative duty be given?

Rehabilitation

Rehabilitation of workers is another important aspect of occupational health care. Management, fellow workers, occupational health professionals and the injured worker have to work together to ensure that suitable alternative duties are provided, and that any work restrictions or physical limitations are understood. There should be clear short and long term goals in rehabilitation, and alternative duties should be meaningful and contribute to production (Australian College of Occupational Medicine & Australian College of Rehabilitation Medicine, 1987). Sometimes, the use of external rehabilitation resources may be needed.

Rehabilitation may also be applied to a wide range of conditions, including occupational skin disorders. For example, a tertiary individual prevention programme for patients with severe occupational skin disorders was shown to produce sustained improvements in disease severity, ability to work, quality of life, and prognosis over a follow up period of 3 years (Brans *et al.*, 2016).

Evaluation of Prevention Programmes

Evidence for the success of prevention programmes has been increasingly documented. There have already been several Cochrane reviews produced on the effectiveness of various preventive strategies in occupational health practice. (Cochrane Reviews are systematic reviews of primary research in human health care and health policy that investigate the effects of interventions for prevention, treatment and rehabilitation.)

These include reviews on interventions for musculoskeletal disorders, smoking, injuries and poisonings, infectious diseases, mental health, and cover primary, secondary and tertiary prevention strategies (Box 2).

Evaluations of incentives to promote occupational safety and health showed that economic incentive schemes were feasible and reasonably effective. The few cases that were considered delivered positive results for large samples. However, analysis regarding the efficiency of such

Box 2. Cochrane Reviews in Occupational Health for Decreasing or Eliminating Hazards (The Cochrane Collaboration, 2020).

Biological Agents

- Personal protective equipment for preventing highly infectious diseases due to exposure to contaminated body fluids in healthcare staff
- Education and training for preventing sharps injuries and splash exposures in healthcare workers (protocol stage)
- Remediating buildings damaged by dampness and mould for preventing or reducing respiratory tract symptoms, infections and asthma
- Devices for preventing percutaneous exposure injuries caused by needles in healthcare personnel
- Gloves, extra gloves or special types of gloves for preventing percutaneous exposure injuries in healthcare personnel
- Behavioural interventions to reduce the transmission of HIV infection among sex workers and their clients in low- and middle-income countries
- Behavioural interventions to reduce the transmission of HIV infection among sex workers and their clients in high-income countries
- Blunt versus sharp suture needles for preventing percutaneous exposure incidents in surgical staff
- Antiretroviral post-exposure prophylaxis (PEP) for occupational HIV exposure

Circadian Rhythm Disruption (e.g. shiftwork)

- Pharmacological interventions for sleepiness and sleep disturbances caused by shift work
- Adaptation of shift work schedules for preventing and treating sleepiness and sleep disturbances caused by shift work (protocol stage)
- Person-directed non-pharmacological interventions for preventing and treating sleepiness and sleep disturbances caused by shift work (protocol stage)

Stress

- Preventing occupational stress in healthcare workers
- Interventions for prevention of bullying in the workplace (protocol stage)

(*Continued*)

Box 2. (*Continued*)

- Psychological debriefing for preventing post-traumatic stress disorder (PTSD)

Other Agents or Exposures

- The psychological effects of the physical healthcare environment on healthcare personnel
- Interventions for preventing voice disorders in adults

Other Preventive Measures to Prevent Occupational Disease Health Examinations

- Pre-employment examinations for preventing injury, disease and sick leave in workers

Policy Measures and Legislation

- Interventions to increase the reporting of occupational diseases by physicians
- Occupational safety and health enforcement tools for preventing occupational diseases and injuries

Other Measures

- Humidification of indoor air for preventing or reducing dryness symptoms or upper respiratory infections in educational settings and at the workplace (protocol stage)
- Web-based stress management for preventing stress and reducing sick leave in workers (protocol stage)
- Workplace interventions for preventing work-related rhinitis and rhinosinusitis (protocol stage)
- Interventions for increasing the uptake of immunisation in healthcare workers (protocol stage)
- Ergonomic interventions for preventing musculoskeletal disorders in dental care practitioners (protocol stage)
- Interventions for preventing the spread of infestation in close contacts of people with scabies
- Vaccines for preventing hepatitis B in health care workers

schemes was generally scarce and there were also deficits in the quality of evaluations in many instances (Elsler *et al.*, 2010).

An evaluation of a programme could comprise comparison of pre- and post-intervention health outcomes, as Case Study 7 demonstrates.

Case Study 7: Prevention Programme for Beryllium Exposure

A preventive programme, which emphasised skin and respiratory protection, workplace cleanliness, and beryllium migration control in lowering beryllium sensitisation, was evaluated. Sensitisation prevalence and incidence were 8.9% and 3.7/1000 person-months for the Pre-Programme Group compared to 2.1% and 1.7/1000 person-months for the Programme Group.

After adjusting for potential selection and information bias, sensitisation prevalence for the Pre-Programme Group was found to be 3.8 times higher (95% CI = 1.5 to 9.3) than the Programme Group. The sensitisation incidence rate ratio of the Pre-Programme Group to the Programme Group was 1.6 (95% CI= 0.8 to 3.6).

It was concluded that the preventive programme reduced the prevalence of beryllium sensitisation, but did not eliminate it altogether (Bailey et al., 2010).

Conclusion

This chapter addresses the relevance of health promotion as well as the prevention of work-related and occupational disease in the working population. In prevention of occupational diseases, the priority should be to effect primary prevention. However, secondary and tertiary prevention activities are also useful complementary measures.

References

American Conference of Governmental Industrial Hygienests. (2020) *Threshold Limit Values for chemical substances and physical agents and Biological Exposure Indices.* Cincinnati, American Conference of Governmental Industrial Hygienests.

Australian College of Occupational Medicine & Australian College of Rehabilitation Medicine. (1987) *Occupational rehabilitation. Guidelines and practice: A report prepared by the joint working party of the Australian College of Occupational Medicine and Australian College of Rehabilitation Medicine*. Australia, The College.

Bailey RL, Thomas CA, Deubner DC, Kent MS, Kreiss K, Schuler CR. (2010) Evaluation of a preventive program to reduce sensitization at a beryllium metal, oxide, and alloy production plant. *J Occup Environ Med* **52**(5): 505–512.

Brans R, Skudlik C, Weisshaar E, Scheidt R, Ofenloch R, Elsner P, Wulfhorst B, Schönfeld M, John SM, Diepgen TL. (2016) Multicentre cohort study rehabilitation of occupational skin diseases — optimization and quality assurance of inpatient management (ROQ): Results from a 3-year follow-up. *Contact Derm* **75**(4): 205–212.

The Cochrane Collaboration. (2020) *Cochrane reviews about occupational safety and health*. [Online] Available from: http://work.cochrane.org/cochrane-reviews-about-occupational-safety-and-health. [Accessed on 27 Aug 2020].

Elsler D, Treutein D, Rydlewska I, Frusteri L, Krüger H, Veerman T, Eeckelaert L, Roskams N, Van Den Broek K, Taylor TN. (2010) A review of case studies evaluating economic incentives to promote occupational safety and health. *Scand J Work Environ Health* **36**(4).

European Chemicals Agency. (2020) *Understanding prior informed consent*. [Online] Available from: https://echa.europa.eu/regulations/prior-informed-consent/understanding-pic. [Accessed on 27 Aug 2020].

Feltner C, Peterson K, Weber RP, Cluff L, Coker-Schwimmer E, Viswanathan M, Lohr KN. (2016) The effectiveness of total worker health interventions: A systematic review for a national institutes of health pathways to prevention workshop. *Ann Intern Med* **165**(4): 262–269.

International Labour Organization. (2013) *The prevention of occupational diseases*. Geneva, International Labour Organization. [Online] Available from: https://www.ilo.org/wcmsp5/groups/public/---ed_protect/---protrav/---safework/documents/publication/wcms_208226.pdf. [Accessed on 18 Aug 2020].

National Institute for Occupational Safety and Health. (2016) *Hierarchy of controls*. [Online] Available from: https://www.cdc.gov/niosh/topics/hierarchy/default.html. [Accessed on 18 Aug 2020].

Occupational Safety and Health Administration. (1995) *Personal protective equipment*. United States Department of Labour. OSHA 3077.

United Nations Environment Programme Rotterdam Convention. (2020) *Prior informed consent circulars.* [Online] Available from: http://www.pic.int/Implementation/PICCircular/tabid/1168/language/en-US/Default.aspx. [Accessed on 27 Aug 2020].

Vlaanderen J, Moore LE, Smith MT, Lan Q, Zhang L, Skibola CF, Rothman N, Vermeulen R. (2010) Application of OMICS technologies in occupational and environmental health research; current status and projections. *Occup Environ Med* 67(2): 136–143.

Wolf J, Prüss-Ustün A, Ivanov I, Mudgal S, Corvalán C, Bos R, Neira M. (2018) *Preventing disease through a healthier and safer workplace.* [Online] Available from: https://apps.who.int/iris/bitstream/handle/10665/272980/9789241513777-eng.pdf?ua=1. [Accessed on 27 Aug 2020].

Index

www.ingramcontent.com/pod-product-compliance
Ingram Content Group UK Ltd.
Pitfield, Milton Keynes, MK11 3LW, UK
UKHW020356150926
8624IPUK00004B/190